RECENT ADVANCES IN ARTHROPLASTY

Edited by **Samo K. Fokter**

Recent Advances in Arthroplasty
Edited by Samo K. Fokter

Published by InTech
Janeza Trdine 9, 51000 Rijeka, Croatia

Publishing Process Manager Adriana Pecar

Technical Editor Teodora Smiljanic

Cover Designer InTech Design Team

Additional hard copies can be obtained from orders@intechopen.com

Recent Advances in Arthroplasty, Edited by Samo K. Fokter
p. cm.
ISBN 978-953-307-990-5

For EU product safety concerns:
IN TECH d.o.o., Prolaz Marije Krucifikse Kozulić 3, 51000 Rijeka, Croatia,
info@intechopen.com or visit our website at intechopen.com.

Meet the editor

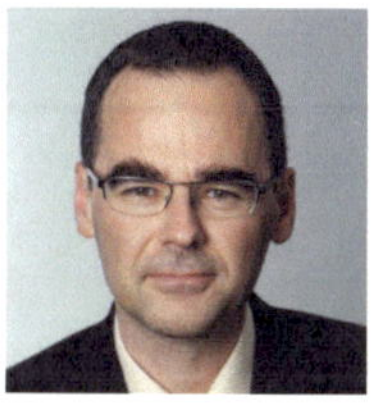

Dr. Samo K. Fokter obtained his medicine degree in 1985 at the Medical Faculty of Ljubljana University, Slovenia, where he also completed his residency in orthopaedics. He was a research fellow at the Orthopaedic Clinic of Zagreb, Croatia, visiting fellow in Basel, Switzerland, and Koeln, Germany. He is currently appointed as Assistant Professor of Surgery at the Medical Faculty of Maribor University and Assistant Professor of Orthopaedic Surgery at the Medical Faculty of Ljubljana University. He works as Head of Department of Orthopaedic Surgery and Sports Trauma at Celje Teaching Hospital, and is current Immediate Past President of the Slovenian Orthopaedic Society at Slovenian Medical Association. He is a Board member of European Association of Research Groups for Spinal Osteosynthesis (ARGOSPINE) and an Assistant Editor in Chief of European Journal of Orthopaedic Surgery and Traumatology (EJOST). He dedicated a large part of his free time to active voluntary work at the Mountain Rescue Service of Slovenia.

Contents

Preface

The purpose of this book is to offer an exhaustive overview of the recent insights into the state-of-the-art in arthroplasty. The tremendous long-term success of Sir Charnley's total hip arthroplasty has encouraged many researchers, physicians, surgeons, and technicians to search for new applications, designs, technology, and surgical exposures to treat pain, improve function and create solutions for higher quality of life.

Indeed, the success story was repeated very soon with knee arthroplasty. Moreover, the number of knee arthroplasties has shown almost exponential growth worldwide and has exceeded the number of total hip arthroplasties in many clinics in the Western countries in the past decade. Besides, and as described in a special chapter of this book, arthroplasty of the upper extremity joints and spine is an emerging field.

However, there are complications involved in bringing any foreign design into the unique and wonderful system of the human body. First, opportunistic germs try to win the ever-ongoing war with their host in the cover of the prosthesis. In the chapter on infections we endeavor to provide a comprehensive, up-to-date analysis and description of the surgical and medical management of this difficult problem. Secondly, the immune system is suddenly faced with a strange material coming in huge amounts of micro-particles from the tribology code for an extended period of time. Therefore, great attention has been given to the problem of aseptic loosening in special chapters on loosening and materials.

Each chapter includes an extensive review of the literature as well as current techniques and philosophies. We have been as fortunate as to have an outstanding group of arthroplasty specialists from all over the world contributing to this publication. Some current topics have been discussed by several authors; therefore some repetition has been inevitable. However, as the problems are illuminated from different points of view, this only brings an added value to the book.

We especially wish to acknowledge the contributing authors, without whom a work of this magnitude would clearly not be realizable. We thank them for allocating much of their very scarce time to this project. Not only do we appreciate their participation but also their adherence as a group to the time parameters set for this publication.

Dr. Samo K. Fokter, MD,
Assist. Professor and Chairman,
Dept. for Orthopaedic Surgery and Sports Trauma,
Celje Teaching Hospital
Slovenia

Part 1

Introduction

1

Postoperative Cognitive Dysfunction (POCD) and Markers of Brain Damage After Big Joints Arthroplasty

Dariusz Tomaszewski
Military Institute of Medicine
Poland

1. Introduction

Brain dysfunction can manifest itself either as focal laesions or mental impairment (Roach et al., 1996). In orthopedic patients, in comparison to any other group of hospitalized people, cognitive dysfunction was present more often. It included a deterioration of perception, memory, information analysis, attentional focus as well as of concentration and decreased patients' response (L. S. Rasmussen, 1998). When occurring after a surgery, the symptoms were defined as Postoperative Cognitive Dysfunction (POCD) (Newman, Stygall, Hirani, Shaefi, & Maze, 2007) and were nonspecific signs of brain disorders resulting from cellular abnormalities. Very often the dysfunction's nature was subclinical and no changes in diagnostic imaging were present (Wu, Hsu, Richman, & Raja, 2004). As a consequence, the hospitalization time was longer, the outcome and quality of life were worsened as well as prolonged medical and social assistance were necessary (Gao et al., 2005; Veering, 1999). The problem concerned up to 26% of elderly patients during the first week after a non-cardiac surgery (Rohan et al., 2005). Amongst 60-year-old patients who underwent major surgical procedures under general anesthesia lasting over 2 hours, 10% suffered from memory impairment and concentration problems for more than 3 months after the surgery. The disorder occurs twice more often in 70 – 80-year-old people in comparison to 60 – 70-year-olds (Harwood, 2000). According to statistic data, about 70% of the patients with POCD die within 5 years compared to about 35% of the patients without postoperative delirium (Fodale, Santamaria, Schifilliti, & Mandal, 2010).
All above data were alarming, but the problem seemed to be more complex. The diagnosis of POCD depends on performing a proper assessment of the cognitive function before and after the surgery through a battery of neuropsychological tests, so the incidence of POCD varies. According to the work of Blaise et al., the variability can result from nonstandardization of neuropsychological tests performed at different times of the day, lack of a control group, differences in significance levels between studies as well as from the so-called "learning effect", as when the same test is applied to the same person many times (Blaise, Taha, & Qi, 2007). Another question concerns the time at which the diagnosis of POCD was made. Different drugs administered in the perioperative period can affect patients' cognition. Thus some authors believe that the diagnosis of POCD should be made not earlier than 2 weeks after the surgery (Blaise, et al., 2007)

2. Surgery induced stress response and risk factors of POCD

Surgery induced stress response leads to [1] the activation of the sympathetic nervous system, [2] increased secretion of pituitary hormones, and [3] immunological as well as hematological changes (Desborough, 2000).

Activation of the sympathetic nervous system leads to an increased secretion of catecholamines from the adrenal medulla and of norepinephrine from presynaptic nerve terminals. It results in such cardiovascular effects as tachycardia and hypertension (Desborough, 2000).

The secretion of adrenocorticothropic hormone (corticotrophin, ACTH), growth hormone (GH) and arginine vasopressin (AVP) increases; the secretion of thyroid-stimulating hormone (TSH) as well as of follicle-stimulating hormone (FSH) and luteinizing hormone (LH) may increase or decrease. As a result, the secretion of cortisol and aldosterone increases; that of insulin often decreases, while that of glucagone usually decreses; and, finally, decreases, and the secretion of thyroxine and tri-iodothyronine decreases. All those changes influence the metabolism of carbohydrates, proteins and fat as well as that of salt and water (Desborough, 2000).

Immunological and hematological changes include cytokine production, acute phase reaction, neutrophil leucocytosis and lymphocyte proliferation (Desborough, 2000). Cytokines - mainly interleukin-1 (IL-1), tumor necrosis factor-α (TNF-α) and IL-6, released from activated leukocytes, fibroblasts and endothelial cells - play an important role in the systemic inflammatory reaction (Desborough, 2000). Some authors (Blaise, et al., 2007; Singh & Antognini, 2010; Van Munster et al., 2009) suggest that inflammation plays a substantial role in the pathogenesis of POCD. Their claim was supported by the observation that cyclooxygenase-2 (COX-2) inhibitors protect the amyloid β-induced memory disturbances in mice (Blaise, et al., 2007). The animal studies also showed that the development of POCD in rats was associated with glial activation and the expression of proinflammatory cytokines within the hippocampal region (Blaise, et al., 2007). Some studies revealed the role of interleukin-18 (IL-18) in the neuroinflammation and neurodegeneration of the central nervous system. Patients with a defect in the IL-18 cytokine promoter gene had a higher concentration of serum amyloid peptides (Fodale, et al., 2010). The amyloid β peptide concentration was related to learning and memory deficiences as well as to neurodegeneration. Continuous infusion of amyloid β peptide in rats resulted in learning and memory impairments. Higher levels of amyloid β peptide in the hippocampus were observed in older rats when compared to those in younger ones (Fodale, et al., 2010). Some anesthetic agents can influence the amyloid β production. Isoflurane increases the amyloid β production through an alteration in the processing of amyloid precursor protein; desflurane also causes an increase, but only in the presence of hypoxia. Propofol and thiopental do not significantly change the amyloid precursor protein (Fodale, et al., 2010).

The following were counted as risk factors of POCD in an early postoperative period: advanced age, a general anesthesia rather than a regional one, an increasing duration of anesthesia, poor education, re-operation, postoperative infections, postoperative respiratory complications, lower preoperative level of consciousness, and treatment with cholinergic drugs and benzodiazepines, but also sleep deprivation, isolation, noise, bright light and such physiologic disturbances as hyponatremia or hypoalbuminemia as well as male sex, depression or reduced activity in daily life (Blaise, et al., 2007; Canet et al., 2003; Fines & Severn, 2006; Kyziridis, 2006; Singh & Antognini, 2010; Veering, 1999). Oddly enough, there

was no evidence that hypoxemia is associated with the development of POCD (Fines & Severn, 2006). Some studies found that hypotension was the only intraoperative risk factor responsible for postoperative delirium (Kyziridis, 2006). However, other authors did not support that observation (Fines & Severn, 2006).
Some authors discussed the role of genetic factors in the pathogenesis of neurodegenerative disorders. They found an association between the apolipoprotein ε4 (APO-ε4) allele and Alzheimer's disease (Blaise, et al., 2007), so the APO-ε4 gene could be a predictor of postoperative cognitive disorders (Fodale, et al., 2010).

3. Etiology of POCD

The high incidence of cognitive dysfunction in orthopedic patients can result (apart from the above mentioned risk factors) from long bone fractures, prolonged immobilization, and partially from perioperative stress (Wu, et al., 2004) or a surgery technique. Colonna et al. concluded that the incidence of cerebral embolization after lower extremities arthroplasties was up to 40 - 60% (Colonna et al., 2002). Thromboembolic events played an important etiological role. There were described fatal cerebral embolizations that constituted complications accompanying long bones fractures (Riding et al., 2004), total knee replacements (Jenkins, Chung, Wennberg, Etchells, & Davey), hip arthroplasties (Fallon, Fuller, & Morley-Forster, 2001), and vertebroplasties (Scroop, Eskridge, & Britz, 2002) in which the embolic material passed into the brain through an open foramen ovale (Sukernik, Mets, & Bennett-Guerrero, 2001), although postmortem examinations did not reveal it (Colonna, et al., 2002).

3.1 Biomarkers of brain damage

Biochemical tests are useful diagnostic tools in the examinations of functional brain disorders. Elevated serum concentrations of the markers of brain damage indicate that there has been a neuronal and/or glial injury. The biomarkers are released as a consequence of either transient ischemia or ultimate cell degradation, and their serum concentration depends on the localization of pathological changes, the degree of tissue damage and the time that has passed since the onset of changes.
The ideal marker of brain damage should be: [1] highly specific, [2] highly sensitive, [3] released in cases of an irreversible damage to cerebral neurons only, [4] possible to detect in the blood and/or cerebrospinal fluid within a short period of time after the injury, and [5] released in well-known time sequences after the injury; furthermore, it ought to be [6] age- or sex-independent, [7] easily detectable in the blood since frequent drawing of cerebrospinal fluid samples is impractical, and [8] its concentration should be easily measureable in laboratory tests (Ingebrigtsen T). Many compounds were investigated for this purpose of founding such a marker. In the '70s, it was lactic dehydrogenase (LDH) and aspartate aminotransferase (AspAT); in the '80s, creatine kinase BB isoenzyme (CK-BB); and later, the S100B protein and neuron-specific enolase (NSE). Nowadays, glial fibrillary acidic protein (GFAP) seems most promising (Ingebrigtsen & Romner, 2003). The latter three (the S100B protein, NSE and GFAP) were the best known biomarkers of brain damage (Ingebrigtsen & Romner, 2003; L. E. Pelinka, 2004). Of these the S100B protein is thought to correspond the best to the optimal indicator of a neuronal injury (Ingebrigtsen & Romner, 2003).

3.2 S100B protein

In 1965, Moore isolated from the bovine brain a fraction containing brain specific proteins (Kleindienst & Ross Bullock, 2006). Since then, our knowledge about the above mentioned compounds has increased. Currently, the S100B proteins family consist of 24 members, with similar structures and like functions (Marenholz, Heizmann, & Fritz, 2004).

They play different roles in the human body and are present in many types of cells and tissues (Eckert et al., 2003). Some members of the S100 protein family are specific for certain localizations (Heizmann, 2004). High S100B protein concentrations were present inside the brain, mainly in astroglial and Schwann cells (Ali, Harmer, & Vaughan, 2000; L. E. Pelinka, 2004) as well as in adipocytes, chondrocytes and melanocytes (L. E. Pelinka, 2004; Raabe et al., 2003). The S100B protein can be either actively released into the extracellular space or passively excreted after cell death (L. E. Pelinka, 2004). An animal study revealed high S100B concentrations in cerebral regions injured by chronic ischemia (Ohtani et al., 2007).

In 2003, there was published a review of 18 clinical studies (involving 1085 patients) of the S100B protein as a marker of brain damage (Kleindienst & Ross Bullock, 2006). In 2004 and 2005, another 6 papers appeared (involving more than 600 adults) on the correlations between an elevated concentration of the S100B protein and poor outcome after brain injury (Kleindienst & Ross Bullock, 2006). The highest S100B protein serum level was observed just after an injury (Ingebrigtsen & Romner, 2003), then normalized within 24 hours, even in patients with poor outcome (Kleindienst & Ross Bullock, 2006). The study of Raabe and Seifert showed an increased concentration of the S100B protein on the 6th day after head trauma, probably as a result of a secondary injury (Kleindienst & Ross Bullock, 2006). The elevated posttraumatic S100B protein concentration was also demonstrated in an animal model (Kleindienst & Ross Bullock, 2006).

The increased concentration of the S100B protein can be a result of an increased permeability of the blood-brain barrier, regardless of cerebral damage (Kleindienst & Ross Bullock, 2006). The results of animal studies suggested that S100B protein levels correlated with the degree of shock: in moderate shock they were higher than in a severe one (L. E. Pelinka, 2004). The S100B protein concentration was increased just after bilateral long bones fractures as well as after local ischemia and the reperfusion of the liver, gut and kidneys (L. E. Pelinka, 2004). Elevated levels of S100B protein were shown in basketball and hockey players after competitions as well as in runners, boxers (Stalnacke, Tegner, & Sojka, 2003), swimmers and soccer players; although in the latter there was a correlation between an increased protein concentration and the frequency of head injury (Stålnacke, Ohlsson, Tegner, & Sojka, 2006). There was a possibility that some amounts of the S100B protein were released from red cells, melanocytes and steatocytes. The protein's origin – whether it was extra- or intracerebral - remains unclear. If it was of cerebral origin, the question is whether it was released due to an astroglial injury or activation, or as an effect of the blood-brain barrier impairment (Stalnacke, et al., 2003). Stress and physical effort can lead to an increased permeability of the blood-brain barrier (Stålnacke, et al., 2006). In some cases, a raised plasma level of the S100B protein was an effect of long bones fractures, multiple traumas and surgical procedures. It also occurred in melanoma patients (Salama, Malone, Mihaimeed, & Jones, 2008) and in sepsis-associated encephalopathy (Piazza, Russo, Cotena, Esposito, & Tufano, 2007).

The possibility that the S100B protein could be released from extracerebral localizations as well confines its utility as a marker of brain damage, which, nonetheless, still ranges from 70 to 80% (Raabe, et al., 2003). The S100B protein was a very useful biochemical tool because of its short (below 30 minutes) half-life (Ingebrigtsen & Romner, 2003; Raabe, et al., 2003) as well as sex and age non-dependent serum concentrations (Ingebrigtsen & Romner, 2003). Neither alcohol overdose nor hemolysis altered its concentration (Raabe, et al., 2003). The S100B protein was stable in solution, there was no need to centrifuge and freeze its samples (Raabe, et al., 2003). Contemporary biochemical tests measure either S100B or S100A1B and S100BB serum levels. Because S100BB is considered to be the most brain-specific unit, its determination could eliminate the influence of the extracerebrally released S100B protein (Raabe, et al., 2003).

3.3 S100B protein in orthopedic patients

There were a few papers on the S100B protein in orthopedics only.
Kinoshita et al. (Kinoshita et al., 2003) examined 14 patients; half of them underwent total knee arthroplasty (TKA) with bone cement, the other half underwent intramedullary nail stabilization of the tibia. All the procedures were performed with tourniquet and ischemia. In the TKA group, in blood samples withdrawn 15 minutes after tourniquet release, there was a statistically significant elevation of the S100B serum level in comparison to the group where tibial fracture was stabilized with an intramedullary nail. The authors suggested that the increase was due to a transient injury of brain tissues caused by bone cement (Kinoshita, et al., 2003).
An increased serum concentration of the S100B protein was observed after injuries which did not include brain damage. The highest levels were noted in patients with long bones fractures (Anderson, Hansson, Nilsson, Dijlai-Merzoug, & Settergren, 2001). Studies on people with isolated bone fractures without brain injury revealed that patients with hip, radius or tibia fractures had significantly higher concentrations of the S100B protein, but those with phalanges, hand or foot fractures did not (Undén et al., 2005). In animal studies there were increased S100B serum levels after bilateral femur fractures in rats (L. Pelinka et al., 2003). These results indicated that bone marrow could be a potential source of the S100B protein.
During orthopedic cement was used for fixing the elements of the prosthesis to the bone basis. The use of cement can lead to hemodynamic instability, a decrease in cardiac output, heart contractility, systemic vascular resistance and blood pressure, i.e. to the so-called bone cement implantation syndrome (Donaldson, Thomson, Harper, & Kenny, 2009). Hemodynamic changes have an impact upon cerebral perfusion, as in the relation between the S100B concentration and the degree of shock that has been discussed above (L. E. Pelinka, 2004). Although the presence of bone cement inside the medullar cavity itself did not produce hypotension, hemodynamic instability is often observed when hammering the prosthesis stem into the bone (Sharrock, Beckman, Inda, & Savarese) - the pressure inside the marrow cavity increases. The higher the pressure, the better the penetration of the cement into the bone and the greater the strength of osteosynthesis. But due to the increased pressure, the translocation of the cellular material originating at the site of the surgery into the systemic circulation was facilitated, and the said material could reach the lungs via the bloodstream. The diameter of the lung capillaries is about 8 μm. In 1956, Niden and Aviado showed that there was a possibility of transferring glass spheres up to 420 μm in diameter through the pulmonary vessels (Nunn, 1981). The second way of going round the pulmonary filter was via the foramen ovale. In 1/3 of the population it is closed only functionally. Thus, it is a way for transferring the embolic material into the brain. The presence of cellular material from the site of the surgery in the circulation can be shown with an ultrasound examination as a "snow flurry." In the work of Hayakawa et al.

(Hayakawa, Fujioka, Morimoto, Okamura, & Kemmotsu, 2001), the "snow flurry" was observed from the beginning of the reaming of the femoral canal until the end of the surgery and it intensified especially while the cemented prosthesis stem was being inserted into the bone. This was not noted during procedures without bone cement use. A histological examination of the elements forming the "snow flurry" revealed the presence of amorphic eozynophilic particles with fibrin attached to their surface. The same was noted in patients who had undergone cemented hip arthroplasty during the whole procedure, either before or after bone cement use. In none of the samples were fat particles or bone marrow detected; the authors thought that they had examined "bone dust" particles with attached fibrin fibers (Hayakawa, et al., 2001). The work was limited to a relatively small group: only 7 patients were examined. In the study of Kim et al., the histological examination of samples from the right atrium revealed the presence of fat particles in 34 and 44% as well as of bone marrow cells in 13 and 11% of the procedures, with and without bone cement use, respectively (Kim, Oh, & Kim, 2002). The contribution of bone cement to the etiology of thromboembolic events was suggested (Scroop, et al., 2002). Clark and al. showed a transient, but statistically significant, decrease of cardiac output, by 33%, and of stroke volume, by 44%, during procedures with bone cement use; before the use of bone cement there were no changes between the two (the cemented and the cementless) groups. Because embolic material was released either before or after bone cement use, the decrease in cardiac output and stroke volume might have been followed by the embolic material originating from bone marrow or a vasodilatation caused by a monomer (Clark, Ahmed, Baxendale, & Moran, 2001). Dog studies showed that an intravenous injection of the acrylic acid monomer does not affect the partial pressures of oxygen and carbon dioxide in the arterial blood. Mild and transient hypotension was observed while monomer concentration in the pulmonary artery was much higher than that noted in usual clinical situations (Concepcion, 1998).

The author of the present chapter examined changes in S100B protein levels in patients who underwent total hip arthroplasty, with or without bone cement use. In both groups of patients the mean preoperative concentration of the S100B protein was comparable to that in healthy subjects and reached its maximum just after the operation. In the cemented group its level was significantly higher than in the cementless one and normalization was slower. The operation technique in both types of hip arthroplasty was similar. The elevated serum S100B protein levels may be a result of the S100B protein release from bone marrow as well as of the transfer of cellular materials from the site of the surgery with the bloodstream into the brain (Edmonds, Barbut, Hager, & Sharrock, 2000; Ozelsel et al., 1998; Sukernik, et al., 2001). Because all patients with intraoperative mean blood pressure dropping below 50 mmHg were excluded from the study, it ruled out hypotension as a possible cause of the elevation of the S100B concentration. We concluded that the most probable cause of an increased S100B protein was bone cement use (Kinoshita, et al., 2003; Scroop, et al., 2002). The exothermic polymerization reaction is not always complete because the monomer particles' mobility decreases with the progression of this process. After its completion, 2 to 6% of the monomer remains; it yields to late polymerization to a limited degree, partially transferring into the circulation (Kuhn, 2005). Due to which, the normalization of the elevated S100B protein level in the cemented group was slower.

3.4 POCD and anesthesia

There were discussions on the influence of different types of anesthesia (general vs. regional) on elderly patients. Neither had advantages for the recovery of cognitive functions in geriatric patients during the first three days after the surgery (Dahn et al., 1999). Randomized clinical studies did not show a prevalence of any special kind of anesthesia in POCD prevention (Wu, et al., 2004). Moreover, in 2009, Avidan et al. (Avidan et al., 2009), in his retrospective cohort study including 575 patients, did not find a long-term cognitive impairment due to surgery and illness. But in the ISPOCD study a higher incidence of postoperative cognitive dysfunction was observed after total hip and knee arthroplasties. In both these groups the serum level of the S100B protein was significantly higher, regardless of the diagnosis of POCD in the postoperative period (Linstedt et al., 2002).

Such was the conclusion from both statistic and bibliographic data. However, the central cholinergic system has been identified as the basic system of neurotransmitters taking part in the regulation of the level of conscience, memory and learning (Fodale, et al., 2010), and the interactions between anesthetic drugs and this system may be important in the pathogenesis and development of POCD. There are two main classes of cholinergic receptors: nicotinic and muscarinic. Nicotinic acetylcholine receptors (nAChRs) are ligand-gated cation channels and muscarinic acetylcholine receptors (mAChRs) are ligand-gated K^+ channels, divided into five subtypes (M1 - M5). The agonists of central mAChRs and nAChRs may improve, while the antagonists might impair performance in cognition, learning and memory (Fodale, et al., 2010). Volatile anesthetics and ketamine are potent inhibitors of nAChRs. Desflurane selectively binds the M1 subtype, sevoflurane depresses the M1 and M2 subtypes, whereas isoflurane interferes with the M3 subtype only. All barbiturates are competitive antagonists of mAChRs. Propofol acts on mAChRs and nAChRs, but in concentrations higher than those used clinically. Fentanyl and morphine inhibit signals mediated by both types of receptors and remifentanyl does not change the release of acetylcholine from cholinergic nerves. Furthermore, for example neuromuscular blocking agents or neostigmine administered during general anesthesia can influence cholinergic transmission. The interactions between anesthetics and amyloid β peptide have been discussed above. Thus, it is possible that general anesthesia could be a factor in the pathogenesis of POCD (Fodale, et al., 2010). However, in his study, Hudetz et al. (J. Hudetz et al., 2009; J. A. Hudetz et al., 2009) found that a single administration of ketamine, 0.5 mg/kg, during the induction of anesthesia reduced the incidence of POCD to one week after a cardiac surgery. The authors concluded that it was due to the anti-inflammatory properties of ketamine.

In some cases, an increased concentration of the S100B protein was an effect of an increased permeability of the blood-brain barrier (Kleindienst & Ross Bullock, 2006). In such cases regional anesthesia with intravenous sedation can be effective in limiting surgery-induced stress and the inflammatory reaction of the human organism. In reducing stress it diminished a possible cause of the elevated S100B protein concentration. Regional anesthesia decreased mortality and the incidence of POCD in the early postoperative period (L. Rasmussen et al., 2003; Williams-Russo, Sharrock, Mattis, Szatrowski, & Charlson, 1995). That was confirmed by the observations made by patients under general anesthesia; those with lower values of the Bispectral Index (BIS) had lesser disturbances in cognitive functions, especially in information processing, between the 4th and 6th weeks after the surgery (Farag, Chelune, Schubert, & Mascha, 2006). But there still remained the question concerning the influence of anesthesia and sedation - particularly of anticholinergic therapy (1st generation of antihistaminics) and long-lasting benzodiazepines - on postoperative cognitive functions. An increased S100B protein serum level was observed during a therapy with β-adrenergic agonists and phosphodiestease inhibitors (Linstedt, et al., 2002).

According to Sharrock et al. (Sharrock et al., 2005), there occurred a worsening of test-evaluated cognitive functions occurred during the first hour after the surgery, with significant improvement during the second hour. However, in patients aged over 70 years the problem can last longer (Sharrock, et al., 2005), probably due to the influence of centrally acting analgesics administered after the operation. Insufficient postoperative analgesia, hypoglycemia, hypotension and hypoxaemia may all be important.

There were studies (Herrmann et al., 2001; Kilminster, Treasure, McMillan, & Holt, 1999; Snyder-Ramos et al., 2004) showing that an elevated serum S100B protein correlated with a worsening of the results of neuropsychological tests, while in some papers those correlations (Anderson, 2002) were not observed. Patients after cardiac surgery with an increased serum S100B concentration who showed any signs of brain injury had a shorter time of survival (Johnsson, 2000); thus, an elevated level of the S100B protein may reflect subclinical brain damage. Linstedt et al.(Linstedt, et al., 2002) did not observe any differences in S100B protein serum concentrations in urological patients, irrespective of the presence (or absence) of signs of POCD, but in all the patients after hip or knee arthroplasty an increased serum level of the S100B protein was noted, regardless of the presence (or absence) of POCD. An elevated concentration of the S100B protein may partially reflect a release of the protein from an extracerebral localizations, e.g. from bone marrow. During bone cement use, however, one of the reasons of an increased S100B protein level may be a thermal bone marrow injury, or an injury to the brain or red blood cells.

4. Summary

Cognitive dysfunctions in hospitalized patients were important clinically and socially, but difficult to analyze methodologically. Disturbances at the cellular level can manifest themselves as mood disorders and lead to a deterioration in the patients' functioning and their social assessment. It is very difficult to define either the normal state or the pathology of cognitive functions.

Although there was no agreement as to the correlation between an increased serum concentration of the S100B protein and the results of neuropsychological tests, we know that the measurement of the S100B protein as a single parameter was not sufficient to anticipate the occurrence of POCD in the postoperative period following orthopedic procedures.

The identification of patients with preexisting risk factors of POCD, shortening the period of time preceding the surgery and a proper technique of the procedure as well as physical and intellectual exercises, nutrition and medication (Blaise, et al., 2007) play an important role in decreasing the incidence of neurocognitive deficits in the elderly.

5. References

Ali, M. S., Harmer, M., & Vaughan, R. (2000). Serum S100 protein as a marker of cerebral damage during cardiac surgery. *Br J Anaesth, 85*(2), 287.

Anderson, R. E. (2002). No correlation between serum concentrations of S100B and cognitive function. *Acta Anaesthesiol Scand, 46*(9), 1179. doi: aas460922_7 [pii]

Anderson, R. E., Hansson, L. O., Nilsson, O., Dijlai-Merzoug, R., & Settergren, G. (2001). High serum S100B levels for trauma patients without head injuries. *Neurosurgery, 48*(6), 1255.

Avidan, M. S., Searleman, A. C., Storandt, M., Barnett, K., Vannucci, A., Saager, L., . . . Morris, J. C. (2009). Long-term cognitive decline in older subjects was not attributable to non-cardiac surgery or major illness. *Anesthesiology, 111*(5), 964-970.

Blaise, G., Taha, R., & Qi, Y. (2007). Postoperative Cognitive Dysfunction (POCD). *Anesthesiology Rounds, 6*(4), 1-6.

Canet, J., Raeder, J., Rasmussen, L., Enlund, M., Kuipers, H. M., Hanning, C., . . . Dodds, C. (2003). Cognitive dysfunction after minor surgery in the elderly. *Acta Anaesthesiol Scand, 47*(10), 1204-1210.

Clark, D., Ahmed, A., Baxendale, B., & Moran, C. (2001). Cardiac output during hemiarthroplasty of the hip: A prospective, controlled trial of cemented and uncemented prostheses. *Journal of Bone and Joint Surgery-British Volume, 83*(3), 414.

Colonna, D. M., Kilgus, D., Brown, W., Challa, V., Stump, D. A., & Moody, D. M. (2002). Acute brain fat embolization occurring after total hip arthroplasty in the absence of a patent foramen ovale. *Anesthesiology, 96*(4), 1027-1029.

Concepcion, M. (1998). Anesthesia for orthopedic surgery. In J. Tinker, G. E. Morgan Jr & D. E. Longnecker (Eds.), *Principles and practice of anesthesiology* (Vol. II, pp. 2113-2137): Mosby.

Dahn, J., Oster, M., Möltner, A., Wöhrle, C., Rätzer-Frey, A., van Ackern, K., . . . Segiet, W. (1999). Anesthesia in geriatric patients. The determination of physiological variables for cognitive function in geriatric patients after regional or general anesthesia]. *Der Anaesthesist, 48*(6), 379.

Desborough, J. (2000). The stress response to trauma and surgery. *Br J Anaesth, 85*(1), 109-117.

Donaldson, A., Thomson, H., Harper, N., & Kenny, N. (2009). Bone cement implantation syndrome. *Br J Anaesth, 102*(1), 12.

Eckert, R. L., Broome, A. M., Ruse, M., Robinson, N., Ryan, D., & Lee, K. (2003). S100 proteins in the epidermis. *Journal of Investigative Dermatology, 123*(1), 23-33.

Edmonds, C. R., Barbut, D., Hager, D., & Sharrock, N. E. (2000). Intraoperative cerebral arterial embolization during total hip arthroplasty. *Anesthesiology, 93*(2), 315.

Fallon, K. M., Fuller, J. G., & Morley-Forster, P. (2001). Fat embolization and fatal cardiac arrest during hip arthroplasty with methylmethacrylate. *Can J Anaesth, 48*(7), 626-629.

Farag, E., Chelune, G. J., Schubert, A., & Mascha, E. J. (2006). Is depth of anesthesia, as assessed by the bispectral index, related to postoperative cognitive dysfunction and recovery? *Anesth Analg, 103*(3), 633.

Fines, D. P., & Severn, A. M. (2006). Anaesthesia and cognitive disturbance in the elderly. *Continuing Education in Anaesthesia, Critical Care & Pain, 6*(1), 37.

Fodale, V., Santamaria, L., Schifilliti, D., & Mandal, P. (2010). Anaesthetics and postoperative cognitive dysfunction: a pathological mechanism mimicking Alzheimer's disease. *Anaesthesia, 65*(4), 388-395.

Gao, L., Taha, R., Gauvin, D., Othmen, L. B., Wang, Y., & Blaise, G. (2005). Postoperative Cognitive Dysfunction After Cardiac Surgery. *Chest, 128*(5), 3664-3670.

Harwood, T. N. (2000). Optimizing outcome in the very elderly surgical patient. *Curr Opin Anaesthesiol, 13*(3), 327-332.

Hayakawa, M., Fujioka, Y., Morimoto, Y., Okamura, A., & Kemmotsu, O. (2001). Pathological evaluation of venous emboli during total hip arthroplasty. *Anaesthesia, 56*(6), 571-575. doi: 10.1111/j.1365-2044.2001.1913-2.x

Heizmann, C. W. (2004). S100B protein in clinical diagnostics: assay specificity. *Clinical Chemistry, 50*(1), 249.

Herrmann, M., Curio, N., Jost, S., Grubich, C., Ebert, A., Fork, M., & Synowitz, H. (2001). Release of biochemical markers of damage to neuronal and glial brain tissue is associated with short and long term neuropsychological outcome after traumatic brain injury. *Journal of Neurology, Neurosurgery & Psychiatry, 70*(1), 95.

Hudetz, J., Iqbal, Z., Gandhi, S., Patterson, K., Byrne, A., Hudetz, A., . . . Warltier, D. (2009). Ketamine attenuates post operative cognitive dysfunction after cardiac surgery. *Acta Anaesthesiol Scand, 53*(7), 864-872.

Hudetz, J. A., Patterson, K. M., Iqbal, Z., Gandhi, S. D., Byrne, A. J., Hudetz, A. G., . . . Pagel, P. S. (2009). Ketamine attenuates delirium after cardiac surgery with cardiopulmonary bypass. *J Cardiothorac Vasc Anesth, 23*(5), 651-657.

Ingebrigtsen T, R. B. Biochemical serum markers for brain damage: a short review with emphasis on clinical utility in mild head injury. *Restorative Neurology and Neuroscience 2003; 21: 171 - 176.*

Ingebrigtsen, T., & Romner, B. (2003). Biochemical serum markers for brain damage: a short review with emphasis on clinical utility in mild head injury. [Review]. *Restor Neurol Neurosci, 21*(3-4), 171-176.

Jenkins, K., Chung, F., Wennberg, R., Etchells, E. E., & Davey, R. Fat embolism syndrome and elective knee arthroplasty.

Johnsson, P. (2000). Markers of brain cell damage related to cardiac surgery. *Critical Care, 4*, 1-2.

Kilminster, S., Treasure, T., McMillan, T., & Holt, D. W. (1999). Neuropsychological change and S-100 protein release in 130 unselected patients undergoing cardiac surgery. *Stroke, 30*(9), 1869-1874.

Kim, Y.-H., Oh, S.-W., & Kim, J.-S. (2002). Prevalence of Fat Embolism Following Bilateral Simultaneous and Unilateral Total Hip Arthroplasty Performed with or without Cement : A Prospective, Randomized Clinical Study. *J Bone Joint Surg Am, 84*(8), 1372-1379.

Kinoshita, H., Iranami, H., Fujii, K., Yamazaki, A., Shimogai, M., Nakahata, K., . . . Hatano, Y. (2003). The use of bone cement induces an increase in serum astroglial S-100B protein in patients undergoing total knee arthroplasty. *Anesth & Analg, 97*(6), 1657.

Kleindienst, A., & Ross Bullock, M. (2006). A critical analysis of the role of the neurotrophic protein S100B in acute brain injury. [Review]. *J Neurotrauma., 23*(8), 1185-1200.

Kuhn, K.-D. (2005). Properties of bone cement: what is bone cement? In H. Malchau & S. J. Breutsch (Eds.), *The well-cemented total hip arthroplasty* (pp. 66-73). Heidelberg: Springer Medizin Verlag.

Kyziridis, T. C. (2006). Post-operative delirium after hip fracture treatment: a review of current literature. *GMS Psycho-Social-Medicine, 3*, 1-12.

Linstedt, U., Meyer, O., Kropp, P., Berkau, A., Tapp, E., & Zenz, M. (2002). Serum concentration of S 100 protein in assessment of cognitive dysfunction after general anesthesia in different types of surgery. *Acta Anaesth Scand, 46*(4), 384-389.

Marenholz, I., Heizmann, C. W., & Fritz, G. (2004). S100 proteins in mouse and man: from evolution to function and pathology (including an update of the nomenclature). *Biochemical and Biophysical Research Communications, 322*(4), 1111-1122.

Newman, S., Stygall, J., Hirani, S., Shaefi, S., & Maze, M. (2007). Postoperative cognitive dysfunction after noncardiac surgery: a systematic review. *Anesthesiology, 106*(3), 572-590. doi: 00000542-200703000-00023 [pii]

Nunn, J. F. (1981). *Kliniczna fizjologia oddychania ze szczególnym uwzględnieniem anestezjologii.* Warszawa: PZWL.

Ohtani, R., Tomimoto, H., Wakita, H., Kitaguchi, H., Nakaji, K., & Takahashi, R. (2007). Expression of S100 protein and protective effect of arundic acid on the rat brain in chronic cerebral hypoperfusion. *Brain Research, 1135*, 195-200.

Ozelsel, T., Tillmann Hein, H., Marcel, R. J., Rathjen, K. W., Ramsay, M., & Jackson, R. W. (1998). Delayed neurological deficit after total hip arthroplasty. *Anesth Analg, 87*(5), 1209.

Pelinka, L., Szalay, L., Jafarmadar, M., Schmidhammer, R., Redl, H., & Bahrami, S. (2003). Circulating S100B is increased after bilateral femur fracture without brain injury in the rat. *Br J Anaesth, 91*(4), 595.

Pelinka, L. E. (2004). Serum markers of severe traumatic brain injury: Are they useful? *Indian Journal of Critical Care Medicine, 8*(3), 190.

Piazza, O., Russo, E., Cotena, S., Esposito, G., & Tufano, R. (2007). Elevated S100B levels do not correlate with the severity of encephalopathy during sepsis. *Br J Anaesth, 99*(4), 518.

Raabe, A., Kopetsch, O., Woszczyk, A., Lang, J., Gerlach, R., Zimmermann, M., & Seifert, V. (2003). Serum S-100B protein as a molecular marker in severe traumatic brain injury. *Restorative Neurology and Neuroscience, 21*(4), 159-170.

Rasmussen, L., Johnson, T., Kuipers, H. M., Kristensen, D., Siersma, V. D., Vila, P., . . . Silverstein, J. (2003). Does anaesthesia cause postoperative cognitive dysfunction? A randomised study of regional versus general anaesthesia in 438 elderly patients. *Acta Anaesth Scand, 47*(3), 260-266.

Rasmussen, L. S. (1998). Defining postoperative cognitive dysfunction. *Eur J Anaesthesiol, 15*(6), 761-764.

Riding, G., Daly, K., Hutchinson, S., Rao, S., Lovell, M., & McCollum, C. (2004). Paradoxical arterial embolization. An explanation for fat embolism syndrome. *J Bone Joint Surg [Br], 86-B*, 95-98. doi: 10.1302/0301-620x.86b1.14108

Roach, G. W., Kanchuger, M., Mangano, C. M., Newman, M., Nussmeier, N., Wolman, R., . . . Ley, C. (1996). Adverse cerebral outcomes after coronary bypass surgery. *N Engl J Med, 335*(25), 1857-1864.

Rohan, D., Buggy, D. J., Crowley, S., Ling, F. K. H., Gallagher, H., Regan, C., & Moriarty, D. C. (2005). Increased incidence of postoperative cognitive dysfunction 24h after minor surgery in the elderly. *Can J Anaesth, 52*(2), 137-142.

Salama, I., Malone, P., Mihaimeed, F., & Jones, J. (2008). A review of the S100 proteins in cancer. *European Journal of Surgical Oncology (EJSO), 34*(4), 357-364.

Scroop, R., Eskridge, J., & Britz, G. W. (2002). Paradoxical cerebral arterial embolization of cement during intraoperative vertebroplasty: case report. *AJNR Am J Neuroradiol, 23*(5), 868-870.

Sharrock, N. E., Beckman, J. D., Inda, E. C., & Savarese, J. J. Anesthesia for orthopedic surgery. In R. D. Miller (Ed.), *Miller's Anesthesia* (Vol. II, pp. 2417).

Sharrock, N. E., Fischer, G., Goss, S., Flynn, E., Go, G., Sculco, T. P., & Salvati, E. A. (2005). The early recovery of cognitive function after total-hip replacement under hypotensive epidural anesthesia. *Reg Anesth Pain Med, 30*(2), 123-127.

Singh, A., & Antognini, J. F. (2010). Perioperative pharmacology in elderly patients. *Curr Opin Anesthesiol, 23*(4), 449-454.

Snyder-Ramos, S. A., Gruhlke, T., Bauer, H., Bauer, M., Luntz, A. P., Motsch, J., . . . Bottiger, B. W. (2004). Cerebral and extracerebral release of protein S100B in cardiac surgical patients. *Anaesthesia, 59*(4), 344-349. doi: 10.1111/j.1365-2044.2004.03663.x ANA3663 [pii]

Stålnacke, B., Ohlsson, A., Tegner, Y., & Sojka, P. (2006). Serum concentrations of two biochemical markers of brain tissue damage S-100B and neurone specific enolase are increased in elite female soccer players after a competitive game. *British Journal of Sports Medicine, 40*(4), 313.

Stalnacke, B. M., Tegner, Y., & Sojka, P. (2003). Playing ice hockey and basketball increases serum levels of S-100B in elite players: a pilot study. *Clinical Journal of Sport Medicine, 13*(5), 292.

Sukernik, M. R., Mets, B., & Bennett-Guerrero, E. (2001). Patent Foramen Ovale and its Significance in the Perioperative Period. *Anesth Analg, 93*(5), 1137-1146.

Undén, J., Bellner, J., Eneroth, M., Alling, C., Ingebrigtsen, T., & Romner, B. (2005). Raised serum S100B levels after acute bone fractures without cerebral injury. *J Trauma, 58*(1), 59.

Van Munster, B. C., Korse, C. M., De Rooij, S. E., Bonfrer, J. M., Zwinderman, A. H., & Korevaar, J. C. (2009). Markers of cerebral damage during delirium in elderly patients with hip fracture. *BMC Neurology, 9*(1), 21.

Veering, B. T. (1999). Management of anaesthesia in elderly patients. *Curr Opin Anaesthesiol 12*(3), 333-336.

Williams-Russo, P., Sharrock, N. E., Mattis, S., Szatrowski, T. P., & Charlson, M. E. (1995). Cognitive effects after epidural vs general anesthesia in older adults. *JAMA: The Journal of the American Medical Association, 274*(1), 44.

Wu, C. L., Hsu, W., Richman, J. M., & Raja, S. N. (2004). Postoperative cognitive function as an outcome of regional anesthesia and analgesia. *Reg Anesth Pain Med, 29*(3), 257-268. doi: 10.1016/j.rapm.2003.11.007

2

The Stress Response and Its Functional Implications in the Immune Response After Surgery in Patients with Chronic Inflammation Undergoing Arthroplasty

Barbara Lisowska
Institute of Rheumatology, Warsaw, Poland

1. Introduction

Surgical injury evokes an injury response involving immunologic mechanisms. Alterations in the immune response after surgery are recognized as physiological reactions of the organism to restore its homeostasis. The immune responses are characterized by the release of cytokines, inflammatory mediators and acute-phase proteins. The activation of immune cells is followed by the release of various cytokines as well as by a migration of leukocytes into inflamed tissues. Cytokines play roles in the immune response, inflammatory reaction and homeostasis maintaining. Alternations of cytokines concentration in patients with normal immune system function are probably not sufficient and temporary to cause the relevant immune problems postoperative. Moreover, this response is characterized by proper balance between pro-and anti-inflammatory cytokines. Conversely, in patients with chronic inflammatory state the surgery stimulated immune response can be an additional aggravating factor that can contribute to the weakening or pathological intensification of the response.

The surgery is associated with trauma-related immunological changes. The level of these immunological changes directly correlates with the degree of tissue damage. Both surgery and anesthesia are immunosuppressive factors, but regional anesthesia seems to be less than general anesthesia.

Rheumatoid arthritis is an autoimmune disorder characterized by immune-mediated chronic inflammation including a degradation of the connective tissue and bone. The chronic inflammatory state is related with a strong prolonged stimulation of the immune system including a release of the complete cytokines cascade and inflammatory mediators targeted against self cells. So suddenly and unexpectly the friend turns into the enemy with a excited powerful destructive force.

2. The short overview of the immune system and stress response to a surgery

The surgery-associated tissue damage leads to the activation of the immune system and the inflammatory response. The bidirectional relationship between the neuroendocrine and

immune systems with the participation of common mediators seems be essential for the mechanisms of the chronic inflammatory state including hormonal and immune changes. The tight coexistence the autonomic nervous system and the hypothalamic-pituitary adrenal axis (HPA axis) is extremely important for damping as well as hastening the reaction of the immune system. The presence of the chronic inflammatory state is exactly with the dysfunction of the neuroendocrine-immune system. The crucial aims of the immune system are the organism protection by recognition and elimination of the antigens which are usually different various components but generally are infectious agents such as bacteria, viruses and fungi.
Two types of immunity can be distinguished from the immune system: the nonspecific (innate) and the specific (acquired) response. There are two forms of acquired response the humoral and the cell mediated.

2.1 The innate immunity

The innate immunity contains the following elements such as: the Langerhans cells inside the skin, the submucosal tissues of the respiratory and alimentary tracts, the complement system, the phagocytic cells (granulocytes and macrophages) and the glial cells. Lymphocytes, granulocytes and macrophages are responsible for the elimination of antigens. The initiation of the immune response has its own essential origin in the mononuclear phagocyte system (MPS) which is represented by monocytes and macrophages (both type of cells accumulate in the site of surgery). During the first step of immune response the antigen is absorbed by MPS cells and degraded into peptides in the intracellular compartments. The pathogen-associated molecular patterns (PAMPs) are the molecules associated with microorganisms which can be recognized by sophisticated presentation to the pattern-recognition receptors (PRR) and the Toll-like receptors (TLRs) situated on the membrane surface or inside of various cells. They have unique ability of the triggering innate immune responses. Toll like receptors (TLR) belong to the PRR family and play key role whilst the induction of the immune response. The TLRs are also expressed by immune cells and various other cells such as endothelium, muscle cells and adipocytes. It can be said they participate while both types of immune response especially during the induction and the regulation of T and B lymphocytes activates (Majewska & Szczepanik 2006).

2.2 The cells and mechanism of the acquired immunity

When the innate mechanisms are not enough to inactive microorganisms then the proteins from pathogenic antigens are presented to molecules expressed on B or T cells becoming their activators. The process called the antigen processing and the presentation leads to the proliferation of the activated lymphocytes and is typical for the acquired immunity.
As the after-consequence of the response to signals from the mononuclear phagocytes the B lymphocytes differentiate into plasma cells. Moreover, T lymphocytes become active and starts to release soluble factors known as cytokines (Stevenson et al., 1990).
Contrasted with innate **the acquired response** is more sophisticated form of the immunity and requires longer activation period. The main cells of the **acquired immunity** are both type of lymphocytes and also the antigen presenting cells (APC) such as dendritic cell. Chronic inflammatory state can modify these elements and delay the triggering of the both mechanism of the immune response. The primary role of the **B**

lymphocytes/ plasma cells is the synthesis and the secretion of antibodies associated with the components of the humoral response.

Immunoglobulins (antibodies) are formed by - two identical light (L) and the two identical heavy (H) chains. The main form of the immunoglobulins are described: one of them is presented on the membrane surface of the B cells as the antigen specific receptor (BCR). However, the other one exists as the soluble form and is produced by plasma cells. The biologic results of the antigen-antibody reactions include many consequences such as agglutination with soluble antigen, as well as precipitations and activation of complement that results in the neutralization of bacterial toxins and microorganisms activity.

The activation of the B cells starts through the B cell receptor (BCR) at the cell membrane and triggers the intracellular signaling pathways regulating the transcription of antibodies and cytokines genes (Coico & Sunshine 2009). The BCR has the exceptional ability to react with many different types of antigens such as peptides DNA, lipids and carbohydrates.

The T lymphocytes are a part of the **cell-mediated** immunity and their role is the cytokines production and support of the B cells activation. The T lymphocytes are divided into following subsets: h*elper (Th), cytotoxic (CCTL), regulatory (T reg) and memory (Tm).* Similarly B cells and the T cells also have the antigen binding receptor on their surface (TCR) but in contrast to the BCR, the TCR interacts with small fragments of antigenic proteins called peptides which are presented on APC in association with class I and class II molecules included MHC.

The major histocompatibility complex (MHC) in the humans called human leukocyte antigen (HLA) has many different diverse immunological and non-immunological functions. The MHC is divided into two types of molecules encoded by the MHC classes: MHC class I and MHC class II. Both of them are recognized by different subsets of the T cells. The MHC class I molecules have the crucial task of the presentation of an antigenic protein to the T Cytotoxic lymphocytes (CD8+) while MHC class II presents an antigen to T Helper lymphocytes (CD4+). Molecules of MHC class I are found on the surface of all nucleated cells of human body while molecules of MHC class II are found on the surface of the APC (Coico & Sunshine 2009). The MHC complex includes the most polymorphic genomes in the human genomes with many consequences related to the transplantation and the autoimmune disease. It turned out that the human leukocyte antigen HLA-B27 is tightly correlated with the frequency of the spondylarthritis (Cauli et al., 2002; Jin & Wang, 2003). The adhesion molecules CD4+ and CD8+ are necessary to enhance the binding of the T cells and the APC. The expression of CD4+ and CD8+ is variable on the T cells. The normal ratio of CD4+ T cell to CD8+ T cells is approximately 2:1 in healthy population.

The dendritic cells (DC) are classical, the most potent APC and by this way they contribute to connection between the innate and acquire immune systems. The dendritic cells present the ability to initiate several immune responses such as stimulation of T and B lymphocytes and the resistance against various infections and cancer cells (Bodey et al., 1997).

Cytokines are produced by all cells of the human immune system. Cytokines form a complex network secretory molecules which exert their effects on the phases of the immune response. Cytokines are immensely responsible for the transduction of information among the immune system cells and are the very important components of the bi-directional communication between the immune and the neuroendocrine systems (Lisowska et al., 2008). Depending on the prevailing effects of inflammatory response they are called as a pro-inflammatory or anti-inflammatory. The pro-inflammatory cytokines are mainly represented by interleukins: IL-1, IL-6, TNF, IL-2, IL-6, IL-8, IL-15. The examples of the anti-inflammatory cytokines are interleukins IL-4, IL-10, TGF-β. Cytokines may act locally or systemically by cell to cell signaling. The action of cytokines can be described as autocrine, paracrine or endocrine. Some cytokines are known to act in either synergistic or antagonistic way. Cytokines may affect the action of each other which may give synergistic or antagonistic effect on the targeted cells. Both the synthesis and activity of cytokines are regarded at different levels. Different type of antagonistic molecules (e.g. soluble receptor, cytokine binding proteins, molecules that compete with cytokine for binding to the receptors) are produced to restrict they activities. The potent pro-inflammatory activities of cytokines are restricted by three major systems that can prevent uncontrolled excessive production of cytokines. These relates to their synthesis and release membrane receptors and intracellular signal transduction (Weber et al., 2010). Both overproduction and underproduction of cytokines and their receptors take place in many diseases with prevailed acute or chronic inflammatory state.

2.3 The interdependence between the neuroendocrine and the immune system whilst direct response to surgery stress

The surgical stress" can be described as a various alterations inside organism undergoing surgical procedure. The tissue damage caused by surgery leads to activation of the immune system and the early inflammatory response and directly correlates with the degree of tissue damage. A full-fledged systemic inflammatory reaction results in stimulation of the four major programs: the acute-phase reaction, the sickness syndrome, the pain program and the stress response, mediated by the hypothalamic-pituitary-adrenal axis and the sympathetic nervous system. The cooperation between the autonomic nervous system and the hypothalamic-pituitary adrenal axis (HPA axis) is important to dampen the reaction of the immune system.

The response to trauma consists of the hormonal as well as the immunological and the metabolic responses. The host response is mainly characterized by increased secretion of various hormones such as: cortisol, catecholamines, ADH (antidiuretic hormone), glucagon and growth hormone.

The direct afferent impulses from surgery site release several factors which strongly activate hypothalamus for corticotropin releasing hormone (CRH) secretion which in turn stimulates the pituitary gland to release its typical hormones. The potent correlation exist between concentration of hormones such as ACTH, cortisol, ADH and intensity of the surgical stress. The neurogenic stimuli from surgery site can be ceased by central blockade such as the spinal and the epidural anesthesia. The immune system and the neuroendocrine system influence each other via molecules and receptors shared by both systems. Activation of the neuroendocrine system results in alteration of the host homeostasis and the immune response including cytokine production.

Somatostatin and catecholamines are the basic examples of the mentioned correlation. Somatostatin (SS) is an endogenous peptide widespread distribute related with five known somatostatin receptors (sst1-5) which are usually expressed on the surface of the immune cells and on central and peripheral neurons as well. The SS is found in the central nervous system, the gastrointestinal tract and endocrine glands. Moreover, macrophage, endothelial cells and lymphocytes express high affinity receptors for the somatostatin (Armani et al., 2007; Dalm et al., 2003; Ferone et al., 2006).

Norepinephrine and dopamine can also increase the activation and the proliferation of T cells. Moreover, norepinephrine modulates the innate immune response e.g. by the inhibition of tumor necrosis factor (TNF) synthesis. TNF and IL-1β are classical pro-inflammatory cytokines secreted mostly by monocytes (Torres et al., 2005).
The different types of stress is associated with high production of catecholamines and corticosteroids cause immunosupression. Both hormones can inhibit the production of interferon gamma (IFN-γ) and simultaneously stimulate the production of the anti-inflammatory cytokines: IL-4, IL-10 by the T helper cells via adrenergic receptors. The stimulation of the β2-adrenergic receptors on CD4(+) T lymphocytes cause the inhibition of their proliferation and the cytokines secretion (Riether et al., 2011; Salicrú et al., 2007).
The another example of bidirectional correlation between the immune and the neuroendocrine system is the ghrelin secreted primarily by the stomach and intestine cells. Although, it should be noted that the hypothalamus, the pituitary gland and the other peripheral organs can also be the source of the ghrelin. The ghrelin acts on the other, however expresses many immunological functions through the growth hormone receptor expressed in many immune cells include the T lymphocytes,the B lymphocytes, monocytes and neutrophils. In addition, the ghrelin is known as the anti-inflammatory mediator and seems to have an opposite effects to the TNF while modulation of the immune response (Baatar et al., 2009; Hattori, 2009).
Ghrelin acts on other immune cells such as the T lymphocytes, the B lymphocytes, monocytes and neutrophils via the growth hormone receptor via and shows the anti-inflammatory action in inflammatory response (Himmerich & Sheldrick, 2010).
Metabolic response is also induced by the surgery trauma: However, depressed during first hours after the surgery in next phase is characterized by increase of catabolism and hypermetabolism with gluconeogenesis lasting 3-4 days. Metabolic changes induced by the surgery trauma are the part of the systemic reaction that includes a wide range of endocrinological, immunological and hematological effects. Perioperative metabolic changes described as the hypermetabolism include rapid increased oxygen consumption. Postoperatively, hypermetabolism is associated with increased glucose serum level, lactates and free fatty acids. The electrolytes disturbance takes important part while the metabolic response. Lower serum potassium level is the predictor of a serious perioperative arrhythmia and hypoproteinemia as well as it can disturb the process of wound healing (Blackburn, 2011; Jakob & Stanga, 2010; Wahr, 1999).

2.4 The inflammatory response

The inflammatory response is the fundamental type of response against various situation like e.g. trauma or infection and it is focused on stimulation of various parameters which are essential for the wound healing, the protection against infection and the maintenance of homeostasis. The acute inflammatory response to surgery trauma can be prescribed as the combination of the neurological stimulation with the metabolic changes trigger release of the molecules of the local inflammation such as histamine, kinins and prostaglandins with increasing capillary permeability which allows leucocytes and lymphocytes the infiltration into injury site. The pro-inflammatory cytokines such as IL-1, IL-6, TNF-α are released from immune cells, their concentration correlate with the length of surgery therefore they are considered as an indicator of stress severity (Cruickshank et al., 1990; Norman & Fink, 1997). The function of cytokines focusing on communication between cells in both the paracrine and the endocrine way. Pro-inflammatory cytokines (IL-6, TNF, IL-1) are potent

inducers of acute phase proteins (APPs). Among some (e.g. C-reactive protein (CRP), complement factors, fibrinogen, plazminogen CAPPs) are up- regulated while production of others (albumin, transferrin, antitrombin) decreased (Engler, 1995).
The long-lasting inflammatory process called chronic inflammatory response, itself is a organism wasting disease. The presence of the chronic inflammatory state is immensely associated with the dysfunction of the neuroendocrine-immune system. The neuroendocrine -immune disturbances also play an crucial role in the development of human autoimmune diseases such as the rheumatoid arthritis and the systemic lupus erythematous and the others. During the chronic inflammatory stage all these systems have become deficient.

3. The short overview of the role of cytokines in rheumatoid arthritis

Inflammatory diseases such as arthritis share some common clinical characteristics including the degradation of the connective tissue and bone. The rheumatoid arthritis (RA) is the chronic inflammatory state characterized by synovial inflammation and progressive joint cartilage and bone destruction. The chronic inflammatory process with the continuous stimulation of synoviocytes directly leads to the hypertrophy of the synovial membrane and bone resorption. The development of RA is associated with the uncontrolled production of pro-inflammatory cytokines by the activated synoviocytes and the antigen stimulated lymphocytes. The cytokines mentioned below play significant role while both the development of the RA and the surgical stress response
Interleukin -1 (IL-1) is produced by macrophages, monocytes and endothelial cells. The secretion of IL-1 is triggered by many factors including TNF and complements. The interleukin 1 (IL-1) family includes two forms of IL-1 (IL-1α, IL-1β), IL-1 receptors (RI, RII) and IL-1 receptor antagonist (IL-1Ra). Interestingly, the recent results of studies suggested that the interleukin-1α (IL-1α) plays the neuroprotective role inside the damaged brain cells (Clausen et al. 2011). During the early stages of shock, the IL-1β is secreted from liver cells after the stimulation of noradrenalin, which may be the example of the relationship between neuro-immune systems (Zhou et al., 2005). In rheumatoid arthritis patients, the plasma and the synovial fluid concentrations of IL-1 are elevated and are correlated with various parameters of disease severity. The production of endogenous IL-1Ra appears to be insufficient to counteract IL-1 activity (Pritchard et al., 2008). It is also appeared that IL-1β has a significant impact on the process of damage and degradation of the cartilage in the pathogenesis of arthritis (Aida et al., 2006).
Interleukin -6 (IL-6) is secreted by many cells types. In RA joints synoviocytes are the major source of IL-6. The production of IL-6 is induced by IL-1 and TNF. IL-6 is involved in development of immune response, inflammation and haemotopoiesis. For instance, it regulates the growth and differentiation of the lymphocytes T and is considered as the a critical factor for B cells proliferation and stimulation of the immunoglobulin production. The serum elevation of IL-6 is noticeable in face of infections, inflammation and injury when IL-6 induces fever and production of acute phase proteins. Silverman et al. (28) recently demonstrated that IL-6 can directly stimulate the corticosteroid secretion from the adrenal cortex and there is evidence suggesting that it can also stimulate ACTH secretion from the pituitary gland (Silverman et al., 2004). IL-6 has also anti -inflammatory function by stimulation of monocytes to release anti inflammatory cytokines such as IL-10, IL-1Ra.

The receptor for IL-6 consists of two proteins: the chain α, that can be expressed on membrane cell or in soluble form and subunit gp130 that belongs to proteins receptor for IL-6 in membrane cells. In contrast to most cytokines (e.g. TNF) soluble IL-6 acts as agonist but not antagonist.

IL-6 play important role in many inflammatory diseases. RA is characterized by the overproduction of IL-6. The very high level of IL-6 in the serum and synovial fluid is involved and correlated with clinical and laboratory indices (Lisowska et al., Dec 2007; Nishimoto, 2006).

The secretion of both, described cytokines (IL-1, IL-6) is stimulated by tumor necrosis factor (TNF).

Tumor necrosis factor - is produced by monocytes, macrophages, neutrophils, mast cells, fibroblasts, and the activated T cells.

TNF is a number of TNF family. The binding of TNF to its receptors TNFR1 and TNFR2 cause multiple effects including: the increase of inflammatory mediators (e.g. nitric oxide (NO), arachidonic acid pathway, the platelet activating factor (PAF) and intracellular adhesion molecules (ICAM)) (Lenzab et all., 2007; Lenz et al., 2007).

The increased expression of TNF occurs in the synovium of rheumatoid arthritis patients with following induction of its cells activities. TNF is thought to play the role key role in the local activation of immune cells and joint cartilage and bone destruction. Together with IL-1 TNF-α also induce an expression of adhesion molecules on the surface of the endothelial cells which is particularly important during the first stages of inflammation, because it enables the infiltration of leukocytes from the bloodstream into the tissues.

Transforming growth factor -β (TGF-β) belongs to the TGF family cytokines. The TGF-β plays crucial role in inhibition of the inflammatory reaction and autoimmune diseases. The TGF-β plays the essential role in control and regulation of the lymphocytes proliferation, differentiation and survival. The TGF function including the antiproliferation activity on the T, B lymphocytes that can initiate and aggravate the disease. The TGF-β is also an important regulator of the B cell activation and differentiation (Li et al., 2006) Most of the produced cytokines are not stored at all. Nevertheless there are produced and released as needed. However, transforming growth factor β is stored inside the mast cells and platelets (Sheran & Hall, 1997).

4. The influence of regional anesthesia for stress surgery response

The choice of anesthesia type as well as technique relates to influence on the immune response and may be important in patients with immunological disorders. This situation occurs in patients with immune system deficiency. Patients suffer from immune system disturbances, due to autoimmune or cancer diseases, appear to require special consideration. Among this group of patients should be expected the pathological reaction of immune system or significant immunosupression caused by the surgery trauma.

The imbalanced immune system can modulate the neuroendocrine system and inflammatory responses to the surgery trauma in terms of production of cytokines, immunoglobins, proliferation of lymphocytes, and phagocytosis monocytes/macrophages. The choice of regional anesthesia techniques allow to avoid the supply of volatile/ intravenous anesthetics agents and the controlled ventilation procedures. Furthermore , the afferent nerves blockade is associated with attenuation of the hormonal response to the surgery stress. The regional anesthesia techniques have a significant effect on the immune

system which depends on both the nerve blockade and the administrated local anesthetic drugs (Lisowska, 2008).
The results of study revealed the influence of the bupivacaine presence for the reduction of the synthesis of immunoglobin IgG, IgM, IgA and enhancing the granulocytes phagocytosis. The epidural anesthesia with bupivacaine was associated with lower serum concentration of gammaglobulins (IgG, IgM, IgA) and the complement components C3 and C4 (Gajdosz, 1994).
Bupivacaine is the most popular, long acting local anesthetic with a wide range of administration for peripheral and central nerves blockades. Ropivacaine is also a long acting local anesthetic drug similar to bupivacaine in terms of pharmacological activity, but in contrast to is characterized by the lower cardiotoxity. Lidocaine is the most often and widely used local anesthetic for the peripheral nerves blockades especially in the combination with the bupivacaine for more beneficial balance of duration and onset. Lidocaine is also classified as an anti-arrhythmic agent. Bupivacaine in comparison with the lidocaine shows more potent effect on the function of leukocytes. However, the ropivacaine has been shown its anti-inflammatory properties related to the inhibition of leukocyte function such as the rolling/ adhesion which accompanies the early stage of the local inflammatory response. Moreover, both the ropivacaine and lidocaine could inhibit the CD11b/CD18 up-regulation and the L-selectin down-regulation on neutrophils migration between endothelial cells. There has been found that the effect of the lidocaine was 2.5 times lower than the ropivacaine (Martinsson et al., 1997; Zhang et al., 2000).
The extent of nerves blockade, occurs due to regional anesthesia, appears to have an influence on the neuro-endo-immune response intensity. The endocrine - metabolic stimulation following the surgical procedure can be inhibited by the afferent nerves blockade. The blockade of motor, sensory and afferent sympathetic fibers leads to resulted in predominance of parasympathetic system resulting changes in circulation The intensified circulation may reduce the release of cytokines associated with the tissue ischemia and hypoxia but from the other site a marked low perfusion triggers cytokines burs following hypoxia. The degree of blood flow distribution is directly related to the level of the blockade. It was shown that usage of continuous epidural anesthesia reduced the hormonal stress response and improved the protein metabolism, but it didn't play any significant role in the stimulation of inflammatory response (Kehler, 2000). Although in comparison with general anesthesia, the epidural anesthesia demonstrate less effect on the activity of natural killer cell (NK), T and B cells (Tonnesen et al., 1988).
The spinal anesthesia is considered as the standard procedure for the orthopedic surgery. The choice of the central blockade is influenced with many benefits such as reduced risk of the postoperative cardiovascular, pulmonary and thromboembolic complications. The prolonged analgesia which spreads onto post operative period is also worth to be emphasized. The patients who underwent surgery with the spinal anesthesia would require greatly less opioids which action is not neutral to the immune system. Further advantages of the regional anesthesia, especially in the RA patients, has ability to avoid the difficult and traumatic intubation. The majority of patients with advanced RA demonstrated the atlanto-axial instability with the great risk of spinal cord compression (Lisowska et al., Jan 2007; 2008).
Many studies have revealed that the regional anesthesia can attenuate the perioperative immunosuppression related to the stress surgery. There are evidences demonstrating a greater number of the Th1 compare to Th2 (CD4+ T and CD8+ T cells) and increased the

neutrophil activity in patients with the spinal anesthesia compare to general anesthesia. The Th1/T2 (CD4+ T/ CD8+ T) balance is necessary for the immune response - both the humoral and the cell-mediated. The Th1 cells produce the interferon gamma and are responsible for the cell-mediated immunity. The Th2 cells produce interleukin-4 and are more effective in inducing the humoral immunity. Cytokine concentration is altered during the surgery as well as anesthesia, which may effects the Th cell predominance with consequences for immune responses.

The advances in the knowledge on the T helper 1 (Th1) and T helper 2 (Th2) cells revealed that the Th1 cells produce cytokines that stimulate the proliferation of CTLs while Th2 cells produce cytokines that are responsible for the activation of the humoral immune response in healthy people. The use of regional anesthesia allows the weakening of the immunosuppression caused by the operational trauma, which is evidenced by studies demonstrating a greater proportion of the Th1 to Th2 and increased neutrophils activity in patients received spinal anesthesia (Erskine et al., 1992; Erskine et al., 1994; Le-Cras et al., 1998).

It has also been demonstrated the beneficial effect of the spinal anesthesia on the immune system regards with its activity and the relationship with the incidence of cancer metastasis. Compared with the general anesthesia using volatile agents, the spinal anesthesia caused significantly less immunosuppressive effects with less postoperative incidences of metastasis in patients underwent surgery. That confirms the beneficial effects of the regional anesthesia on the immune system and the relationship between its activity and the incidence of cancer (Bar- Yosef et al., 2001; Wada et al., 2007).

5. The stress response and its functional implications in the immune response after surgery in patients with chronic inflammation (clinical study)

The connection between the surgery stress and the immune system has been presented in numerous publications and while many aspects of the subject have been discussed, most research has been devoted mainly to patients whose immune system works properly. In the available literature there is little information on the impact of the surgery stress on the immune system in patients with a chronic inflammation which in the light of the accepted hypothesis should contribute to the modulation of the immune system response to the surgery stress. Therefore it can be assumed that the development of the stress surgery response should be altered by abnormalities of immune system associated with chronic inflammation. The previous results had reported by author et al. partially helped to confirm the chronic inflammatory state ability to modify of the response of the immune system to surgery trauma (Lisowska et al., 2008). In view of the fact that many of earlier evaluated patients presented significant advanced chronic inflammatory process that reflected in the high activity disease being evaluated the Disease Activity Score-28 (DAS28) based European League Against Rheumatism (EULAR) response criteria (Fransen & van Riel, 2009). DAS28 seems to be correlated with severity of inflammation; therefore, the immune response to surgery was evaluated in the patients with the different disease activity.

5.1 Material and methods

Patients:

The 37 patients with long term rheumatoid arthritis scheduled for knee arthroplasty under spinal anesthesia. Hyperbaric bupivacaine in dose 4 mg was used in all cases.

Standard monitoring including continuous electrocardiogram, nonivasive automated blood pressure and pulse oxymetry. Cardiovascular and respiratory monitoring was continued at the time following surgery. All patients were transferred in the postoperative care unit after the operation.
Crystalloids, colloids were used perioperatively. Homologous blood was used for transfusion depending on the patient's requirements.
Patients with long-term steroids therapy received additional steroid doses during postoperative period in a predefined regiment.
Thromboprophylaxis with low-molecular weight heparin was given.
All patients received antibiotic prophylaxis with Cephazolin 1g on induction and 1 g eight-hourly within 3-5 days.
For postoperative pain relief, they were given standard analgesic drug consisting of opioid and paracetamol.
The tourniquet was used in all patients. Tourniquet pressure was 350 mmHg.
Exclusion criteria included an ASA≥3, BMI>30 (obesities), Hb≤9g/dl, treatment with biologic agents, allergy to local anesthetics, contraindications to spinal anesthesia.
The duration of RA was evaluated and the Disease Activity Score-28 (DAS28) was calculate for all patients before operation. The set of questionnaires was used, the Disease Activity Score-28 was assessed by the number of swollen and tender joints, erythrocyte sedimentation rate (ESR, mm/h) and general health assessment on a visual analog scale (VAS).
During observation the normally physical examination of respiratory system was performed in all patients. No patient had significant tachycardia, tachypnea or other symptoms of atelectasis. Moreover, none of patient complained of sharp pain burning sensation in urine tract that might be a sign of infection and no patient had documented wound complication during observations.
Patients were divided into two groups depending on the activity of the disease being evaluated DAS28. The patients with DAS-28 score lower than 5.0 were classified into the group 1 (G1) and the patient with DAS28 score≥5 were classified into the group 2 (G2).

Blood samples:

Samples of venous blood were taken before induction of anesthesia (a baseline sample-0 h) and at 6, 12, 24, 36 hours (6h, 12h, 24h, 36h) after the end of surgery. Blood was collected in 5 ml pyrogen -free tube, the samples were centrifuged at 3000 rpm for 10 min then serum was separated and stored at -70°C for future analysis.
The serum concentration of interleukins IL-6, TGF-β and C-reactive protein (CRP) were determined in all patients. Serum CRP was determined rapidly after obtaining.
The serum concentration of IL-6 was determined with a commercially available using ELISA kits (R&D System).
TGF-β was determined with using DuoSet ELISA kits (R&D System). All determinations were performed according to the manufacturer's instructions.
CRP was determined using routine diagnostic test (dry chemistry) in analizator Vitros 250.
Statistical analysis of results was performed using a standard computer application Statistica version 9. Continuous parametric data were assessed using one-way analysis of variance (ANOVA). Statistical significance was considered at the $p \leq 0{,}05$
The study was approved by the medical Ethics Committee of the Institute of Rheumatology and informed written consent was obtained from each patient all the patients.

5.2 Results

The study population consisted of 37 patients (35 women, 2 men) with a primary diagnosis of rheumatoid arthritis underwent total knee arthoplasty under spinal anesthesia. ASA physical status II.

Patients were divided into two groups depending on the activity of the disease being evaluated DAS-28. Group 1 (G1) DAS-28 <5, group 2 (G2) DAS-28≥5

	Group 1	Group 2	P value
Number of patients	17	20	
Age (yr)	56. 56.8±11.2	61.4±5.9	0.02
RA duration (yr)	18.5±7.3	20.2±8.2	0.61
DAS-28	4.09±0.59	5.9±0.75	0.39
Intravenous fluids (ml)	crystaloids: 3300± 376	crystaloids: 3300±316.0	0.5
	coloids: G1 500	coloids: 530±129	1.0
Tourniquet duration (min)	86.6±14.6	95.3±13.5	0.77

Data are mean ±SD or n

Table 1. Characteristics and surgical data of patients divided into DAS-28 groups (G1, G2)

Details of 37 patients studied are shown in Table 1. The significant difference was observed in relation to age between groups. By contrast, there were no significant differences between groups in terms of volume given fluids and tourniquet duration.

With regard to the DAS, the difference between groups is not statistically significant but this difference is particularly shown in the clinical observation.

No significant differences were observed with cardiovasculary parameters between groups during observation: MAP (p=0.61) and SaO2 (p=0.98). MAP: G1: 89.6±11, G2: 86.7±10.2 and SaO2: G1 97.2±1.3 G2 96.5±1.3, the values are mean ±SD.

Analysis of concentration level of IL-6 shown statistically significant difference between groups ($F_{v1=1,\ v2=171}$ =41.23, p<0.0001). The was no found significant differences in concentration level of IL-6 in time segments ($F_{v1=4,\ v2=171}$ =0.13, p=0.9721). No interaction time and groups for IL-6 ($F_{v1=4,\ v2=171}$ =0.15, p=0.9650).

The concentration of IL-6 before operation was particularly higher in patients in G2. Moreover, a comparison of value of IL-6 concentration thirty-six hours after surgery with baseline value indicated small increase of IL-6 in patients in this group.

Taking into consideration the range of IL-6 value it can be concluded that the concentration of IL-6 was kept on the similar levels after operation.

There were none changes in concentration of IL-6 during observation in patients in G1 (Fig. 1).

In terms of TGF-β concentration, the analysis of results shown no statistically significant variation of mean value across time ($F_{v1=4,\ v2=168}$ =0.29, p=0.8867). There was no found the significant difference between groups ($F_{v1=2,\ v2=168}$ =2.79, p=0.0966). However, in opposition to IL-6, in both group the values of TGF-β measured at 36 hour were lower in comparison with preoperative values (Fig.2).

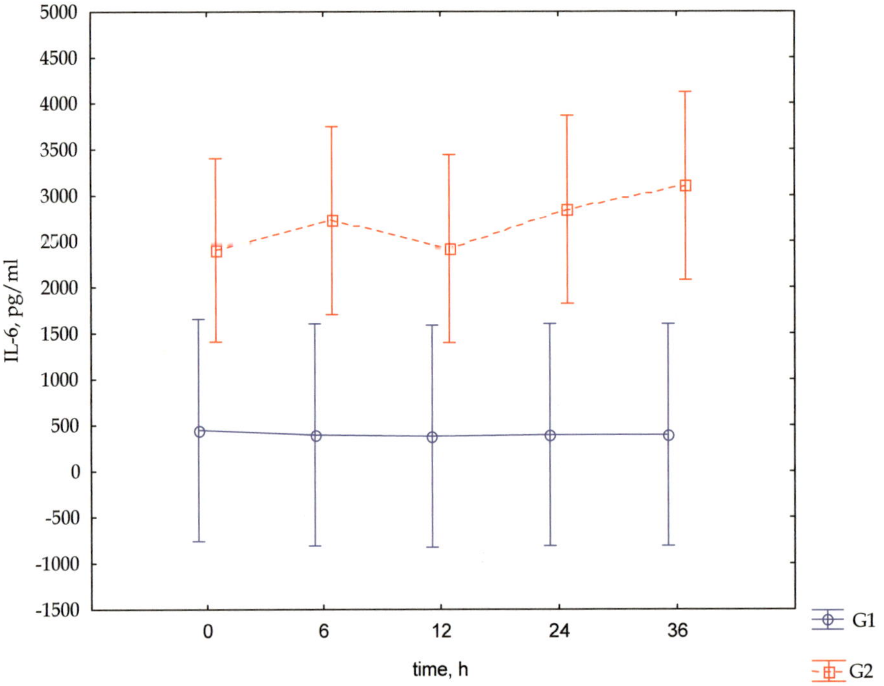

Fig. 1. Changes in serum IL-6 level against time in group G1 and G2. Presented values are mean.

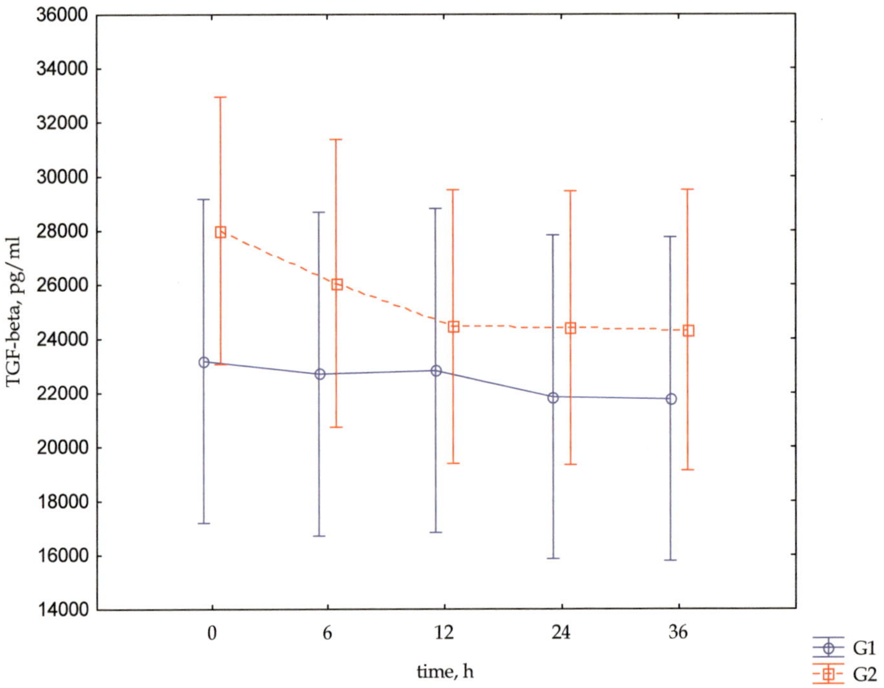

Fig. 2. Mean serum levels of TGF-β at predefined time in group G1 and G2.

The analysis of results of serum CRP concentration shown statistically significant variation $p<0.005$ across time ($F_{v1=4, v2=160}=26.56$, $p<0.0001$) in both groups.
No significant difference was observed in CRP serum concentration between groups across time ($F_{v1=2, v2=160}=4.10$, $p=0.0446$). In all patients the concentration of CRP systematically increased during observation with the peak level at 36 hour (Fig. 3).

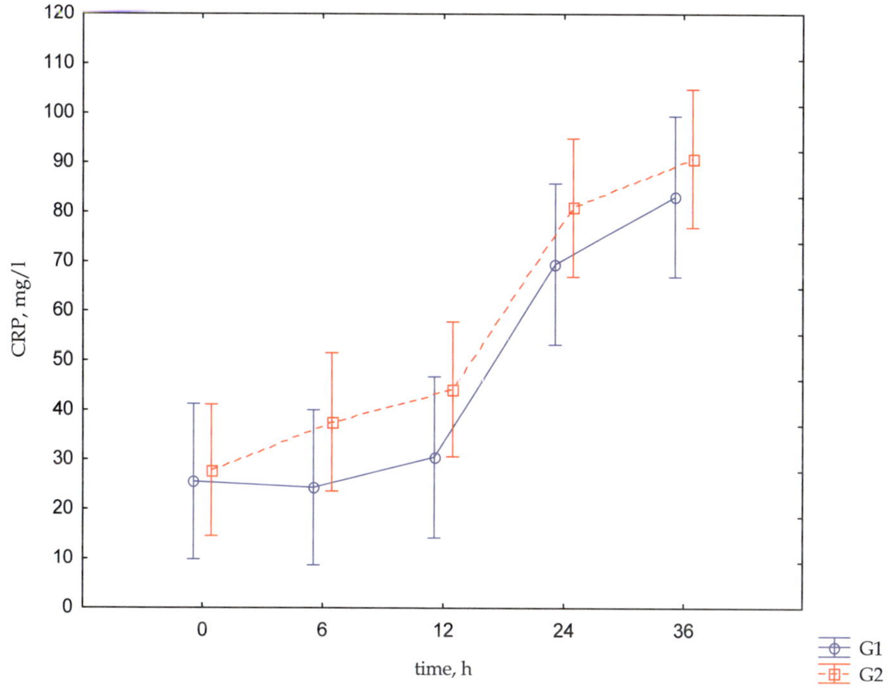

Fig. 3. Changes in serum CRP concentration against time in group G1 and G2. Data are mean

5.3 Discussion

No significant difference (p>0.05) in DAS 28 was shown between groups. However, these differences were strongly marked in a clinical picture. The patients with higher DAS 28 demonstrated significantly more swollen and painful joint counts that related to disability and progression of joint damage.
High, as well as the very high, the cytokines concentration such as IL-6 and TGF-β was observed in all patients before the surgery. The disease severity common with degenerative joint changes were directly influence on the high cytokines concentrations. This also consistent with previous publications demonstrated the high serum IL-6 level in patients with chronic inflammatory disease (Kaneko et al., 2000; Desgeorges et al., 1997). The preoperative stress has also been proposed as one of factor could affect the IL-6 level (Hirano et al. 1988; Tanno et al., 2004). However, taking into consideration the very high baseline level of IL-6 the stress factor did not seem play significant role in this study. Besides that, the preoperative stress response was reduced with midanium premedication in all patients before the surgery. The autoimmune disease severity, as well as joint cartilage

catabolic damages could directly influence on the very high preoperative serum TGF-β1 level. The cytokines familiar with the growth factors group are major factors responsible for the metabolic processes of chondrocytes, consequently for their homeostasis (Shin-Han et al. 2009). TGF-β have role in recruiting immune cells to site of injury and facilitates wound healing by influence for connective tissue remodeling relates with fibroblast proliferation and the synthesis of a number of extracellular matrix proteins (Cutroneo, 2007). Data on dynamic changes of postoperative serum concentration of tested cytokines showed not significant differences ($p>0.05$). Indeed, the postoperative results of cytokines concentration (IL-6 and TGF-β) revealed the insignificant changes in both groups of patient, regardless the disease severity. The one of possibly explanation for this finding is the significant impairment of inflammatory response due to autoimmune disease. In contrast, many reports have demonstrated the dynamics of the IL-6 increase after surgery in groups of patients with normal immune system (Minetto et al., 2006; Demura et al., 2006; Cruickshank et al., 1990).

The CRP levels significantly increased after surgery. The peak level occurred at 36 hour. The changes were similar for both groups. CRP is most important factor involved in inflammatory response and may reflect the surgical magnitude. Its concentration is normally less than 10 mg/L. In this study, the elevated levels of CRP before surgery could be evidence of confirm the chronic inflammatory state. The concentration of CRP revealed no significant differences between groups.

Regional anaesthesia decreases the neuroendocrine response but does not influence on the inflammatory response (Moor et al., 1994; Naito et al., 1992; Høgevold et al., 2000). Both, the regional and general anaesthesia does not significantly influence on the postoperative immunosuppression decrease [Kawasaki et al., 2007). As the matter of fact, the postoperative changes demonstrated in this study may reflect the modulation of immune response to stress surgery due to the chronic inflammatory response.

The tourniquet time seemed not to have an influence on the serum cytokines level dynamic changes. The average tourniquet time was 86.6 in group 1 and in group 2 was 95.3 minutes. The tourniquet time longer than 105 minutes was found as statistically significant according to the results of previous study (Tak et al., 2000).

6. Conclusion and future research

Data on the dynamic changes of postoperative serum concentration of tested cytokines revealed the impairment response of the immune system to surgical stress, regardless of the intensity of disease activity.

Together, the evidence presented above suggests that it may be possible to identify patients likely to develop a more intensive problems with wound healing and postoperative complications. In conclusion the abnormal immune system with chronic inflammatory process due to autoimmune disease can attenuate the cytokines response to surgery.

The future experiments has to be enlarged on the other immunological response factors evaluations including endothelial dysfunction factors. The chronic inflammatory response influence on the wound healing process has to be evaluate in details. Thus, the major role of the growth factors while fibroblastic proliferation reactions as the key pathogenic factor during rheumatoid arthritis has to be initially evaluated.

7. Acknowledgment

The immunological and laboratory tests have been done in the Department of Immunopathology and the Diagnostic Laboratory of the Institute of Rheumatology.
Author is extremely grateful to Professor Ewa Kontny for her consultations on the immunological problems.

8. References

Aida, Y., Maeno, M., Suzuki, N., Namba, A., Motohashi, M., Matsumoto, Makimura M. & Matsumura, H. (2006). The effect of IL-1beta on the expression of inflammatory cytokines and their receptors in human chondrocytes. Life Sci, 79, 8, (Jul 2006), pp. 764-771 ISSN 0024-3205

Armani, C., Catalani, E.†, Balbarini, A.*, Bagnoli, P.,‡ & Cervia, D. (2007). Expression, pharmacology, and functional role of somatostatin receptor subtypes 1 and 2 in human macrophages Journal of *Leukocyte Biology*, 81 (March 2007), pp. 845-855. ISSN 0741-5400

Baatar, D., Patel, K. & Taub, DD. (2011). The effects of ghrelin on inflammation and the immune system. *Mol Cell Endocrinol*, 20, 340 (1), (June 2011), pp. 44-58.

Bar-Yosef, S., Melamed, R., Page, GG., Shakhar, G., Shakhar, K. & Ben-Eliyahu, S. (2001). Attenuation of the tumor-promoting effect of surgery by spinal blockade in rats. *Anesthesiology*, Vol.94, No6, (June 2001), pp. 1066-1073 ISSN 0003-3022

Blackburn, GL. (2011). Metabolic considerations in management of surgical patients. *Surg Clin North Am*, 2011, Vol.91, No.3, (April 2011), pp. 467-80.

Bodey, B., Bodey, B. & Jr, Kaiser, HE. (1997). Dendritic type accessory cells within the mammalian thymic microenvironment. Antigen presentation in the dendritic neuro-endocrine-immune cellular network. *In Vivo*, 11, (4), (Mar-Jun 2000), pp. 351-70, online ISSN 1791-7549, n.d. Available from www.ncbl.nlm.nih.gov/pubmed

Cauli, A., Dessole, G., Fiorillo, MT., Vacca, A., Mameli, A., Bitti P., Passiu, G., Sorrentino, R. & Mathieu, A. (2002). Increased level of HLA-B27 expression in ankylosing spondylitis paties compared with healthy HLA-B27-positive subjects: a possible further susceptibility factor for the development of disease. *Rheumatology* (Oxford), 41, (12), issue 12, (December. 2002), pp. 1375-9, online ISSN 1462-0332, n.d. Available from www.ncbl.nlm.nih.gov/pubmed

Clausen, F., Hånell, A., Israelsson, C., Hedin, J., Ebendal, T., Mir AK, Gram, H. & Marklund, N. (2011). Neutralization of interleukin-1â reduces cerebral edema and tissue loss and improves late cognitive outcome following traumatic brain injury in mice. *Eur J Neurosci*, 30, (Epub ahead of print) online ISSN 1460-9568, May 2011 Available from www ncbl.nlm.nih.gov/pubmed

Coico, R.; Sunshine, G. (2009-6th ed.) *Immunnology a short course* Wiley J & Sons, Inc. (Ed.) 107-124, ISBN 978-0-470-08158-7, Hoboken, New Jersey, USA

Cruickshank, AM., Fraser, WD., Burns, HJ., Van Damme, J &, Shenkin, A. Response of serum interleukin-6 in patients undergoing elective surgery of varying severity.

Clin Sci (Lond), Vol.79, No.2, (August 1990), pp. 161-5 online ISSN 1470-8736, Available from www.ncbl.nlm.nih.gov/pubmed

Cutroneo, KR. (2007). TGF-beta-induced fibrosis and SMAD signaling: oligo decoys as natural therapeutics for inhibition of tissue fibrosis and scarring. *Wound Repair Regen,* 15 Suppl 1 (September-October 2007), pp. 54-60. Available from www.ncbl.nlm.nih.gov/pubmed

Dalm, VA., van Hagen, PM., van Koetsveld, PM., Achilefu, S., Houtsmuller, AB., Pols, DH., van der Lely, AJ., Lamberts, SW. & Hofland, LJ.(2003). Expression of somatostatin, cortistatin, and somatostatin receptors in human monocytes, macrophages, and dendritic *cells Am J Physiol Endocrinol* Metab, 285, 2, (August 2003), pp. 344-53. ISSN 0193-1849

Demura, S., Takahashi, K., Kawahara, N., Watanabe, Y. & Tomita, K. (2006). Serum interleukin-6 response after spinal surgery: estimationof surgical magnitude. *J Orthop Sci,* Vol. 11, pp.241-247 ISSN 1436-2023 Available from http://www.springer.com/medicine/orthopedic/journal

Desgeorges, A., Gabay, C., Silacci, P., Novick, D., Roux-Lombard, P., Grau, G., Dayer, JM., Vischer, T. & Guerne, PA. (1997) Concentrations and origins of soluble interleukin 6 receptor-alpha in serum and synovial fluid. *J Rheumatol,* Vol.24, No.8, (August 1997), pp. 1510-1516 ISSN 0315-162X

Engler, R. (1995). Acute-phase proteins in inflammation. *Soc Biol Fil,*189(4), pp. 563-78 Available from www.ncbl.nlm.nih.gov/pubmed

Erskine, R., Janicki, PK., Ellis, P. & James, MF. (1992). Neutrophils from patients undergoing hip surgery exhibit enhanced movement under spinal anaesthesia compared with general anaesthesia. *Can J Anaesth,* Vol.39 No.9: (November 1992), pp. 899-904

Erskine, R., Janicki, PK., Neil, G. & James MF. (1994). Spinal anaesthesia but not general anaesthesia enhances neutrophil biocidal activity in hip arthroplasty patients. *Can J Anaesth,* Vol.41, No.7, (July 1994), pp. 632-638

Ferone, D., Boschetti, M., Resmini, E., Giusti, M., Albanese, V., Goglia, U., Albertelli, M., Vera L., Bianchi, F. & Minuto, F. (2006). Neuroendocrine-immune interactions: the role of cortistatin/somatostatin system. *Ann N Y Acad* Sci, (June 2006),1069,129-44, online ISSN pp. 1749-6632, n.d. Available from www.ncbl.nlm.nih.gov/pubmed

Fransen, J., & van Riel, PL. (2009). The Disease Activity Score and the EULAR response criteria. *Rheum Dis Clin North Am.* Vol.35, No.4, (November 2009), pp. 745-57, Available from http://www.rheumatic.theclinics.com/issues.

Gajdosz, R. Ocena wpływu analgezji przewodowej na wybrane wskaźniki układu odpornościowego człowieka. Folia -Med.-Cracov 1994, 35 (1-4), pp. 69-86 ISSN 0015-5616

Grisanti, LA., Evanson, J., Marchus, E., Jorissen, H., Woster, AP., DeKrey, W., Sauter, ER., Combs, CK &, Porter, JE. (2010). Pro-inflammatory responses in human monocytes are beta1-adrenergic receptor subtype dependent. *Mol Immunol,* 47, 6, (March 2010), pp. 1244-54, ISSN 0161-5890

Hattori ,N. (2009). Expression, regulation and biological actions of growth hormone (GH) and ghrelin in the immune system. *Growth Horm IGF Res,* 19 (3), (June 2009), pp. 187-97. ISSN 1096-6374

Himmerich, H.& Sheldrick, AJ. (2010). TNF-alpha and ghrelin: opposite effects on immune system, metabolism and mental health. *Protein Pept Lett,* Vol.17, No.2, (February 2010), pp. 186-96. ISSN 0929-8665

Hirano, T., Matsuda, T., Turner, M., Miyasaka, N., Buchan, G., Tang, B., Sato, K., Shimizu, M., Maini R., Feldmann, M. et al. (1988). Excessive production of interleukin 6/B cell stimulatory factor-2 in rheumatoid arthritis. *Eur J Immunol,* Vol.18, No.11, (November 1988), pp. 1797-1801, Available from http://onlinelibrary.wiley.com/journal ISSN 1521-4141

Høgevold, HE., Lyberg, T., Kähler, H., Haug, E. & Reikerås, O. (2000). Changes in plasma IL-1beta, TNF-alpha and IL-6 after total hip replacement surgery in general or regional anaesthesia. *Cytokine,* Vol.12, No.7 (July 2000), pp. 1156-1159.

Jakob, SM. & Stanga Z. (2010). Perioperative metabolic changes in patients undergoing cardiac surgery. *Nutrition,* Vol.26, No.4, (January 2010), pp. 349-53. ISSN 1475-2891

Jin P. & Wang E. Polymorphism in clinical immunology - From HLA typing to immunogenetic profiling. *J Transl Med,* 2003 Nov 18;1(1):8. Available from www.ncbi.nlm.nih.gov/pubmed

Kaneko, S., Satoh T., Chiba, J., Ju C., Inoue, K. & Kagawa, J. (2000). Interleukin-6 and interleukin-8 levels in serum and synovial fluid of patients with osteoarthritis. *Cytokines Cell Mol Ther,* Vol.6, No.2, (June 2000) pp. 71-79, ISSN 138-4736

Kawasaki, T., Ogata, M., Kawasaki, C., Okamoto, K. & Sata, T. (2007). Effects of epidural anaesthesia on surgical stress-induced immunosuppression during upper abdominal surgery. *Br J Anaesth,* Vol.98, No.2, (February 2007), pp. 196-203. Available from http://bja.oxfordjournals.org/content/98/2.toc ISSN 1471-6671

Kehlet, H. (2000). Manipulation of the metabolic response in clinical practice. *World J Surg,* Vol.24, No.(6), pp. 690-695, (June 2000), ISSN 0364-2313

Le-Cras, AE., Galley, HF. & Webster, NR. (1998). Spinal but not general anesthesia increases the ratio of T helper 1 to T helper 2 cell subsets in patiens undergoing transurethral resection of the prostate. *Anesth Analg,* Vol.87, No.6, pp.1421-1425. ISSN 0003-2999

Lenzab, A., Franklinab, GA. & Cheadlea, WG. (2007). Systemic inflammation after trauma *Injury,* Vol.38, No.12, (December 2007), pp. 1336-1345, ISSN 0020-1383

Li, M., Wan, Y., Sanjabi, S., Robertson, A. & Flavell, R. (2006). Transforming growth factor -β regulation of immune responses. *Annu. Rev. Immunol,* Vol 24, pp. 99-146

Lenz, A., Franklin, G. & Cheadle, (2007). Systemic inflammation after trauma. *Injury,* 38, pp. 1336-1345, ISSN 0020-1383

Lisowska, B. (2008). The effect of trauma surgery on selected parameters of immune system in patients with osteoarthitis and rheumatoid arthritis. *Reumatologia,* Vol.46, No.1, pp.1-69 ISSN 0034-6223

Lisowska, B., Rutkowska-Sak, L., Małdyk, P. & Ćwiek R. Anaesthesiological problems in patients with rheumatoid arthritis undergoing orthopedic surgeries. *Clinical Rheumatology,* No.27, January 2007, pp. 553-556 ISSN 1434-9949

Lisowska, B., Maśliński, W., Małdyk, P. (2008). Perioperative inflammatory response In patients with rheumatoid arthritis undergoing orthopaedic surgery. *Arch Med Sci,* Vol.5, No.2, (April 2008), pp.248-254 ISSN 1734-1922

Maddali, S., Stapleton, PP., Freeman, TA., Smyth, GP., Duff, M. & Yan, Z, Daly, JM., (2004). Neuroendocrine responses mediate macrophage function after trauma. *Surgery,* 136, 5, (November 2004), pp. 1038-46. ISSN 0039-6060

Majewska, M. & Szczepanik, D. (2006). The role of toll-like receptors (TLR) in innate and adaptive immune responses and their function in immune response regulation *Postepy Hig Med Dosw,* (online), Vol.60, pp. 52-63, ISNN 1732-2693, Available from www,phmd.pl

Martinsson, T., Oda, T., Fernvik, E., Roempke, K, Dalsgaard, CJ. & Svensjo, E. (1997). Ropivacaine inhibits leukocyte rolling, adhesion and CD11b/CD18 expression. *J Pharmacol Exp Ther,* 283(1), (October 1997), pp. 59-65 Available from www.ncbl.nlm.nih.gov/pubmed ISSN 1521-0103

Minetto, MA., Oprandi, G., Saba, L., Mussino, A., Aprato, A., Masse, A., Angeli, A. & Gallinaro, P. (2006). Serum interleukin-6 response to elective total hip replacement surgery. *International Orthopaedics,* Vol.30, pp. 172-176

Moore, CM., Desborough, JP., Powell, H., Burrin, JM. & Hall, GM. (1994). Effects of extradural anaesthesia on intreleukin-6 and acute phase response to surgery. *Br J Anaesth,* Vol.72, No.3, (March 1994), 272-279, ISSN 0007-0912

Naito, Y., Tamai, S. 7 Shingu, K. (1992). Responses of plasma adrenocorticotropic hormone, cortisol and cytokines during and after upper abdominal surgery *Anesth,* Vol.77, pp. 426-43, ISSN 0003-2999

Nakashima, Y., Sun, DH., Trindade, MC., Maloney, WJ., Goodman, SB., Schurman, DJ. & Smith, RL. (1999). Signaling pathways for tumor necrosis factor-alpha and interleukin-6 expression in human macrophages exposed to titanium-alloy particulate debris in vitro. *J Bone Joint Surg Am,* Vol.81, No.5, (May 1999), pp. 603-615, Available from www.ncbl.nlm.nih.gov/pubmed ISSN 1535-1386

Nishimoto N. (2006). Interleukin-6 in rheumatoid arthritis. *Curr Opin Rheumatol,* Vol.18, No.3, (May 2006), pp. 277-81, ISSN 1040-8711

Norman, JG. & Fink, GW. The effects of epidural anesthesia on the neuroendocrine response to major surgical stress: a randomized prospective trial. *Am Surg,* Vol.63, No.1, (January 1997) pp. 75-80

Pritchard, S., Votta, BJ., Kumar, S. & Guilak, F. (2008). Interleukin-1 inhibits osmotically induced calcium signaling and volume regulation in articular chondrocytes. *Osteoarthritis Cartilage,* 16, 12, (May 2008), 1466-73 Available from www.ncbl.nlm.nih.gov/pubmed

Riether, C., Kavelaars, A., Wirth T., Pacheco-López, G., Doenlen, R., Willemen, H., Heijnen, CJ., Schedlowski, M. & Engler, H. (2011). Stimulation of β2-adrenergic receptors inhibits calcineurin activity in CD4(+) T cells via PKA-AKAP interaction. *Brain Behav Immun,* 25 (1), (Jan 2011), pp. 59-66. ISSN 0889-1591

Salicrú, AN., Sams, CF. & Marshall, GD. (2007). Cooperative effects of corticosteroids and catecholamines upon immune deviation of the type-1/type-2 cytokine balance in favor of type-2 expression in human peripheral blood mononuclear cells. *Brain Behav Immun*, 21 (7), (October 2007), pp. 913-20. ISSN 0889-1591

Sheran, P. & Hall, G.M. (1997). Cytokines in anaesthesia. *Br J Anaesth*, 78, pp. 201-219. ISSN 0007-0912

Shin-Han, T., Ming-Thau, S., Yu-Chih, L., Hsiu-Tan C.,, Sheng-Shiung, F. & Chien-Ho, C. (2009) TGF-β inhibits IL-1β-activated PAR-2 expression through multiple pathways in human primary synovial cells. *J Biomed Sci*, 23;16:97 (October 2009), ISSN 1423-0127

Silverman, MN., Miller, AH., Biron CA. & Pearce, BD. (2004). Characterization of an interleukin-6 and adrenocorticotropin-dependent, immune-to-adrenal pathway during viral infection. *Endocrinology*, 145, pp. 3580–9, (Mars 2004), Available from www.ncbl.nlm.nih.gov/pubmed ISSN 1945-7170

Stevenson, GW., Hall SC., Rudnick, S., Seleny FL, & Stevenson HC. (1990) The effect of anesthetic agents on the human immune response. *Anesthesiology*, 72(3) (March 1990), pp. 542-52, ISSN 0003-3022

Tak, PP. & Brenishan, B. (2000) The pathogenesis and prevention of joint damage in rheumatoid arthritis. *Arthritis Rheum*, Vol.43, pp. 2619–2633

Tanno, M., Nakajima A., Ishiwata, T., Naito Z. & Yoshino, S. (2004). Effect of general anesthesia on the abnormal immune response in patients with rheumatoid arthritis. *Clin Exp Rheumatol*, Vol.22, No.6, (November-December 2004), pp. 727-732. Available from http://www.clinexprheumatol.org/a.asp?IDArchivio=54 ISSN 1593-098X

Tonnesen, E. & Wahlegreen, C. (1988) Influence of extradual and general anaesthesia on natural killer cell activity and lymphocyte subpopulations in patients undergoing hysterectomy. *Br J Anaesth*, Vol.60, pp. 500-7, ISSN 0007-0912

Torres, KC., Antonelli, LR., Souza, AL., Teixeira, MM., Dutra, WO. & Gollob, KJ.(2005). Norepinephrine, dopamine and dexamethasone modulate discrete leukocyte subpopulations and cytokine profiles from human PBMC. *J Neuroimmunol*. 166, 1-2, (September 2005), pp. 144-57. ISSN 0165-5728KC

Wada, H., Seki, S., Takahashi, T., Kawarabayashi, N., Higuchi, H., Habu, Y., Sugahara, S. & Kazama, T. (2007). Combined spinal and general anesthesia attenuates liver metastasis by preserving TH1/TH2 cytokine balance. *Anesthesiology*, Vol.106, No.3, (March 2007), pp. 499-506. Available from www.ncbl.nlm.nih.gov/pubmed ISSN 1528-1175

Wahr, JA., Parks, R., Boisvert, D., Comunale, M., Fabian J., Ramsay, J. & Mangano DT. (1999). Preoperative serum potassium levels and perioperative outcomes in cardiac surgery patients. Multicenter Study of Perioperative Ischemia Research Group. *JAMA*, 16, 281(23), (June 1999), pp. 2203-10, ISSN 1538-3598, Available from www.ncbl.nlm.nih.gov/pubmed

Weber, A., Wasiliew, P. & Kracht, M. (2010). Interleukin-1 (IL-1) pathway. *Sci Signa, Vol.3,* No.105, (January 2010) pp. 1934-9145, Available from http://stke.sciencemag.org/content/vol3/issue105 ISSN 1937-9145

Zhang, XW. & Thorlacius H. (2000) Inhibitory actions of ropivacaine on tumor necrosis factor-alpha-induced leukocyte adhesion and tissue accumulation in vivo. *Eur J Pharmacol*, Vol.24, No.392(1-2), pp. 1-3, (March 2000), ISSN 0014-2999

Zhou, M., Das, P., Simms, HH. & Wang, P. (2005). Gut-derived norepinephrine plays an important role in up-regulating IL-1beta and IL-10. *Biochim Biophys Acta*, Vol.10, No.1740(3), (June 2005), pp. 446-452

3

Provider Volumes and Surgical Outcomes in Total Hip and Knee Replacement

S. Rodriguez-Elizalde, R. Jenkinson, H. Kreder and J.M. Paterson
Division of Orthopaedic Surgery, Sunnybrook Health Sciences Centre, University of Toronto; and the Institute for Clinical Evaluative Sciences
Canada

1. Introduction

There has been much discussion of the role of provider (both surgeon and hospital) surgical volumes and their effect on patient outcomes after total joint replacement (TJR)[1-14]. Common sense would suggest that individuals and institutions with greater experience should demonstrate reduced rates of complications and improved outcomes, however, in the setting of surgical outcomes, the question remains: does practice really make perfect? As medical costs continue to rise, institutions look for ways to optimize outcomes while decreasing complication rates and their associated financial and legal liabilities. There is ongoing debate as to whether the centralization of hospital resources to create large volume regional specialty centers and the sub-specialization of surgeons to increase their procedure volumes is an effective means of reducing cost and complications[2,5,7,12]. Potential disadvantages of such centralization include increased wait times and travel distances for patients, and the possible closure of viable institutions. While most would likely agree that a volume exists below which procedure performance is suboptimal, where this threshold lies with respect to surgeon and institutional volumes in the field of hip and knee arthroplasty has yet to be defined.

Much of the literature on surgical volume-outcome associations comes from our colleagues in cardio-vascular, thoracic surgery and general surgery[15]. The early studies in this field were landmark in that they demonstrated a clear-cut reduction in mortality for procedures performed in specialized centers and by high volume surgeons[15]. In the past few decades, the frequency of total hip and knee arthroplasty has increased dramatically and these procedures are now considered among the most successful and reproducible medical procedures routinely performed [5,14]. Overall, complication rates are low and consequently demonstrating volume-outcome associations requires enormous sample sizes[4,8].

Previous studies of the effect of provider volumes on the outcomes of hip and knee replacement have shown mixed results with respect to both surgeon volume and institutional volume[1-14]. Furthermore, difficulty arises when attempts are made to compare the results of studies across different institutions and countries due to the different methods used for defining procedure volumes, as well as for handling case complexity and patient comorbidities. This lack of consistency coupled with differences in health care delivery have contributed to inconsistent findings.

Below we review and comment on the key TJR volume-outcome studies from England and North America, where most TJR surgeries are performed. Results from the American and Canadian studies are summarized in Tables 1 and 2.

2. The American experience

Literature emerging from the United States has provided both the largest volume of data and greatest variation in results. The landmark study by Kreder et al[1] examining outcomes of total hip arthroplasty (THA) in Washington state between 1987-1991 demonstrated that low-volume surgeons experienced higher rates of mortality, infection, and revision arthroplasty when compared to high-volume surgeons. Low volume surgeons were defined as those performing less than 2 THA/year and high-volume surgeons as those performing greater than 10 THA/year. Complication rates were adjusted for patient age, comorbidity, gender and diagnosis. Patients of low-volume surgeons also had a longer acute duration of hospitalization, which was 0.8 days longer than patients of high-volume surgeons. However, this effect was reversed with respect to institutional volume with low-volume hospitals demonstrating a shorter duration of hospital stay. This could be due to a variety of factors, such as low volume centers (which do not have inpatient rehabilitation services) having to discharge patients to outpatient rehabilitation facilities. It is also possible that high volume centers have more complex cases or patients with a greater number of comorbidities - factors which may not have been fully accounted for in data analysis. Interestingly, average costs for hospital services were found to be greater in low-volume centers, due primarily to relatively higher charges for implants and the operations as a whole. Overall, the majority of THAs in this study were performed by low-volume surgeons who comprised 170 of 494 (34.4%) of the study population. The cut-off for center volumes was less than 16 for low-volume, and greater than 65 for high volumes. Volume categories for both surgeons and institutions were derived from the quartiles of the volume distributions. The second and third quartiles were collapsed into one group for comparison. Perhaps one of the most surprising results from this study is that over one third of all practicing surgeons performed an average of 2 or fewer THA/year. With such low average volumes, it is therefore not surprising that the complication rates among this group were significantly higher. Given the steady rise in rates of THA in the past decade, it is likely that the average numbers of low volume surgeons and centers have experienced a similar and parallel upward trend, possibly narrowing the difference in complication rates between the lowest and highest quartile surgeons.

Katz et al, who have extensively published on the volume-outcome relationship, studied the association between procedure volume and primary and revision THA outcomes in Medicare patients operated on in 1995-1996[2]. Rather than use the data distributions to define procedure volume categories, hospital and surgeon volumes were stratified into what the authors described as clinically sensible categories. In their analysis, it was revealed that 52% of primary THAs and 77% of revisions were performed by surgeons doing 10 or fewer procedures a year. A strong association was found between low surgical volumes and increased complications. Surgeons in the low volume group (<12/year) compared to those in a high volume group (>50/year) experienced higher rates of all complications examined including death, pneumonia, pulmonary embolism, myocardial infarction and deep infection with significant lower rates of dislocation and deep hip infection. Perhaps one of the most striking observations was the discrepant mortality rate for patients who underwent primary or revision THA by a surgeon performing greater than 10, as opposed to fewer than 3, procedures per year. After adjusting for patient comorbidities, mortality rates for primary THA by a high volume surgeon were 0.7% versus 1.3% for low-volume surgeons. Mortality for revision THA was 1.5% for high volume surgeons as compared to 3.1% for low-volume surgeons. Similar increased complication rates were found for low volume surgical centers (<25 TKA/year) when compared to high volume centers (>200/year). While this study demonstrated a clear trend toward better outcomes with higher volumes, no specific recommendations were given on what might constitute an acceptable minimum number of procedures.

Shortly thereafter, Katz's group used Medicare data from 1995-1997 to study rates of revision within 3 years of primary THA[6]. Hospitals were stratified into 4 volume groups: low (<25/year), medium (26-50/year and 51-100/year) and high (>100/year). Low volume surgeons were defined as those performing fewer than 12 primary THA/year. At the time of the study, 75% of all total hip replacements in the US were performed by surgeons doing less than 25/year, with centers performing over 100 cases a year accounting for only 10% of all hip replacements done. Comparing high volume surgeons (>12/year) in high volume hospitals (>100/year) to low volume surgeons (<12/year) and low volume centers (<25/year), the early failure rates were 3.3% vs 4.9%, or approximately a 50% increase in revision surgery. The highest rates of revisions for low volume surgeons were found within the first 18 months.

SooHoo and Lieberman examined the effect of hospital volume on outcomes of total knee arthroplasty (TKA) in California from 1991-2001[8]. They divided hospitals into three groups: low volume (bottom 40th percentile), intermediate volume (middle 40th percentile) and high volume (top 20th percentile). Interestingly, the lowest volume centers (which accounted for 40% of the hospitals examined) averaged only 13 (standard deviation (SD) 5) TKA/year. This is in stark contrast to the intermediate group (50, SD 15) and high volume group (145, SD 47). Outcome measures included complications within the first 90 days and 365 days post-operatively. Statistically significant higher complication rates were found for low-volume centers across the outcomes measured, including mortality, readmission for infection, pulmonary embolism and thromboembolism.. The largest difference between the low and high volume centers was for infection (1.13% versus 0.65%, respectively; $p = 0.004$). However, the overall postoperative complication rates remained relatively low, even among low-volume centers, leading authors to question the rationale behind regionalization for TKA.

Hervey et al examined provider volumes and patient outcomes in an analysis of primary and revision TKAs[3]. Using the Healthcare Cost and Utilization Project Nationwide Inpatient Sample (HCUP-NIS), they were the first to create a national data set from multiple states and hospital settings in order to generate more comprehensive and robust estimates. Hospitals were divided by volume cutoffs into 4 groups: those performing <85, 85-149, 150-250, and >250 TKA/year. Surgeons were stratified from lowest to highest volumes into 4 groups: those performing <15, 15-30, 30-59, and >60 procedures/year. Interestingly, surgeons performing 30 or fewer primary TKAs/year were responsible for nearly half the surgical volume of knee replacements in the US. Using multivariate regression analysis, higher volume surgeons and hospitals had lower mortality rates. Rates of other complications were elevated in the low volume groups, but did not differ statistically from those in the highest-volume groups. The other major finding was that low volume surgeons and centers tended to discharge patients later than their higher volume counterparts, in contrast to the early findings of Kreder et al[1].

Finally, Katz et al analyzed Medicare data on TKAs performed in Tennessee, Ohio, Illinois and North Carolina in 2000 to examine the effect of provider volume on patient function post-operatively[7]. Using a random sample of TKAs from various hospitals, patients were sent questionnaires capturing both self-reported WOMAC scores and surgery satisfaction scores. Poor WOMAC functional status scores (< 60) were noted to be more frequent among patients of surgeons who performed fewer than 12 TKA/year (20%), and centers performing fewer than 10 TKA/year (19%), as compared to their higher-volume counterparts (12% and 10% amongst high-volume surgeons and hospitals, respectively). These findings were consistent across the country, even after adjusting for medical comorbidities and age.

Overall, the American experience is quite unique in that across the country there is a virtual myriad of low volume centers that coexist with some of the largest and highest volume centers in the world. The current body of data indicates that despite increasing volume trends for THA and TKA, the majority of these procedures in the United States are still being performed by surgeons who perform fewer than 30/year and centers performing fewer than 100/year. Several studies have demonstrated increased complications rates, including increased risk of infection, revision, and mortality among low-volume surgeons and centers. In particular, it is evident that very low provider volumes (fewer than 10/year) are more frequently associated with increased morbidity and mortality. However, consensus on a minimum individual or institutional volume threshold for optimal patient outcomes has not been reached. The data are less conclusive with respect to the relationship between provider volumes and length of hospital stay, with early studies showing shorter stays in low-volume centers and subsequent studies the reverse. Little has been published on the financial costs of care in high versus low-volume centers. Further such studies are needed.

3. The English experience

Judge et al examined the effects of hospital surgical volumes and teaching center status on the outcomes of total joint replacement between 1997 and 2002 in the United Kingdom, looking at over 280,000 hip and 211,000 knee replacements[11]. They used National Health Service Hospital Episode Statistics and defined hospital volume groups of <51, 51-100, 101-250, 251-500 and >500 procedures/year. They observed a decrease in patient mortality for both hip and knee replacement as volumes increased. Training institutions also had better THA outcomes, but no such effect was observed for TKA. Lower volume centers had longer lengths of stay.

This study demonstrated that overall, in contrast to the US, most arthroplasty surgery in England was being done in proportionally higher-volume centers. This was true for each of the six years studied. This finding is not surprising as it is easier to consolidate health care resources in a geographically smaller country. Further, over 80% of surgical services in the UK are publicly insured.

4. The Canadian experience

Results from Canadian volume-outcome studies have been mixed. Compared to their southern neighbors, Canadians have a more centralized medical delivery system, with more limited access to surgeons. On average, Canadian surgeons perform higher volumes than their American counterparts, resulting in relatively greater average annual procedure volumes among both surgeons and institutions. For example, surgeons performing greater than 25 procedures a year in Canada account for nearly 75% of the THA and TKA surgical volume[14] whereas in the US, only one third of arthroplasties are performed by those doing over 25 procedures a year[6].

Kreder et al performed a study of THA using Ontario data from 1992[12]. Surgeons and institutions were divided into 3 groups defined by the procedure volume distributions: <40th, 40-80th, and >80th percentile. The low surgeon volume group performed on average 9 THAs compared to the high volume group who performed on average over 27 THAs /year. Low volume centers performed <40 annual THAs compared to >80/year in the high volume groups. Though Kreder attempted to use the procedure volume cut-offs from his earlier Washington study[1], Canadian provider volumes were such that the vast majority of Canadian surgeons would have been labeled high-volume (>10 procedures/year). The major finding of this study was that higher volume surgeons and centers discharged their patients much earlier (2.4 days earlier). No volume-outcome associations were found.
Kreder et al later looked at provider volume-outcome relations in Ontario TKAs from 1993-1996 using similar methods to the above study[10]. Again, patients of lower-volume surgeons had longer lengths of stay in hospital. They also had double the risk of reoperation.
Finally, Paterson et al performed a more recent, larger study of Ontario patients including over 20,000 THA patients and 27,000 TKA patients[14]. In the 10 years since Kreder's previous analysis,[12?] hip replacement volumes had grown by 50%, and total knee replacement volumes by 100%. The number of arthroplasty surgeons during that time period also increased, but at a much slower rate, resulting in an increased volume of cases per individual surgeon.
In this study, low-volume hip surgeons performed an average of 2-25 cases per annum, compared to 2-35 cases per annum for low-volume knee surgeons. This contrasted to the high-volume groups which were greater than 60 cases per annum for hip and greater than 71 cases per annum for knee. Of note, extremely low volume surgeons (defined as those performing less than 2 procedures/year) and low volume centers (defined as those performing less than 10 procedures/year) were excluded from analysis. The results of this study corroborated those of Kreder's earlier work in that no consistent relationships were found between complication rates and hospital volumes for either TKA or THA. Surgeons in the lowest volume quartile demonstrated a 30% increased rate of complications for THA but no similar relationship was seen for TKAs. Surgeon volume was also related to increased risk of revision for THA but not for TKA. Again, patients of lower-volume surgeons had relatively longer lengths of stay in hospital, although no similar relation was observed with hospital volumes.
Overall, the Canadian experience with respect to TJR surgical volume-outcome relationships is mixed. The differences in adverse outcome as related to provider volumes is much less pronounced than in the US, with the most recent Canadian study showing essentially no relations for TKA and inconsistent findings for THA. The one consistent finding among the Canadian studies is that, adjusting for hospital volume, patients of higher-volume surgeons have relatively shorter lengths of hospital stay.

5. Discussion

In summary, while the literature suggests that lower surgeon and hospital procedure volumes are associated with poorer short-term patient outcomes after TJR,[1-3,6,7,8,10,12,14] this relationship appears to exist only when provider volumes are extremely low. The data among moderate and high volume providers is otherwise inconsistent with no clear relationship between surgeon or center experience and patient outcomes. Shorter hospital stays have also been observed among high volume surgeons and to a lesser extent among high volume centers[1,10,12,14].

These findings raise several points for consideration. The fact that extremely low provider volumes are associated with higher complication rates supports the notion of some minimum number of procedures that surgeons and surgical centers should perform in order to optimize outcomes. However, exactly where this threshold lies is difficult to determine from published reports. The fact that Canadian studies, where individual surgeons and centers perform relatively more procedures on average, generally fail to demonstrate a link between provider volumes and adverse outcomes suggests that few Canadian providers fall below this unidentified threshold. The association between surgeon procedure volume and decreased length of hospital stay (even after adjustment for hospital volume) does seem to be a reproducible finding and may be associated with lower costs for acute hospital care. It has been hypothesized that high volume surgeons and centers have more streamlined post-operative protocols and better access to rehabilitation and other ancillary services that could act to facilitate more rapid discharge[1]. Further research is needed to demonstrate whether there is a cost benefit to performing joint replacements in higher volume settings.

There is a global trend toward increasing surgeon and center procedure volumes in an effort to accommodate the fast-growing needs of an aging population. This increasing demand for joint replacement surgery has lead to the introduction of practice standards and protocols for everything from intake assessments, pre-operative work-up, surgical techniques, post-operative pain management and rehabilitation, which serve to streamline the care process and have contributed to significantly lower complication rates than seen in the previous two decades. The fact that complication rates are so low makes it harder to detect significant differences in outcomes related to provider volumes and also raises the question of whether small statistical differences in complication rates are of sufficient clinical importance to warrant the closure of low-volume centers in favor of high-volume regionalized centers of excellence. While small differences in outcomes, such as mortality, are likely to be important to patients, these must be weighted against potentially competing priorities such as access to service, inconvenience, and quality of life.

Other factors that may be contributing to heterogeneity among volume-outcome study findings are differences in the data used and patients studied. Most American studies have used Medicare data. In the US, Medicare covers selected patients (including those aged 65 years). This contrasts the Canadian and British public health insurance systems, which are universal. Consequently, it is likely that US Medicare patients undergoing TJR are, on average, older than Canadian and British TJR recipients. Furthermore, the US studies' reliance on Medicare data means that many private, high-volume clinics are excluded. When such centers are included, Medicare patients typically comprise a small percentage of total clinic and surgeon volumes. Thus, relative to Canadian and British studies, the American studies may be biased toward poorer outcomes, making volume-outcome relationships potentially easier to detect.

In summary, the relationship between TJR provider volumes and patient outcomes is complex. Based on intuition, it seems logical that surgeons and institutions that perform few procedures should have higher rates of complications, given the lack of familiarity, practice and available resources, such as rehabilitation and other ancillary services. US studies support this notion. However, there is no consensus regarding the number of procedures below which adverse patient outcomes (and possibly increased costs) would justify a change in policy. Further research and debate are needed to determine whether such a threshold exists and if so, where it lies.

Author	Year	Databases	Methods	Volume Categories	Results
Kreder et al[1]	1997	CHARS computerized data set of Washington State Health Department	Examined 7936 primary THA between 1988-1991	3 groups: low <40 %ile, medium 40-80 %ile and high >80 %ile Surgeons: Low: <2/yr Medium: 2-10/yr High: >10/yr Hospitals: Low: <16/yr Medium: 16-65/yr High: >65/yr	Low volume surgeons experienced higher rates of mortality, infection, revision operations and serious complications during initial hospital stay High volume surgeons demonstrates shorter length of hospital stay High volume centers had longer average length of hospital stay Average cost per procedure higher in low volume centers
Katz et al[2]	2007	Medicare claims data	Examined 58,521 primary THA and 12,956 revision THA between July 1995-June 1996	Surgeon volume: Low: 1-3/yr Medium: 4-10/yr High: >10/yr Hospital volume: 1-5/yr 6-10/yr 11-25/yr 26-50/yr >50/yr	Higher hospital volume associated with lower rates of mortality and dislocation following primary THA Higher surgeon volume associated with lower rate of dislocation and deep hip infection Similar results for revision THA Steady trend toward better outcome associated with higher volume but no discrete volume thresholds identified
Hervey et al[3]	2003	Healthcare Cost and Utilization Project Nationwide Inpatient Sample	Examined 50,874 primary TKA and 4636 revision TKA performed in 1997	Created 4 volume groups for surgeon and hospital volume to attain approximately equal percentages in each category Surgeon volume: <15/yr, 15-29/yr, 30-59/yr and >60/yr Hospital volume:	Higher surgeon and hospital volumes associated with lower mortality Surgeons performing <15/yr category associated with increased DVT risk and post-operative infection risk No other relationship between volume and outcome

				<85/yr, 85-149/yr 150-249/yr and >250/yr No clear definition of low versus high volume	
Katz et al[5]	2004	Medicare claims data	Examined 78,745 primary TKA performed between January and August 2000	Surgeon volume: 1-12/yr, 13-25/yr, 26-50/yr and >50/yr Hospital volume: 1-25/yr, 26-100/yr, 101-200/yr and >200/yr No clear definition of low versus high volume	Highest volume centers had lower risk of pneumonia, dealth, PE acute MI and infection when compared to lowest volume centers Highest volume surgeons compared to lowest volume surgeons had lower risks of pneumonia and any adverse outcome
Losina et al[6]	2003	Medicare claims data	Examined 76,627 primary THR between July 1995 and June 1996	Surgeon volume: Low: <12/yr Hospital volume: 1-25/yr 26-50/yr 51-100/yr >100/yr	Only looked at rate of early failure requiring revision surgery Patients of low volume surgeons more likely to need revision THA compared to high volume surgeons Strongest association within first 18 months suggesting technical cause as mechanism of early failure Higher hospital volume independently associated with lower failure rates
Katz et al[7]	2006	Medicare claims data	Examined functional status of 932 patients who underwent primary TKA	Surgeon volume: Low: ≤6/yr Hospital volume: Low: ≤25/yr	Patients of low volume surgeons and centers were 2X as likely to report poor functional score compared to high volume surgeons and centers Lowest volume group 2X as likely to have decreased range of motion

					No difference in pain or level of satisfaction
SooHoo et al[8]	2006	California's Office of Statewide Health Planning and Development records	Examined discharge data for 222,684 primary TKA between 1991-2001	Hospital volume: Low (<40%ile): 13/yr Intermediate (40-80%ile): 50/yr High (>80%ile): 145/yr	Low volume hospitals had higher mortality in 90 days post discharge and higher 90-day readmission rate for infection, pulmonary embolism and thrombophlebitis

Table 1. Summary of American TJR Volume-Outcome Studies

Author	Year	Databases	Methods	Volume Categories	Results
Kreder et al[12]	1998	Canadian Institute for Health Information (CIHI) Hospital Discharge Abstracts and Ontario Health Insurance Plan (OHIP) Physician Service Claims	Examined 3645 patient with elective THA in Ontario in 1992	Volumes stratified based on percentiles into 3 categories – low (<40%ile), medium (40-80%ile) and high (>80%ile) Surgeon volume: Low: <9/yr Medium: 9-27/yr High: >27/yr Hospital volume: Low: <42/yr Medium: 42-107/yr High: >107/yr	No difference in complication rate between low and high volume categories Patients of high volume surgeons had shorter length of hospital stay with lowest volume group averaging 2.4 days longer in hospital than highest volume group Hospital volume not related to length of stay
Kreder et al[10]	2003	CIHI Hospital Discharge Abstracts and Ontario Health Insurance Plan	Examined 14,352 patients with elective TKA between 1993-1996	Volumes stratified based on percentiles into 3	No effect of provider volume on infection or mortality Low volume groups (both surgeon and center) had longer

		(OHIP) Physician Service Claims		categories – low (<40%ile), medium (40-80%ile) and high (>80%ile) Low: <14/yr Medium: 14-42/yr High: >42/yr Hospital volume: Low: <48/yr Medium: 48-120/yr High: >120/yr	hospital stays Higher revision rates seen in low volume hospitals No association between revision rate and surgeon volume
Paterson et al[14]	2010	CIHI Hospital Discharge Abstracts and Ontario Health Insurance Plan (OHIP) Physician Service Claims	Examined 20,290 THA and 27,217 TKA patients between April 2000-March 2004	Hospital and surgeon volumes divided based on quartile distribution Surgeon volume: 2-25/yr, 26-40/yr, 41-60/yr and >60/yr Hospital volume: 10-110/yr, 111-150/yr, 151-225/yr and >225/yr Extremely low volume groups (surgeons <2/yr and hospitals <10/yr) excluded	Higher volume surgeons had relative shorter length of hospital stay for both TKA and THA No association between hospital volume and length of stay for either procedure No relationship found between hospital volume and rate of complications Lowest volume surgeons only had increased complication rates for THA but not TKA Low volume surgeons had higher rates of revision for THA

Table 2. Summary of Canadian TJR Volume-Outcome Studies

6. References

Gawande, A. (2003). Complications: a surgeon's notes on an imperfect science. Metropolitan Books.

Hagen, T.P., Vaughan-Sarrazin, M., & Cram, P. (2010). Relation between hospital orthopaedic specialization and outcomes in patients aged 65 and older:retrospective analysis of US Medicare data. *Br Medical J*. Pp. 340:c165.

Hervey, S.I., Purves, H.R., Guller, U., Toth, A.P., Vail, T.P., & Pietrobon, R. (2003). Provider Volume of Total Knee Arthroplasties and Patient Outcomes in the HCUP-Nationwide Inpatient Sample. *J Bone Joint Surg Am*. Pp. 85:1775-83.

Judge, A., Chard, J., Learmonth, I., & Dieppe, P. (2006). The effects of surgical volumes and training centre status on outcomes following total joint replacement: analysis of the Hospital Episode Statistics for England. *J of Public Health*..

Katz, J.N., Losina, E., Barrett, J., Phillips, C.B., Mahomed, N.N., Lew, R., Guadagnoli, E., Harris, W.H., Poss, R., & Baron, J.A. (2001). Association Between Hospital and Surgeon Procedure Volume and Outcomes of Total Hip Replacement in the United States Medicare Population. *J Bone Joint Surg Am*. Pp 83:1622-29.

Katz, J.N., Barrett, J., Mahomed, N.N., Baron, J.A., Wright, J., & Losina, E. (2004). Association Between Hospital and Surgeon Procedure Volume and the Outcomes of Total Knee Replacement. *J Bone Joint Surg Am*. Pp. 86:1909-16.

Katz, J.N., Mahomed, N.N., Baron, J.A., Barrett, J.A., Fossel, A.H., Creel, A.H., Wright, J., Wright, E.A., & Losine, E. (2007). Association of Hospital and Surgeon Procedure Volume With Patient-Centered Outcomes of Total Knee Replacement in a Population-Based Cohort of Patients Age 65 Years and Older. *Arthritis and Rheumatism*.Pp. 56(2):568-574.

Kreder, H.J., Deyo, R.A., Koepsell T., Swiontkowski, M.F., & Kreuter, W. (1997). Relationship between the Volume of Total Hip Replacement Performed by Providers and the Rates of Postoperative Complications in the State of Washington. *J Bone Joint Surg Am*. Pp 79:485-94.

Kreder, H.J., Williams, J.I., Jaglal, S., Hu, R., Axcell, T., & Stephen, D. (1998). Are Complication Rates for Elective Primary Total Hip Arthroplasty in Ontario Related to Surgeon and Hospital Volumes? A Preliminary Investigation. *Can J Surg*. Pp. 41(6):431-7.

Kreder, H.J., Grosso, P., Williams, J., Jangial, S., Axcell, T., Wai, E.K., & Stephen, D.J.G. (2003). Provider volume and other predictors of outcome after total knee arthroplasty: a population study in Ontario. *Can J Surg*. Pp. 46(1):15-21.

Losina, E., Barrett, J., Mahomed, N.N., Baron, J.A., & Katz, J.N. (2004). Early Failures of Total Hip Replacement. *Arthritis and Rheumatism*. Pp. 50(4):1338-43.

Mahomed, N.N., Barrett, J.A., Katz, J.N., Phillips, C.B., Losina, E., Lew, R.A., Guadagnoli, E., Harris, W.H., Poss, R. & Baron, J.A. (2003). Rates and Outcomes of Primary and Revision Total Hip Replacement in the United States Medicare Population. *J Bone Joint Surg Am*. Pp. 85:27-32.

Patterson, J.M., Williams, J.I., Kreder, H.J., Mahomed, N.N., Gunraj, N., Wang, X., & Laupacis, A. (2010). Provider volumes and early outcomes of primary total joint replacement in Ontario. *Can J Surg*. Pp. 53(3):175-83.

SooHoo, N.F., Zingmond, D.S., Lieberman, J.R., & Ko, C.Y. (2006). Primary Total Knee Arthroplasty in California 1991 to 2001. *J of Arthroplasty*. Pp. 21(2):199-205.

Zhan, C., Kaczmarek, R., Loyo-Berrios, N., Sangl, J., & Bright, R.A. (2007). Incidence and Short-Term Outcomes of Primary and Revision Hip Replacement in the United States. *J Bone Joint Surg Am*. Pp. 89:526-33.

4

Gait Analysis in Patients with Gonarthrosis Treated by Total Knee Arthroplasty (TKA)

Katarzyna Ogrodzka[1] and Tadeusz Niedźwiedzki[2]
[1]*Rehabilitation In Traumatology Unit, Rehabilitation Clinical Department, University School of Physical Education in Cracow*
[2]*Orthopedics And Traumatology Clinic, Collegium Medicum UJ Cracow*
Poland

1. Introduction

The aim of the studies was an attempt to evaluate the variability of kinematic parameters of the lower limb joints of subjects before and after total knee replacement in gait with natural speed. Angular values changes in the knee, ankle, and hip joints were studied in three planes of movement.

2. Gait analysis

Walking and running are natural ways of human locomotion which are shaped during phylogenetic development. According to Zembaty (1987) the walking cycle involves "activities and movements performed by a walking person between the contact of one of the heels with the ground and its subsequent contact with the ground", another definition assumes that gait means "locomotion consisting in moving the body weight, focused at the centre of gravity, in space, along a rout requiring the least energy expenditure" (Basmajian, 1976).

There are a lot of more definitions which have been devised over several dozen years when thorough research over the methods of human movement was started. First reports on this issue date back to the 1830s when the Weber brothers performed an analysis of time and space parameters of gait, while the locomotion pattern was first determined by means of a photographic technique by Marey and Muybridge (Andriacchi et al. 2000).

On the basis of these long-term and numerous studies individual gait phases were distinguished, their duration was determined and dependencies between gait phases and their mutual changes induced by changing conditions under which motion is executed.

2.1 Gait phases

The constant and characteristic gait feature includes its cyclicity, i.e. the alternating occurrence of two phases (Bober, 1985):

- single support - only one lower limb has contact with the ground, the support time is approx. 0.53 s.
- double support – both feet have contact with the ground, the support time is approx. 0.15 s.

In each gait cycle the alternating phases of lower extremity movements listed in Table 1 can be distinguished.

General division	Detailed division	Indirect positions
support	shock-absorption	initial contact
		mid stance
	rebound	toe off
swing	pre swing	pre swing
		mid swing
	terminal swing	terminal swing

Table 1. Step phases (Bober, 1985)

The first application of gait analysis for clinical needs was described at Rancho Los Amigos Medical Center in Los Angeles. Dr Jacqueline Perry used film cameras and a dynamometric platform to determine the gait stereotype in children with lower extremity orthopedic problems, such as the monitoring of surgical treatment results (Minns 2004). It was also there that a gait division system commonly used today was devised (Fig. 1) (Perry, 1992).

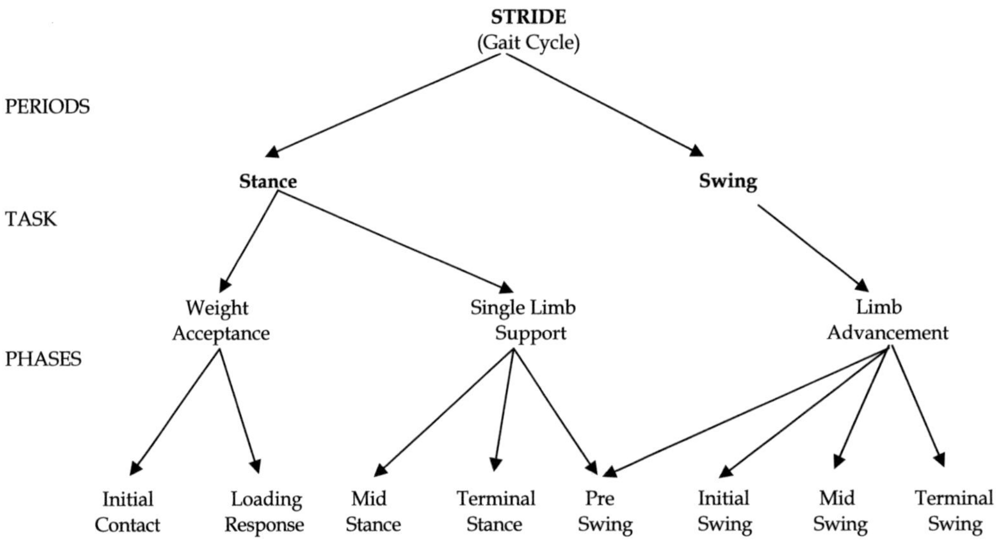

Fig. 1. Gait phases worked out by Rancho Los Amigos Medical Center (Perry, 1992)

On the basis of this division, the gait cycle is divided into the support phase and the swing phase. The support phase consists of:

- the weight acceptance period which includes the initial contact period, which lasts approx. 0-2% of the gait cycle and the loading response period, which lasts 0-10% of the gait cycle. It begins when the heel comes in contact with the ground and ends when the other leg is lifted up and enters the limb advancement period;
- during the single limb support phase the midstance period is distinguished, which lasts for 10-30% of the gait cycle. This period starts when the other leg is lifted from the ground and it ends when the forefoot touches the ground and, next, it enter the terminal stance period. This period lasts 30-50% of the gait cycle and it starts when the

lateral and medial ankles are lifted and it ends when the other foot touches the ground. This is the end of the support phase.

- The swing phase:
- the limb advancement period including the last support period (preswing) (50-60% of the gait cycle); this is the moment when both feet have contact with the ground;
- the initial swing period (60-73% of the gait cycle) begins at toe off and ends when the leg is at the level of the support foot);
- the midswing phase (73-87%) begins when the foot is at the level of the support foot and ends when the tibia is vertical to the ground (the knee and the hip in flexed position);
- the terminal swing period (87-100%) constitutes the continuation of the previous period and ends when the heel touches the ground;

While describing gait periods attention should also be paid to the changing range of motion in the individual lower extremity joints (Fig. 2):

- initial contact *(F1)* – 20° hip joint flexion, extended knee joint, slightly dorsi-flexed foot;
- loading response *(F2)* – hip and ankle joints in flexed position, plantar flexion of the foot until the forefoot is placed on the ground;
- mid stance *(F3)* – hip and ankle joints in extended position, dorsi-flexed foot – approx. 20°;
- terminal stance *(F4)* – extended hip joint, flexed knee joint;
- preswing *(F5)* – hip in intermediate position, flexed knee joint, plantar flexion of the foot;
- initial swing (F1) – hip and knee joints in flexed position, dorsi-flexed foot;
- midswing *(F7)* – hip joint flexion, extended knee joint, slightly dorsi-flexed foot;
- terminal swing *(F8)* – slight hip flexion, extended knee joint, foot in intermediate position (Fig. 2)

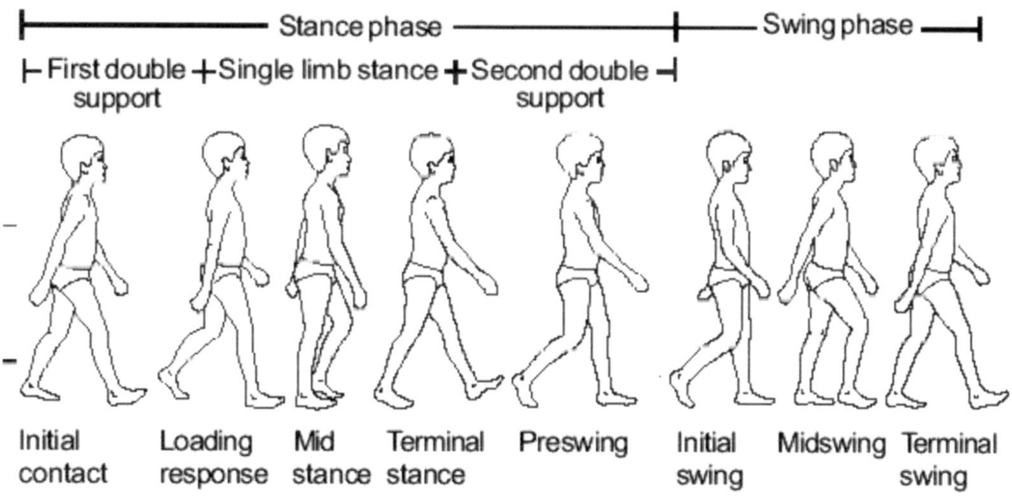

Fig. 2. Angular placing of joints during gait cycle (Perry, 1992).

3. Gait analysis in patients with gonarthrosis before and after total knee arthroplasty based on own research

The literature on the subject (Baliunas et al. 2002, Manetta et al. 2002. Fantozzi et al. 2003, Wu et al. 2007) provides a broad description of the work of the knee joint before and after knee replacement, but these studies are mostly limited to the presentation of the joint movement in the saggital plane, without considering the other planes or the influence of the disease on the ankle and hip joints and the side which was not operated on. Therefore, research was undertaken to assess the change in kinematic parameters of the gait of persons with degenerative knee joint changes before and after arthroplasty of the joint, to present the three planes of the operated and unoperated knee - in search of compensation mechanisms and to devise a biokinematic chain of the lower limb before and after the surgical procedure.

3.1 Material and method

27 patients participated in the study, including 20 women (74%) and 7 men (26%), aged 60 to 74 (average of the age 66,29 (±5,2)), qualified for knee arthroplasty due to degenerative changes of the joint. X-ray tests performed within the framework of pre-operative diagnostics at the Clinic did not reveal degenerative changes in hip joints. The gonarthrosis evoked an apparent flexion contraction in the affected knee joint in all patients (mean angle value:6°)

Locomotion tests included measurements of biomechanical parameters of the gait on the basis the three-dimensional analysis using the Vicon system. The analysis took into account angular changes in the three planes of knee joint motion and in the saggital plane of the ankle and hip joints, as well as time and spatio-temporal parameters.

First examination was done before knee arthroplasty and the second 6 months after the operation when patients mobile without orthopedic support devices.

The control group consisted of 30 healthy persons aged 50-70 (18 women and 12 men) in whom no significant neurological diseases or orthopaedic injuries which might affect the individual gait pattern were found.

Results of control group are a part of a conducted research project through Dr. Wiesław Chwała, being aimed at creating the norm of the locomotion of healthy persons in an all sorts age brackets.

Locomotion tests were conducted at the Biokinetics Laboratory, Department of Anthropomotorics, University School of Physical Education in Cracow.

The research project was approved by the Bioethics Committee at the Regional Chamber of Physicians.

The gait was examined using the Vicon 250 computer system for three-dimensional gait analysis. This system consists of five cameras with a set of luminescent diodes and a data station. The cameras work in the infrared band, and the speed of image recording depends on the setting and type of camera. The frequency of camera operation is 120 images per second. The recorded two-dimensional image from one of the cameras is then transmitted to the data station, where, after being combined with the images from the other cameras, it creates a three-dimensional representation of markers.

The data station is a specialised computer which collects and processes the data recorded by the cameras. Markers are plastic balls with a diameter of 25 mm covered with fluorescent material. The system determines the three-dimensional location of the markers in the form of points and registers their changes in space. The so-called passive markers are glued directly on the patient's skin. Their arrangement reflects the pattern of the biomechanical model. They are glued along the joint axes at an appropriate distance from the centre of the joints and at characteristic points on the head, chest and pelvis. In this way, it is possible to create a spatial representation of these segments of the body and to measure the individual parameters - the dimensions of the pelvis and the span of the chest.

It is important to place the markers of the head, trunk and the lower half of the body in a precise manner. Anterior head markers define the beginning and the scale of the head as a body part, and the posterior markers indicate its location in space. Trunk markers (C7, CLAV, TH10, STRN), together with head markers, determine the axes of the coordinate system of the trunk. The pelvic markers (LASI, RASI), together with the sacrum marker, define the axes of the coordinate system of the pelvis. The marker of the sacrum should be placed in the plane perpendicular to the line joining the ASIS markers (LASI i RASI). It is very important to place the knee markers and the thigh and crus markers in the proper manner.

The Microsoft Excel software and the statistical package SPSS 14 were used for statistical analysis of the research results. The statistical analysis of the data collected was performed on the basis of descriptive and mathematical methods of statistics.

Descriptive methods of statistics were used to present the results in tables containing arithmetic means, standard deviations (s) and the range (min-max).

Mathematical methods of statistics involved significance analysis of the means for repeated measurements by means of Student's t-test for repeated measures.

Both of the aforementioned techniques assumed that the dependent variable distribution is not distant from normal. However, the legitimacy of this assumption cannot be verified using such a small sample. Therefore, it was decided to use parametric tests as the application of non-parametric tests (which do not require a normal distribution) would additionally reduce the strength of the analysis and, in this way, also the chance of obtaining statistically significant results.

4. Results

4.1 Comparsion of angular changes in knee joint in sagittal plane

The values of the range of angular changes in the knee are presented in figures 3-7 in three planes of motion (saggital, frontal and transverse), in patients before and after knee arthroplasty. The grey ribbon in each diagram shows the variability of the results in the healthy population (the mean + 2sd). In the saggital plane, both in the operated and unoperated leg, a limitation of the knee extension at the stance phase is distinctly marked in the 1st and 2nd examination, while insufficient flexion can be noticed at the swing phase. (Fig. 3)

I bad op - examination before arthroplasty, operated knee

I bad n/op - examination before arthroplasty, not operated knee

II bad op - examination after arthroplasty, operated knee

II bad n/op - examination after arthroplasty, not operated knee

Ext - extension, Flex - flexion

Angle (degrees) - angular degrees in the knee joint (in degrees)

Normalised (percent) - normalised time of the gait cycle (in percentages)

Norm - angular changes during normal gait in the comparative group (mean value±SD)

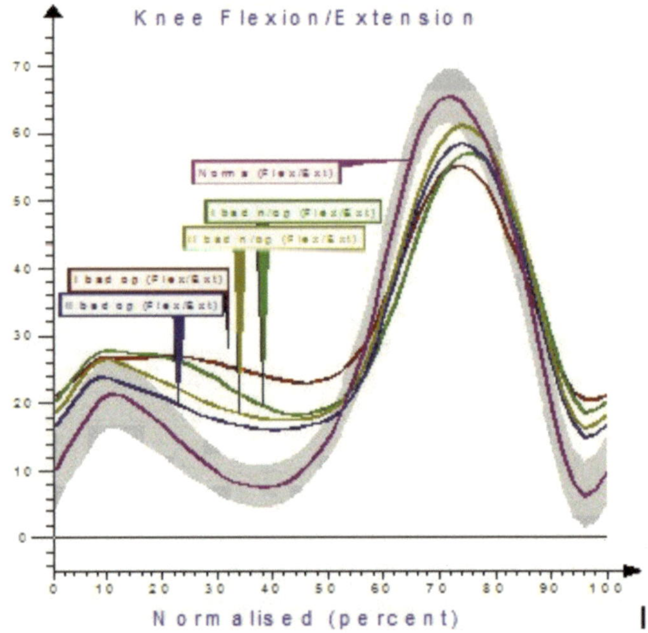

Fig. 3. Angular changes in the knee joints in the sagittal plane

4.2 Comparsion of angular changes in knee joint in frontal plane

During the 1st examination excessive genu varum is revealed at the stance and swing phases. After the procedure this position changes slightly. On the operated side, increased

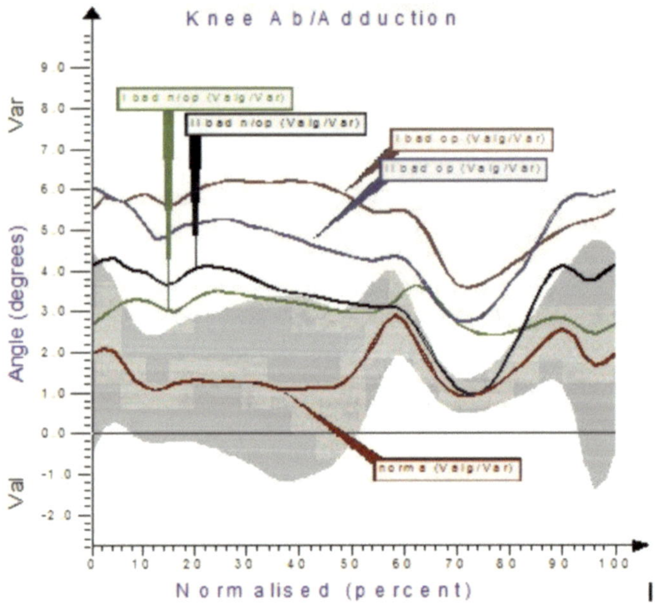

Var - varus knee, Val - valgus knee

Fig. 4. Angular changes in the knee joints in the frontal plane

genu varum is marked during the mid stance, intial swing and mid swing periods. After the procedure, genu varum deteriorated during mid stance period; however, it improved during the swing period (Fig. 4).

4.3 Comparsion of angular changes in knee joint in transversal plane

As a result of the disease external rotation is marked on the operated side during the initial contact and loading response periods and throughout the swing phase. After the treatment, on the other hand, the crus undergoes external rotation throughout the stance phase and the internal rotation is insufficient at the swing phase.

Distinct external rotation appeared on the unoperated side throughout the gait cycle, crus rotation occurred after the procedure towards proper internal rotation (Fig. 5).

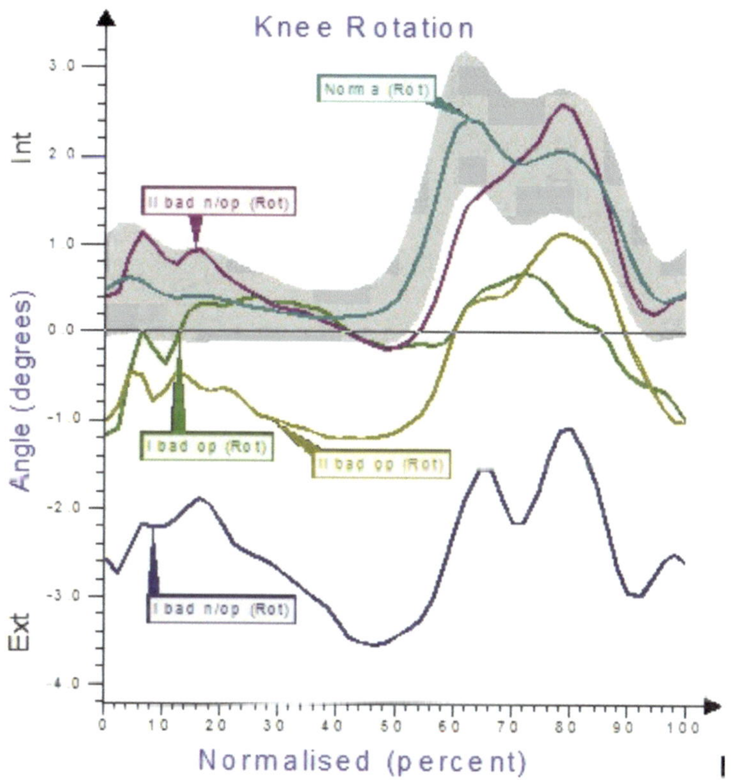

Ext – external rotation, Int – internal rotation

Fig. 5. Angular changes in the knee joints in the transversal plane

4.4 Comparsion of angular changes in ankle joint in sagittal plane

The 1st and 2nd examinations revealed that the position of the ankle joints was correct at the stance phase, while no plantar flexion of the joints occurred during the preswing period (Fig. 6).

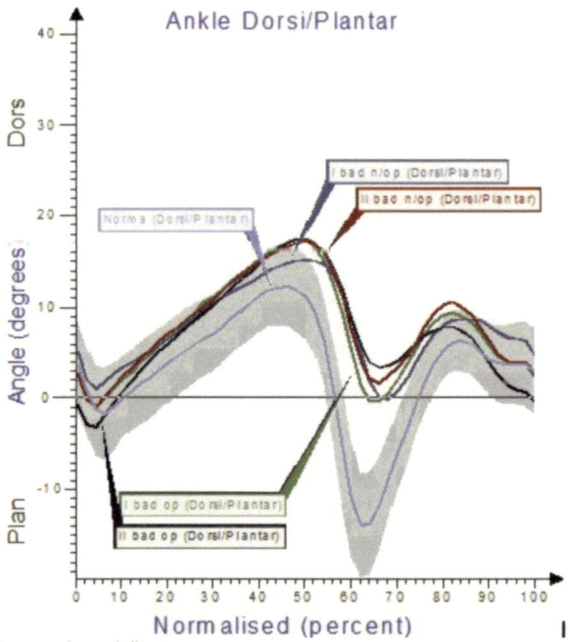

Plan - plantar flexion, Dors - dorsal flexion

Fig. 6. Angular changes in the ankle joints in the transversal plane

4.5 Comparsion of angular changes in hip joint in sagittal plane

Flexion contracture of the hip joints was marked on both sides in the 1st and 2nd examination. It was slightly reduced after the procedure (Fig. 7).

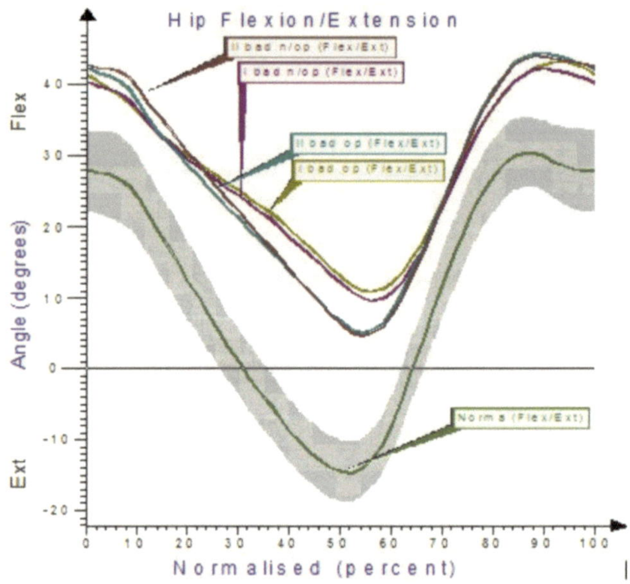

Ext - extension, Flex - flexion

Fig. 7. Angular changes in the hip joints in the transversal plane

4.6 Analysis of spatio-temporal parametres

The table below presents a comparison of the average values of time and space parameters obtained before and after the endoprosthetic replacement for the control group.(Tab.2)

The following parameters were measured for all perosns:

Cadence - number of steps within the minute
DS - double support
Foot Off - end of stance phase
SS - single support
StrL - stride lenght
StrT - stride time
WS - walking speed

spatio-temporal parametres	I examination		II examinaton		control group
	operated knee	not operated knee	operated knee	not operated knee	
Cadence [steps/min]	87,0	86,7	88,8	87,9	112,0
Foot Off [%]	68,3	70,7	68,0	68,5	62,8
DS [s]	0,6	0,6	0,5	0,5	0,3
SS [s]	0,4	0,4	0,4	0,5	0,4
StrL [m]	0,8	0,8	0,9	0,9	1,3
StrT [s]	1,5	1,5	1,4	1,4	1,0
WS [m/s]	0,6	0,6	0,7	0,7	1,2

sides: operated knee - knee before and after arthroplasty; not operated knee - healthy knee

Table 2. Comparing temporary-spatial values at patients before and after the arthroplasty with results of the control group

On the basis of the analysis of the time and space parameters it can be noticed that patients move with a reduced frequency of steps and at a slower rate. Thus, the double support phase and cycle duration are longer for them; similarly, the stance phase ends later.

Time and space parameters were also compared between the operated and unoperated side in the 1st and 2nd examination. Tables 3 & 4.

Statistical analysis also revealed a significant difference between the operated and unoperated side for the Foot Off parameter in the 1st and 2nd examination. No statistically significant differences between the analyzed parameters were found in the 2nd examination.

I examination									
spatio-temporal parametres	operated knee				not operated knee				statistical significant differences (p)
	x	s	min	max	x	s	min	max	
Cadence [steps/min]	87,0	18,8	34,4	118,0	86,7	18,8	34,2	117,4	0,622
DS [s]	0,6	0,4	0,3	2,3	0,6	0,4	0,2	2,2	0,318
Foot Off [%]	68,3	5,5	59,8	81,8	70,7	5,4	63,6	84,3	0,013
SS [s]	0,4	0,05	0,3	0,5	0,4	0,1	0,3	0,8	0,194
StrL [m]	0,8	0,2	0,6	1,3	0,8	0,2	0,5	1,2	0,630
StrT [s]	1,5	0,5	1,0	3,5	1,5	0,5	1,0	3,5	0,932
WS [m/s]	0,6	0,2	0,2	1,0	0,6	0,2	0,2	1,0	0,639

sides: operated knee – knee before and after arthroplasty; operated knee – healthy knee

Table 3. Comparing temporary-spatial values at patients before the arthroplasty on the operated and not operated side.

II examination									
spatio-temporal parametres	spatio-temporal parametres				spatio-temporal parametres				spatio-temporal parametres (p)
	x	s	min	max	x	s	min	max	
Cadence [steps/min]	88,8	18,4	46,8	115,5	87,9	18,6	45,9	116,7	0,188
DS [s]	0,5	0,3	0,3	1,4	0,5	0,3	0,3	1,4	0,585
Foot Off [%]	68,0	4,5	52,8	78,3	68,5	6,2	60,6	84,3	0,500
SS [s]	0,4	0,08	0,3	0,8	0,5	0,1	0,3	0,8	0,342
StrL [m]	0,9	0,2	0,6	1,2	0,9	0,2	0,5	1,3	0,169
StrT [s]	1,4	0,4	0,7	2,6	1,4	0,4	0,7	2,6	0,208
WS [m/s]	0,7	0,3	0,2	1,4	0,7	0,3	0,2	1,4	0,943

sides: operated knee – knee before and after arthroplasty; operated knee – healthy knee

Table 4. Comparing temporary-spatial values at patients after the arthroplasty on the operated and not operated side

5. Discussion

5.1 Locomotion of patients with gonarthrosis

Gait analysis in osteoarthritis patients indicates that as a result of degenerative knee disease, limitation of hip joint movement occurs - marked flexion contracture can be observed in these patients.

On the basis of the research conducted by the present authors, it can be concluded that the patients taking part in the study walk with their knees bent. Additionally, the joints assume the genu varum position and are considerably externally rotated. There is no plantar flexion of the ankle joints occurs at the beginning of the limb advancement period.

Considerable bow-leggedness is also observed in the authors' own research, especially on the affected side.
Similar results were obtained by Gök et al. 2002 who analyzed the gait of 13 patients suffering from knee arthritis. Their results were compared with 13 healthy persons. The analysis was performed using the Vicon 370 system and it involved kinetics, kinematics and time and space parameters of the gait. Significant movement limitation was discovered in the saggital plane, as well as genu valgum at the support phase.
One of the reasons may be the patients' reduced daily physical activity caused, among other things, resulting in lower flexibility and reduced active range of motion in the joints.
On the basis of the research conducted it can also be concluded that due to pain the support phase is extended and thus, the limb advancement period is shortened in patients suffering from degenerative knee disease. A similar conclusion was reached by Andriacchi et al. (1997) who found that an extended gait cycle can be observed in patients waiting form endoprosthetic replacement. The knee function was not completely restored, despite good clinical results, which is confirmed by the authors' own research.
Astephen et al. (2007), on the basis of locomotion tests of persons with degenerative changes of knee joints, concluded that changes in ankle and knee joints are marked in the saggital plane. However, they did not determine the direction of the changes in the joints.
Similar results for the saggital plane were obtained by Baliunas et al. [21], who discovered there existed a restriction of the range of motion throughout the gait cycle.
This is yet another confirmation of the results of the author's own studies, where a clear restriction of the active range of motion was found in the knee joint in the saggital plane.
Manetta et al. (2002), on the other hand, examined 10 persons suffering from degenerative knee joint disease and compared the results with the control group. They determined the kinetics and kinematics of the gait on the basis of a motion analysis system. It turned out that the maximum flexion at the support stage was lower in the patients. As the values of the maximum flexion at the support phase were similar among the patients compared to the norm and no weakening of the quadriceps femoris muscle was observed, they concluded that this pattern was caused by a compensatory reduction in gait speed.
These reports are not fully consistent with the results of the author's own research, as extension limitation was observed in the examined patients (increased flexion) at the support phase.
Results similar to Manetta et al. 92002), and not fully consistent with the results of the author's own research, were obtained by Childs et al. (2004), who found that flexion during loading response was limited in patients suffering from articular disease compared to the norm.
Bajek et al. (2006a) analyzed the gait of 20 patients suffering from degenerative knee disease and compared with a control group consisting of 20 persons. The analysis included the time and space parameters and the range of motion in the saggital plane of the knee and hip joints in both legs and the three-dimensional pelvic function.
The results obtained indicate a considerably higher limitation of flexion during the limb advancement period than the results of the present authors' research. Flexion contracture of the hip joints was also visible, which confirms the results of the authors' own research.
The authors assumed that the limitation of motion in the affected knee joint will be compensated by an increased range of motion in the hip joint, however, the results of their research show that this range of motion becomes reduced, in particular, on the side of the affected joint.

Similar results are presented in this study. However, on the basis of the present authors' own research it can be concluded that the reason for such position of the hip joints is the flexion contracture in the knee joints, which leads to excessive hip flexion potentially accompanied by increased anterior pelvic tilt.

No study describing the gait stereotype before and after endoprosthetic knee replacement presents such an interpretation.

A change in the leg axis is a characteristic feature of degenerative disease. Changes located within the medial range cause a varus deformity of the leg, while changes in the lateral section lead to its valgosity (Wierusz-Kozłowska et al. 2004, Kwiatkowski et al. 2004). This alignment results in a dominating varum or valgum deformity. In the present study, a varus deformity of knee joints was observed both before and after the arthroplasty procedure. The fact that the situation does not change after the procedure may result from changes in lower extremity biomechanics consolidated as a result of the disease.

Similar conclusions were reached by Rudolph et al. (2007), who, while evaluating the gait pattern in patients, found that a varum deformity of the knees and the weakening of the quadriceps femoris is a characteristic feature.

A study by Al-Zahrani et al. (2002) describes the influence of the disease on the gait stereotype. The analysis involved the function of the lower extremity joints in the saggital plane, time and space parameters and the bioelectric activity of the knee joint muscles. The test was performed using an optoelectronic system for three-dimensional gait analysis combined with a dynamometric platform and an electromyograph. 58 persons participated in the study. The results were compared with a control group consisting of 25 (average age: 69).

Gait analysis performed in the patients revealed a restriction of the active range of motion was found in the knee joint in the saggital plane. All these results corroborate the findings of previous studies and are interpreted as the result of pain and a change of the joint prioprioception. However, the weakening of the prioprioception of the knee joint is not a fully objective explanation of the changes in the gait stereotype. Despite the fact that the prioprioception of the joint was not studied directly, no neurological changes were found in any of the patients.

Marks et al. (1993) concluded that there was no relationship between the locomotion possibilities in patients suffering from degenerative disease and the weakening of the proprioceptive function of the joint. Differences in the gait kinematics between the patients and the control group may also result from different gait speed, however, the authors did not study this influence. Many authors emphasize the importance of proprioception changes both before and after the procedure. Proprioception decreases with age and causes a change in the muscle pattern when the joint is under load, thus contributing to the development of degenerative disease (Cash et al. 1996, Barret et al. 1991, Sharma et al. 1997).

5.2 Locomotion of patients after arthroplasty

After arthroplasty gait parameters do not change significantly. A slight improvement is marked in the range of motion of the knee joints – the flexion contracture decreased during the mid stance and terminal stance periods. External rotation of the joint became more marked with a simultaneous reduction of the varus deformity on the operated side.

No distinct changes in the ankle joint function were observed – the restriction of plantar flexion during the initial swing period increased slightly.

Thus, knee arthroplasty changes the three-dimensional picture of the joint function but these changes do not fully correspond to the biomechanical norm. This may be caused by the fact that the second locomotion examination was performed only 6 months after the procedure, when the previously developed compensation mechanisms still persisted and the results obtained are just an intermediate stage before returning to the correct values (Ogrodzka et al. 2008). It also needs to be emphasized that all patients were rehabilitated for only 2 weeks after the procedure. Thus, it turns out that it is too short a period for the disease-induced changes in the gait stereotype to subside. Therefore, it is important to underline that long-term rehabilitation (emphasizing the correct gait function) after the procedure could accelerate the patient's return to full mobility.

Lack of the required range of motion in the knee joints in the saggital plane while walking before and after arthroplasty results in a lack of plantarflexion in the ankle joints at the initial swing phase and persistent contracture of the hip joints. This makes it possible to move the lower extremity without "catching" the ground.

Slight changes in the patients' gait stereotype before knee arthroplasty may primarily result from their long-standing locomotor habits. Increasing pain makes the patients change their way of walking – if the knee joint is straightened, the pressure on the joint surface increases and the pain becomes more intense. As a result, these patients try to avoid straightening of the joint, which is characteristic for the beginning and end of the stance phase. Flexion contracture of knee joints is the results of long-term knee flexion.

As degenerative disease is progressive in nature the procedure will not bring about sudden changes in the joint position. Despite good clinical results, the patient's consolidated habits prevent a quick change of the gait stereotype.

Consequently, tests performed 6 months after the procedure make it possible to capture the direction of the changes, but this period is still to short to determine the locomotion stereotype in this group of patients in an unambiguous manner.

Such conclusions are also supported by the literature on the subject (Chao et al. 1980, Andriacchi et al. 1982, Kramers-de Quervain et al. 1997 and Sukru Solak et al. 2005).

A comparison of the results of the authors' own research with reports found in the literature it can be concluded that there exist certain similarities in the results obtained, but also some conclusions differ.

It was found in the authors' own research that patients walk with their knees bent - hip joints are excessively flexed at the support phase and this flexion is insufficient during the advancement period.

Ishii et al. (1998) examined locomotion at natural walking speed using an eletrogoniometer attached to the knee joint. In this way, they obtained information about three-dimensional knee function in 20 patients (11 with posterior cruciate ligament retention and 9 with PCL removal) after arthroplasty. The analysis was performed 18-20 months after the procedure.

On this basis a conclusion was formulated that in persons after total knee replacement (in both groups) the range of motion of the knee joints is limited, mostly in the saggital and transverse planes.

They also found that despite correct passive range of motion in the joint, limited flexion during the limb advancement period is clearly marked in the gait, which may result from the consolidated gait stereotype from before the procedure which has not improved to date.

Such conclusions partly corroborate the results of the authors' own research where insufficient flexion of the knee joint was also observed during the limb advancement period.

Bőrjesson et al. (2005) and Astephen et al. (2005) also confirm that, as a result of the disease, changes in the gait stereotype occur, but despite good results they continue to walk more slowly and do not regain the correct gait stereotype after the procedure.
Such an interpretation also confirms the results of the present study, as, despite satisfactory results, the biomechanical picture of the knee joints during gait changed only slightly.
Total knee replacement improves the function of the hip joints only slightly - the contracture is reduced mostly during the terminal stance and preswing periods.
Numerous authors conclude that the gait stereotype after arthroplasty does not change despite reduced pain and the achievement of sufficient range of motion. This is probably caused by patients' habits developed before the procedure, as well as by changes in proprioceptive sensations in the joint occurring before and after the operation, which also corresponds to the results of this study; however, no significant lengthening of the support phase was observed before or after the procedure in the authors' own research.
On the basis of the results of the authors' own research conducted after the total knee replacement it can be concluded that, despite good clinical conditions, the pattern of the lower extremity joint function changes to an insignificant degree during gait. The range of motion in the individual planes improves, but consolidated habits developed before the operation do not allow for a complete change of the gait stereotype in this group of patients.
Such conclusions are presented by, among others, Sukru Solak et al. (2005), who assessed the locomotion of 24 women with the average age of 67/ The examination was performed before the procedure and 1 and 2 years after the procedure. There were no differences between the examination 1 and 2 years after the procedure.
The authors concluded that the limitation of the range of motion after total knee arthroplasty (TKA) results from the joint contracture consolidated before the procedure. Andriacchi et al. (1982) and Chao et al. (1980) are of a similar opinion. They believe that the stereotype of the patients' gait after the TKA procedure results from the locomotion method consolidated before the procedure, caused by pain, changes in the joint proprioception and lack of full extension which would protect the patients' against pressure on joint surfaces and, in consequence, pain avoidance.
Kramers-de Quervain et al. (1997) analyzed the gait of 5 patients after bilateral total knee replacement. The authors conclude, that despite the procedure, the changed locomotion pattern persists, just like disturbed proprioception of the joint.
In another study of the locomotion of patients after knee replacement, Wu et al. (2007) discovered that the range of knee flexion is reduced throughout the gait cycle. Reduced plantar flexion of the ankle joint at the end of the preswing period was also observed, compared to the unaffected leg and the control group.
The results of the authors' own research also revealed limitation of the range of motion of knee joints and considerably reduced plantar flexion of ankle joints during the preswing period. The limitation of plantar flexion may caused by the fact that patients do not achieve sufficient flexion at the knee joint, so to be able to move the limb under the pelvis they must flex the foot to compensate for this.
16 persons (average age: 69) after arthroplasty were examined (Wilson et al. 1996). The analysis encompassed the gait and isokinetic measurement of flexors and extensors (Cybex 6000 dynamometer). The Vicon system with 5 cameras was used for gait analysis. The patients walked at their natural walking speed.

No statistically significant differences were observed in the results of time and space parameters, however, significantly lowered (statistically significant) values were noted for gait kinematics - limited range of motion of the knee joints in the saggital plane throughout the gait cycle.

67° range of motion is required while walking, which becomes reduced as a result of knee joint degeneration. In the research conducted by Dorr et al. (1988) the range of motion after the procedure was 52° and similar results were obtained by Steiner et al. (1989). In a study by Wilson et al. (1996) the range of motion was 53°. The restriction of the range of motion after the treatment may result from both the structure of the prosthesis and the weakening of the muscles, a change in the proprioception or a locomotion pattern consolidated before the procedure.

In the authors' own research the maximum knee joint flexion was approx. 58° on the operated side and 60° on the unoperated side, so these values are higher than those obtained by other authors, but they are still lower than the correct values, so the change in the range of motion in other joints will compensate for deficiencies of the knee joint position. However, the interpretation of these results may be similar to the interpretation presented by Wilson et al. (1996).

McClelland et al. (2006, 2007) and Smith et al. (2006) as well as Webster et al. (2003) found that patients after the procedure walk with restricted range of motion in the knee joint compared to the norm. The flexion is reduced both at the support and swing phase. The results of the authors' own research are confirmed again, as, according to them, patients do not achieve full knee flexion during the limb advancement period, but also it can be noticed that the results are diversified if we consider the function of the knee joint at the stance phase – the patients' knees are excessively bent compared to the biomechanical norm.

Benedetti et al. (2003) analyzed the gait of 15 persons after the knee endoprosthesis procedure. No degenerative changes were observed in any of the patients in the other joints, each person underwent a rehabilitation treatment after the procedure, during which continuous passive movement, exercises of flexors and extensors of the knee joint and proprioception exercises were used, the patients were able to put their weight on the leg after two weeks. The locomotion test was performed 6, 12 and 24 months after the procedure.

Despite rehabilitation, changes in the patients' gait persisted. The results of the tests show that 6 months after the procedure the length of the cycle is reduced and restricted flexion of the knee joint persists during the loading response period.

These results are slightly different from the results obtained in this study. No restriction of knee flexion was observed during the loading response period and the length of the cycle after the procedure increased.

5.3 Three-dimensional stereotype of the move of joint of lower limbs before and after the treatment

The literature does not refer to results similar to the results obtained in the authors' own research in which it was attempted to evaluate the position of knee joints in the saggital and transverse planes before and after an arthroplasty procedure.

While devising a biomechanical gait pattern in persons before and after knee replacement it is important to take into account all planes of motion. This allows to present the stereotype of motion in a spatial way and, at the same time, it draws attention to the existing, pathological position of the joints, which may lead to other strains and diseases of the locomotor system. On the basis of test results presented in this study, it can be concluded that three-dimensional gait analysis determines the scope of changes in lower extremity joints and their dysfunctions in the three planes of motion in an unambiguous way.

The interpretation of other authors' results presented above confirms that the determination of the locomotion pattern in patients before and after knee arthroplasty on the basis of the description of movement only in the saggital plane is not sufficient. Before and after the procedure patients develop their own way of walking adjusted to their needs. Therefore, to be able to determine the scope of changes and deviations from correct values, the gait stereotype must be analyzed in all three planes. Such an analysis is presented in the present study, which broadly describes biomechanics of lower extremities during gait.

Due to a very small number of reports on the joint function in the unoperated leg, one of the aims of this study was to determine the biomechanical chain of the unoperated side.

Other authors (Wilson et al. 1996, Al-Zahrani et al. 2002) limit their conclusions to the statement that the range of motion in the unoperated knee joint is also restricted and the ankle joint works properly (Wu et al. 2007). In their study, Bajek et al. (2006a) also describe flexion contracture in hip joints.

These are, however, only statements which are narrow in their scope and which do not take into account the function of all joints in the unoperated leg during all gait periods.

On the basis for the first part of the discussion of the unoperated leg movement analysis throughout the gait cycle, it can be concluded that:

- the function of the hip joint on the unoperated side does not differ from the operated side - considerable flexion contracture of the joint.
- the knee joint in the saggital plane both before and after the procedure works in a similar way and its function is not different from the operated joint
- the varum deformity is considerably smaller in the frontal plane (close to normal values)
- the biggest differences were revealed in the transverse plane – the unoperated joint was positioned in considerable external rotation before the procedure, after the treatment the external rotation of the opposite joint changed into correct internal rotation (such differences were not observed on the operated side)
- the ankle joint on the unoperated side worked in a way similar to the ankle joint on the operated side.

On this basis it can be concluded that as a result of degenerative knee changes, the joints of the other leg begin to function in a different way. The direction of these changes corresponds to the changes in the affected leg (mostly in hip and ankle joints), apart from the transverse plane of the knee joint where the rotation values are significantly higher than the rotation on the operated side.

After the knee replacement procedure the change of the gait stereotype is slight, which results from the patterns consolidated before the procedure, but the direction of these changes is similar to the changes on the operated side. The biggest difference is marked again in the transverse plane of the knee joint, where correct internal rotation has already appeared.

This kind of analysis has not been presented in the literature.

5.4 Spatio-temporal parameters

The analysis of time and space parameters revealed that before the treatment the patients' step frequency was reduced, the length of the cycle was lowered and their walking speed was lower, while the double support phase and the cycle duration were lengthened.

On the basis of the statistical analysis performed in the authors' own research, no statistically significant differences were found - apart from the StrL parameter (length of the cycle) - between the mean values of the time and space parameters in the 1st and 2nd examination on the operated side. On the unoperated side, on the other hand, statistically significant differences occurred between the DS (double support time), StrL (length of the cycle) and the WS (walking speed) parameters. No such differences were observed for the remaining values.

Time and space parameter values were also compared between the operated and unoperated side in the 1st and 2nd examination. Statistical analysis also revealed a significant difference between the operated and unoperated side for the Foot Off parameter in the 1st and 2nd examination. No statistically significant differences between the analyzed parameters were found in the 2nd examination.

It was also attempted to evaluate the strength of the relationship between time and space parameters before and after the knee replacement procedure.

Moderate correlation is revealed between the 1st and 2nd examination as regards the single support time (SS). Considerable dependence was discovered among the other parameters and this dependence was very strong for step frequency values.

Moderate correlation also occurred on the unoperated side in the SS parameter values (single support time). High correlation also occurred for the cycle length and duration and the walking speed parameters, while very high correlation was observed between step frequency and the values of double support time.

Correlation was also analyzed between the operated and unoperated side in the 1st and 2nd examination.

Moderate correlation was observed between the sides in the 1st examination as regards the values of the single support time (SS) and the Foot Off parameters. The correlation was very high for the remaining parameters.

After the operation significance dependence occurred between the sides for the SS variable (single support time). Very high correlation was revealed in the evaluation of the strength of the relationship between the parameters step frequency, double support time, cycle length walking speed on both sides.

This may mean that the gait pattern of both legs under analysis, both in the 1st and in the 2nd examination, are mutually dependent and changes occurring in one leg must be compensated by the other leg.

These results are consistent with the majority of the existing studies on the locomotion in persons with degenerative knee joint changes (Kaufman et al. 2001, Manetta et al. 2002, Astephen et al. 2005, Bejek et al. 2006b, Ogrodzka et al. 2007).

Gök et al. (2002) also studied time and space parameters in their work. The authors observe reduced values of the walking speed, step frequency, length of the cycle and automatically extended duration of the cycle and the double support phase. Based on their result, Andracchi et al. (1982) conclude that reduced walking speed and length of the cycle as well as the delay of the Foot Off period are a part of an adaptation mechanism aimed at pain reduction. Additionally, authors conclude that the shortened length of the cycle may result from the avoidance of full load, which is typical of gonarthrosis patients.

Al-Zahrani et al. (2002) performed a gait analysis in patients suffering from degenerative knee disease which showed that the length of the cycle and the walking speed were reduced for such persons while the support phase is extended.
After the procedure the values of time and space parameters improved only slightly, which may be corroborated by a study by Bőrjessona et al. (2005) who found that patients suffering from degenerative knee disease walk at a lower speed, with lower step frequency and the single support phase is shortened. Despite good results they continue to walk more slowly and do not regain the correct gait stereotype after the procedure.
Similar results, pointing to slight changes in time and space parameters before and after the procedure were observed in research conducted by Sukru Solak et al. (2005).
Fantozzi et al. (2003) studied locomotion in two groups - endoprosthesi with PCL retention and with PCL removal. The extension of the DS period and a reduced walking speed were observed in both groups, compared to the control group.
The results obtained by these authors confirm the results of the authors' own research presented in this study.
Wu et al. (2007) found in their study of patient locomotion after knee replacement that the walking speed is reduced, which is connected with the reduction of the length of the cycle and a reduction in step frequency, especially in the operated leg. The DS period was lengthened.
However, the results were not compared before and after the procedure. Such an analysis presented in this study shows a clear improvement of these parameters after the procedure and their values become close to the control group.

6. Significance of the three-dimensional gait analysis in therapy of patients with gonarthrosis before and after arthroplasty

Degenerative changes in the knee joint lead to its deformation resulting in genu varum or genu valgum. They also cause changes in intra- and peri-articular soft tissues. Cruciate ligaments, collateral ligaments, the quadriceps femoris and other lower extremity muscles influencing the joint function under incorrect conditions. Compensation mechanisms are developed to make it possible for the system to function under normal conditions. All this causes nerve impulses from the end organs of the ligaments of the joint capsule, and especially those responsible for the proper position of the joint surface and joint kinematics reach the central nervous system from damaged locations or from locations which do not function properly. In this way, the stimuli reaching the central nervous system consolidate incorrect patterns of motion.
During the knee replacement procedure, the cruciate ligaments are removed, fat is removed from the joint capsule, the condyles of the femur and tibia are trimmed together with the subcartilage layer. Main end organs informing the central nervous system about the position of the joint are removed. A prosthesis without nerve connections is implanted.
After the surgical procedure, the central nervous system is not properly informed about the position of the individual elements of the joint, so, during gait, it uses the patters consolidated during the disease.
It is important to capture all deviations caused by the developing disease in the gait analysis performed before the procedure. As both legs are used for walking, changes occurring in the affected joint often influence the function of the healthy joint.

All deviations captured in the gait analysis performed before the procedure should be used for the planning of rehabilitation treatment to eliminate them after the operation.
Kinezytherapy planning should emphasize the use of end organs in the remaining joint structures which are responsible for proprioception to open a new rout for information flowing from these elements to the central nervous system.
Selection of appropriate exercises may help eliminate motion patterns consolidated before the procedure to achieve the correct gait pattern. Without being familiar with locomotion patterns before the procedure it will be difficult, which is confirmed by results of research conducted even two years after the procedure.
The patients taking part in the study were rehabilitated for only two weeks after the procedure and the results of locomotion examination show that changes consolidated in the gait stereotype resulting from the progressive nature of the disease were not considerably improved after the procedure. Thus, on the basis of the research conducted it should be concluded that physiotherapeutic procedures should include changes in the gait pattern and should be conducted until normal values are reached in follow-up examinations. The rehabilitation program should include elements of correct gait learning, dominated by exercises teaching the correct function of the pelvis and the lower extremity joints. This will make it possible to reconstruct the biomechanical locomotion pattern changed as a result of the disease. This will also extend the endoprothesis life.
Compensation mechanisms developing in the locomotor system due to disease make it possible to reduce pain, however, they cause strain changes in other locomotor segments with time - in the pelvis, ankle and hip joints. Knee replacement reduces articular pain, however, it will not reverse these mechanisms. It will be possible only by proper rehabilitation based on three-dimensional gait analysis.
The gait analysis presented in this study may be an example of locomotor disturbance examination in a group of patients before and after knee replacement. Thus, the application of more and more accurate measuring instruments in gait analysis becomes a necessity to achieve the best clinical results. On the basis of the presented three-dimensional gait analysis, a change in the locomotor pattern in patients after joint replacement can be noticed and the degree and scope of these dysfunctions can be determined. So one of the possibilities offered by the method is the monitoring of the treatment after surgical procedures. The results obtained can be used to evaluate and verify the effectiveness of the treatment methods used.
Owing to the application of three-dimensional gait analysis it is possible to adjust the therapeutic programme to individual changes in the locomotor stereotype and to monitor the direction of the rehabilitation as well as walking reeducation processes.
Advanced gonarthrosis affects significantly gait stereotype with a limitations in function of a patients. Knee arthroplasty is a method of therapy which allows to improve the gait pattern, although it demands time and proper rehabilitation to record correct pattern. A detailed analysis of gait cycle is necessary of optimal results, since it illustration and presents various disturbances in individual gait pattern. This can be reached in 3D notion analysis, which presents spatial arrangement of body segments in three planes of motion
Application of more and more exact hardware for motion analysis is necessary to obtain best clinical results. Changes in gait pattern is apparent in 3D analysis of patients motion after arthroplasty of knee join, estimation of these changes and range of dysfunction can thus be measured. As so, one of applications of the presented method is monitoring of the

patients after the surgery. The obtained result can be used for validation and verification of the efficacy of applied therapy.

7. References

Al-Zahrani K., Bakheit A. (2002). *A study of the gait characteristics of patients with chronic osteoarthritis of the knee.* Disability and Rehabilitation, Vol.24, No.5, pp.275-280, ISSN 0963-8288

Andriacchi T.P., Galante J., Fermier R. (1982). *The influence of total knee-replacement design on walking and stair climbing.* The Journal of Bone & Joint Surgery. Vol.64A, pp. 1328-1335, ISSN: 1535-1386

Andriacchi T.P., Hurwitz D.E. (1997). *Gait biomechanics and the evolution of total joint replacement,* Gait and Posture, No.5, pp. 256-264, ISSN 0966-6362

Andriacchi T.P., Alexander E. J. (2000). *Studies of human locomotion: past, present and future,* Journal of Biomechanics, No.33, pp. 1217-1224, ISSN 0021-9290

Astephen J.L., Deluzio K.J. (2005). *Changes in frontal plane dynamics and the loading response phase of the gait cycle are characteristic of severe knee osteoarthritis application of a multidimensional analysis technique.* Clinical Biomechanics, No. 20, pp. 209-217, ISSN 0268-0033.

Astephen J.L., Deluzio K.J., Caldwell G.E., Hubley-Kozey C.L., Dunbar M.J. (2007). *Gait and neuromuscular changes associated with knee OA severity.* Journal of Biomechanics, *No.*40(S2), pp. 287-294, ISSN: 0021-9290

Baliunas A.J., Hurwitz A.B., Ryal A.B., Karrar A., Case J.P. (2002). *Increased knee joint loads during walking are present in subjects with knee osteoarthritis,* Osteoarthritis and Cartilage, No. 10, pp. 573-579, ISSN 1063-4584

Barret D., Cobb A., Bentley G. (1991). *Joint proprioception in normal, osteoarthritic and replaced knees.* The Journal of Bone & Joint Surgery, No. 73, pp. 53-56, ISSN: 1535-1386

Basmajian JV (1976) The human bicycle. In: Biomechanics V-A (Komi PV, ed), pp 297-302, University Park Press: Baltimore

Bejek Z., Paróczai R., Illyés Á., Kocsis L., Kiss R. (2006a) *Gait parameters of patients with osteoarthritis of the knee joint.* Facta Universitatis: Physical Education and Sport, Vol.4, No.1, pp. 9-16, ISSN 1451 740X

Bejek Z., Paróczai R., Illyés Á., Kiss R. (2006b). *The influence of walking speed on gait parameters in healthy people and in patients with osteoarthritis.* Knee Surgery, Sports Traumatology, Arthroscopy, Vol. 14, No.7, pp. 612-622, ISSN 0942-2056

Benedetti M.G., Catani F., Bilotta T.W., Marcacci M., Mariani E. (2003). *Muscle activation pattern and gait biomechanics after total knee replacement.* Clinical Biomechanics, No.13, pp. 871-876, ISSN 0268-0033.

Bober T. (1987). *Biomechanika chodu i biegu,* ISBN 83-89156-38-5, AWF Wrocław

Bőrjesson M., Weidenhielm L., Mattsson E., Olsson E. (2005). *Gait and clinical measurements in patients with knee osteoarthritis after surgery: a prospective 5 – year follow – up study.* The Knee, No.12, pp. 121-127, ISSN 0968-0160

Cash R., Gonzales M., Garst J., Barmada R., Stern S. (1996). *Proprioception after arthroplasty.* Clinical Orthopaedics and Related Research, No.331, pp. 172-178, ISSN 0009-921X

Chao E., Laughman R., Stauffer R. (1980). *Biomechanical gait evaluation of pre and postoperative total knee replacement patients.* Archives of Orthopaedic and Trauma Surgery, No.97, pp. 309, ISSN 1434-3916

Childs J., Sparto P., Fitzgerald K., Bizzini M., Irrgang J. (2004). *Alterations in lower extremity movement and muscle activation patterns in individuals with knee osteoarthritis.* Clinical Biomechanics, No.19, pp. 44-49, ISSN 0268-0033.

Dorr L.D., Ochsner J.L., Gronley J., Perry J. (1988). *Functional comparsion of posterior cruciate-retained versus cruciate-sacrificed total knee arthroplasty.* Clinical Orthopaedics and Related Research, No.336, pp. 36-45, ISSN 0009-921X

Fantozzi S., Benedetti M.G., Leardini A., Banks S.A., Cappello A. (2003). *Fluoroscopic and gait analysis of functional performance i stair ascent of two total knee replacement designs.* Gait and Posture, No.17, pp. 225-234, ISSN 0966-6362

Gök H., Ergin S., Yavuzer G. (2002). *Kinetic and kinematic characteristics of gait in patients with medial knee arthrosis.* Acta Orthopaedica Scandinavica, Vol.73, No.6, pp. 647-652, ISSN 0001-6470

Ishii Y., Terajima K., Koga Y., Takahashi H.E., Bechtold J.E. (1998). *Gait analysis after total knee arthroplasty. Comparison of posterior cruciate retention and substitution.* The Journal of Orthopaedic Science No.3, pp. 310-317, ISSN 1436-2023

Kaufman K.R., Huges C., Morrey B.F., Morrey M., An K – N. (2001). *Gait characteristics of patients with knee osteoarthritis.* Journal of Biomechanics, No. 34, pp. 907-915, ISSN: 0021-9290

Kramers-de Quervain A., Stussi E., Muller R., Drobny T., Munzinger U. (1997). *Quantitative gait analysis after bilateral total knee arthroplasty with two different systems within each subject.* Journal of Arthroplasty, Vol.12, No.2, pp. 168-179, ISSN 1532-8406

Kwiatkowski K., Płomiński J. (2004) *Choroba zwyrodnieniowa stawu kolanowego – patomechanizm i rozpoznawanie,* Polski Merkuriusz Lekarski, Vol.17, No.100, pp. 415 – 419, ISSN 1426-9686

Manetta J., Franz L.H., Moon C., Perell K.L., Fang M. (2002). *Comparison of hip and knee muscle moment in subject with and without knee pain.* Gait and Posture, No.16, pp. 249-254, ISSN 0966-6362

Marks R., Quiney H., Wessel J. (1993). *Proprioceptive sensibility in woman with normal and osteoarthritic knee joints.* Clinical Rheumatology, No.12, pp. 170-175, ISSN 0770-3198

McClelland J., Webster K., Feller J. (2006). *A comparison of gait patterns in patients following total and unicompartmental knee replacement surgery* Gait and Posture, No.24S, pp. 139-140, ISSN 0966-6362

McClelland J., Webster K., Feller J. (2007). *Gait analysis of patients following total knee replacement: A systematic review.* The Knee, No.14, pp. 253-263, ISSN 0968-0160

Minns R.J. 2005. *The role of gait analysis in the management of the knee.* The Knee, Vol.12, No.3, pp. 157-162, ISSN 0968-0160

Ogrodzka K., Chwała W., Niedźwiedzki (2007). T. *Three-dimensional pattern of the knee movement of subjects with gonarthrosis.* Ortopedia Traumatologia Rehabilitacja, Vol.9, No.6, pp. 605-614, ISSN 1509-3492

Ogrodzka K., Niedźwiedzki T. (2008). *The variability of kinematic parameters of the lower limb joints of subjects before and after total knee replacement.* The Journal of Orthopaedics Trauma Surgery and Related Research, Vol.1, No.9, pp. 25-30, ISSN 1897-2276

Otsuki T., Nawata K., Okuno M. (1999). *Quantitative evaluation of gait pattern in patients with osteoarthrosis of the knee before and after total knee arthroplasty. Gait analysis using a pressure measuring system.* The Journal of Orthopaedic Science, No.4, pp. 99-105, ISSN 1436-2023

Perry J. (1992) Gait analysis: normal and pathological function. Thorofare, SLACK Incorporated, ISBN 1-55642-192-3, New Jersey

Rudolph K.S., Schmitt L.C., Lewek M.D. (2007). *Age-related changes in strength, joint laxity and walking patterns: are they related to knee osteoarthritis?* Physical Therapy, Vol.87, No.11, pp. 1422-1432, ISSN 0031-9023

Sharma L., Pai Y. (1997). *Impaired proprioception and osteoarthritis.* Current Opinion in Rheumatology. No.9, pp. 253-258, ISSN 1040-8711

Smith A., Lloyd D., Wood D. (2006). *A kinematic and kinetic analysis of walking after total knee arthroplasty with and without patellar resurfacing.* Clinical Biomechanics, No.21, pp. 379-386, ISSN 0268-0033

Steiner M.E., Simon S.R., Pisciotta J.C. (1989). *Early changes in gait and maximum knee torque following knee arthroplasty.* Clinical Orthopaedics and Related Research, No.238, pp. 174-180, ISSN 0009-921X

Sukru Solak A., Kentel B., Ates Y. (2005). *Does bilateral total knee arthroplasty affect gait in women? Comparison of gait analyses before and after total knee arthroplasty compared with normal knees.* Journal of Arthroplasty, Vol.20, No.6, pp. 745-750, ISSN 1532-8406

Webster KE., Wittwer JE., Feller JA. (2003). *Quantitative gait analysis after medial unicompartmental knee arthroplasty for osteoarthrosis* Journal of Arthroplasty, Vol.18, No.6, pp. 751-759, ISSN 1532-8406

Wierusz-Kozłowska M., Markuszewski J. (2004). *Choroba zwyrodnieniowa stawów,* In: Wiktora Degi ortopedia i rehabilitacja pod red. Marciniak W., Szulc A., PZWL, Warszawa. Tom 2, ISBN 978-83-200-3792-0

Wilson S., McCann P., Gotlin R., Ramakrishnan H., Wootten M., Insall J. (1996). *Comprehensive gait analysis in posterior-stabilized knee arthroplasty.* Journal of Arthroplasty, Vol.11, No.4, pp. 359-367, ISSN 1532-8406

Wu W., Huang H., Chen C. (2007). *Quantitative gait analysis after unilateral knee arthroplasty for patients with bilateral knee osteoarthritis.* Journal of Biomechanics, No. 40(S2), pp. 502, ISSN 0021-9290

Zembaty A. (1987). *Fizjoterapia.* PZWL, Warszawa, ISBN 83-910437-4-6

5

Hip-Spine Relations: An Innovative Paradigm in THR Surgery

Jean Yves Lazennec[1,2], Adrien Brusson[1] and Marc-Antoine Rousseau[1,2]
[1]Department of Orthopaedic Surgery, Hôpital Pitié Salpétrière Assistance Publique - Hôpitaux de Paris (AP-HP), Paris
[2]Biomechanics Lab, Arts et Métiers ParisTech, Centre National de la Recherche Scientifique (CNRS), Unités Mixtes de Recherche (UMR), Paris
France

1. Introduction

The sagittal balance of the trunk is considered to be a key point for spinal fusion and disc replacement. This balance is the manifestation of a postural strategy conditioned by anatomic and functional characteristics that can differ greatly from one person to another (Duval-Beaupere et al., 1992). The role of the pelvic area is evident for spinal surgeons in their planning and analyses; they pay special attention to the sacral slope, which is closely related to the pelvic tilt (Chanplakorn et al., 2011; Dorr et al., 1983; Jackson & McManus, 1994; Kobayashi et al., 2004; Murray, 1993; Vialle et al., 2005). Dubousset underlined this concept as early as 1984, in treating the pelvis as a "pelvic vertebra" (Dubousset, 1984).

Although the concept of spinopelvic balance is well accepted today (Lazennec et al., 2004), conventional imagery underestimates the influence of the coxofemoral joint and explains it inadequately. The EOS imaging system (Dubousset et al., 2008), by optimizing radiologic data in functional situations, is revolutionizing our understanding of hip-spine relations (Lazennec et al., 2011b).

These anatomic and functional considerations often remain foreign to hip surgeons, who focus on the bone landmarks of the pelvis for their navigation, individualized adjustments, and failure analyses (Woo & Morrey, 1982; Woolson & Rahimtoola, 1999). Although the hip is a highly mobile joint, surgical concepts are still based on the static AP view of the pelvis in standing or supine position to assess cup orientation, which is an essential risk factor for prosthesis instability and wear (Kennedy et al., 1998). Influenced by the classic anatomic culture of cross-sectional slices, they consider the CT scan a reference tool for the "horizontal" assessment of the coxofemoral joints (Ackland et al., 1986; Dorr et al., 1983; Kennedy et al., 1998; Murray, 1993; Seki et al., 1998; Wan et al., 2009). Nonetheless, as this chapter will show, lateral views of the hips and the evaluation of sitting position provide new information about "normal" hip function and THR failures.

The concept of cumulative anteversion between the acetabular cup and the femur is considered a key factor in the stability of the hip prosthesis. This concept, however, is based on the measurements taken by computed tomography in a supine position, which do not take into account the functional dimension of the problem.

Degeneration of the spinopelvic balance, often associated with spinal aging or hip dysfunction, can generate a cascade of mechanical events that involve the relation between the hips and spine and in particular the adaptive capacities of the hips (Itoi, 1991). These problems have become more acute today, with patients' ever greater functional demands after hip arthroplasty (**Fig. 1**). Hip-spine relations must therefore be better investigated in planning total hip arthroplasties (THAs), as lumbosacral orientation plays a critical role in the function of the hip joints.

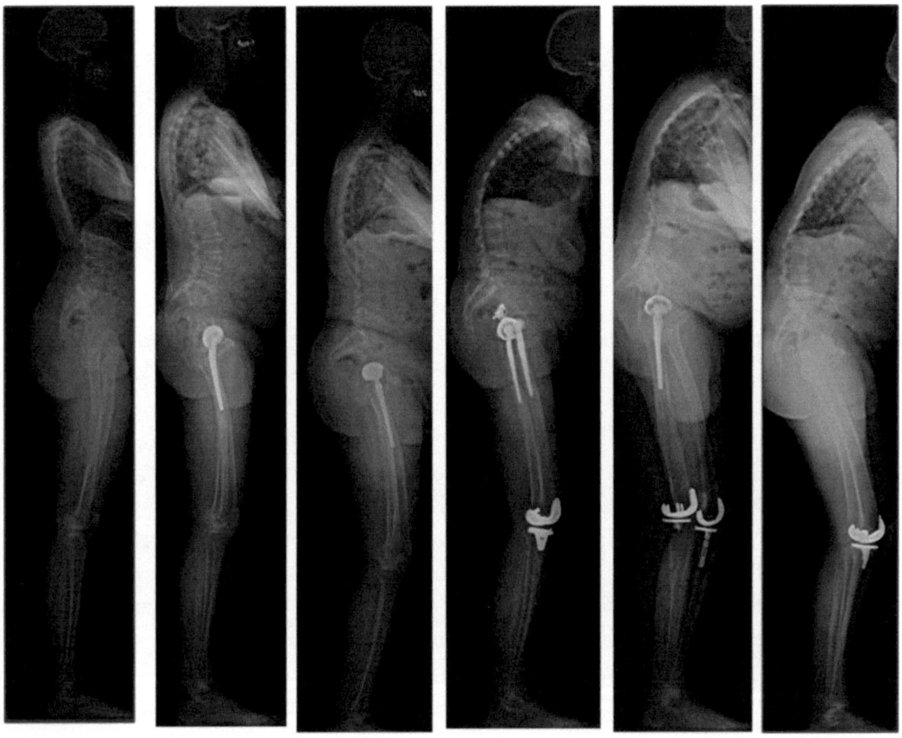

Fig. 1. Degeneration of the sagittal spinopelvic balance : loss of spinal curvatures and modifications of pelvis orientation

2. Anatomic bases of lumbopelvic balance: The importance of sagittal spinopelvic balance in standing position

The most important radiographic parameters of spinopelvic balance in upright posture have been well defined (Tassin, 2004; Vaz et al., 2002; Vialle et al., 2005). The sacral slope (SS, 41° ± 8.4°) is the angle between the horizontal line and the cranial sacral endplate tangent (Vialle et al., 2005).

The pelvic tilt (PT, 13° ± 6°) is the angle between the vertical line and the line joining the middle of the sacral endplate and the center of the bicoxofemoral axis (the line between the geometric center of both femoral heads) (Vialle et al., 2005).

The pelvic incidence (I, 55° ± 10.6°) is the angle between the line perpendicular to the middle of the cranial sacral endplate and the line joining the middle of this endplate to the center of the bicoxofemoral axis (Vialle et al., 2005).

Each subject is characterized by this "morphologic" parameter, which schematically represents pelvic thickness. The adaptation of other functional factors, such as pelvic tilt, and the spinal parameters (sacral slope, lumbar lordosis, and thoracic kyphosis) makes it possible to position the center of gravity of the component specifically so that it is supported by the femoral heads relative to the pelvic base, to maintain balance with only a minimal muscular effort (Duval-Beaupere et al., 1992; Legaye et al., 1998; Rillardon et al., 2003; Roussouly et al., 2005) **(Fig. 2).**

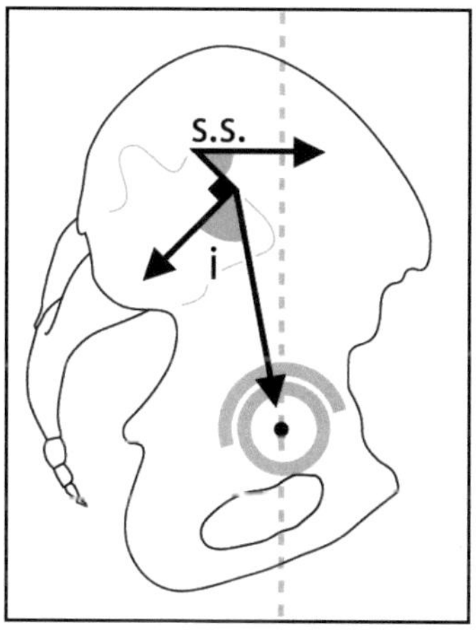

Fig. 2. Definition of sacral slope (S.S.) and pelvic incidence angle (i)

Pelvic incidence (I, a morphologic and anatomical parameter) is associated with the sacral slope (SS) and pelvic tilt (PT) (positional parameters) in a geometric relation: I = SS + PT (1) **(Fig. 3).** A sequence of significant correlations has been reported between pelvic incidence and the functional indicators, sacral slope (r = 0.98) and lordosis (r = 0.9) (Boulay et al., 2006; Rillardon et al., 2003; Vialle et al., 2005). A high pelvic incidence corresponds to a sharp sacral slope and strong lordosis, while a small pelvic incidence corresponds to a low sacral slope and flatter lordosis. The borderline balance conditions and spinopelvic balance in seated positions are less known, in particular, for patients with hip prostheses.

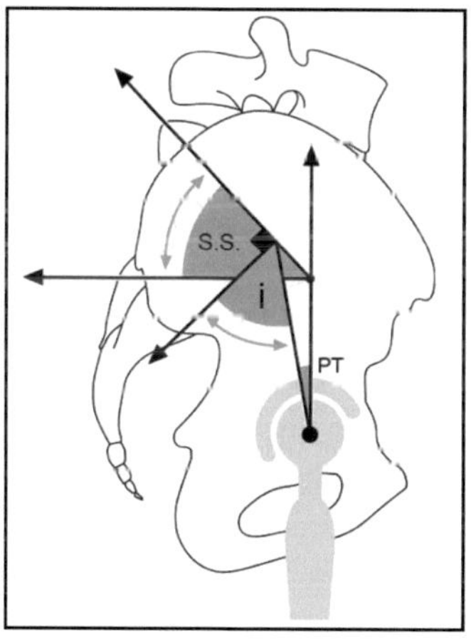

Fig. 3. Pelvic incidence (I) is associated with the sacral slope (S.S.) and pelvic tilt (PT) in a geometric relation: I = SS + PT

The pelvis moves, rotating around the bicoxofemoral axis, leading to both anterior tilt (where the upper portion of the pelvis tips forward) and posterior tilt (upper portion of the pelvis tips backward). The variations in the angles of the sacral slope determine the range of this pelvic tilt, and its variations in turn influence the orientation of the anterior pelvic plane or the Lewinnek plane classically used as a reference for navigation of the acetabular components in THAs **(Fig. 4)** (Lewinnek et al., 1978). The surprising consequences of some spinal arthrodeses or stiffening on the hips and the difficulties of adjusting prostheses below stiffened spines illustrate the importance of these anatomic-functional parameters.

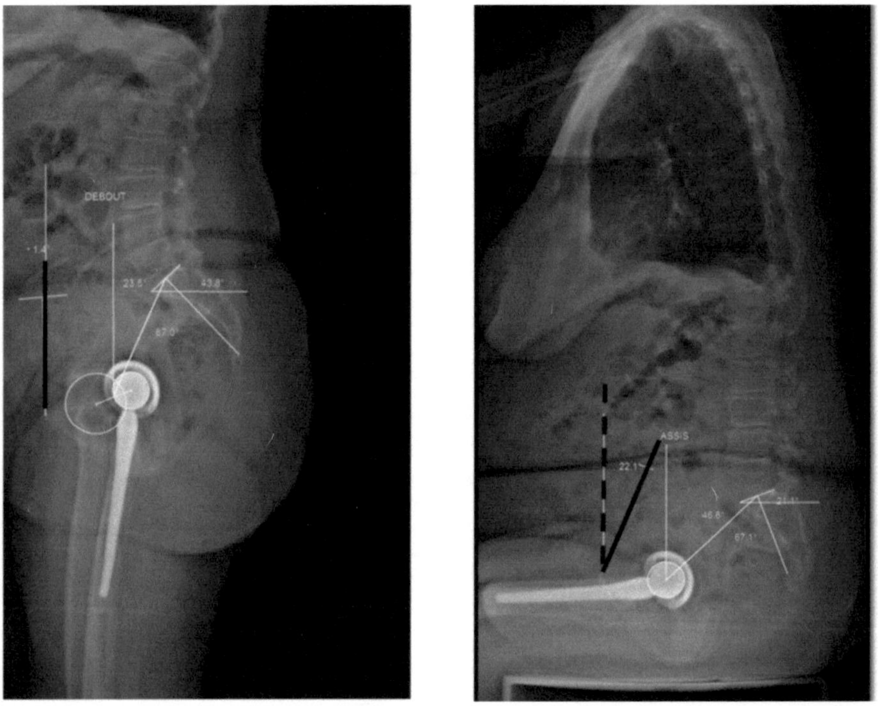

Fig. 4. The pelvis moves, rotating around the bicoxofemoral axis, the anterior tilt (where the upper portion of the pelvis tips forward) is observed in standing position and posterior tilt (upper portion of the pelvis tips backward) in seated position.

2.1 The standing position

Fig. 5 corresponds to a forward tilt of the pelvis as a whole. In this situation, the upper endplate of S1, viewed laterally, makes an angle of approximately 35° to 45° between the sacral slope and the horizontal (Lazennec et al., 2000; Lazennec et al., 2011c). Some subjects have a small sacral slope angle in standing position: we talk then about posterior pelvic tilt (or pelvic retroversion or pelvic extension) and the sacrum seen on a lateral image appears more vertical than usual (Fig. 6a). On the contrary, other subjects have a very horizontal sacrum in standing position with a sacral slope angle sometimes much greater than 50° (anterior pelvic tilt, pelvic anteversion or pelvic flexion) (Fig. 6b).

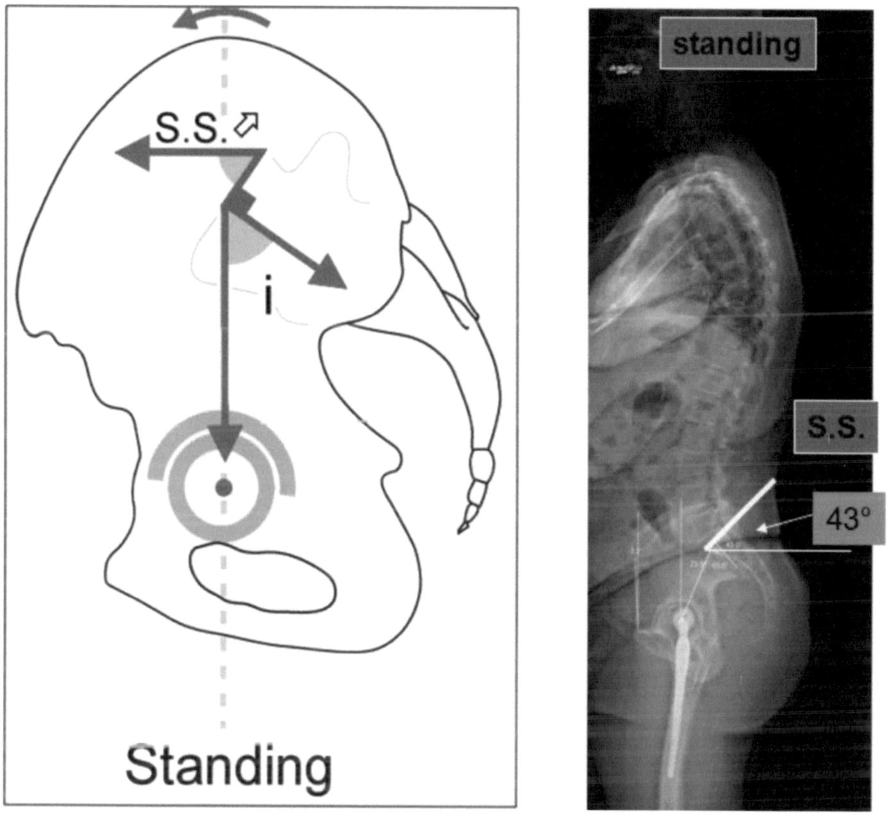

Fig. 5. The standing position corresponds to a forward tilt of the pelvis: the upper endplate of S1, viewed laterally, makes an angle of approximately 35° to 45 between the sacral slope and the horizontal

2.2 In the supine position

When the lower limbs are extended, the sacral slope is often greater than in standing position. The measurement of its angle with the vertical often exceeds 45° (Lazennec et al., 2011a; Lazennec et al., 2004). This can be seen on scout views of pelvic CT scans. This additional pelvic tilt may not be well tolerated in the case of a stiff or deformed spine since the dorsal decubitus position deepens lumbar lordosis. Sometimes a limitation of the available extension of the hips or posterior osteoarthritis makes a strict decubitus position unbearable, at least without a slight compromise flexion of the coxofemoral joints.

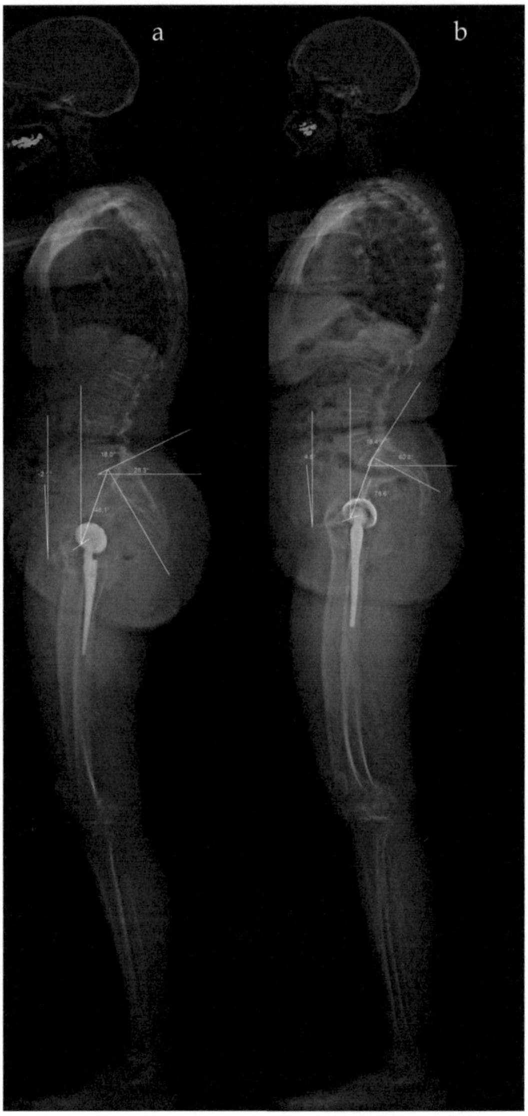

Fig. 6. a: Some subjects have a small sacral slope angle in standing position: the sacrum appears more vertical than usual (posterior pelvic tilt , pelvic retroversion or pelvic extension), 6. b: Some subjects have a very horizontal sacrum in standing position with a greater sacral slope angle (anterior pelvic tilt, pelvic anteversion or pelvic flexion)

2.3 In a sitting position

The phenomenon is inversed **(Fig. 7)**. The pelvis tilts backwards as it progresses toward a sitting position. The sacral slope diminishes, to values of 20° to 25° on average (Lazennec et al., 2011a; Lazennec et al., 2011c). This slope may still be slightly positive (by 5 to 10°) or even sometimes negative. As a function of the height of the seat, the subject's morphology or any associated spinal disease, we observe pelvic posterior tilt (pelvic retroversion or pelvic extension) more or less accentuated with a sacrum more or less vertical. The difference in the values of the sacral slope between standing and seated positions makes it possible to define the available flexion associated with the lumbosacral joint (extrinsic available pelvic flexion) by opposition to the potential for flexion associated with the coxofemoral joint (intrinsic available pelvic flexion).

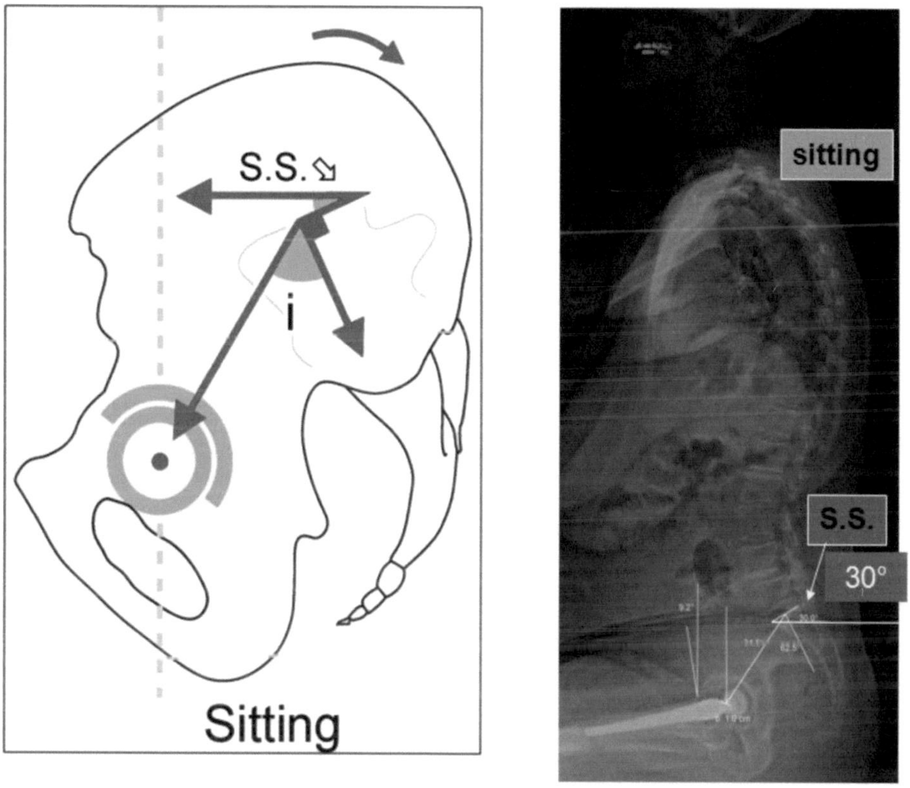

Fig. 7. In sitting position, the pelvis tilts backwards. The sacral slope diminishes. The difference in the values of the sacral slope between standing and seated positions is about 20°

2.4 Progression from standing to sitting positions

Causes considerable modification in the orientation of the anterior pelvic plane, today considered the reference for adjusting the acetabular cups (D'Lima et al., 2000; Herrlin et al., 1988; Rousseau et al., 2009). These variations must concern us. Lewinnek's plane (the anterior pelvic plane) is evaluated in the dorsal decubitus position to collect morphologic data for planning the hip prosthesis (Lewinnek et al., 1978). The information obtained must extrapolated prudently because it is not necessarily vertical in standing positions, and its tilt is highly variable in sitting positions (Philippot et al., 2009; Rousseau et al., 2009). Accordingly, for mean values of 3° in standing positions, the values reported while sitting were 17.5° (Lazennec et al., 2011c) **(Fig. 8).**

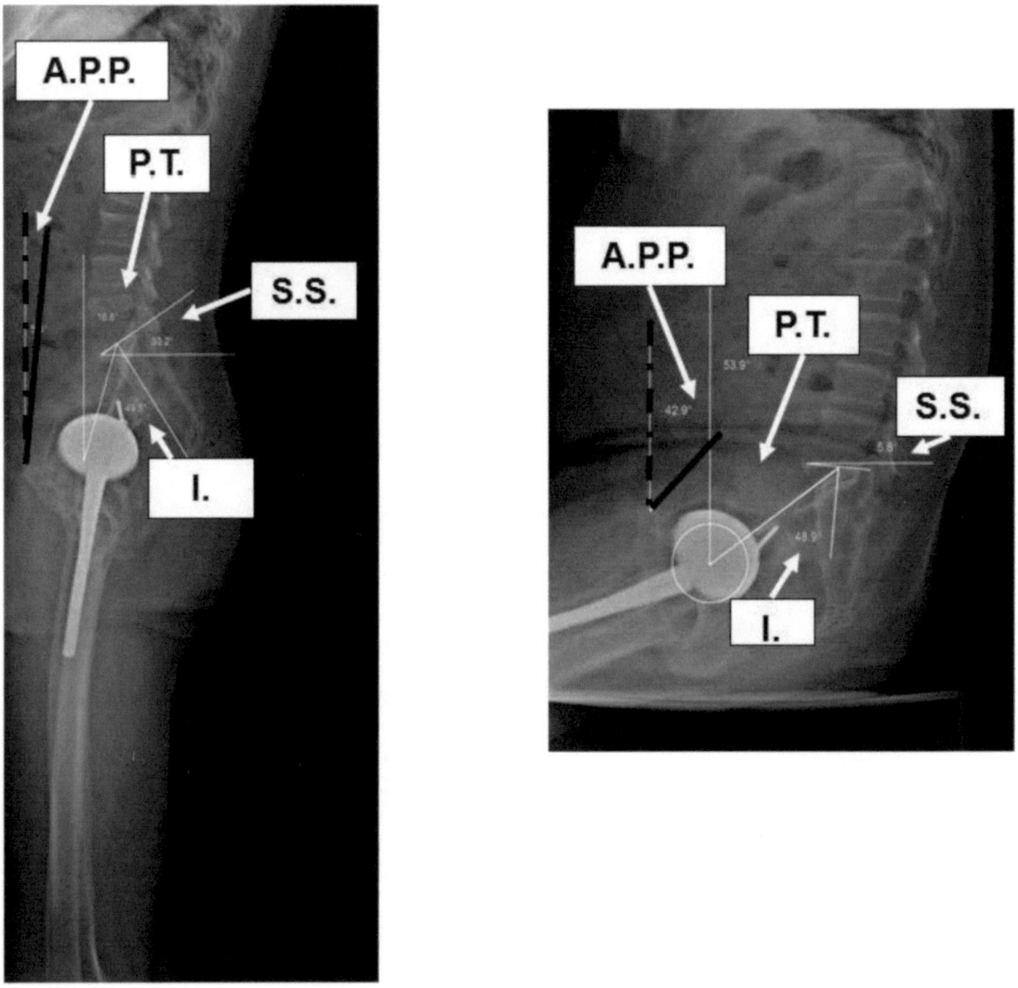

Fig. 8. Progression from standing to sitting positions causes considerable modification in the orientation of the anterior pelvic plane (A.P.P. or Lewinnek plane)

3. Influence of sagittal posture on the frontal and sagittal acetabular orientation in functional situations

3.1 Anatomic foundations

Most surgeons use only AP X radiograms of the pelvis to assess the cup orientation in standing position, measuring the frontal inclination angle or abduction angle (AA). The lateral view is little used in the literature. Acetabular tilt is assessed by the SIA (sagittal inclination angle between the horizontal and the axis of the cup ellipse, also called the sagittal tilt (Lazennec et al., 2011a) **(Fig. 9)**.

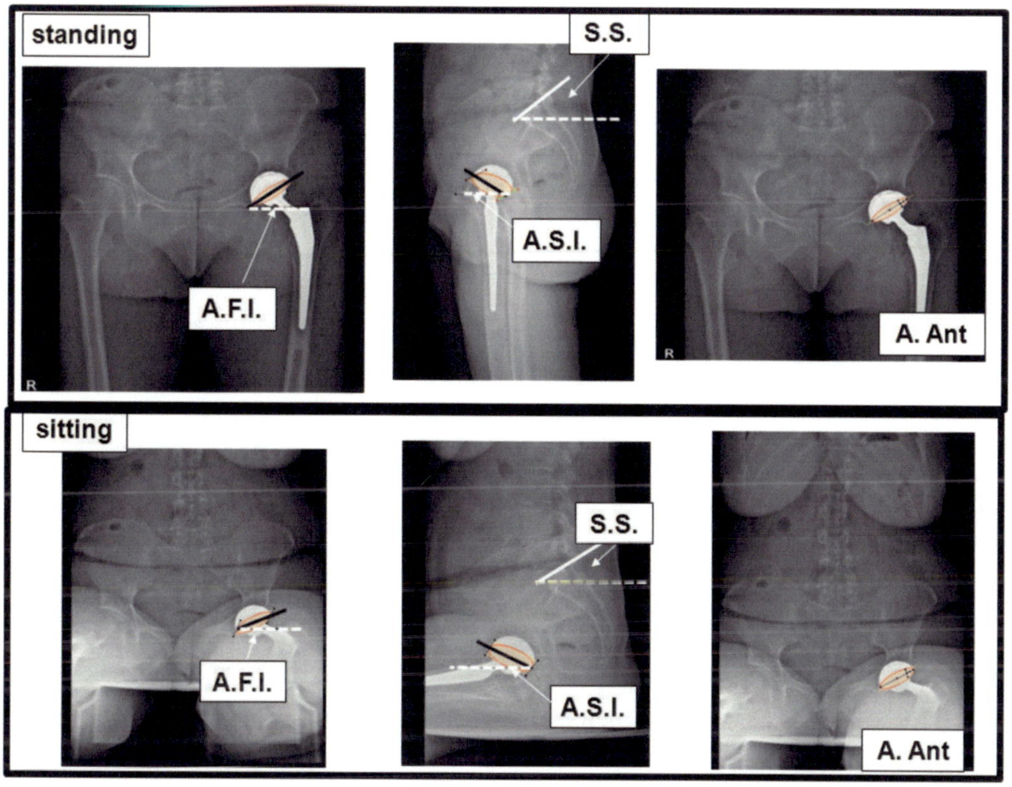

Fig. 9. AP and lateral images provide a global evaluation of the pelvis and cup orientations in standing or seated positions

Because of basic trigonometric relations in three dimensions, the SIA has the same value as the operative anteversion described by Murray (Murray, 1993), although it is a different angle. But sitting and even squatting are critical positions, as they address most of instability or impingement situations. The abduction and sagittal inclination angles of the cup are functional parameters with significant variations between the standing, sitting, and supine positions (Lazennec et al., 2011b). The interdependence between the sagittal tilt or **AST** of the cup and the sacral slope is obvious when reading lateral images, seated or standing, of the lumbosacral joint (Bolger et al., 2007). This interrelation is expressed by the value of the sacroacetabular angle **(SAA)**, defined by the axis of the acetabular ellipse viewed laterally (which defines the acetabular sagittal tilt, **AST**, with the horizontal) and the tangent to the sacral endplate. This is a fixed angle, imposed by the surgeon empirically at implantation (Lazennec et al., 2007) **(Fig. 10)**.

In a standing position, the value of the sacral slope is high and the angle of the acetabular tilt is small. Inversely, in a seated position, the sacral slope diminishes and the acetabular tilt increases. From both AP and lateral positions, the THA cup appears more vertical in seated than in standing positions. Observational series of THA from diverse institutions (Lazennec et al., 2011a; Lazennec et al., 2011c) report mean values of 49° to 52° for the frontal cup inclination in standing position and 57° to 64° while seated. At the same time the sagittal inclination is 36° to 47° standing and 51° to 58° seated. These variations in acetabular tilt contribute to modifying the "anterior opening" of the acetabulum and therefore the orientation of the functional "mobility cone" generated by the coxofemoral joint **(Fig. 11 a and b)** (Kummer et al., 1999; Lazennec et al., 2011a) (Pradhan, 1999).

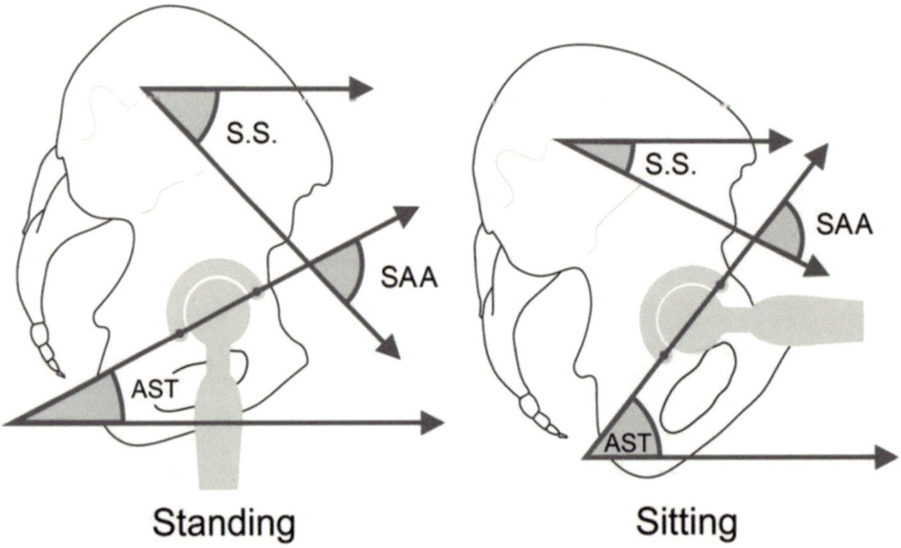

Fig. 10. The interdependence between the sagittal tilt or AST of the cup and the sacral slope is expressed by the value of the sacroacetabular angle (SAA)

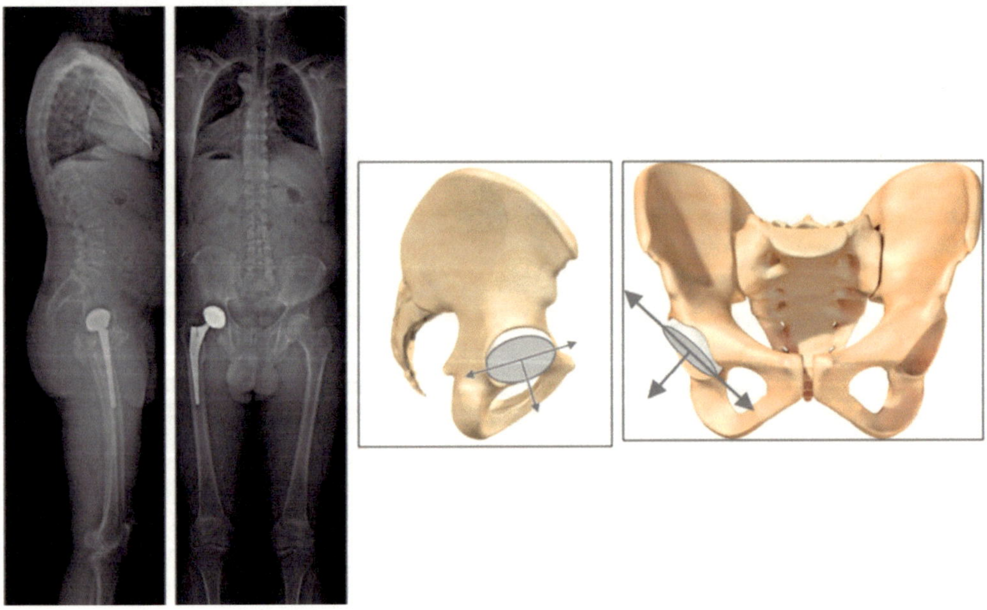

Fig. 11. a: The variations in acetabular tilt in standing and seated positions contribute to modifying the "anterior opening" of the acetabulum and therefore the orientation of the functional "mobility cone" generated by the coxofemoral joint

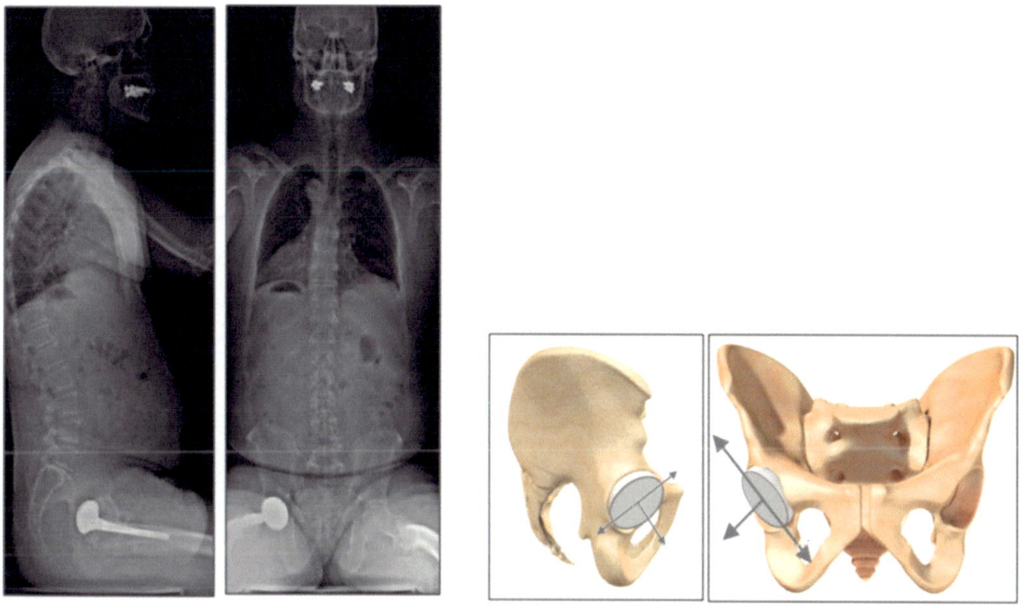

Fig. 11. b: The variations in acetabular tilt in standing and seated positions contribute to modifying the "anterior opening" of the acetabulum and therefore the orientation of the functional "mobility cone" generated by the coxofemoral joint

Modifications in the acetabular orientation produce consequences for the stability of hip arthroplasties and for all aspects of their tribology in the intermediate and long term (Lazennec et al., 2007; von Knoch et al., 2002; Woo & Morrey, 1982; Yamaguchi et al., 1997). The acetabular parameters in a supine position are highly correlated with those in a standing position but poorly correlated with those in a sitting position (Lazennec et al., 2011a). These correlations underline the importance of specific studies of the seated position in work-ups of prostheses that malfunction and of screening subjects at risk before surgery.

3.2 Disruptions can come from atypical postures

These considerations illustrate the consequences of spinal fusions regarding hip function and the possible difficulties in adjusting acetabular cup implantation in cases of an unusually stiff or unbalanced spine (Watanabe et al., 2002). Excess posterior tilt of the pelvis is often associated with postural imbalance to compensate for a forward tilt of the entire trunk. This postural adaptation verticalizes the cup from both the AP and lateral views and places the hips in a hyperextended position when standing. This solicitation of the available hip extension can lead to a posterior impingement. A typical example is posterior impingement of the hip prosthesis in standing position even though the cup was placed perfectly in accordance with the pelvic bone landmarks **(Fig. 12).** This situation can be encountered in native hips in the case of excessive posterior tilt of the pelvis (abnormal posture, trunk aging and induced posterior coxarthrosis) (Hammerberg & Wood, 2003; Itoi, 1991; Lafage et al., 2009; Offierski & MacNab, 1983).

Analysis of these situations can be difficult because they involve simultaneously diseases of the spine and hips. Assessment of the available hip extension is thus essential to distinguish true and false inability to extend the hip fully **(Fig. 13).** This analysis can be performed easily with EOS® technology, which makes it possible to individualize the available extension associated with the lumbosacral joint, that is, the extrinsic available extension, as well as the intrinsic available extension of each coxofemoral joint. Inversely, excess anterior tilt of the pelvis in a seated position can cause anterior impingement **(Fig. 14)**. In some cases, the anterior tilt of the acetabulum is also excessive in a standing position: the acetabulum is "horizontalized" from both AP and lateral views, as if the hips are permanently flexed when the subject is standing. This type of mechanism is suggested on native hips in anterior impingements, especially in some repetitive athletic or occupational movements.

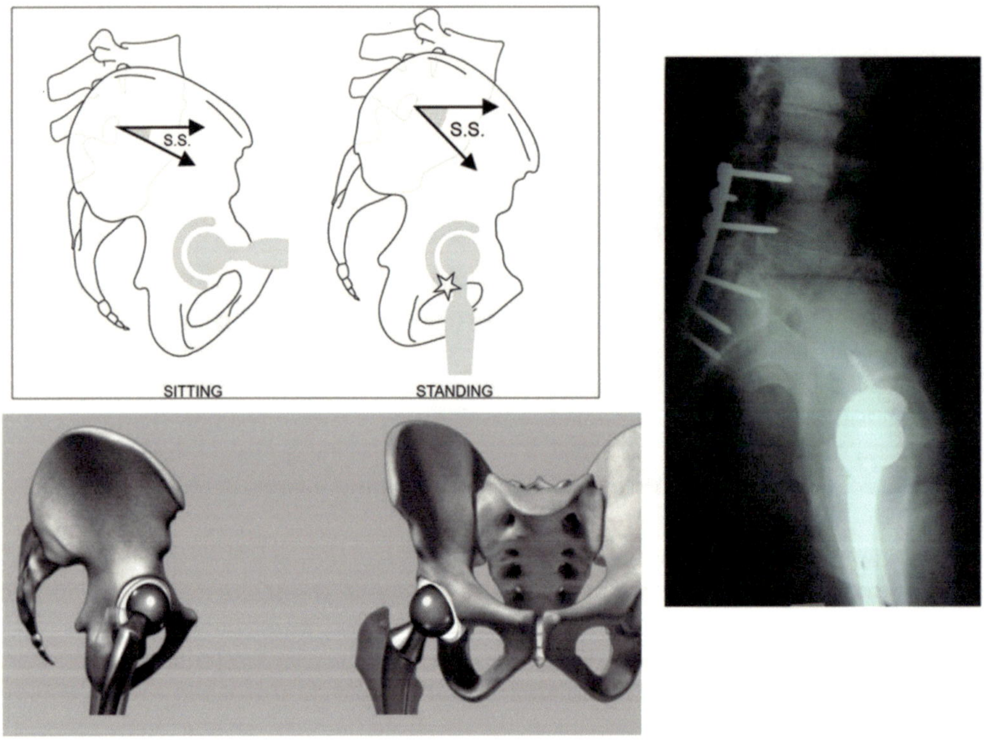

Fig. 12. Excess posterior tilt of the pelvis is often associated with postural imbalance to compensate for a forward tilt of the entire trunk. A typical example is posterior impingement of the hip prosthesis in standing position even though the cup was placed perfectly in accordance with the pelvic bone landmarks (no impingement in sitting position).

We also observed a mechanism of specific adaptation in hips that could not be fully extended secondary to coxarthrosis. The loss of range of motion of the abnormal hip results in a forward tilt of the pelvis when the patient tries to straighten up. When possible, the spine adapts by increasing lumbar lordosis, thus causing low back pain. Frequently, only one hip is involved. The test for available extension allows us to assess the phenomenon selectively.

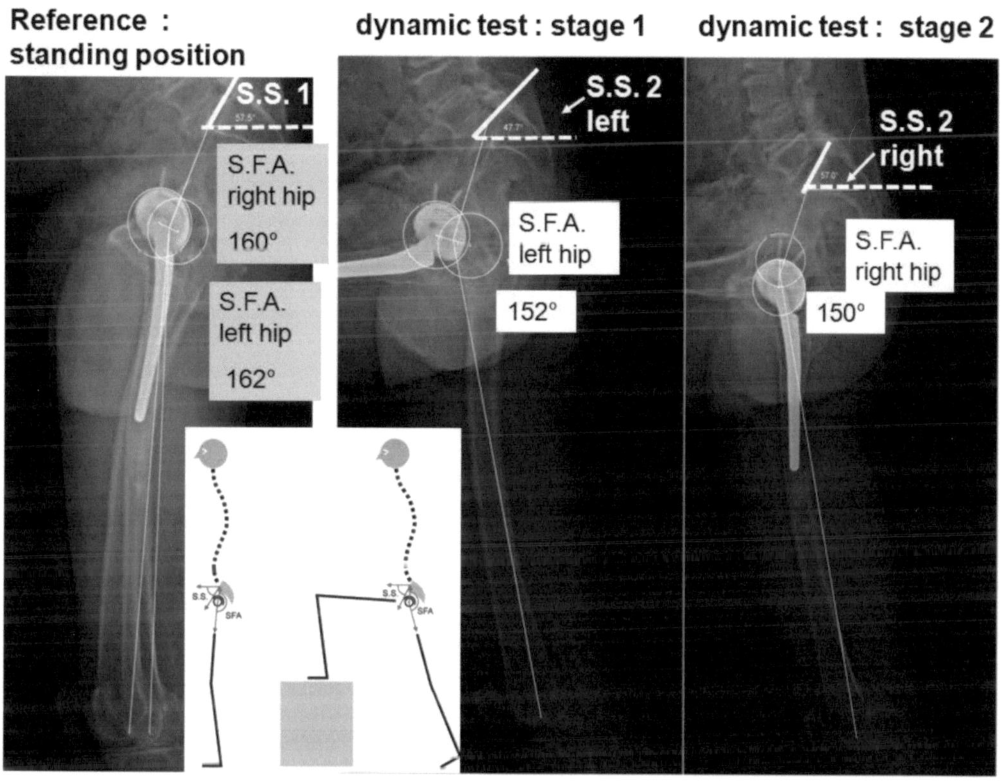

Fig. 13. EOS® technology makes it possible to individualize the available extension associated with the lumbosacral joint (the extrinsic available extension) as well as the intrinsic available extension of each coxofemoral joint. Each hip is assessed in its maximum range of extension in standing position, placing the contralateral lower limb on a step such that it is in a position of maximum flexion of the coxofemoral joint. The extrinsic available extension is measured by the capacity to increase the sacral slope (SS 2 – SS 1). The intrinsic available extension is measured by the variation of the sacro-femoral angle (SFA). In this example: the available extension is 10° for the 2 hips.

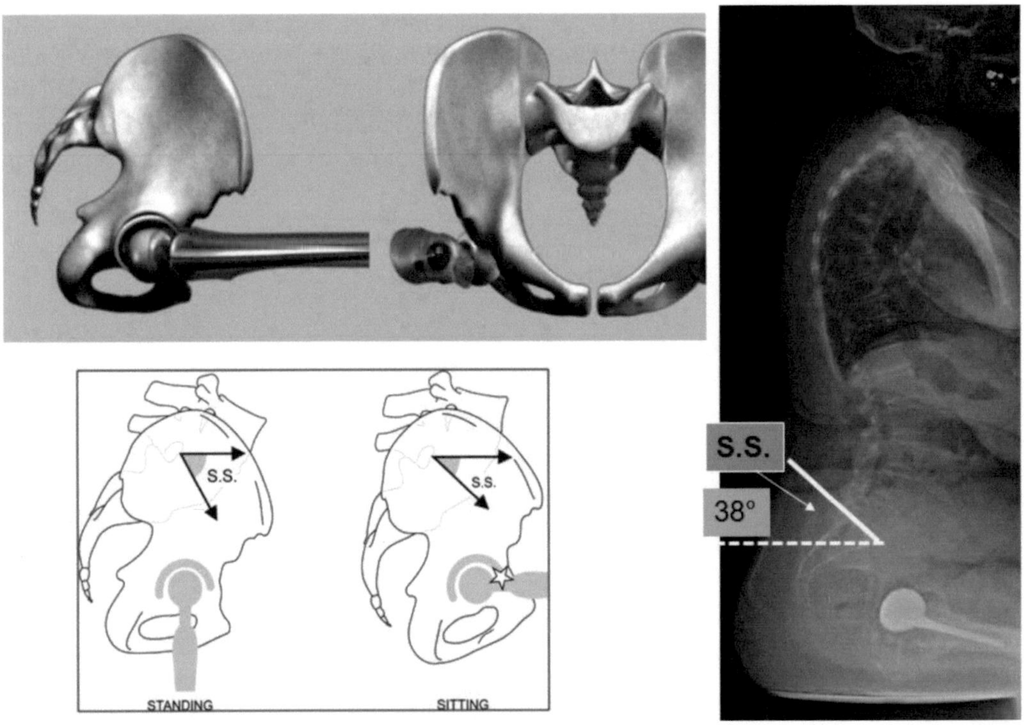

Fig. 14. Excess anterior tilt of the pelvis in a seated position can cause anterior impingement; no impingement in standing position

3.3 Disturbances can come from atypical morphotypes

The angle of incidence is the morphologic parameter determinant for the adaptation of sagittal spinopelvic balance. Two types of population require specific attention relative to those with a normal incidence. In subjects with a high angle of pelvic incidence, theoretical lumbar lordosis is greater as the range of adaptation of the sacral slope may also be, according to the formula I= SS +PT. The femoral heads are projected forward relative to the sacrum and the acetabular anterior opening is less marked. The coxofemoral joints of these subjects have a greater theoretical available extension and therefore a better ability to adapt. The range of pelvic tilt and sacral slope adaptation is higher. On the other hand, these patients are risky for spine surgeons in cases of spinal arthrodesis: the surgical achievement of adequate lordosis is technically challenging and tolerance of residual flat back is very poor.

Inversely, in subjects with a low pelvic incidence angle, there is less theoretical lumbar lordosis and the adaptability of the sacral slope and pelvic tilt may be more limited. The femoral heads are embedded under the sacrum and the anterior opening of the acetabulum is more marked. Theoretically, these subjects have less available hip extension and a weaker capacity to adapt to sagittal imbalance **(Fig. 15).** In standing position, their hips are naturally in extension, which means they cannot increase the posterior range of motion significantly. Due to potential posterior impingements, these patients can experience anterior dislocation or subluxation in standing position. Compensatory mechanisms may involve hips and knee flexion (Vialle et al., 2005). Accordingly, these subjects are more easily subject to a global and unstable imbalance because of their small margin for adaptation.

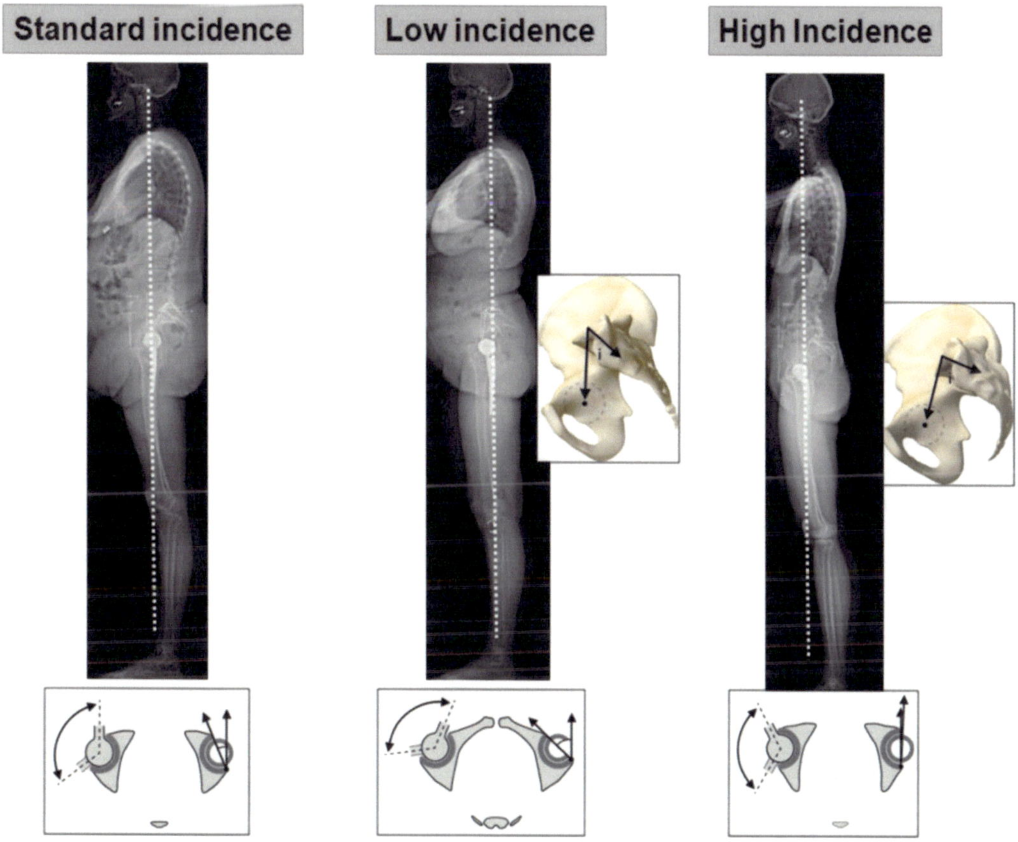

Fig. 15. In subjects with a high angle of pelvic incidence, lumbar lordosis is greater and the coxofemoral joints have a greater theoretical available extension and a better ability to adapt.In subjects with a low pelvic incidence angle, there is less lumbar lordosis and the adaptability of the sacral slope and pelvic tilt may be more limited

4. Influence of sagittal posture on cross-sectional acetabular cup orientation: Anatomic and functional anteversion

4.1 Standard data

The transverse orientation of the acetabulum is expressed by its anterior opening angle or anteversion. Anatomical acetabular anteversion is a restrictive concept as it is defined as the anterior opening according to the pelvic frame. According to Murray, "anatomical" or "morphological "anteversion is the angle between the AP pelvic axis and the acetabular axis when this is projected on to the transverse reference plane perpendicular to the longitudinal axis and the midsagittal plane of the pelvis (Murray, 1993).

In current practice, anteversion is measured on CT scans: this angle is often considered to be anatomical anteversion, leading to some confusion because the angle value depends on the pelvic orientation in the lying position.

That is, the orientation of the cross-sectional slices in relation to the sagittal plane is left to radiologists to assess without any specific criterion for standardization, although it has a critical effect on the values of the angles measured. Fortuitously, they can be strictly perpendicular to the longitudinal axis of the pelvic bone frame. Most of the time these slices, perpendicular to the plane of the examination table, do not correspond to the anatomic plane because the position of the supine subject has a more or less marked sagittal pelvic tilt (Lazennec et al., 2011a). Therefore this angle is only a "functional" supine anteversion, reflecting the projected anterior opening of the acetabulum in a specific position.

The variation in the anteversion measured is approximately 0.5° for 1° of rotation of the plane of the slice in relation to the pelvis (Anda et al., 1990; Lazennec et al., 2004; Muller et al., 2005). The literature also reports measurements of anatomic acetabular anteversion on CT, according to a plane perpendicular to the anterior pelvic plane (Lewinnek's plane)(McKibbin, 1970). In this case, the cut plane analyzes the acetabulum according to the same orientation, regardless of the subject's position. The anteversion value measured refers exclusively to the pelvic bone landmarks without taking into account the variations of position in standing, seated and squatting positions. It is fixed, regardless of the subject's position **(Fig. 16).**

Anatomic or morphologic anteversion can also be measured reliably relative to the table or machine stand by using the reference transverse plane (Aubry et al., 2005; Lazennec et al., 2004; Lazennec et al., 2007) through the upper sacral endplate (the sacral transverse plane). This technique is easier to implement than the preceding method, but the acetabulum is not analyzed according to the same angle, and the angle values are different **(Fig. 17).**

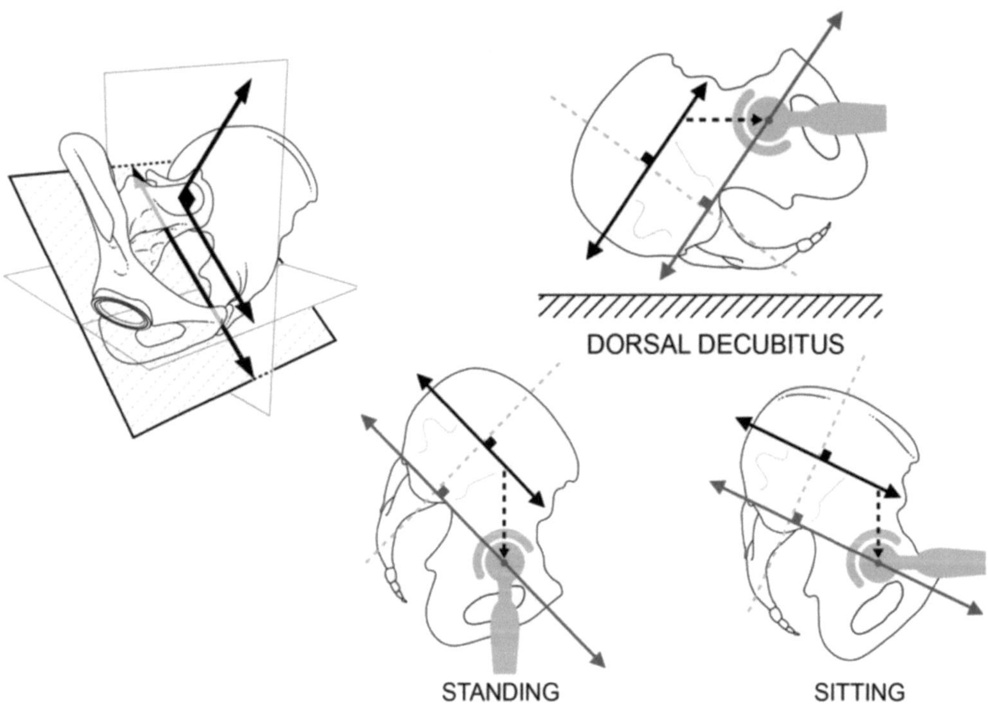

Fig. 16. Anatomic acetabular anteversion can be measured on CT scans according to a plane perpendicular to the anterior pelvic plane (Lewinnek's plane): the cut plane analyzes the acetabulum according to the same orientation, regardless of the subject's position. The anteversion value is the same in all of the positions

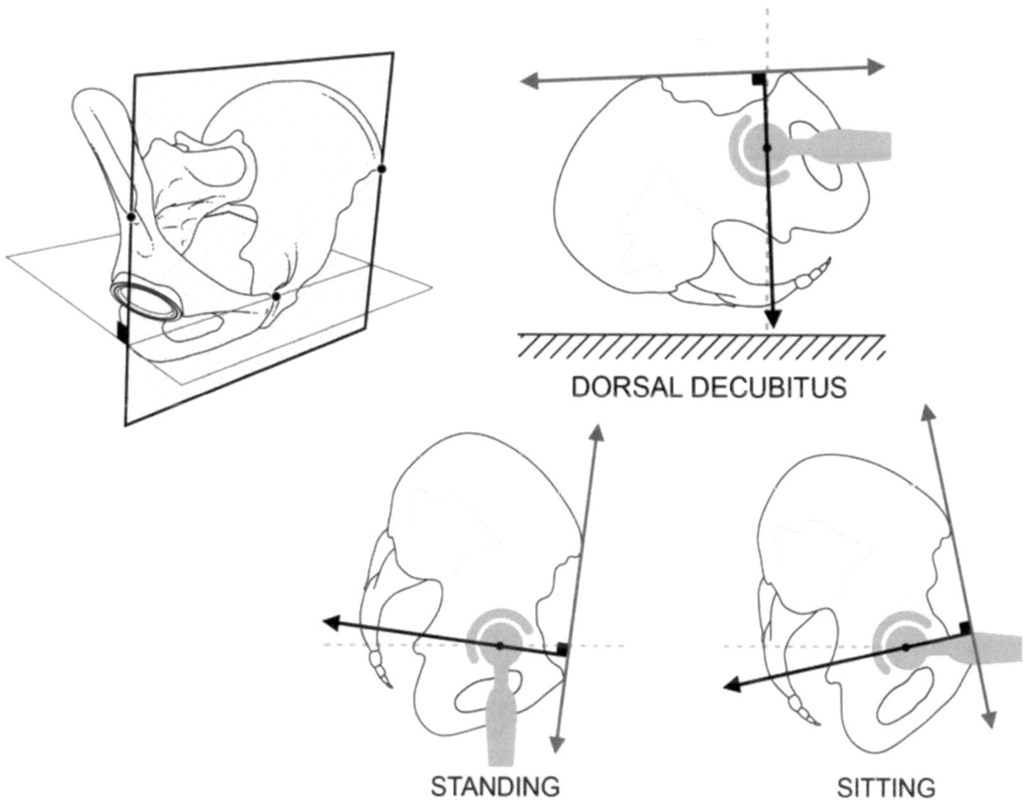

Fig. 17. Anatomic or morphologic anteversion can be measured reliably by using the reference transverse plane through the upper sacral endplate (the sacral transverse plane): the anteversion value refers exclusively to the pelvic bone landmarks without taking into account the variations of position. The anteversion value is the same in all of the positions

4.2 The concept of functional anteversion

An accurate understanding of lumbosacral posture and its influence on cup tilt shows us that the measurement of anteversion must not be linked to an arbitrary orientation of the slices to the machine stand (Anda et al., 1990). This point is essential for assessing the real acetabular anteversion of THA in terms of instability, especially when the lumbosacral joint is stiffened or in an atypical position (Eddine et al., 2001; Lembeck et al., 2005; Terver et al., 1982). The concept of functional standing and sitting anteversion has been defined to address this problem. The functional anteversion values are the projected angles measured in the horizontal transverse plane, for any of the positions of the pelvis, reflecting the different amount of anterior opening which varies as a function of pelvic tilt **(Fig. 18a and b).**

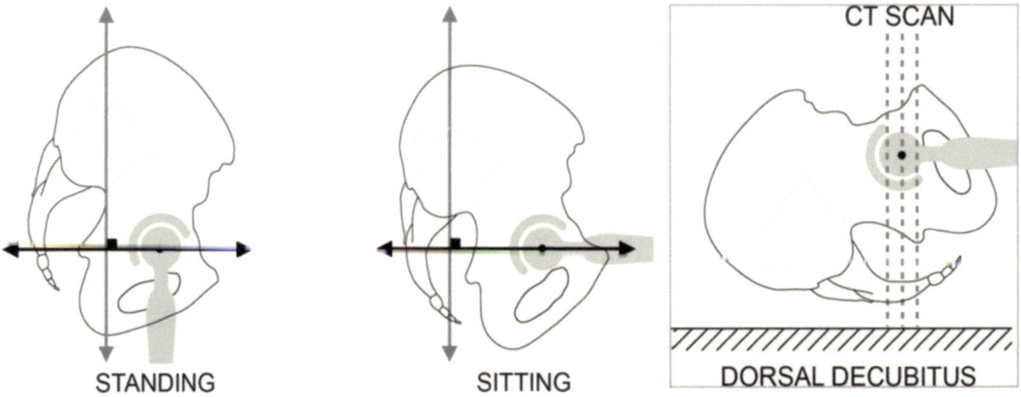

Fig. 18. a: The horizontal transverse plane can be used as a reference plane; the relation with the acetabulum is different according to the standing or seated positions. In current practice, anteversion is measured on CT scans but the angle value depends on the pelvic orientation in the lying position. Fortuitously, the cross-sectional slices, perpendicular to the plane of the examination table, can also be strictly perpendicular to the longitudinal axis of the pelvic bone frame. But, most of the time, these slices do not correspond to this anatomic plane because the position of the supine subject has a more or less marked sagittal pelvic tilt

It is calculated from the CT scan slices taken as a function of the sacral slope measured on the initial standard lateral image. In a plane with the upper sacral endplate, these slices reconstitute the sacral tilt angle, measured in a standing, sitting, or supine position. They make it possible to observe important changes in the cup orientation and improve our understanding of some coxofemoral joint dysfunctions.

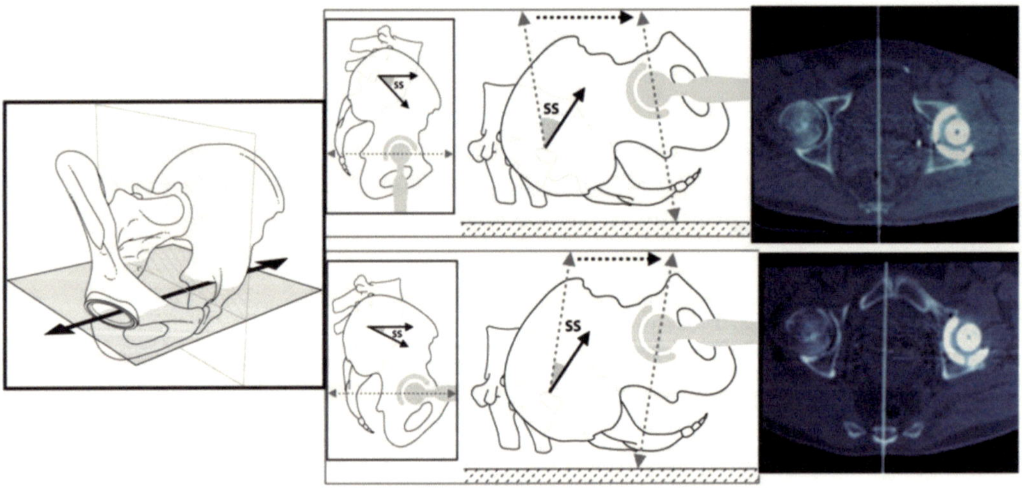

Fig. 18. b: The functional anteversion values are the projected angles measured in the horizontal transverse plane, for any of the positions of the pelvis, reflecting the different amount of anterior opening which varies as a function of pelvic tilt. The measurement of the functional anteversion corresponding to standing and sitting positions can be done using CT scan : it requires an adjustment of the sectional plane following the value of the SS on lateral radiographs with the patients in standing and sitting positions

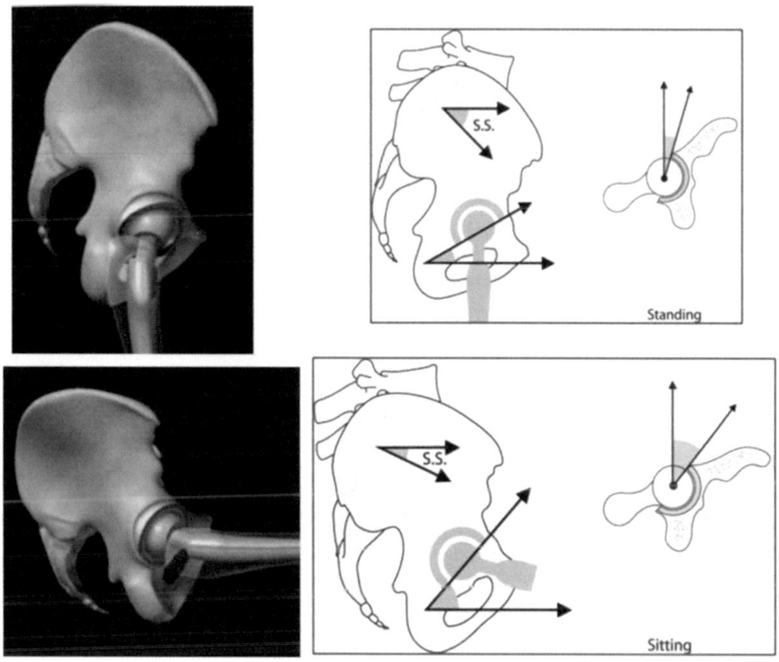

Fig. 19. In standing positions, there is less cross-sectional anteversion than in sitting positions, where the cup opens completely forward, thus favoring flexion of the hip and avoiding impingement at the femoral neck

In standing positions, there is less cross-sectional anteversion than in sitting positions, where the cup opens completely forward, thus favoring flexion of the hip and avoiding impingement at the femoral neck **(Fig. 19).** In supine positions, with the lower limbs extended, the pelvic tilt is often greater than in standing positions, lordosis more accentuated and anteversion still more reduced than when standing. In a series of 328 THAs, we reported a mean anteversion of 31.7° standing, 38.8° seated , and 24.2° supine (Lazennec et al., 2011a). The strong correlation observed between the supine and standing measurements suggests that the classic CT assessment of the anatomic acetabular anteversion is still a relevant source of information in cases of anterior THA dislocation and subluxation. But poor correlations have been reported between the supine and sitting positions; they demonstrate that the usual CT scan protocol is biased and not fully appropriate in an investigation of posterior THA dislocation, which occurs in hip flexion (Lazennec et al., 2011a)
Globally, the "standard" CT scan measurements tend to overestimate anteversion in standing positions and to underestimate it in seated positions. More or less, 1° of pelvic tilt affects acetabular anteversion by 0.5 to 1°, depending on the specific study (Anda et al., 1990; Lazennec et al., 2004). Some subjects have completely stiff lumbosacral joints, and this significantly reduces the variations in acetabular anteversion between seated and standing positions. Such stiffening of the pelvis, in either a relative anterior or posterior tilt, may lead to a reproducible impingement situation. This phenomenon has been documented in the literature for deformities of the sagittal plane in spondylarthritis, in poorly adjusted lumbosacral arthrodesis (flat back), and especially in spinal aging (During et al., 1985; Fogel & Esses, 2003; Hammerberg & Wood, 2003; Itoi, 1991; Lazennec et al., 1997; Offierski &

MacNab, 1983). In these cases, we observed a reduction in lordosis and the appearance of an adaptive posterior pelvic tilt. The patient is standing, as if he were seated. This phenomenon reduces adaptation in the lumbosacral area and deviates the functional mobility cone of the coxofemoral joints towards flexion. The cup is permanently in hyper-anteversion, which is not bothersome during hip flexion but creates a problem of posterior impingement, especially in a standing position: the person progressively loses his or her available extension **(Fig. 20)**.

The compensating hyperextension of the hips often has a limited impact in these patients, especially those who are elderly or have hip disorders. The last adaptation to attempt to improve balance is thus flexion of the knees, which enables additional posterior tilt of the pelvis. This phenomenon explains prosthesis dislocation after several years, following an overall sagittal disruption of the lumbo-pelvic-femoral complex (Legaye, 2009; Rousseau et al., 2009; Tang et al., 2007).

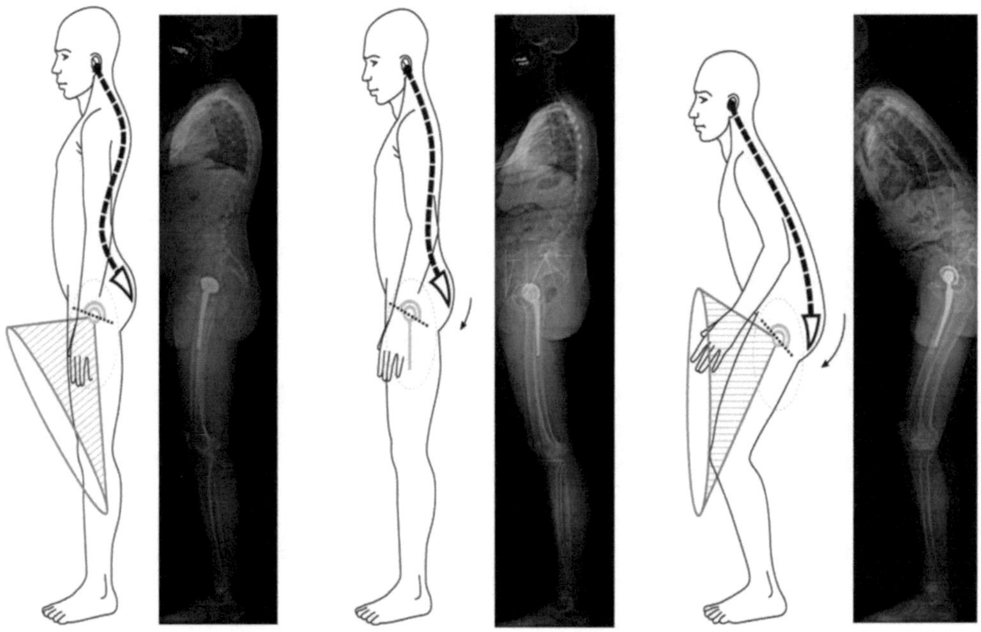

Fig. 20. Reduction in lordosis and the appearance of an adaptive posterior pelvic tilt has been documented in deformities of the sagittal plane in spondylarthritis, in poorly adjusted lumbosacral arthrodesis (flat back), and especially in spinal aging : This phenomenon reduces adaptation in the lumbosacral area and deviates the functional mobility cone of the coxofemoral joints towards flexion

5. Influence of axial rotation of the pelvis and the lumbopelvic region

Hip surgeons define a "normal" pelvic posture for imaging work-ups of subjects in a strictly anatomic position, with the two iliac wings projecting exactly and symmetrically, compared with the longitudinal axis of the trunk. Spine surgeons have been made aware of the three-dimensional view of the spine and the phenomenon of vertebral rotation that disturbs analysis of the lateral view. In this framework, the concept of the pelvic vertebra leads us to integrate pelvic rotation into the analysis of the overall trunk posture (Dubousset et al., 2007). The use of standing and seated EOS® images in the subject's "usual" position is particularly instructive. Our database of complete EOS® acquisitions, both standing and seated, from more than 2500 patients reveals the frequency of cases involving a forward hemipelvis and therefore a backward contralateral hemipelvis. This is expressed on the AP image by asymmetry of the projection of the iliac wings; the "forward" wing appears thinner than the other. Laterally, the two femoral heads and the two iliac wings are not superimposed **(Fig. 21).**

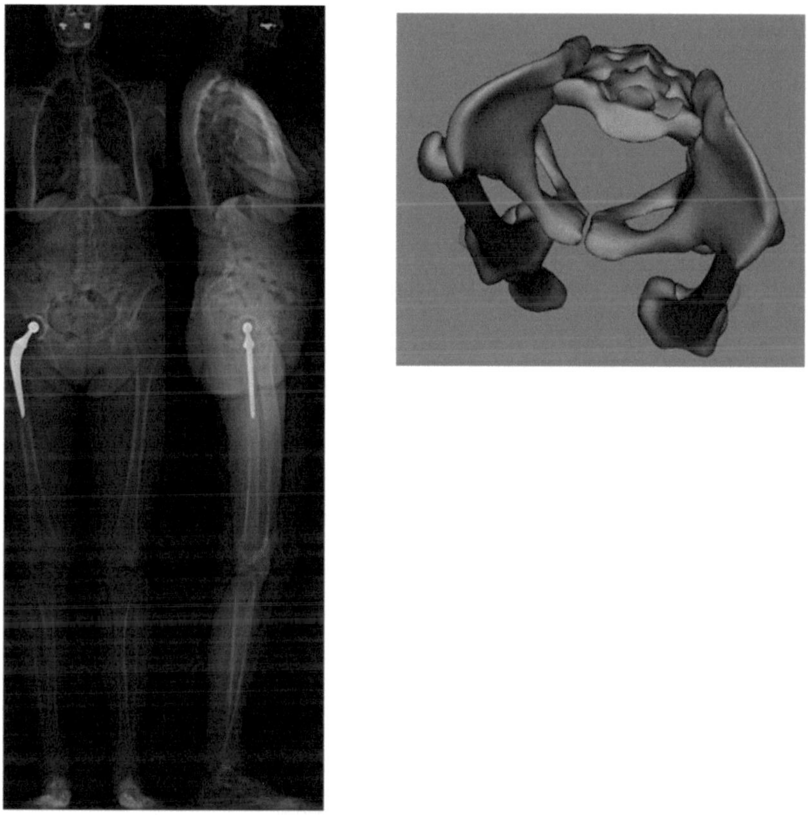

Fig. 21. This "twisting" phenomenon of the pelvis is expressed on the AP image by asymmetry of the projection of the iliac wings; the "forward" wing appears thinner than the other. Laterally, the two femoral heads and the two iliac wings are not superimposed

This "twisting" phenomenon is difficult to quantify with standard radiography because of the cone-shaped distribution of X-rays, which distorts interpretation of the image of the femoral head furthest from the scanner source. On the other hand, it is well analyzed by EOS® images in both the standing and seated positions, and 3D visualization of the pelvic position is possible. This situation of pelvic rotation is pushed to extremes in cases of scoliosis with the pelvic vertebrae included in the deformity **(Fig. 22).** The consequences on cup orientation can be significant, in particular for patients with THA, because of the induction of changes in functional anteversion, in both standing and seated positions (Tannast et al., 2005).

The impact of pelvic rotation and of the pelvic tilt on acetabular orientation raises the question of the choices of guidelines for pre- and postoperative evaluation in cases of hip replacement surgery. The use of guidelines depending on the pelvic bone (anterior pelvic plane, sacral transverse plane, axis through the femoral heads) neglects these two essential phenomena (Lazennec et al., 2007; Tannast et al., 2005). The use of the horizontal transverse plane (or the horizontal plane in space) makes it possible to integrate pelvic tilt into the assessment of acetabular anteversion, which can thus be envisioned "functionally" and not only restrictively as a simple fixed morphologic parameter. Pelvic rotation must be considered and assessed just like vertebral rotation, as analyzed by spine surgeons, compared with a vertical plane of reference perpendicular to the horizontal transverse plane.

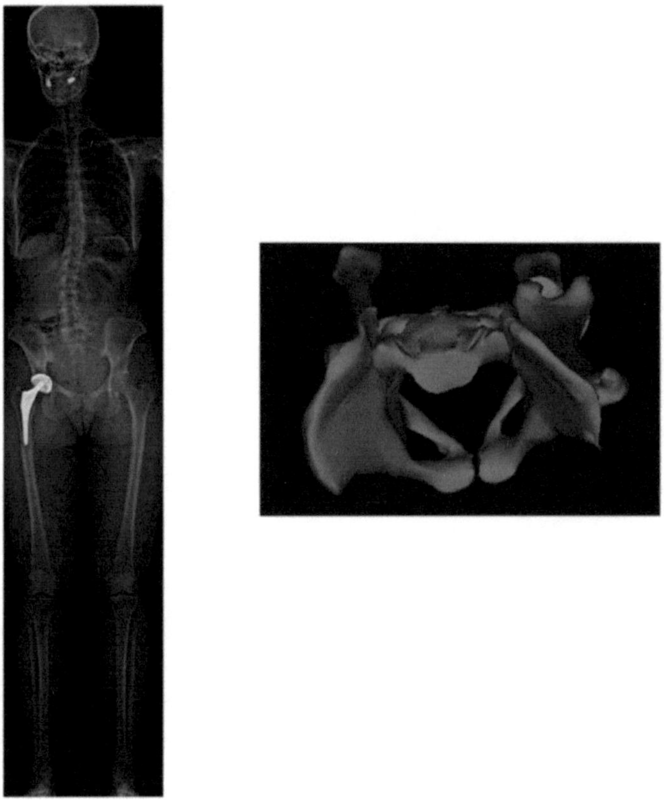

Fig. 22. Pelvic rotation is pushed to extremes in cases of scoliosis with the pelvic vertebrae included in the deformity

6. Conclusions

Comprehensive analysis of the pelvic and subpelvic sectors as part of the sagittal, frontal and cross-sectional balance of the trunk sheds new light on some spinal diseases and their relation to the pelvis. Stiffness in the lumbar spine and lumbosacral fusion, both seen in everyday practice, are significant risk factors for THA subluxation and dislocation due to the lack of variation in the acetabular anteversion from a standing to a sitting position. This

concept is not yet well defined, but our data suggest that taking spinal flexibility into account is important when planning a THA implantation, or at least identifying the unusual patients who have an abnormal pelvic (i.e. acetabular) posture.
Knowledge of the biomechanics of the lumbosacral joint is relevant for the hip surgeon performing hip replacements in elderly subjects or in those with abnormal sagittal, frontal or rotational posture and/or a large reduction in functional range of motion. Analysis of sagittal balance must therefore be individual and integrated into the comprehensive evolution of the subject over time, because the phenomenon of an aging spine is frequently associated with the process of aging hips.
The analysis of acetabular orientation cannot be limited to the frontal orientation of the acetabular cup on the AP view and the lateral view of the hip should be considered: standing, sitting, and squatting positions correspond to changes in spinal orientation and acetabular sagittal tilt. The relation between the position of the spine and the acetabulum has a direct influence on the real functional range of motion of the hips. Anterior pelvic plane, pelvic tilt and sacral slope variations are relevant parameters for planning and navigation.
The mobility of the lumbosacral junction is a crucial parameter in the mechanical function and the stability of THAs, especially in elderly populations. With the increase of the survival of THA, spinal aging and progressive pelvic posterior version must now to be taken into account. Late dislocations of mechanical origin have been reported: modifications of the biomechanics of the spine, transmitted to the hip, may be responsible. The standard measurement of anatomic acetabular anteversion on CT scan images in a supine position should be carefully interpreted as it can induce a false or approximate analysis of the acetabular cup position from a functional standpoint. The analysis of pelvic morphology based on the incidence angle may provide new information about THR dysfunction and abnormal wear, especially in patients with unusual postures.

7. References

Ackland, M.K., Bourne, W.B., & Uhthoff, H.K. (1986). Anteversion of the acetabular cup. Measurement of angle after total hip replacement. *J Bone Joint Surg Br*, 68, 409-413.

Anda, S., Svenningsen, S., Grontvedt, T., & Benum, P. (1990). Pelvic inclination and spatial orientation of the acetabulum. A radiographic, computed tomographic and clinical investigation. *Acta Radiol*, 31, 389-394.

Aubry, S., Marinescu, A., Forterre, O., Runge, M., & Garbuio, P. (2005). [Definition of a reproducible method for acetabular anteversion measurement at CT]. *J Radiol*, 86, 399-404.

Bolger, C., Kelleher, M.O., McEvoy, L., Brayda-Bruno, M., Kaelin, A., Lazennec, J.Y., et al. (2007). Electrical conductivity measurement: a new technique to detect iatrogenic initial pedicle perforation. *Eur Spine J*, 16, 1919-1924.

Boulay, C., Tardieu, C., Hecquet, J., Benaim, C., Mouilleseaux, B., Marty, C., et al. (2006). Sagittal alignment of spine and pelvis regulated by pelvic incidence: standard values and prediction of lordosis. *Eur Spine J*, 15, 415-422.

Chanplakorn, P., Wongsak, S., Woratanarat, P., Wajanavisit, W., & Laohacharoensombat, W. (2011). Lumbopelvic alignment on standing lateral radiograph of adult volunteers and the classification in the sagittal alignment of lumbar spine. *Eur Spine J*, 20, 706-712.

D'Lima, D.D., Urquhart, A.G., Buehler, K.O., Walker, R.H., & Colwell, C.W., Jr. (2000). The effect of the orientation of the acetabular and femoral components on the range of motion of the hip at different head-neck ratios. *J Bone Joint Surg Am,* 82, 315-321.

Dorr, L.D., Wolf, A.W., Chandler, R., & Conaty, J.P. (1983). Classification and treatment of dislocations of total hip arthroplasty. *Clin Orthop Relat Res,* 151-158.

Dubousset, J. (1984). Le bassin « os intercalaire ». . *Monographie du GES,* 15-22.

Dubousset, J., Charpak, G., Skalli, W., de Guise, J., Kalifa, G., & Wicart, P. (2008). [Skeletal and spinal imaging with EOS system]. *Arch Pediatr,* 15, 665-666.

Dubousset, J., Charpak, G., Skalli, W., Kalifa, G., & Lazennec, J.Y. (2007). [EOS stereo-radiography system: whole-body simultaneous anteroposterior and lateral radiographs with very low radiation dose]. *Rev Chir Orthop Reparatrice Appar Mot,* 93, 141-143.

During, J., Goudfrooij, H., Keessen, W., Beeker, T.W., & Crowe, A. (1985). Toward standards for posture. Postural characteristics of the lower back system in normal and pathologic conditions. *Spine (Phila Pa 1976),* 10, 83-87.

Duval-Beaupere, G., Schmidt, C., & Cosson, P. (1992). A Barycentremetric study of the sagittal shape of spine and pelvis: the conditions required for an economic standing position. *Ann Biomed Eng,* 20, 451-462.

Eddine, T.A., Migaud, H., Chantelot, C., Cotten, A., Fontaine, C., & Duquennoy, A. (2001). Variations of pelvic anteversion in the lying and standing positions: analysis of 24 control subjects and implications for CT measurement of position of a prosthetic cup. *Surg Radiol Anat,* 23, 105-110.

Fogel, G.R., & Esses, S.I. (2003). Hip spine syndrome: management of coexisting radiculopathy and arthritis of the lower extremity. *Spine J,* 3, 238-241.

Hammerberg, E.M., & Wood, K.B. (2003). Sagittal profile of the elderly. *J Spinal Disord Tech,* 16, 44-50.

Herrlin, K., Selvik, G., Pettersson, H., Kesek, P., Onnerfalt, R., & Ohlin, A. (1988). Position, orientation and component interaction in dislocation of the total hip prosthesis. *Acta Radiol,* 29, 441-444.

Itoi, E. (1991). Roentgenographic analysis of posture in spinal osteoporotics. *Spine (Phila Pa 1976),* 16, 750-756.

Jackson, R.P., & McManus, A.C. (1994). Radiographic analysis of sagittal plane alignment and balance in standing volunteers and patients with low back pain matched for age, sex, and size. A prospective controlled clinical study. *Spine (Phila Pa 1976),* 19, 1611-1618.

Kennedy, J.G., Rogers, W.B., Soffe, K.E., Sullivan, R.J., Griffen, D.G., & Sheehan, L.J. (1998). Effect of acetabular component orientation on recurrent dislocation, pelvic osteolysis, polyethylene wear, and component migration. *J Arthroplasty,* 13, 530-534.

Kobayashi, T., Atsuta, Y., Matsuno, T., & Takeda, N. (2004). A longitudinal study of congruent sagittal spinal alignment in an adult cohort. *Spine (Phila Pa 1976),* 29, 671-676.

Kummer, F.J., Shah, S., Iyer, S., & DiCesare, P.E. (1999). The effect of acetabular cup orientations on limiting hip rotation. *J Arthroplasty,* 14, 509-513.

Lafage, V., Schwab, F., Patel, A., Hawkinson, N., & Farcy, J.P. (2009). Pelvic tilt and truncal inclination: two key radiographic parameters in the setting of adults with spinal deformity. *Spine (Phila Pa 1976),* 34, E599-606.

Lazennec, J.Y., Boyer, P., Gorin, M., Catonne, Y., & Rousseau, M.A. (2011a). Acetabular Anteversion with CT in Supine, Simulated Standing, and Sitting Positions in a THA Patient Population. *Clin Orthop Relat Res,* 469, 1103-1109.

Lazennec, J.Y., Charlot, N., Gorin, M., Roger, B., Arafati, N., Bissery, A., et al. (2004). Hip-spine relationship: a radio-anatomical study for optimization in acetabular cup positioning. *Surg Radiol Anat,* 26, 136-144.

Lazennec, J.Y., Ramare, S., Arafati, N., Laudet, C.G., Gorin, M., Roger, B., et al. (2000). Sagittal alignment in lumbosacral fusion: relations between radiological parameters and pain. *Eur Spine J,* 9, 47-55.

Lazennec, J.Y., Riwan, A., Gravez, F., Rousseau, M.A., Mora, N., Gorin, M., et al. (2007). Hip spine relationships: application to total hip arthroplasty. *Hip Int,* 17 Suppl 5, S91-104.

Lazennec, J.Y., Rousseau, M.A., Rangel, A., Gorin, M., Belicourt, C., Brusson, A., et al. (2011b). Pelvis and total hip arthroplasty acetabular component orientations in sitting and standing positions: Measurements reproductibility with EOS imaging system versus conventional radiographies. *Orthop Traumatol Surg Res.*

Lazennec, J.Y., Rousseau, M.A., Rangel, A., Gorin, M., Belicourt, C., Brusson, A., et al. (2011c). Pelvis and total hip arthroplasty acetabular component orientations in sitting and standing positions: Measurements reproductibility with EOS imaging system versus conventional radiographies. *Orthop Traumatol Surg Res,* 97, 373-380.

Lazennec, J.Y., Saillant, G., Saidi, K., Arafati, N., Barabas, D., Benazet, J.P., et al. (1997). Surgery of the deformities in ankylosing spondylitis: our experience of lumbar osteotomies in 31 patients. *Eur Spine J,* 6, 222-232.

Legaye, J. (2009). Influence of the sagittal balance of the spine on the anterior pelvic plane and on the acetabular orientation. *Int Orthop,* 33, 1695-1700.

Legaye, J., Duval-Beaupere, G., Hecquet, J., & Marty, C. (1998). Pelvic incidence: a fundamental pelvic parameter for three-dimensional regulation of spinal sagittal curves. *Eur Spine J,* 7, 99-103.

Lembeck, B., Mueller, O., Reize, P., & Wuelker, N. (2005). Pelvic tilt makes acetabular cup navigation inaccurate. *Acta Orthop,* 76, 517-523.

Lewinnek, G.E., Lewis, J.L., Tarr, R., Compere, C.L., & Zimmerman, J.R. (1978). Dislocations after total hip-replacement arthroplasties. *J Bone Joint Surg Am,* 60, 217-220.

McKibbin, B. (1970). Anatomical factors in the stability of the hip joint in the newborn. *J Bone Joint Surg Br,* 52, 148-159.

Muller, O., Lembeck, B., Reize, P., & Wulker, N. (2005). [Quantification and visualization of the influence of pelvic tilt upon measurement of acetabular inclination and anteversion]. *Z Orthop Ihre Grenzgeb,* 143, 72-78.

Murray, D.W. (1993). The definition and measurement of acetabular orientation. *J Bone Joint Surg Br,* 75, 228-232.

Offierski, C.M., & MacNab, I. (1983). Hip-spine syndrome. *Spine (Phila Pa 1976),* 8, 316-321.

Philippot, R., Wegrzyn, J., Farizon, F., & Fessy, M.H. (2009). Pelvic balance in sagittal and Lewinnek reference planes in the standing, supine and sitting positions. *Orthop Traumatol Surg Res,* 95, 70-76.

Pradhan, R. (1999). Planar anteversion of the acetabular cup as determined from plain anteroposterior radiographs. *J Bone Joint Surg Br,* 81, 431-435.

Rillardon, L., Levassor, N., Guigui, P., Wodecki, P., Cardinne, L., Templier, A., et al. (2003). [Validation of a tool to measure pelvic and spinal parameters of sagittal balance]. *Rev Chir Orthop Reparatrice Appar Mot,* 89, 218-227.

Rousseau, M.A., Lazennec, J.Y., Boyer, P., Mora, N., Gorin, M., & Catonne, Y. (2009). Optimization of total hip arthroplasty implantation: is the anterior pelvic plane concept valid? *J Arthroplasty,* 24, 22-26.

Roussouly, P., Gollogly, S., Berthonnaud, E., & Dimnet, J. (2005). Classification of the normal variation in the sagittal alignment of the human lumbar spine and pelvis in the standing position. *Spine (Phila Pa 1976),* 30, 346-353.

Seki, M., Yuasa, N., & Ohkuni, K. (1998). Analysis of optimal range of socket orientations in total hip arthroplasty with use of computer-aided design simulation. *J Orthop Res,* 16, 513-517.

Tang, W.M., Chiu, K.Y., Kwan, M.F., & Ng, T.P. (2007). Sagittal pelvic mal-rotation and positioning of the acetabular component in total hip arthroplasty: Three-dimensional computer model analysis. *J Orthop Res,* 25, 766-771.

Tannast, M., Langlotz, U., Siebenrock, K.A., Wiese, M., Bernsmann, K., & Langlotz, F. (2005). Anatomic referencing of cup orientation in total hip arthroplasty. *Clin Orthop Relat Res,* 144-150.

Tassin (2004). Equilibre sagittal du rachis. *Cahier d'enseignement de la SOFCOT,* 85, 241-269.

Terver, S., Dillingham, M., Parker, B., Bjorke, A., Bleck, E.E., Levai, J.P., et al. (1982). [True orientation of the acetabulum as determined by CAT scan. Preliminary results (author's transl)]. *J Radiol,* 63, 167-173.

Vaz, G., Roussouly, P., Berthonnaud, E., & Dimnet, J. (2002). Sagittal morphology and equilibrium of pelvis and spine. *Eur Spine J,* 11, 80-87.

Vialle, R., Levassor, N., Rillardon, L., Templier, A., Skalli, W., & Guigui, P. (2005). Radiographic analysis of the sagittal alignment and balance of the spine in asymptomatic subjects. *J Bone Joint Surg Am,* 87, 260-267.

von Knoch, M., Berry, D.J., Harmsen, W.S., & Morrey, B.F. (2002). Late dislocation after total hip arthroplasty. *J Bone Joint Surg Am,* 84-A, 1949-1953.

Wan, Z., Malik, A., Jaramaz, B., Chao, L., & Dorr, L.D. (2009). Imaging and navigation measurement of acetabular component position in THA. *Clin Orthop Relat Res,* 467, 32-42.

Watanabe, W., Sato, K., Itoi, E., Yang, K., & Watanabe, H. (2002). Posterior pelvic tilt in patients with decreased lumbar lordosis decreases acetabular femoral head covering. *Orthopedics,* 25, 321-324.

Woo, R.Y., & Morrey, B.F. (1982). Dislocations after total hip arthroplasty. *J Bone Joint Surg Am,* 64, 1295-1306.

Woolson, S.T., & Rahimtoola, Z.O. (1999). Risk factors for dislocation during the first 3 months after primary total hip replacement. *J Arthroplasty,* 14, 662-668.

Yamaguchi, M., Bauer, T.W., & Hashimoto, Y. (1997). Three-dimensional analysis of multiple wear vectors in retrieved acetabular cups. *J Bone Joint Surg Am,* 79, 1539-1544.

X-Ray Digital Linear Tomosynthesis Imaging of Arthoroplasty

Tsutomu Gomi[1], Hiroshi Hirano[2] and Masahiro Nakajima[3]
[1]*School of Allied Health Sciences, Kitasato University*
[2]*Department of Radiology, Shinshu University Hospital*
[3]*Department of Radiology, Dokkyo Medical University Hospital*
Japan

1. Introduction

Interest in tomosynthesis and its clinical applications has been revived by recent advances in digital X-ray detector technology. Conventional tomography technology provides planar information of an object from its projection images. In tomography, an X-ray tube and X-ray film receptor are positioned on either side of the object. The relative motion of the tube and film is predetermined based on the location of the in-focus plane (Ziedses des plate 1932). A single image plane is generated by a scan, and multi-slice computed tomography (CT) scans are required to provide a sufficient number of planes to cover the selected structure in the object. Tomosynthesis acquires only one set of discrete X-ray projections that can be used to reconstruct any plane of the object retrospectively (Grant 1972). This technique has been investigated in angiography and imaging of the chest, hand joints, lungs, teeth, and breasts (Stiel et al 1993 , Duryea et al 2003 , Sone et al 1995 , Niklason et al 1997 , Dobbins et al 2003).

2. Performance of tomosynthesis

2.1 General tomosynthesis reconstruction methods

Existing tomosynthesis algorithms can be divided into three categories: (1) backprojection algorithms, (2) filtered backprojection (FBP) algorithms, and (3) iterative algorithms. The Fig.1 view shown here highlights the difficulty in visualizing three-dimensional (3D) information in X-ray radiography. In the Fig.2 view it turns an acquisition direction to avoid superimposition of an object. The three resulting projection images may be shifted and added (SAA) so as to bring either the circles or triangles to coincide (i.e., focus), with the complementary object smeared out. The basis for FBP is the backprojection of data acquired in projections acquired over all angles. This procedure is performed for each pixel in a projection, and for all possible angles of the projected data, then one has created a simple backprojection image of the object (Fig.3). The backprojection algorithm is referred to as "SAA", whereby projection images taken at different angles are electronically SAA to generate an image plane focused at a certain depth below the surface. The projection shift is adjusted so that the visibility of features in the selected plane is enhanced while that in other planes is blurred. Using a digital detector, image planes at all depths can be retrospectively reconstructed from one set of projections. The SAA algorithm is valid only if the motion of the X-ray focal spot is parallel to the detector.

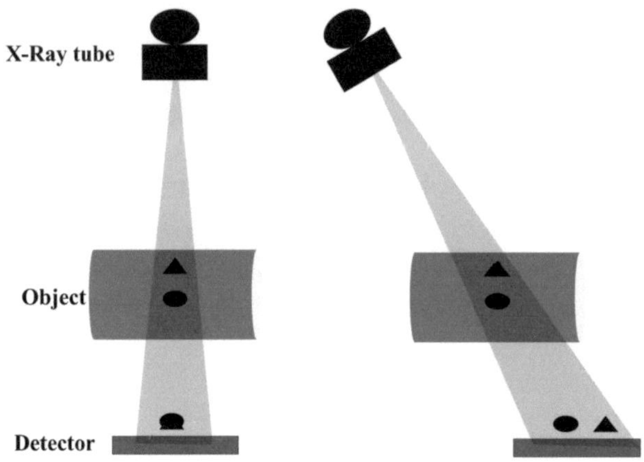

Fig. 1. Overview of the conventional radiography method.

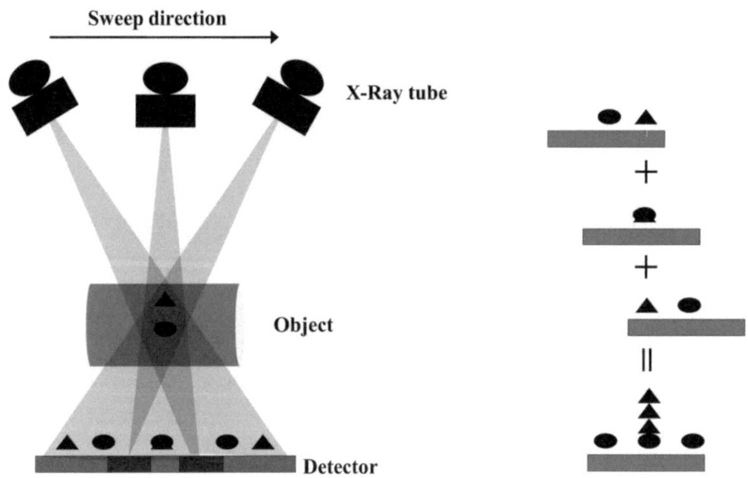

Fig. 2. Overview of the shifted and added (SAA) algorithm.

FBP algorithms are widely used in CT in which many projections acquired at greater than 360 degrees are used to reconstruct cross-sectional images. The number of projections typically ranges between a few hundred to about one thousand. The Fourier central slice theorem is fundamental to the FBP theory. In two-dimensional (2D) CT imaging, a projection of an object corresponds to sampling the object along the direction perpendicular to the X-ray beam in the Fourier space (Kak et al 1988). For many projections, information about the object is well sampled and the object can be restored by combining the information from all projections. In 3D cone-beam imaging, the information about the

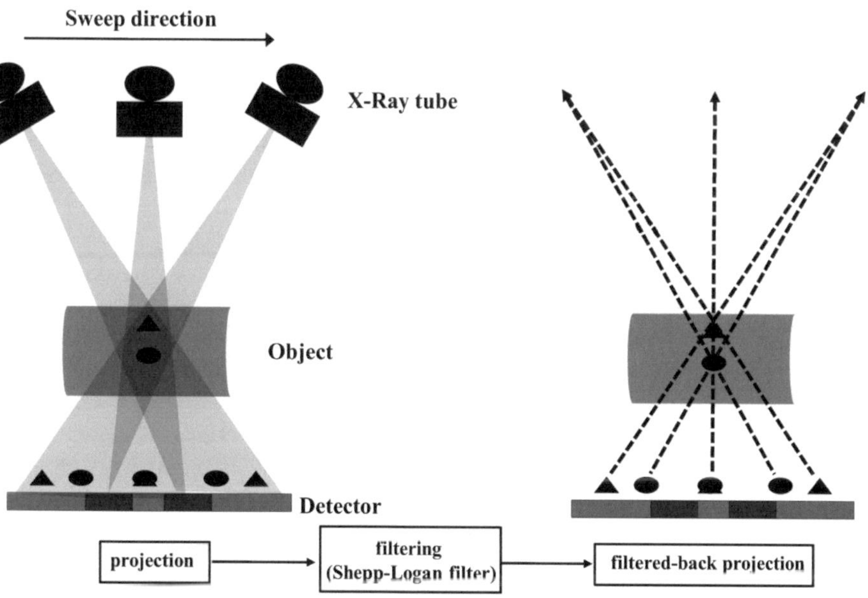

Fig. 3. Overview of the filtered backprojection (FBP) algorithm.

object in Fourier space is related to the Radon transform of the object. The relationship between the Radon transform and cone-beam projections has been well studied and solutions to the cone-beam reconstruction have been provided (Smith 1985).The FBP algorithm generally provides a high degree of precision for 3D reconstruction images when an exact type algorithm is employed (Feldkamp et al 1984) (see Appendix). Therefore, this method has been adopted for image reconstruction of 3D tomography and multi-detector cone-beam CT.

An iterative algorithm performs the reconstruction in a recursive fashion (Ruttimann et al 1984 , Bleuet et al 2002), unlike the one-step operation in backprojection and FBP algorithms. During iterative reconstruction, a 3D object model is repeatedly updated until the model converges to the solution that optimizes an objective function. The objective function defines the criteria of the reconstruction solution. The objective function in the maximum likelihood (ML) algorithm is the likelihood function, which is the probability of getting the measured projections in a given object model. The solution of the ML algorithm is an object model that maximizes the probability of getting the measured projections.

2.2 Radiography vs. tomosynthesis

Anteroposterior (AP) radiograph of these joints demonstrate the excellent visualization of the prostheses in this view. AP radiograph is difficult to visualize 3D information in an AP radiograph as shown (Fig.4). An alternative approach to tomosynthesis imaging is to determine the number of views that can be acquired given imaging constraints (e.g., time restrictions from patient motion, dose restrictions of the detector). The tomographic angle can be selected to yield images with an acceptable level of artifacts. This is certainly the case with FBP algorithm and is suspected to be the case with simple backprojection (or the SAA algorithm). It is possible, however, that this restriction could be reduced by the use of an alternative reconstruction scheme.

2.3 CT vs. tomosynthesis

Imaging by X-ray CT has improved over the last three decades and is now a powerful tool in medical diagnostics. CT imaging has become an essential noninvasive imaging technique since the advent of spiral CT imaging in the 1990s, which led to shorter scan times and improved 3D spatial resolution. CT provides high resolution in the tomographic plane but limited resolution in the axial direction. However, the quality of images generated by a CT scanner can still be reduced due to the presence of metal objects in the field of view. Imaging of patients with metal implants, such as marker pins, dental fillings, or hip prostheses, is susceptible to artifacts generally in the form of bright and dark streaks, cupping and capping, etc. This artifact susceptibility is mostly due to quantum noise, scattered radiation, and beam hardening (Hsieh 1995). Metal artifacts influence image quality by reducing contrast and by obscuring details, thus impairing the ability to detect structures of interest and possibly leading to misdiagnosis. In addition, CT values are impaired, which can lead to errors when using these data e.g., for attenuation correction in positron emission tomography (PET)/CT imaging (Kamel et al 2003). The metallic components of arthroplasty devices are high-contrast objects that generate artifacts when imaged using CT scans. These artifacts can make it extremely difficult or impossible to interpret images obtained by devices. The presence of artifacts along with partial volume effect (PVE) severely limits the potential for objective quantification of total joint replacement with CT.

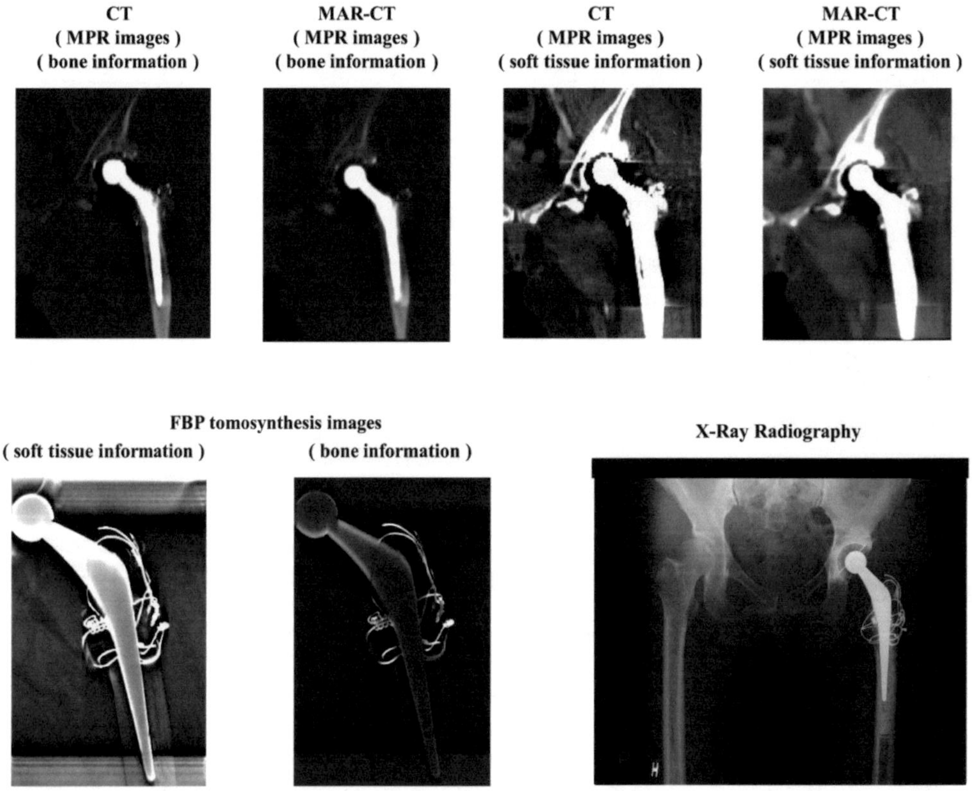

Fig. 4. Patient (52-year-old woman; total hip arthroplasty; THA). Anteroposterior (AP) radiographs of the hip joint prostheses are demonstrated.

Methods for reduction of metal artifacts aim to improve the quality of images affected by these artifacts. In recent years, modified iterative (Wang et al 1996 , 1999 , 2000 , Man et al 2000) or wavelet reconstruction techniques have produced promising results. However, these methods cannot be combined with the fast and robust FBP algorithm, which is the standard reconstruction technique (Robertson et al 1997) implemented in modern CT scanners.

Digital linear tomosynthesis using the FBP algorithm shows adequate overall performance, but its effectiveness depends strongly on the region of the image. Digital linear tomosynthesis using FBP algorithm images gives good results independent of the type of metal present in the patient and shows good results for the removal of noise artifacts, especially at greater distances from metal objects. Application of digital linear tomosynthesis to the imaging of hip prostheses appears promising. In addition, flexibility in the choice of digital linear tomosynthesis imaging parameters based on the desired final images and generation of high quality images may be beneficial.

In Fig.4, Coronal slice images (multi-planar reconstruction; MPR) of the hip prosthesis at center heights on metal artifact reduction (MAR) CT (MAR-CT) and non MAR-CT scans at approximately the same level. Remarkable metal artifacts can be seen occurring in the neighborhood of the hip prosthesis. However, MAR-CT processing reduced the metal artifacts. Tomosynthesis images of the prostheses at center heights at the same level. The new diagnostic information that could not be acquired from CT images is provided. Reduction in metal artifacts was obtained in the images as shown here. The use of tomosynthesis allowed better visualization of the prosthesis caused by the blurring of anatomic structures above and below the visualized planes.

The FBP tomosynthesis was compared to MAR CT, and non-MAR CT scans of a prosthesis case. The effectiveness of this method in enhancing visibility of a prosthesis case was quantified in terms of the signal-to-noise ratio (SNR), and removal of ghosting artifacts in a prosthesis case was quantified in terms of the artifact spread function (ASF). The SNR in the prosthetic case was determined. The SNR is defined as $\frac{N_1 - N_0}{\sigma_0}$, where N_1 is the mean pixel value in the region of interest (ROI) within the object, N_0 is the mean pixel value in the ROI in a background area, and σ_0 is the standard deviation of pixel values in the background ROI. Throughout these results, σ_0 includes structure noise that can obscure the object, in addition to photon statistics and electronic noise. Wu et al. proposed an ASF metric to quantify artifacts observed in planes outside the focus image plane (Wu et al 2003). The artifacts are generated from real features located in the focus image plane, and resemble the real feature. The artifacts exhibited in image planes are defined by the ASF as $\frac{N_{artifact}(z) - N_{BG}(z)}{N_{artifact}(z_0) - N_{BG}(z_0)}$, where z_0 is the location of the in-focus plane of the real feature, z is the location of the off-focus plane, and $N_{artifact}(z_0)$ and $N_{BG}(z_0)$ are the average pixel intensities of the feature and the image background in the in-focus plane, respectively, $N_{artifact}(z)$ and $N_{BG}(z)$ are the average pixel intensities of the artifact and the image background in the off-focus plane, respectively.

The effectiveness of this method in enhancing visibility of a prosthesis case was quantified in terms of the SNR, and removal of ghosting artifacts in a prosthesis case was quantified in terms of the ASF. In the near in-focus plane, the contrast is greater in the MAR CT or FBP tomosynthesis relative to the non-MAR CT (Fig.5).

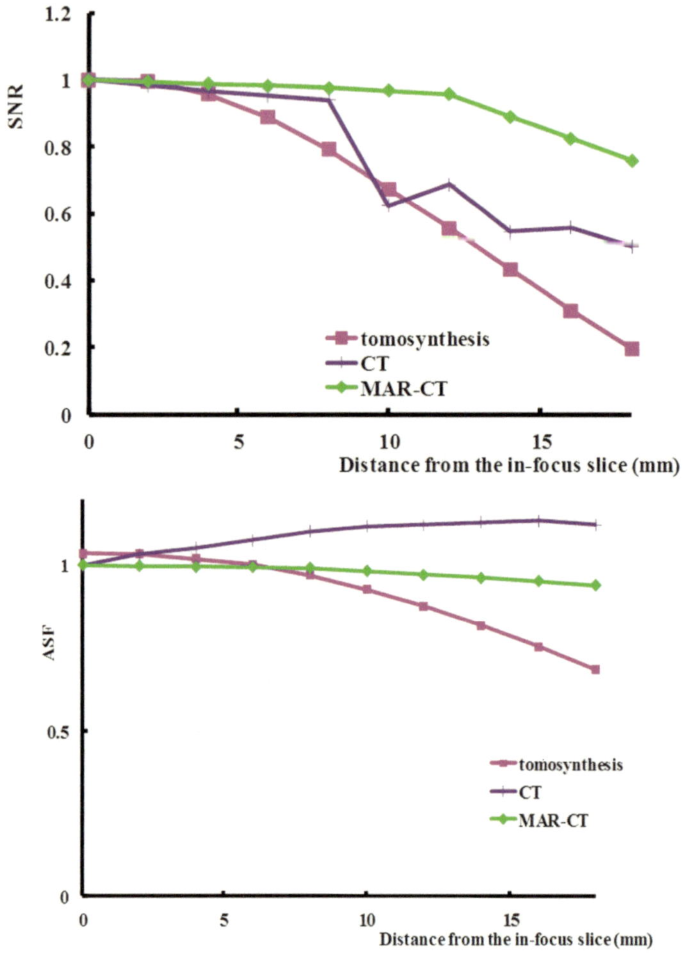

Fig. 5. Metal artefact reduction computed tomography (MAR-CT) with in-focus plane is best for signal-to-noise ratio (SNR) optimization, whereas MAR-CT with off-focus plane is best for SNR optimization. It seems that number of the projection, total exposure dose, and pixel size of detector in MAR-CT gives better results than FBP tomosynthesis. Artifact spread function (ASF) chart demonstrates that FBP tomosynthesis results in maximum removal of metal artifacts.

2.4 Evaluation of artifact reduction for prosthesis imaging

Metal artifacts influence image quality by reducing contrast and obscuring detail, thus impairing the ability to detect structures of interest and making diagnosis impossible. The objective of this report is to evaluate the clinical application of digital linear tomosynthesis in imaging a phantom and hip prosthesis using a relatively new tomosynthesis instrument and applying a selection of reconstruction algorithms. Tomosynthesis images were compared with the results from artifact reduction processing and a FBP algorithm.

Artifacts caused by high-attenuation features in hip prostheses were observed in digital linear tomosynthesis reconstruction as a result of the small number of projections and narrow angular range typically employed in tomosynthesis imaging. Gomi et al. (Gomi et al 2008 , 2009) developed artifact reduction methods based on a modified Shepp–Logan reconstruction filter kernel by taking into account the additional weight of direct current components in the frequency domain space. Processing leads to an increase in the ratio of low frequency components in an image (see appendix). Artifact reduction processing was performed with a basic and FBP algorithm. Artifact reduction processing provides a method of filtering that can be used in combination with the backprojection algorithm to yield sliced images with desired properties by means of tomosynthesis.

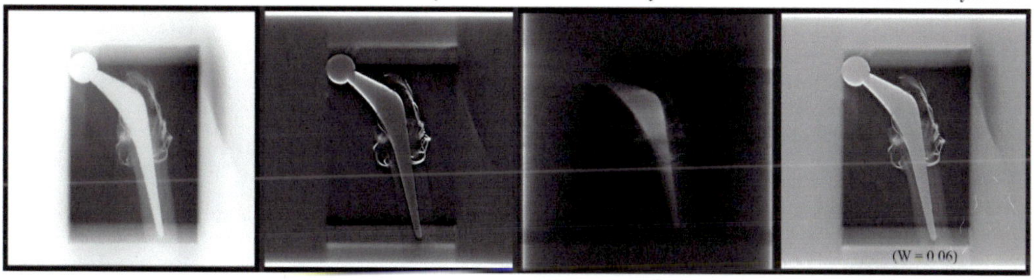

Fig. 6. Comparison of images obtained from artifact reduction tomosynthesis (W= 0.06), FBP tomosynthesis, SAA tomosynthesis, and maximum likelihood tomosynthesis (ML, four subsets & 15 iterations) of the center plane. Artifact reduction tomosynthesis provided better visualization of the hip prosthesis by eliminating blurring and reducing artifacts above and below visualized planes.

The quality of CT images is governed by the strength of artifacts, which depends on numerous factors such as size, shape, density, atomic number and position of metal objects, patient size, and patient's cross-section shape. For small implants manufactured from relatively light metals (e.g., titanium), the effects of beam-hardening and scattering are low. Therefore, the corrupted CT values as well as noise-induced streaking artifacts that pose a major problem to image quality can be neglected. In such cases, the digital linear tomosynthesis approach to artifact reduction processing appears to be promising for the reduction of artifacts stemming from metals with a relatively high atomic number (Fig.6). Improvement of an artificial image (part of undershooting) by an artifact reduction processing is accepted (Fig.7). The effectiveness of the artifact reduction processing method in enhancing the visibility of a prosthetic case was quantified in terms of removal of artifacts. The potential of artifact reduction processing for digital linear tomosynthesis in the evaluation of hip prostheseswas demonstrated. Artifact reduction processing tomosynthesis realize that an especially normal bone and adhesion of an artificial bone become observable (Fig.8-9).

2.5 Potential artifacts

Ideally, structures in a given plane of interest should be clearly displayed in the corresponding tomosynthesis reconstruction plane, whereas structures located outside of that plane should not be visible. Essentially, the limited angular range of the tomosynthesis image acquisition geometry dictates that the spatial resolution is limited in the dimension perpendicular to the detector plane. As a result, out-of-plane structures cannot be completely removed from the reconstruction plane. Out-of-plane structures are present in every reconstruction plane, but most are not visible because the various low-amplitude structures from projections overlap each other in the reconstruction plane, and therefore are blurred. Out-of-plane structures from high-attenuation features cannot be blurred. They appear as multiple replicates of the particular feature in every reconstruction plane except for the one in which the actual high-attenuation feature is located. At one projection angle, these ghosting features are distributed along the line made by the X-ray source and actual feature (Fig.10).

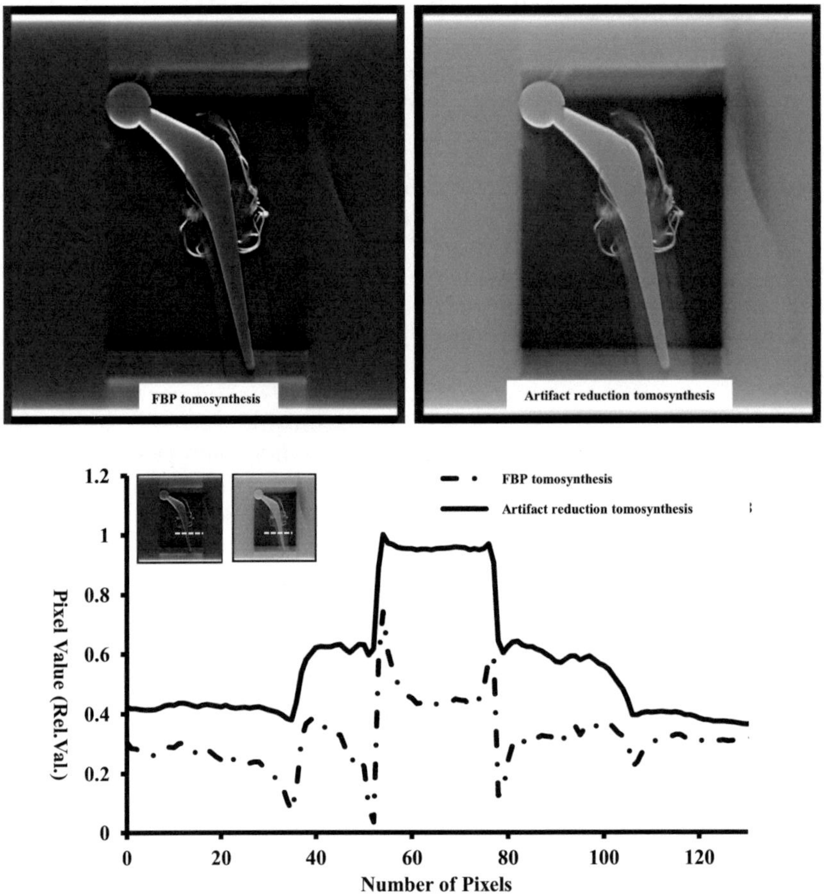

Fig. 7. Comparison of line profiles using artifact reduction processing ($W = 0.06$) and FBP algorithm in the in-focus plane. Artifacts (part of the undershoot) are reduced by artifact reduction processing.

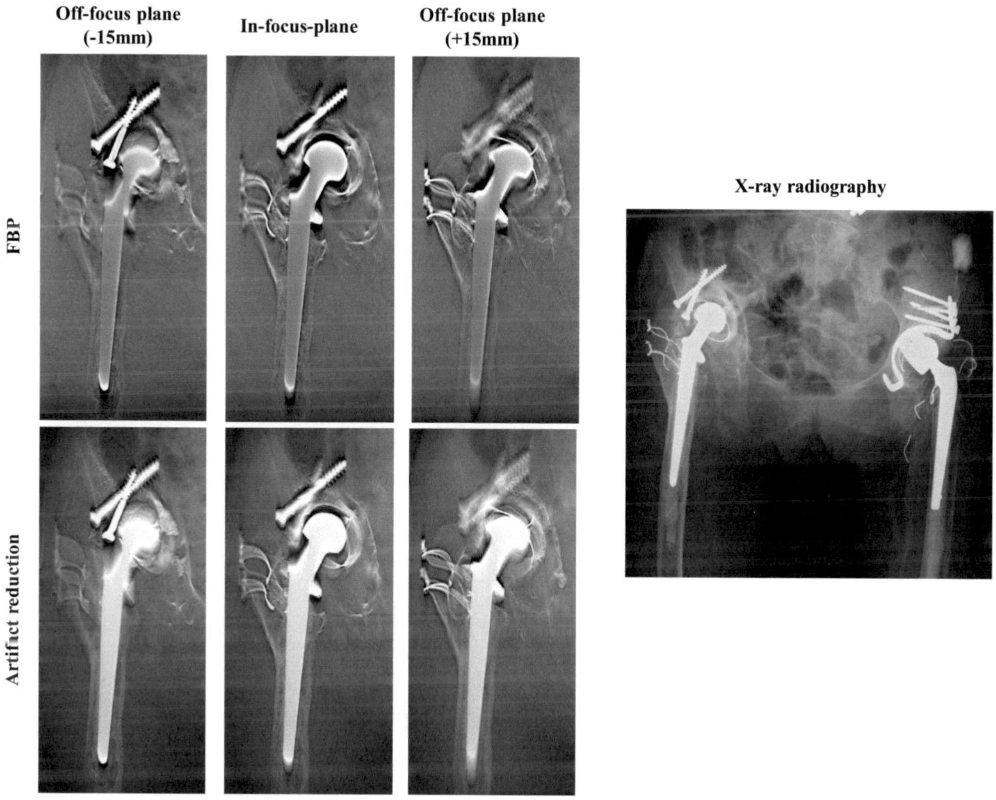

Fig. 8. Case 1 patient (81-year-old woman; Rheumatism, post THA). AP radiographs of the hip joint prostheses are demonstrated. AP radiograph is difficult to visualize 3D information in an AP radiograph as shown. The use of artifact reduction tomosynthesis (w=0.06) allowed better visualization of the right hip joint prosthesis caused by the blurring of anatomic structures above and below the visualized planes.

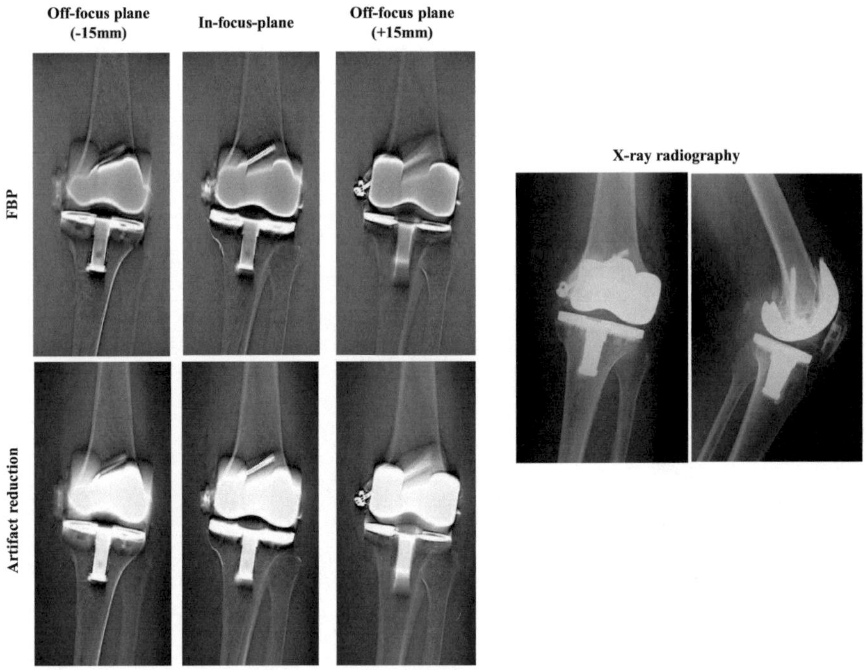

Fig. 9. Case 2 patient (71-year-old woman; Gonarthrosis, post total knee arthroplasty; TKA). AP radiographs of the knee joint prostheses are demonstrated. AP radiograph is difficult to visualize 3D information in an AP radiograph as shown. The use of artifact reduction tomosynthesis (w=0.06) allowed better visualization of the prosthesis caused by the blurring of anatomic structures above and below the visualized planes.

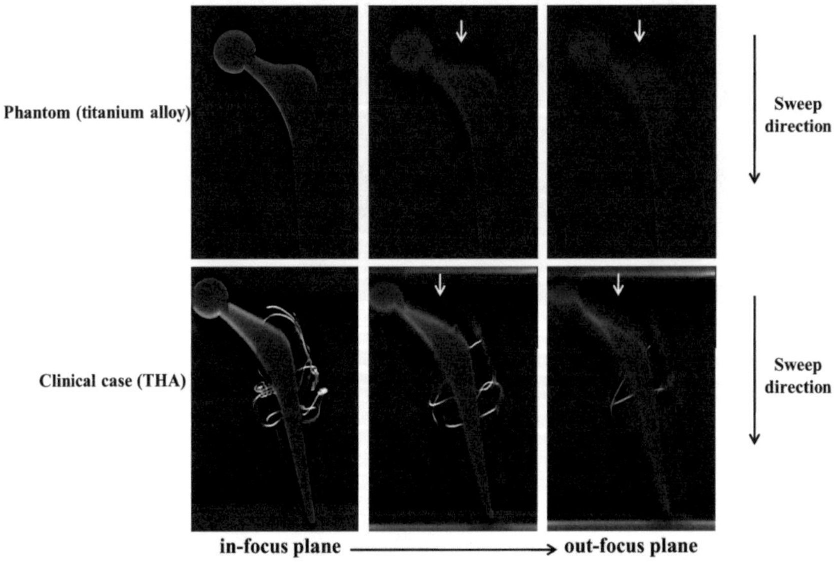

Fig. 10. Blurring occurs along the sweep direction and results from imaging studies show that a high contrast structure exists out of the slice plane that is continuously perpendicular to the sweep direction.

3. Conclusion

The digital linear tomosynthesis images in this review were acquired using linear motion of the X-ray tube and detector. The type of motion used during data acquisition dictates the type of blurring of off-focal-plane objects in the image. Linear motion blurs objects in one dimension only, which leads to linear streak artifacts caused by high-contrast off-focal-plane objects. On the other hand, 3D reconstruction schemes, such as tomosynthesis and CT, require complete knowledge of the X-ray source projection geometry prior to exposure. This limitation precludes much of the potential task-dependent flexibility. This limitation also precludes accurate reconstruction from projections acquired from a patient who moves unpredictably between exposures, as this is geometrically equivalent to not knowing the projection geometry.
Use of digital linear tomosynthesis in imaging of prostheses appears promising. The results of the prosthesis study suggest that digital linear tomosynthesis can improve image quality compared with conventional radiography by removing overlying structures and providing limited 3D information. In addition, the digital linear tomosynthesis method appears to allow for significant improvement of images corrupted by metal artifacts. Digital linear tomosynthesis provided higher quality images than CT. Tomosynthesis is the best solution for cases in which the high-attenuation feature causing the artifacts can be segmented accurately from the projection.
Artifact reduction processing showed an adequate overall performance, but its effectiveness strongly depended on the image region. Digital linear tomosynthesis images gave good results independent of the type of metal present in the patient and showed good results for the removal of noise artifacts, particularly at greater distances from metal objects. The potential for application of digital linear tomosynthesis to the imaging of prostheses appears promising. Flexibility in the choice of imaging parameters in artifact reduction processing based on the desired final images and realistic imaging conditions may be beneficial.

4. Acknowledgment

We wish to thank for Shimadzu Corporation for her helpful research assistance in this work.

5. Appendix

5.1 FBP algorithm

The 3D Fourier transform of the 3D volume data generated by the backprojection is based on the following equation (1):

$$F(\omega_x,\omega_y,\omega_z)=\iiint f(x,y,z)\cdot\exp\{-j(\omega_x\cdot x+\omega_y\cdot y+\omega_z\cdot z)\}dx\cdot dy\cdot dz \quad (1)$$

where $f(x,y,z)$ is the simple backprojection intermediate image, and x, y, and z are real numbers. The meaning of the filtering process performed in 3D Fourier space is described below, and it is mathematically expressed by the following equation (2):

$$FM(\omega_x,\omega_y,\omega_z)=F(\omega_x,\omega_y,\omega_z)\cdot M(\omega_x,\omega_y,\omega_z) \quad (2)$$

where $FM(\omega_x, \omega_y, \omega_z)$ is the filtered 3D Fourier distribution image, and $M(\omega_x, \omega_y, \omega_z)$ is a function representing filter characteristics. The filtering process carried out in 3D Fourier space is to weight the 3D Fourier distribution image of complex data with the real-valued filter function M dependent on the respective frequency values. The weighting function M is compressed in the ω_z direction. $M(\omega_x, \omega_y, \omega_z)$ is expressed by the following equation (3) as a product of three functions representing the filter characteristic:

$$M(\omega_x, \omega_y, \omega_z) = H_{prof}(\omega_z) \cdot H_{spec}(\omega_r) \cdot H_{inverse}(\omega R) \tag{3}$$

$H_{prof}(\omega_z)$ has a low-pass filter characteristic, i.e., a Gaussian characteristic, which is expressed by the following equation (4):

$$H_{prof}(\omega_z) = \exp\left(-0.693 \left[\frac{\omega_z}{CFD} \right]^2 \right) \tag{4}$$

where CFD is the frequency with the Gaussian attenuation halved.
$H_{spec}(\omega_r)$ has a filter characteristic which is expressed by the following equation (5):

$$\begin{cases} H_{spec}(\omega_r) = 1 & \left(case \quad \omega_r < \dfrac{CFR - WFR}{2} \right) \\ H_{spec}(\omega_r) = \dfrac{1 - \sin(\omega_r - CFR) \cdot \pi / WFR}{2} & \left(case \quad \dfrac{CFR - WFR}{2} < \omega_r < \dfrac{CFR + WFR}{2} \right). \\ H_{spec}(\omega_r) = 0 & \left(case \quad \dfrac{CFR + WFR}{2} < \omega_r \right) \end{cases} \tag{5}$$

However, $\omega_r = \sqrt{\omega_x^2 + \omega_y^2 + \omega_z^2}$. The function has a sine wave form with high-frequency components smoothly attenuated. CFR is the cut-off frequency, and WFR is the total transition frequency width of the filter strength. $\dfrac{CFR + WFR}{2}$ is the Nyquist frequency and $\dfrac{CFR - WFR}{2}$ is the no-processing region frequency. This $H_{spec}(\omega_r)$ removes high-frequency components from the origin of the 3D Fourier space. $H_{inverse}(\omega R)$ has a filter characteristic which is expressed by the following equation (6):

$$H_{inverse}(\omega R) = |\omega R| \quad , \quad \omega R = \sqrt{\omega_x^2 + \omega_y^2} \tag{6}$$

The 3D back Fourier transforms the Fourier space data back to 3D volume data, having undergone Fourier space low-pass filtering. The 3D back Fourier transform is expressed by the following equation (7):

$$fm(x, y, z) = \frac{1}{8} \pi^3 \iiint FM(\omega_x, \omega_y, \omega_z) \cdot \exp\{ j(\omega_x \, x + \omega_y \, y + \omega_z \, z) \} \, d\omega_x d\omega_y d\omega_z \tag{7}$$

where equation (7) is the transformation from the frequency domain to the space domain. It is the inverse of the relation described by equation (1).

5.2 Artifact reduction processing

$H_{inverse}(\omega R)$ has a artifact reduction filter characteristic expressed by the following equation (8):

$$\omega_{R\_temp} = W + \sqrt{\omega_x^{\,2} + \omega_y^{\,2}}$$

$$\omega_{R\_norm} = \frac{\omega_{R\_temp}}{\omega_{R\_\max}} \tag{8}$$

$$H_{inverse}(\omega R) = \left|\omega_{R\_norm}\right|$$

where W is the addition of a direct current component. $\omega_{R\_\max}$ is the maximum value of a ω_{R_temp} value. The characteristics in the negative direction along the horizontal axis are omitted because these are in linear symmetry about the vertical axis with the characteristics in the positive direction. $H_{spec}(\omega_r)\cdot H_{inverse}(\omega R)$ is expressed by the following equation (9):

$$\begin{cases} H_{spec}(\omega_r)\cdot H_{inverse}(\omega R) = \dfrac{2_{\rho H}}{\pi}\left|\left|\omega_{R\_norm}\right| + \sin\left(\dfrac{\pi\rho}{2_{\rho H}}\right)\right| & (|\rho| \le \rho H) \\ H_{spec}(\omega_r)\cdot H_{inverse}(\omega R) = 0 & (|\rho| > \rho H) \end{cases} \tag{9}$$

ρH is the Nyquist frequency $\left(\dfrac{CFR + WFR}{2}\right)$ and ρ is the no-processing region frequency $\left(\dfrac{CFR - WFR}{2}\right)$.

The 3D back Fourier transforms the Fourier space data back to 3D volume data, having undergone Fourier space low pass filtering.

6. References

Bleuet P, Guillemaud R, Magin I. Et al. (2002) An adapted fan volume sampling scheme for 3D algebraic reconstruction in linear tomosynthesis. *IEEE transactions on nuclear science*, 49, pp.2366-72, ISSN 0018-9499

Dobbins JT III, Godfrey DJ. (2003) Digital x-ray tomosynthesis: curent state of the art and clinical potential. *Physics in medicine and biology*, 48, R65-106, ISSN 0031-9155

Duryea J, Dobbins JT, Lynch JA. (2003) Digital tomosynthesis of hand joints for arthritis assessment. *Medical Physics*, 30, pp.325-33, ISSN 0094-2405

Feldkamp LA, Davis LC, Kress JW. (1984) Practical cone-beam algorithm. *Journal of the Optical Society of America*, A1, pp.612-619, ISSN 0030-3941

Gomi T, Hirano H, Umeda T. (2009) Evaluation of the X-ray digital linear tomosynthesis reconstruction processing method for metal artifact reduction. *Computerized Medical Imaging and Graphics*, 33, pp.257-274, ISSN 0895-6111

Gomi T, Hirano H. (2008) Clinical potential of digital linear tomosynthesis imaging of total joint arthroplasty. *Journal of Digital Imaging*, 21, pp.312-22, ISSN 0897-1889

Grant DG. Tomosynthesis. (1972) A three-dimensional radiographic imaging technique. *IEEE transactions on bio-medical engineering*, 19, pp.20-8, ISSN 0018-9294

Hsieh J. (1995) computed tomography technology and applications; Image artifacts causes and correction, In: *Medical CT and ultrasound*, LW Goleman, JB Fowlkes, pp.487-518, Advanced Medical Publishing ISBN 1-883526-03-5, Madison

Kak A, Slaney M. (1988) *Principles of computerized tomographic imaging*. IEEE, ISBN 0-89874-494-X, New York

Kamel EM, Burger C, Buck A, et al. (2003) Impact of metallic dental implants on CT-based attenuation correction in a combined PET/CT scanner. *European Radiology*, 13, pp.724-8, ISSN 0938-7994

Man B De, Nuyts J, Dupont P, et al. (2000) Reduction of metal streak artifacts in x-ray computed tomography using a transmission maximum a posteriori algorithm. *IEEE transactions on nuclear science*, 47, pp.997-981, ISSN 0018-9499

Niklason LT, Christian BT, Niklason LE, et al. (1997) Digital tomosynthesis in breast imaging. *Radiology*, 205, pp.399-406, ISSN 0033-8419

Robertson DD, Yuan J, Wang G, et al. (1997) Total hip prosthesis metal-artifact suppression using iterative deblurring reconstruction. *Journal of computer assisted tomography*, 21, pp.293-298, ISSN 0363-8715

Ruttimann U, Groenhuis R, Webber R. (1984) Restoration of digital multilane tomosynthesis by a constrained iteration method. *IEEE transactions on medical imaging*, MI-3, pp.141-8, ISSN 0278-0062

Smith DB. (1985) Image reconstruction from cone-beam projections: necessary and sufficient conditions and reconstruction methods. *IEEE transactions on medical imaging*, M1-4, pp.14-25, ISSN 0278-0062

Sone S, Kasuga T, Sakai F, et al. (1995) Image processing in the digital tomosynthesis for pulmonary imaging. *European Radiology*, 5, pp.96-101, ISSN 0938-7994

Stiel G, Stiel LG, Klotz E et al. (1993) Digital flashing tomosynthesis: A promising technique for angiographic screening. *IEEE transactions on medical imaging*, 12, pp.314-21, ISSN 0278-0062

Wang G, Frei T, Vannier MW. (2000) A fast iterative algorithm for metal artifact reduction in x-ray CT. *Academic Radiology*, 7, pp.607-614, ISSN 1076-6332

Wang G, Snyder DL, O'Sullivan JA, et al. (1996) Iterative debluring for metal artifacts reduction. *IEEE transactions on medical imaging*, 15, pp.657-664, ISSN 0278-0062

Wang G, Vannier MW, Cheng PC. (1999) X-ray cone-beam tomography for metal artifacts reduction and local region reconstruction. *Microscopy and microanalysis*, 5, pp.58-65, ISSN 1431-9276

Wu T, Stewart A, Stanton M, McCauley T, et al. (2003) Tomographic mammography using a limited number of low-dose cone-beam projection images. *Medical Physics*, 30, pp.265-380, ISSN 0094-2405

Ziedses des Plante BG. (1932) Eine neue methode zur differenzierung in der roentgenographie (planigraphie). *Acta radiologica*, 13, pp.182-92, ISSN 0284-1851

7

Blood Transfusion in Knee Arthroplasty

Oscar Ares[1], Montserrat Tio[2], Juan Carlos Martinez Pastor[1], Luis Lozano[1], Josep Maria Segur[1], Francisco Macule[1] and Santiago Suso[1,3]

[1]Orthopedic Department, Knee Unit, Hospital Clinic Barcelona
[2]Anesthesioly Department, Hospital Clinic Barcelona
[3]ICEMEQ Institut
Spain

1. Introduction

Orthopedic surgery is one of most blood-consuming surgical specialties since it is associated with a significant preoperative hemorrhage requiring frequent allogeneic blood transfusions. A special mention needs to be done to hip and knee arthroplasty, complex rachis arthrodesis and tumor-pathology removal. The intervention on older and higher-risk patients has raised the demand on allogeneic blood to such levels that even Blood Banks are unable to attend. Besides the high cost, using allogeneic blood has its risks, such as immunosuppression, patient's wrong identification, transfusion reactions or the possibility of infectious disease transmission. This imbalance between blood demand and availability, together with the awareness about potential risks of blood transfusions and the continuous advances both in technology and pharmaceutics, should lead us to extreme changes in transfusion politics; developing a series of therapeutic measures to reduce blood transfusion to minimum, leaving its use only when it is strictly necessary, especially in scheduled surgery.

PREOPERATIVE STRATEGIES
- Correction of preoperative anemia: iron supplements, erythropoietin, vitamin B12 and folic acid
- Autologous blood pre-donation
INTRAOPERATIVE STRATEGIES
- Individualize transfusion threshold
- Anesthetic measures
- Surgical technique
- Erythrocytes' substitutes
- Pharmaceutical measurements
- Autotransfusion:
• Intraoperative blood savers
• Normovolemic hemodilution
POSTOPERATIVE STRATEGIES
- Autotransfusion of blood from postsurgical drainage
- Iron supplements

Table 1. Blood-saving techniques during perioperative time.

The aim of this chapter is to inform on saving techniques of hematic components and its implantation in scheduled orthopedic surgery, summarized in table 1.

2. Preoperative strategies

2.1 Correction of preoperative anemia

In the preanesthetic evaluation we will provide a guideline for preoperative evaluation and preparation of the patient, and we will include him/she to a **blood-saving program** by stimulating their erythropoietin (EPO) production, giving iron (Fe) or autologous blood predonation. It is important to check on hemoglobin levels, as well as iron deposits (ferritin, soluble transferrin receptor and transferrin saturation) and associated pathologies (comorbidity).

Hemoglobin concentration is one of the most predictive factors for autologous blood transfusion (ABT). Patients with preoperative anemia show an increase in postoperative morbimortality and a decrease in quality of life (Shander et al., 2004). Age is a predisposing factor for anemia and the prevalence of postoperative anemia increases with age (Goodnough et al., 2005; Rosencher et al., 2003). Iron deficiency and chronic inflammation, with or without iron deficiency, are the most frequent causes of preoperative anemia in these patients. Folic acid and vitamin B12 deficiency can also be present, especially in elderly people.

A preoperative anemia must be treated before undergoing surgery, if it is possible, limiting exposure risk to allogeneic blood.

- **Human recombinant erythropoietin (rhEPO)** – For the past several years, we have at our disposal the human recombinant erythropoietin (rhEPO), obtained from genetic engineering, identical to the endogenous, which stimulates erythrocyte production in a dose-dependent way. It was considered that its use in surgical patients would arise preoperative hemoglobin values and/or facilitate autologous blood predonation, and this way decreasing the chances of an allogeneic transfusion. It is used in programmed patients undergoing major orthopedic surgeries in which initial hemoglobin is between 10 and 13 g/dl, and the prediction of perioperative blood loss is significant (Laupacis & Fergusson, 1998).

  Its main function is stimulating the bone marrow's erythropoietic activity, acting on specific receptors of erythrocyte-formation precursor target cells. Plasma levels of EPO do not vary with age or sex. In healthy individuals the rank goes from 5 - 25 mU/ml. EPO's dosage varies according to its indication and it must be supplemented with iron to avoid stimulating an iron-deficient erythropoiesis. After undergoing a preoperative treatment with EPO, ferritin concentration decreases to half. The speed at which iron from this deposits can be activated becomes a limiting factor. Patients with serious cardiovascular disease, poorly controlled hypertension and history of thromboembolic disease or deep vein thrombosis cannot be treated with EPO.
- **Iron, vitamin B12 and folic acid** – So that erythropoiesis works properly, besides EPO, it is necessary an appropriate iron intake (fundamental component in the hemoglobin molecule), as well as vitamin B12 and folic acid. Its deficiency affects the proliferation and cellular differentiation in erythropoiesis resulting in central arregenerative anemia (decreased reticulocytes). Total amount of iron in our organism is approximately 4-5 grams. 65% is found as hemoglobin, whereas 15-30% is stored in the hepatic parenchyma and rethiculoendotelial system as ferritin and the rest of it binds to transferrin in blood plasma. It is absorbed in the small intestine.

Iron-deficiency anemia affects approximately 25% of world population. Furthermore, there is a status defined as 'functional iron-deficient states', which is described as a situation where iron deposits are normal (or even increased), but iron supply to bone marrow is inadequate to satisfy the erythroid precursor demands; and another anemia associated to 'chronic processes' where erythropoiesis is deficient because of proinflammatory cytokines-mediated mechanisms.
Nowadays it has been proven its high profitability and efficiency index, mainly to optimize or as support in the erythropoietin treatment and autologous predonation. Administration of oral iron is effective in decreasing allogeneic blood transfusions and/or the number of transfused patients in orthopedic major surgery (Okuyama et al., 2005). Orally or intravenous use of iron will depend at the moment in which the treatment is taking place, oral iron absorptive capacity and existence of any gastric disease that could contraindicate oral iron treatment (Cuenca et al., 2004). If treatment is done with intravenous iron, once it is finished we must prescribe oral iron.
The total amount of administered iron will depend on initial hemoglobin value and existence of an iron-deficient condition. If using saccharose iron, dosage varies from 100 to 200 mg in alternate days, with a maximum dose of 600 mg per week and 200 mg every 2 days. At present there is also carboxymaltose iron, which contains greater amounts of iron (500-1000 mg) to administer in a single dose. In case of a folic acid and/or vitamin B12 deficiency we must supply substitutive treatment to correct it.

2.2 Autologous blood predonation

This means the presurgical patient's blood predonation or autodonation. Some weeks prior to intervention, a blood extraction (one or more units of blood) is performed to the patient to be used at his/her surgery or postoperatively.
To be included in the program the patient must fulfill both medical and analytical special requirements; hemoglobin levels before starting predonation process above 11 mg/dl, as well as an appropriate programming of surgery to avoid expiration of the predonated units (35 days - maximum time permitted for storage). Due to this fact, quite a reasonable amount of patients who have undergone autologous blood donation preoperatively, reach surgery time with hemoglobin values under their initial levels (before predonation), therefore increasing transfusion requirements. The patient carries out the donations once or more times during the days and weeks prior to intervention. 350-400 mL extractions are made not less than 3-day intervals, which is the time needed for protein synthesis and mobilization and to return to normal. This way, they can benefit from erythropoiesis stimulation with erythropoietin. All patients must receive an appropriate iron supplement.
Despite the fact that this technique was at its peak during the nineties, its use has been diminishing progressively for several reasons. In first place, the high number of blood bags that were dismissed because of an imbalance between extracted bags and transfusion requirements, since a good coordination in surgery programming and between all professionals taking part is needed. This difficulty has made this method a very expensive one in resource-consumption and less effective than it was thought to be at first. On the other hand, the establishment of intravenous iron and erythropoietin, decrease in transfusion threshold and improvement of the surgical method too, have pushed into the background autologous donation preoperatively, leaving it as last option in some cases such as complex spinal surgery with a mass blood loss forecast and those patients whose blood group have compatibility difficulties.

The existence of predonation units increases the likelihood of transfusion, as perception of risk decrease; there is less chance of rejection or blood incompatibility, as well as less infections. Moreover, it is exposed to the same errors in the processes of extraction, storage, identification and reinfusion to the autologous blood transfusion. Predonation of autologous blood has the following contraindications: serious cardiac disease, hepatitis B history and positive markers for HCV, HIV-I/II, HTLV-I/II and active bacterial infection.

3. Intraoperative strategies

To improve its efficiency, they must be associated to a blood-saving protocol during perioperative time.

3.1 Individualize transfusion threshold

A restrictive transfusion strategy (transfusion threshold at hemoglobin 7 g/dl) must be used, taking into consideration anemia risks and the benefits from a transfusion in an individualized way for every patient. Nowadays, rarely does hemoglobin over 10 g/dl get considered for transfusion, whereas it is believed to be strictly necessary when hemoglobin is less than 6 g/dl. In either case, the transfusion threshold must be lowered to try and delay the start of blood transfusion until the surgery ends, making a new assessment after each transfused packed red blood cells. Moreover, the usual practice of transfusing always two units of packed red blood cells (PRBC) is considered incorrect; as to raise the hemoglobin concentration 1 g/dl it takes about 4 ml/kg PRBC, being enough one PRBC.

3.2 Anesthetic measures

These include appropriate blood volume maintenance, dealing with pain, tachycardia and high blood pressure, hyperoxic ventilation to improve oxygen transport in patients with low hemoglobin and maintenance of normothermia. As specific actions in orthopedics we include:

- Regional anesthesia, as several studies have demonstrated decrease of perioperative bleeding when comparing with general anesthesia, which appears to be related to lower blood pressure.
- Optimal position of the patient to reduce venous congestion at the surgical field
- Monitoring low blood pressure is a controversial anesthetic measure, with a relative effectiveness amongst bleeding, used to lower down blood pressure and thus reducing blood loss during surgery. In orthopedic surgery, its use gets relegated to high intraoperative bleeding interventions. Relative contraindications include untreated severe high blood pressure, coronary disease, serious lung disease, severe anemia or significant polycythemia, cerebrovascular disease, pregnancy, considerable hypovolemia and serious kidney or liver dysfunction. There are numerous drugs used to control hypertension. Most frequently used in clinical practice are inhalators (isoflurane, sevoflurane), direct acting vasodilators (nitroglycerin, sodium nitroprusside), beta blockers (labetalol, esmolol), others (urapidil, captopril, etc.)

3.3 Surgical technique

This includes an adequate ischemia (use of tourniquet), adequate hemostasis, minimally invasive surgery, etc. The most important factors are surgical time reduction and well-cared hemostasis. There is a straightforward relationship between hematic loss and surgical time; a longer surgical time is associated to a greater hematic loss. During surgery, local hemostatic agents, such as fibrin sealants, which reduce surgical bleeding, can be used. We will develop this part further on.

3.4 Erythrocytes' substitutes

These are substances able to replace the use of allogeneic blood components. They are obtained from human blood, transgenic animals or recombinant technology. Currently still under development. There are hemoglobin solutions and perfluorocarbonate emulsion.

3.5 Pharmaceutical measurements

Several prohemostatic drugs have been used in order to try reducing or preventing intraoperative bleeding. In orthopedic surgery, antifibrinolytic and desmopressin are the mainly used.

3.5.1 Antifibrinolytics

Perioperative bleeding is partially attributed to the fibrinolytic system activation. Several work groups have administered antifibrinolytics, and as a result observed a decrease in perioperative bleeding and blood bags transfused (Henry et al., 2001). In other recent revisions, which evaluate antifibrinolytics drugs in orthopedic surgery (Kagoma et al., 2009; Zufferey et al., 2006), they conclude that using tranexamic acid or aprotinin reduces the percentage of patients requiring blood transfusions and also are efficient decreasing bleeding. When using epsilon-aminocaproic acid (EACA) there are no signs of a significant reduction in hemorrhagic risk, although not many studies have been done. All of them can have relatively infrequent but very serious side effects, such as arterial thrombosis, renal failure or rhabdomyolysis.

3.5.1.1 Aprotinin

It is a 58 amino acid polypeptide. It is found mainly in mammalian mastocytes and it is commercialized from bovine lung. Aprotinin works inhibiting trypsin, plasmin and tissue and plasma kallikrein. In addition to this, it holds an anti-inflammatory effect attenuating inflammatory response in major surgery, particularly at high-doses. It is the antifibrinolytic drug most widely studied to reduce bleeding and diminish transfusion needs. However, in comparison to tranexamic acid or EACA, it increases mortality risk. After the adverse results in mortality in patients who had undergone cardiac surgery in an observational study over more than 4000 patients (Mangano et al., 2006), and in a randomized double blind trial with over 3000 patients (Fergusson et al., 2008), the drug was withdrawn worldwide.

3.5.1.2 *Synthetic antifibrinolytics*

Synthetic analogs of lysine. Tranexamic acid and EACA are able to block fibrinolysis by competitively antagonizing the binding of plasminogen to fibrin.

Tranexamic acid is 10 times stronger in vitro than EACA. In total knee arthroplasty, prophylactic administration significantly reduces blood loss up to 50% and decreases transfusion requirements without increasing the risk of thromboembolic signs (Alvarez et al., 2008; Cid & Lozano, 2005; Lozano et al., 2008). Optimal technique would be with two tranexamic acid bolus (each of them 10-15 mg/Kg), one before surgery and another when letting the air out of the tourniquet. In total hip prosthesis, tranexamic acid results in a

decrease of intraoperative bleeding when administered prophylactically (Benoni et al., 2001), with no raise in thromboembolic complications incidence (Johansson et al., 2005b). However, it must only be used in those patients of whom a significant blood loss is expected. In spinal surgery, its administration is associated with considerable decrease in perioperative blood loss without side effects coming out (Elwatidy et al., 1976).
The rapid administration causes hypotension and its use is not recommended in patients with thromboembolic history although there is no evidence of an association with thromboembolic complications arising.
Epsilon-aminocaproic acid (EACA), in addition to its antifibrinolytic effect, prevents from platelet receptor degradation by plasmin, preserving platelet function. On the whole, recommended dose is a 150-mg/Kg bolus before surgery, followed by a 15-mg/Kg/h infusion during surgery. In a 2008-published meta-analysis they concluded that it is the most effective antifibrinolytic drug in spinal surgery (Gill et al., 2008). Nevertheless, not many studies have been done regarding this drug as to obtain conclusions. The most frequent side effect is hypotension, which is usually associated to a rapid intravenous administration. There is no evidence that EACA would raise thromboembolic episodes.

3.5.2 Desmopressin acetate

Desmopressin acetate is an antidiuretic hormone synthetic analogue. Besides its antidiuretic effect, it has a hemostatic action that would be based in factor VIII and Von Willebrand factor release to the circulatory system from the existent deposits at the vascular endothelium cells, and its ability for increasing platelet adhesion. In orthopedic surgery its use has been reduced mainly to spinal surgery, with initial encouraging results (Kobrinsky et al., 1987), although not proved in subsequent studies. In hip and knee orthopedic surgery there is no evidence of a decrease in blood loss or erythrocyte volume transfusion. Dose for intravenous administration is 0.3 μg/Kg and its main use would be for Von Willebrand syndrome. Desmopressin side effects include facial redness, severe headache, hypotension and high-speed beating. Its strong antidiuretic effect can produce water retention, hyponatremia and convulsions.

3.6 Autotransfusion

It includes all the procedures by which a patient is transfused with his own blood. These methods have a number of advantages such as lack of infectious diseases transmission, avoids hemolytic disease incidence and several different transfusion reactions, it has immediate availability, as well as compatibility, avoids categorization and cross-matching mistakes, and last of all, decreases hypothermal risk of stored blood. It can be performed by two different methods:

3.6.1 Normovolemic hemodilution

Normovolemic hemodilution consists in extraction and anticoagulation of an established blood volume (4 units maximum) after anesthetic induction and its simultaneous substitution for crystalloids and/or colloids to maintain normovolemia, and thus causing dilutional anemia. Reinfusion is done later on when surgical hemorrhage is under control or even before if necessary. Extracted blood is then anticoagulated at room temperature, which preserves platelet functions. Despite these theoretical benefits, dissolving coagulation factors, hematocrit and platelets causes a microvascular bleeding. Furthermore, excessive crystalloid contribution leads to their accumulation on the interstitial space during postoperative time and it is currently considered as an obsolete technique, mostly because of its inefficiency as a blood-saver method. Nowadays the use of normovolemic hemodilution is not recommended for decreasing allogeneic blood transfusion, nor transfused patient number or bags transfused.

3.6.2 Intraoperative blood savers

Retrieving intraoperative blood involves autologous collection and infusion of autologous red blood cells, which is done by means of a device known as cell saver. It is commonly used in orthopedic surgery (spinal surgery and replacement of hip prosthesis) and provides significant autologous blood volumes. In major orthopedic surgery, perioperative blood retrieval reduces the probability of receiving autologous blood transfusion by 65% (Carless et al., 2004). The devices used recover only 50-60% of lost blood during surgery, which together with the high cost of consumables, makes its use only indicated to those procedures in which intraoperative hemorrhage is predicted to be over 1,000-1,500 ml, or else when it is possible to recover at least one packed red blood cells. This method would also be indicated in those patients whose religious believes contraindicates a blood donor transfusion but permits an autologous transfusion, when no compatible blood donor is available or when the patient is not capable of donating enough amount of autologous blood before surgery.
Despite the devices' costs, retrieved and processed blood can be less expensive than allogeneic blood (Gardner et al., 2000). A clear benefit from perioperative blood reinfusion is the erythrocyte viability in collected blood, which is higher than that from allogeneic blood and oxygen transport capacity, being better than in stored blood (Colwell, Jr. et al., 2002). However, autotransfusion programs are associated with certain organization complexity and a weak cost-benefit relationship when used indiscriminately.
This procedure is contraindicated when there is bacterial contamination at the operating field, neoplastic disease, patients with positive viral-markers, sickle-cell anemia and when certain local hemostatics have been used or else when blood is found to be hemolyzed. Different procedures are available for intraoperative blood recovery. Semicontinuous-flow blood centrifugation system is one of the most commonly used, where blood is retrieved by aspiration, anticoagulated, filtered and sent to a reservoir from where it is pumped to a centrifuge bell which divides and washes the cells to return them to the patient as a saline suspended red blood cells, with a hematocrit value around 50-70%. During this process, plasma is dismissed, as well as toxic products from hemolysis, coagulation factors, platelets and fat.
OrthoPAT® (Orthopedic Perioperative Autotransfusion System, Haemonetics), is an autologous blood retrieval, specifically designed for adapting to intermittent bleeding during and after programmed orthopedic surgery, reducing unnecessary allogeneic transfusions. It is a small device, easy to operate and completely automatized. In prosthetic-hip and spinal surgery it is commonly used for intra and postoperative retrieval, whereas in prosthetic-knee surgery it is preferably used postoperatively. Perioperative use of blood retrievals may significantly reduce allogeneic transfusion risks in a not inconsiderable number of patients with high-risk of being transfused (Pola et al., 2004).

4. Postoperative strategies

4.1 Postoperative autotransfusion

There are certain orthopedic surgical procedures (such as knee arthroplasty), in which postoperative bleeding through postsurgical drainages is very significant due to the completion of most of the surgery with lower extremity ischemia, so that bleeding occurs primarily in the early hours of the postoperative period. For this reason, in this type of surgeries, blood retrieval during postoperative time has been the main instruction and the one that has achieved major performance. Several devices for postoperative blood retrieval have been designed, in order to aspirate, store and retransfuse lost blood through postsurgical drainages.

Reinfused blood is often filtered rather than washed. It would be restricted to orthopedic programmed surgeries where estimated postoperative bleeding is between 750 and 1000 mL, and at least the equivalent to one packed red blood cells can be retrieved. Autotransfused blood must be collected and reinfused within a 4-6 hour-period. Stored blood in surgical drainage holds a better oxygen release to tissues than that from blood bank, although having a lower hematocrit. Furthermore, it owns better rheological characteristics and fewer ionic disturbances than blood bank. Hematocrit is low because it is total blood, which means that with this blood reinfusion we will not be able to raise hematocrit, but we will succeed in not diminishing its value.

Comparison analysis from obtained data in several studies shows that, regarding blood bank, blood from postsurgical drainage in orthopedic surgery, even with lower hematocrit and hemoglobin (8-10 g/dL), has higher concentrations of erythrocytic ATP and 2,3-BPG, less ionic disturbances and possibly, less immunosuppressive action. This blood includes too activated coagulation factors and fibrinogen degradation products, which could be the cause of coagulopathies. However, no significant increase in bleeding has been found, neither coagulation disorders clinically expressive There are no differences in perioperative inflammatory mediators levels between patients receiving unwashed retrieved blood from those who do not get it (Munoz et al., 2005b). Fat particles content, which is the main cause of fat embolism and respiratory distress syndrome, is controlled using a filter between collection and reinfusion container, and dismissing the last 80-100 cc. These methods allow removal of 90% of fat particles in the retrieved blood. The remaining 10% is eliminated by leukodepletion filter. These filters have shown to be effective in dismissing bacteria and tumor cells. In accordance with the abovementioned, unwashed blood must be limited to a maximum 1000 ml reinfusion. This collecting system brings advantages such as minimum contamination risk as it is a closed circuit and greater hemodynamic stability during postoperative period due to the disposal of blood volume, which is reinfunded if necessary. Moreover, it is cheap and can be used in Jehovah's Witnesses, as it is a closed circuit in which blood does not lose total contact with the patient's body.

Contraindications for using postsurgical drains' blood are: renal failure, altered hepatic function, coagulation disorders, infusion of hemostatic agents or inadequate solutions (topic antibiotics, antiseptics, oxygenated water) and neoplastic or septic disease. Retrieval of postoperative blood reduces both patients' percentage that would receive allogeneic blood transfusion and volume of transfusion (Carless et al., 2004).

4.2 Iron supplements

The use of intravenous iron during postoperative of orthopedic-surgical patients, is an effective treatment to increase hemoglobin levels, as shown in five clinical trials randomized controlled; unlike oral iron supply.

5. Surgical aspects and its relationship with bleeding

5.1 Introduction

Transfusion requirements are a matter that concerns doctors not only for disease transmission risk but also for transmission complications and the high-cost of the procedure (Garcia-Erce et al., 2002). There has been a recent trend towards developing a protocol in order to decrease transfusion requirements (Garcia-Erce et al., 2002; Kourtzis et al., 2004). Several options have come up, pharmaceutical as well as transfusion options alternatively to allogeneic transfusion, summed up in table 2.

According to different studies who have studied predictive factors in trauma surgeries, preoperative hemoglobin level and levels of red cell mass are predictors of transfusion needs. The higher the levels of hemoglobin and red cell mass, the less need to transfuse (Garcia-Erce et al., 2002; Lozano et al., 2008).

Occult blood has an outstanding paper regarding blood management in the patient being operated of arthroplastic surgery. Occult blood can reach 50% of the missed blood perioperatively (Sehat et al., 2000).

During surgery there are several options to consider in order of preventing bleeding, such as: use or not have drainages, aspiration pressure and time of aspiration of drainages and the use of ischemia during prosthetic surgery.

SURGICAL VARIABLES
1. Drainages and non-infectious complications
2. Relation between drainage and infection
3. Use of postoperative blood retrieval
4. Number of drainages
5. Aspiration pressure
6. Start / Opening-up / End of drainage
7. Tourniquet
8. Surgical technique

Table 2. Different surgical options to reduce bleeding

5.2 Drainages and non-infectious complications

The use of drainages in orthopedic surgery is a matter of tradition. Its use prevents postoperative hematomas and diminishes postoperative pain, but its use is still controversial (Corpe et al., 2000). Despite several evidence based medical studies, British orthopedists were not following their recommendations in 2003 (Canty et al., 2003).

Drains have been related to the transfusion necessity and infection rate, among others. But some studies, such as Seyfert's et al (Seyfert et al., 2002), prove that placing drainages with suction does not increase transfusion requirements or postoperative course.

On the other hand, there are studies whose results highlight that not using drainages does not avoid transfusions nor does it reduce blood loss. Padala et al. find questionable the use of drainages in primary knee surgery as it increases transfusions (Padala et al., 2004). Some studies hold on to the fact that it is not necessary their use in primary knee arthroplasty (Adalberth et al., 1998; Corpe et al., 2000; Jenny et al., 2001), nor hip or knee (Crevoisier et al., 1998; Niskanen et al., 2000), nor primary hip (Acus, III et al., 1992; Beer et al., 1991; Hadden & McFarlane, 1990; Kumar et al., 2006). Della Valle et al found out in their study more complications in the group with drainages in comparison to the non-drainages group in primary hip arthroplasty (Gonzalez, V et al., 2004). Ovadia et al (Ovadia et al., 1997), as well as other work-groups (Hallstrom & Steele, 1992; Walmsley et al., 2005), find significant the premise that the use of drainages increases transfusion requirements (0.7 units per patient with drainage, in comparison to 0.2 unit per patient without, $p = 0.005$).

Widman et al.(Widman et al., 2002) reveal in their study that the use of drainages in hip surgery does not decrease postsurgical hematoma, analyzed with SPECT, but it does increase transfusion requirements.

Esler et al. (Esler et al., 2003) state that they cannot support the use of suction drainages as the group with suction drainages shows a greater blood loss than the non-drainages group. Nevertheless, they do give support to the use of drainages for reusing blood.

Some authors assert that the use of drainage is not harmful but it is of no use at all (Ashraf et al., 2001; Johansson et al., 2005a). Other authors do not see that using drainages in unicompartmental knee surgery has an adequate cost/benefit ratio, since it increases the cost of the procedure both in labor and equipment expenditure; and furthermore, avoiding postoperative drainage in this kind of procedures does not influence the outcome (Confalonieri et al., 2004).

In their meta-analysis, Parker et al. (Parker et al., 2004) find out that suction drainage increases transfusion requirements after a hip or knee arthroplasty, with no benefits contributed.

A mechanical complication that may occur with Redon-drains is that this can break, thus staying intra-articular. In the knee's joint we may keep an expectant management or else require surgical maneuvers such as arthrotomy (Marmor, 1990) or either arthroscopy surgery to remove the drainage (Kao et al., 2002).

5.3 Relation between drainage and infection

Once we reach the infectious complications, the debate remains open. On the one hand, the fact that drains decrease hematoma, knowing that hematoma is an enabling factor for infection, is an argument for its use. But on the other hand, drainages can increase retrograde infection (Mengal et al., 2001).

Regarding deep infections, studies are controversial. Some authors, e.g. Kim et al., defend that using drainages does not increase infections rate or it even decreases it. These associate drains' use with a non-significant decrease in deep infections (Kim et al., 1998).

On the other hand, many authors present results where drains' use has a positive relation to infection. Minnema et al. (Minnema et al., 2004)have linked the use of suction drains with an increasing rate of surgical wound infection after total knee arthroplasty.

Cultivating the drain's end is not a favorable practice in cost-benefit studies, according to the study published by Weinrauch et al. (Weinrauch, 2005). In spite of Weinrauch's study, several groups have cultivated the drain's tip. Zamora-Navas et al. (Zamora-Navas et al., 1999) analyze the drain's tip observing that drainages removed before 12 hours do not have any contamination, those retired at 24 hours show contamination in 2 out of 12 patients for *Staphylococcus epidermidis*, and those drains removed at 48 hours also present contamination for *S. epidermidis* in 2 out of 12 patients. Clinical evaluations of wound healing were similar in both groups. A different group of study, Willemen's et al. (Willemen et al., 1991), cultivated the catheter's tip of all groups and concluded that culture of the catheter's end that had been removed at 24 hours time, were all-negative cultures. A related study to the

abovementioned is that from Schmitt et al. (Schmitt & Weyand, 1997), in which a greater number of hours maintaining the drainage increases bacterial contamination of the drainage tip. Therefore, Willemen (Willemen et al., 1991), Drinkwater et al. (Drinkwater & Neil, 1995) and Rowe's et al. (Rowe et al., 1993) groups recommend use of drainages up to 24 hours, owing to the relationship between use of drains, microbial contamination in the catheter's tip, risk of prosthetic infection and comfort in early rehabilitation.
Regarding superficial infections, authors such as Saleh et al. (Saleh et al., 2002) and Ovadia et al. (Ovadia et al., 1997), find in their studies that superficial infection is significantly related to use and duration of drainages.

5.4 Use of postoperative blood retrieval

Within the options in saving blood we can use intraoperative and postoperative blood retrieval. Regarding the use of blood retrieval in total knee (Dalen et al., 1996; Gannon et al., 1991; Groh et al., 1990; Handel et al., 2006; Heddle et al., 1992; Hendrych, 2006; Kristensen et al., 1992; Majkowski et al., 1991; Martin et al., 1992; Munoz et al., 2005a; Noain et al., 2005; Simpson et al., 1994; Strumper et al., 2004; Thomas et al., 2001; Wojan et al., 2005; Xenakis et al., 1997) and hip (Gannon et al., 1991;Kristensen et al., 1992) arthroplasty, it is considered to be useful as it decreases blood transfusion necessity, reaching a 48% decrease transfusion requirements.
The use of postoperative retrieval in knee or hip primary surgery, analyzed from a cost-benefit point of view, is a profitable procedure (Dramis & Plewes, 2006; Jones et al., 2004; Thomas et al., 2001; Wojan et al., 2005). However, some authors like Umlas et al. show that the use of a retrieving instrument is not profitable due to its high cost and the small amount of blood retrieved (Umlas et al., 1994). Slagis' group (Slagis et al., 1991) find that using a retrieval is actually associated to a diminishment in costs, but it is not recommended as a systematic manner in all patients undergoing total knee arthroplasty as the amount of blood salvaged is low and they still need blood transfusions.
The amount of blood salvaged in hip arthroplasty surgery is 350-700 mL and 500-800 mL in knee arthroplasty (Dutka et al., 2002), although other groups state that the average transfused amount is around 1000 mL in knee arthroplasty (Breakwell et al., 2000). The study by Han et al. (Han & Shin, 1997) shows that using a retrieval is useful as it is possible to reinfuse 437 mL in hip, 883 mL in knee arthroplasty and 1713 mL in bilateral knee surgery without patients having any air embolism problem, coagulopathy, renal failure or sepsis.
The followed protocol in blood retrieval is the reinfusion of the collected blood within 6 first hours (Dalen et al., 1995). Using blood from postoperative drainage (blood retrieval) in knee arthroplasty does not show important complications (Groh et al., 1990; Sinardi et al., 2005; Wojan et al., 2005), neither inflammatory cell response increase (Altinel et al., 2006; Munoz et al., 2005b; Munoz et al., 2006). According to different studies there are no statistically significant differences within the studied parameters, except for IL-6, which could increase febrile reactions (Handel et al., 2006; Kristiansson et al., 1995). In the study by Bengtson et al. (Bengtson et al., 1990) they found a decrease of anaphylactic toxin and complement activation with no clinical impact. Woda et al. (Woda & Tetzlaff, 1992) describe a case with tracheal edema post-reinfusion of salvaged blood.
The recovered blood culture may be positive in some cases, for this reason Wollinsky et al. recommend antibiotic prophylaxis with cefuroxime to reduce contamination of suction tips and collection bags (Wollinsky et al., 1997). This same study shows that the use of prophylactic cefuroxime limits the transfer of autologous blood products.

Several studies compare the different blood retrievals, finding out that whereas some are easier to use, others have a better suction and that side effects do not present statistically significant differences (Trammell et al., 1991).
Another point of view to look at is that from Mauerhan et al. (Mauerhan et al., 1993) and other authors (Mac et al., 1993; Reize et al., 2006), who find that the use of a recovered blood is not necessary in hip and knee arthroplasty. Faraj et al. show in their study that cost/profit ratio is not profitable when using a blood retrieval (Evans et al., 1993; Faraj & Raghuvanshi, 2006; Jackson et al., 2000).

5.5 Number of drainages

The study by Labek et al. (Labek & Bohler, 1998) links the number of drainages with prosthetic hip bleeding. Their article studies the relationship between number of drainages, its positioning (deep and/or superficial) and its relationship with transfusions needed, wound's exudation, subcutaneous hematoma and thigh edema. Given the possibility of placing three drainages, two drainages, (subcutaneously and subfascial) or one drainage (subcutaneously or subfascial), the conclusion was that using two drainages alone is better rather than 3 drainages or no drainage as there are no more complications with respect to surgical injury and a 47% reduction of blood units was achieved.

5.6 Aspiration pressure

Aspiration pressure is one of many variables when using drains. Cheung et al. state that low suction drains do not increase the number of complications (Cheung & Chiu, 2006). Along the same lines, Benoni et al (Benoni & Fredin, 1997) show that a high aspiration pressure increases drained quantity after knee arthroplasty in a significant way with respect to low-pressure aspiration drainages. The average drained amount in 24 hours is 570 mL in high-pressure aspiration drains and 480 mL in low-pressure ones (p=0,03). At 48 hours, drained quantity had raised to 785 mL and 585 mL (p=0,002) respectively.
Another study regarding aspiration pressure is that from Kirschner et al. (Kirschner et al., 1989) where it is observed that the higher suction pressure increases the risk of secondary hematomas. Martin et al. (Martin et al., 2004), in their study with three groups (no drainages, suction drainages and a third group with non-suction drains), find that the group using non-suction drainages is that with fewer complications and less transfusion requirements.
When studying another variable such as time of aspiration (continuous or discontinuous), and according to Berman et al. (Berman et al., 1990), using continuous aspiration increases drained amount, however it also decreases complications from the surgical wound and transudation through surgical injury. Another study evaluating results from a discontinuous opening of the drain is that from Brueggemann, who shows that clamping the drainages during 55 minutes every hour for the first 6 postoperative hours decreases transfusion needs, without increasing the risk of hematomas or complications from the surgical wound (Brueggemann et al., 1999). Prasad et al. in their study show that an intermittent clamping of drains decreases bleeding, rather than clamping the drainage only initially for 2 hours (Prasad et al., 2005).
Seyfert et al. (Seyfert et al., 2002) compare a group with unicompartmental knee prosthesis with suction drainage and another one with no drainage. The study analyzes bleeding at 12, 24, 36 and 48 hours. Average bleeding in the suction-drainage group was

528 mL, whereas in the non-suction 436 mL. However, difference between both averages was not statistically significant.

5.7 Start/opening-up/end of drainage

If the opening-up of drainage is delayed, the obtained amount through drainage diminishes in a statistically significant manner (Roy et al., 2006; Tsumara et al., 2006). Along the same lines, another study states that delaying the opening-up of drainages 4 hours; drainage decreases in a statistically significant way (Shen et al., 2005).

On the other hand, some authors conclude that clamping drains during first 2 postoperative hours does not influence within drained quantity, nor transfusion number, or mobility, or surgical wound complications (Kiely et al., 2001). Study by Leemann et al. affirms that after 6 hours drainage can be removed as 78% of bleeding has been already drained (Leeman et al., 2006).

Senthil et al. (Senthil et al., 2005) state in their study that 84% of total drain was collected during first 12 hours, and 94% during first 24 hours. The study's conclusion is that articular drainages can be safely removed after first 12 postoperative hours.

The Spanish group headed by Zamora-Navas (Zamora-Navas et al., 1999) study bleeding features in three groups in which drainage is maintained 12, 24 and 48 hours. They observed that the group maintaining drainage for 24 hours had already drained 87% of the total amount at 12 hours time. In the last group (with drainage 48 hours), bleeding at 12 hours corresponded to 91% of the total amount, and bleeding at 24 hours was 97% of the total amount collected after 48 hours.

Regarding when to remove drainage, in the study by Benoni et al. (Benoni & Fredin, 1997) we can observe how the drained amount between 24 and 48 hours is only 215 mL in the high-pressure aspiration drainages, and 105 mL in those with low-pressure aspiration. In conclusion, we can see that aspiration pressure is not more than a variable, as previously seen, and that drained volume between 24 and 48 hours is not as far as important as the bleeding that occurs during first 24 hours.

In the study by Slagis et al., the conclusion of greater volume collected during first operative hours repeats (Slagis et al., 1991). The average collected volume was 493 mL, great part of it being collected during first 4 hours.

Another study showing that prosthetic bleeding is produced during first postsurgical hours is that from Willemen et al. (Willemen et al., 1991), in which they keep drains 48 hours and they observe that 85% of total volume was drained after 24 hours. Between 24 and 48 hours the drain was of only 50 mL.

In our own study (Ares-Rodriguez et al., 2008), we observed that mean of the survival curve for postoperative bleeding time was 16 hours for total knee arthroplasty, and we therefore concluded that drainage in total knee arthroplasty can be safely removed after 18 postoperative hours, with a safety margin.

5.8 Tourniquet

A first study shows that releasing the tourniquet intraoperative (before wound closure) and a correct hemostasis does not reduce total amount of blood lost in total knee arthroplasty (Hersekli et al., 2004). Barwell et al. (Barwell et al., 1997) present in their study that using tourniquet has some side effects and that these can be minimized if removal of tourniquet is done prematurely, together with a thoroughly hemostasis prior to surgical wound closing.

Lotke finds in his study that releasing tourniquet, together with coagulation and immediate start of continuous passive motion (CPM) therapy, increases arthroplasty bleeding (Lotke et al., 1991).

5.9 Surgical technique

Regarding which surgical technique would most reduce postoperative bleeding, several maneuvers have been discussed; such as navigation, sealing the intramedullary femoral canal during femoral preparation in total knee arthroplasty, different prosthetic models and using minimally invasive techniques.
The use of the navigator reduces bleeding through drainage in a statistically significant way, according to the studies by Kalairajah (Kalairajah et al., 2005) and Hinarejos (Hinarejos et al., 2009). On the other hand, groups such as Chang's (Chang CW et al., 2010) or Turajane's (Turajane T et al., 2009) do not find statistically significant differences between minimally invasive surgery with navigation and conventional surgery.
Sealing the intramedullary femoral canal in non-navigated surgery and with intramedullary femoral guide decreases both the fall in hemoglobin and transfusion requirements in a statistically significant way (Ko et al., 2003; Raut et al., 1993). Another study showed a decrease in bleeding through drainages with this technique (Kumar et al., 2000).
Porteous et al. (Garcia-Erce et al., 2002; Porteous and Bartlett, 2003) analyze postoperative drainage in three implant types; cemented, hybrid and uncemented total knee replacement. The statistically significant conclusion is that cemented prosthesis has a lesser bleeding with regard to other two groups during 8 first hours, but this difference decreases after 24-48 hours. Another study states that constrained arthroplasty increases blood loss (Berman et al., 1988).

6. References

Acus, R. W., III, J. M. Clark, I. A. Gradisar, Jr., and M. W. Kovacik, 1992, The use of postoperative suction drainage in total hip arthroplasty: Orthopedics, v. 15, no. 11, p. 1325-1328.

Adalberth, G., S. Bystrom, K. Kolstad, H. Mallmin, and J. Milbrink, 1998, Postoperative drainage of knee arthroplasty is not necessary: a randomized study of 90 patients: Acta Orthop.Scand., v. 69, no. 5, p. 475-478.

Altinel, L., K. C. Kose, and V. Ergan, 2006, Shed blood transfusion and its effect on postoperative fever: a comparative study: Arch.Orthop.Trauma Surg..

Alvarez, J. C., F. X. Santiveri, I. Ramos, E. Vela, L. Puig, and F. Escolano, 2008, Tranexamic acid reduces blood transfusion in total knee arthroplasty even when a blood conservation program is applied: Transfusion., v. 48, no. 3, p. 519-525.

Ares-Rodriguez, O., A. H. Martinez, A. H. Fernandez, E. Castellet, and A. N. Quilis, 2008, Survival curve and factors related to drainage during the first 24 h after total knee arthroplasty: Knee.Surg.Sports Traumatol.Arthrosc., v. 16, no. 6, p. 585-589.

Ashraf, T., S. Darmanis, and S. J. Krikler, 2001, Effectiveness of suction drainage after primary or revision total hip and total knee arthroplasty: Orthopedics, v. 24, no. 12, p. 1158-1160.

Barwell, J., G. Anderson, A. Hassan, and I. Rawlings, 1997, The effects of early tourniquet release during total knee arthroplasty: a prospective randomized double-blind study: J.Bone Joint Surg.Br., v. 79, no. 2, p. 265-268.

Beer, K. J., A. V. Lombardi, Jr., T. H. Mallory, and B. K. Vaughn, 1991, The efficacy of suction drains after routine total joint arthroplasty: J.Bone Joint Surg.Am., v. 73, no. 4, p. 584-587.

Bengtson, J. P., L. Backman, O. Stenqvist, M. Heideman, and A. Bengtsson, 1990, Complement activation and reinfusion of wound drainage blood: Anesthesiology, v. 73, no. 3, p. 376-380.

Benoni, G., H. Fredin, R. Knebel, and P. Nilsson, 2001, Blood conservation with tranexamic acid in total hip arthroplasty: a randomized, double-blind study in 40 primary operations: Acta Orthop.Scand., v. 72, no. 5, p. 442-448.

Benoni, G., and H. Fredin, 1997, Low- or high-vacuum drains in hip arthroplasty? A randomized study of 73 patients: Acta Orthop.Scand., v. 68, no. 2, p. 133-137.

Berman, A. T., D. Fabiano, S. J. Bosacco, and A. A. Weiss, 1990, Comparison between intermittent (spring-loaded) and continuous closed suction drainage of orthopedic wounds: a controlled clinical trial: Orthopedics, v. 13, no. 3, p. 309-314.

Berman, A. T., A. E. Geissele, and S. J. Bosacco, 1988, Blood loss with total knee arthroplasty: Clin.Orthop.Relat Res., no. 234, p. 137-138.

Breakwell, L. M., C. J. Getty, and P. Dobson, 2000, The efficacy of autologous blood transfusion in bilateral total knee arthroplasty: Knee., v. 7, no. 3, p. 145-147.

Brueggemann, P. M., J. K. Tucker, and P. Wilson, 1999, Intermittent clamping of suction drains in total hip replacement reduces postoperative blood loss: a randomized, controlled trial: J.Arthroplasty, v. 14, no. 4, p. 470-472.

Canty, S. J., G. J. Shepard, W. G. Ryan, and A. J. Banks, 2003, Do we practice evidence based medicine with regard to drain usage in knee arthroplasty? Results of a questionnaire of BASK members: Knee., v. 10, no. 4, p. 385-387.

Carless, P., A. Moxey, D. O'Connell, and D. Henry, 2004, Autologous transfusion techniques: a systematic review of their efficacy: Transfus.Med., v. 14, no. 2, p. 123-144.

Chang CW, Wu PT, and Yang CY, 2010, Blood loss after minimally invasive total knee arthroplasty: effects of imageless navigation.: Kaohsiung J Med Sci, v. 26, no. 5, p. 237-243.

Cheung, K. W., and K. H. Chiu, 2006, Effect of drain pressure in total knee arthroplasty: J.Orthop.Surg.(Hong.Kong.), v. 14, no. 2, p. 163-166.

Cid, J., and M. Lozano, 2005, Tranexamic acid reduces allogeneic red cell transfusions in patients undergoing total knee arthroplasty: results of a meta analysis of randomized controlled trials: Transfusion., v. 45, no. 8, p. 1302-1307.

Colwell, C. W., Jr., E. Beutler, C. West, M. E. Hardwick, and B. A. Morris, 2002, Erythrocyte viability in blood salvaged during total joint arthroplasty with cement: J.Bone Joint Surg.Am., v. 84-A, no. 1, p. 23-25.

Confalonieri, N., A. Manzotti, and C. Pullen, 2004, Is closed-suction drain necessary in unicompartmental knee replacement? A prospective randomised study: Knee., v. 11, no. 5, p. 399-402.

Corpe, R. S., J. W. Gallentine, T. R. Young, D. E. Steflik, E. J. Rectinwald, and S. Kusuma, 2000, Complications in total knee arthroplasty with and without surgical drainage: J.South.Orthop.Assoc., v. 9, no. 3, p. 207-212.

Crevoisier, X. M., P. Reber, and B. Noesberger, 1998, Is suction drainage necessary after total joint arthroplasty? A prospective study: Arch.Orthop.Trauma Surg., v. 117, no. 3, p. 121-124.

Cuenca, J., J. A. Garcia-Erce, M. Munoz, M. Izuel, A. A. Martinez, and A. Herrera, 2004, Patients with pertrochanteric hip fracture may benefit from preoperative intravenous iron therapy: a pilot study: Transfusion., v. 44, no. 10, p. 1447-1452.

Dalen, T., S. Skak, K. Thorsen, and H. Fredin, 1996, The efficacy and safety of blood reinfusion in avoiding homologous transfusion after total knee arthroplasty: Am.J.Knee.Surg., v. 9, no. 3, p. 117-120.

Dalen, T., L. A. Brostrom, and K. G. Engstrom, 1995, Cell quality of salvaged blood after total knee arthroplasty. Drain blood compared to venous blood in 32 patients: Acta Orthop.Scand., v. 66, no. 4, p. 329-333.

Dramis, A., and J. Plewes, 2006, Autologous blood transfusion after primary unilateral total knee replacement surgery: Acta Orthop.Belg., v. 72, no. 1, p. 15-17.

Drinkwater, C. J., and M. J. Neil, 1995, Optimal timing of wound drain removal following total joint arthroplasty: J.Arthroplasty, v. 10, no. 2, p. 185-189.

Dutka, J., T. Sorysz, and M. Urban, 2002, [Possibilities and profits of blood saving in orthopedics and traumatology]: Chir Narzadow.Ruchu.Ortop.Pol., v. 67, no. 1, p. 87-92.

Elwatidy, S., Z. Jamjoom, E. Elgamal, A. Zakaria, A. Turkistani, and A. El-Dawlatly, 1976, Efficacy and safety of prophylactic large dose of tranexamic acid in spine surgery: a prospective, randomized, double-blind, placebo-controlled study: Spine (Phila Pa, v. %2008 Nov 15;33, no. 24, p. 2577-2580.

Esler, C. N., C. Blakeway, and N. J. Fiddian, 2003, The use of a closed-suction drain in total knee arthroplasty. A prospective, randomised study: J.Bone Joint Surg.Br., v. 85, no. 2, p. 215-217.

Evans, R. L., H. E. Rubash, and S. A. Albrecht, 1993, The efficacy of postoperative autotransfusion in total joint arthroplasty: Orthop.Nurs., v. 12, no. 3, p. 11-18.

Faraj, A. A., and M. Raghuvanshi, 2006, The role of postoperative blood recovery for patients with femoral neck fracture: Acta Orthop.Belg., v. 72, no. 1, p. 11-14.

Fergusson, D. A. et al., 2008, A comparison of aprotinin and lysine analogues in high-risk cardiac surgery: N.Engl.J.Med., v. 358, no. 22, p. 2319-2331.

Gannon, D. M., A. V. Lombardi, Jr., T. H. Mallory, B. K. Vaughn, C. R. Finney, and S. Niemcryk, 1991, An evaluation of the efficacy of postoperative blood salvage after total joint arthroplasty. A prospective randomized trial: J.Arthroplasty, v. 6, no. 2, p. 109-114.

Garcia-Erce, J. A., S. Manuel, V, J. Cuenca, and P. Ortega, 2002, [Preoperative hemoglobin as the only predictive factor of transfusional needs in knee arthroplasty]: Rev.Esp.Anestesiol.Reanim., v. 49, no. 5, p. 254-260.

Gardner, A., N. Gibbs, C. Evans, and R. Bell, 2000, Relative cost of autologous red cell salvage versus allogeneic red cell transfusion during abdominal aortic aneurysm repair: Anaesth.Intensive Care., v. 28, no. 6, p. 646-649.

Gill, J. B., Y. Chin, A. Levin, and D. Feng, 2008, The use of antifibrinolytic agents in spine surgery. A meta-analysis: J.Bone Joint Surg.Am., v. 90, no. 11, p. 2399-2407.

Gonzalez, D., V, G. Slullitel, R. Vestri, F. Comba, M. Buttaro, and F. Piccaluga, 2004, No need for routine closed suction drainage in elective arthroplasty of the hip: a prospective randomized trial in 104 operations: Acta Orthop.Scand., v. 75, no. 1, p. 30-33.

Goodnough, L. T., A. Shander, J. L. Spivak, J. H. Waters, A. J. Friedman, J. L. Carson, E. M. Keating, T. Maddox, and R. Spence, 2005, Detection, evaluation, and management of anemia in the elective surgical patient: Anesth.Analg., v. 101, no. 6, p. 1858-1861.

Groh, G. I., P. K. Buchert, and W. C. Allen, 1990, A comparison of transfusion requirements after total knee arthroplasty using the Solcotrans autotransfusion system: J.Arthroplasty, v. 5, no. 3, p. 281-285.

Hadden, W. A., and A. G. McFarlane, 1990, A comparative study of closed-wound suction drainage vs. no drainage in total hip arthroplasty: J.Arthroplasty, v. 5 Suppl, p. S21-S24.

Hallstrom, B. R., and J. F. Steele, 1992, Postoperative course after total hip arthroplasty: wound drainage versus no drainage: Orthop.Rev., v. 21, no. 7, p. 847-851.

Han, C. D., and D. E. Shin, 1997, Postoperative blood salvage and reinfusion after total joint arthroplasty: J.Arthroplasty, v. 12, no. 5, p. 511-516.

Handel, M., D. Boluki, O. Loibl, J. Schaumburger, T. Kalteis, J. Matussek, and J. Grifka, 2006, [Postoperative autologous retransfusion of collected shed blood after total knee arthroplasty with the cell saver]: Z.Orthop.Ihre Grenzgeb., v. 144, no. 1, p. 97-101.

Heddle, N. M., W. T. Brox, L. N. Klama, L. L. Dickson, and M. N. Levine, 1992, A randomized trial on the efficacy of an autologous blood drainage and transfusion device in patients undergoing elective knee arthroplasty: Transfusion, v. 32, no. 8, p. 742-746.

Hendrych, J., 2006, [Use of post-operative drainage and auto-transfusion sets in total knee arthroplasty]: Acta Chir Orthop.Traumatol.Cech., v. 73, no. 1, p. 34-38.

Henry, D. A., A. J. Moxey, P. A. Carless, D. O'Connell, B. McClelland, K. M. Henderson, K. Sly, A. Laupacis, and D. Fergusson, 2001, Anti-fibrinolytic use for minimising perioperative allogeneic blood transfusion: Cochrane Database.Syst.Rev., no. 1, p. CD001886.

Hersekli, M. A., S. Akpinar, G. Ozkoc, M. Ozalay, M. Uysal, N. Cesur, and R. N. Tandogan, 2004, The timing of tourniquet release and its influence on blood loss after total knee arthroplasty: Int.Orthop., v. 28, no. 3, p. 138-141.

Hinarejos, P., M. Corrales, A. Matamalas, E. Bisbe, and E. Caceres, 2009, Computer-assisted surgery can reduce blood loss after total knee arthroplasty: Knee.Surg Sports Traumatol.Arthrosc., v. 17, no. 4, p. 356-360.

Jackson, B. R., J. Umlas, and J. P. AuBuchon, 2000, The cost-effectiveness of postoperative recovery of RBCs in preventing transfusion-associated virus transmission after joint arthroplasty: Transfusion, v. 40, no. 9, p. 1063-1066.

Jenny, J. Y., C. Boeri, and S. Lafare, 2001, No drainage does not increase complication risk after total knee prosthesis implantation: a prospective, comparative, randomized study: Knee.Surg.Sports Traumatol.Arthrosc., v. 9, no. 5, p. 299-301.

Johansson, T., M. Engquist, L. G. Pettersson, and B. Lisander, 2005a, Blood loss after total hip replacement: a prospective randomized study between wound compression and drainage: J.Arthroplasty, v. 20, no. 8, p. 967-971.

Johansson, T., L. G. Pettersson, and B. Lisander, 2005b, Tranexamic acid in total hip arthroplasty saves blood and money: a randomized, double-blind study in 100 patients: Acta Orthop., v. 76, no. 3, p. 314-319.

Jones, H. W., L. Savage, C. White, R. Goddard, H. Lumley, F. Kashif, and K. Gurusany, 2004, Postoperative autologous blood salvage drains--are they useful in primary uncemented hip and knee arthroplasty? A prospective study of 186 cases: Acta Orthop.Belg., v. 70, no. 5, p. 466-473.

Kagoma, Y. K., M. A. Crowther, J. Douketis, M. Bhandari, J. Eikelboom, and W. Lim, 2009, Use of antifibrinolytic therapy to reduce transfusion in patients undergoing orthopedic surgery: a systematic review of randomized trials: Thromb.Res., v. 123, no. 5, p. 687-696.

Kalairajah, Y., D. Simpson, A. J. Cossey, G. M. Verrall, and A. J. Spriggins, 2005, Blood loss after total knee replacement: effects of computer-assisted surgery: J.Bone Joint Surg.Br., v. 87, no. 11, p. 1480-1482.

Kao, F. C., K. Y. Hsu, H. N. Shih, C. Y. Cheng, Y. H. Tsai, and R. W. Hsu, 2002, Arthroscopic extraction of a drainage tube: solution for a troublesome problem: Arthroscopy, v. 18, no. 7, p. E36.

Kiely, N., M. Hockings, and A. Gambhir, 2001, Does temporary clamping of drains following knee arthroplasty reduce blood loss? A randomised controlled trial: Knee., v. 8, no. 4, p. 325-327.

Kim, Y. H., S. H. Cho, and R. S. Kim, 1998, Drainage versus nondrainage in simultaneous bilateral total knee arthroplasties: Clin.Orthop.Relat Res., no. 347, p. 188-193.

Kirschner, P., H. Romer, and H. P. Werner, 1989, [Complications of Redon drainage following hip joint replacement operations--an analysis of the causes]: Unfallchirurgie, v. 15, no. 1, p. 24-31.

Ko, P. S., M. K. Tio, Y. K. Tang, W. L. Tsang, and J. J. Lam, 2003, Sealing the intramedullary femoral canal with autologous bone plug in total knee arthroplasty: J.Arthroplasty, v. 18, no. 1, p. 6-9.

Kobrinsky, N. L., R. M. Letts, L. R. Patel, E. D. Israels, R. C. Monson, N. Schwetz, and M. S. Cheang, 1987, 1-Desamino-8-D-arginine vasopressin (desmopressin) decreases operative blood loss in patients having Harrington rod spinal fusion surgery. A randomized, double-blinded, controlled trial: Ann.Intern.Med., v. 107, no. 4, p. 446-450.

Kourtzis, N., D. Pafilas, and G. Kasimatis, 2004, Blood saving protocol in elective total knee arthroplasty: Am.J.Surg., v. 187, no. 2, p. 261-267.

Kristensen, P. W., L. S. Sorensen, and H. C. Thyregod, 1992, Autotransfusion of drainage blood in arthroplasty. A prospective, controlled study of 31 operations: Acta Orthop.Scand., v. 63, no. 4, p. 377-380.

Kristiansson, M., M. Soop, L. Saraste, K. G. Sundqvist, A. M. Suontaka, and M. Blomback, 1995, Cytokine and coagulation characteristics of retrieved blood after arthroplasty: Intensive Care Med., v. 21, no. 12, p. 989-995.

Kumar, S., S. Penematsa, and S. Parekh, 2006, Are drains required following a routine primary total joint arthroplasty?: Int.Orthop..

Kumar, N., J. Saleh, E. Gardiner, V. G. Devadoss, and F. R. Howell, 2000, Plugging the intramedullary canal of the femur in total knee arthroplasty: reduction in postoperative blood loss: J.Arthroplasty, v. 15, no. 7, p. 947-949.

Labek, G., and N. Bohler, 1998, [Blood transfusion in total hip endoprosthesis operations in relation to Redon drainage and pressure bandages. An innovation in surgical method]: Z.Orthop.Ihre Grenzgeb., v. 136, no. 5, p. 433-438.

Laupacis, A., and D. Fergusson, 1998, Erythropoietin to minimize perioperative blood transfusion: a systematic review of randomized trials. The International Study of Peri-operative Transfusion (ISPOT) Investigators: Transfus.Med., v. 8, no. 4, p. 309-317.

Leeman, M. F., M. L. Costa, E. Costello, and D. Edwards, 2006, Timing of re-transfusion drain removal following total knee replacement: Ann.R.Coll.Surg.Engl., v. 88, no. 2, p. 134-135.

Lotke, P. A., V. J. Faralli, E. M. Orenstein, and M. L. Ecker, 1991, Blood loss after total knee replacement. Effects of tourniquet release and continuous passive motion: J.Bone Joint Surg.Am., v. 73, no. 7, p. 1037-1040.

Lozano, M. et al., 2008, Effectiveness and safety of tranexamic acid administration during total knee arthroplasty: Vox Sang., v. 95, no. 1, p. 39-44.

Mac, H. L., M. A. Reynolds, J. Treston-Aurand, and J. A. Henke, 1993, Comparison of autoreinfusion and standard drainage systems in total joint arthroplasty patients: Orthop.Nurs., v. 12, no. 3, p. 19-25.

Majkowski, R. S., I. C. Currie, and J. H. Newman, 1991, Postoperative collection and reinfusion of autologous blood in total knee arthroplasty: Ann.R.Coll.Surg.Engl., v. 73, no. 6, p. 381-384.

Mangano, D. T., I. C. Tudor, and C. Dietzel, 2006, The risk associated with aprotinin in cardiac surgery: N.Engl.J.Med., v. 354, no. 4, p. 353-365.

Marmor, L., 1990, Suction drainage tube entrapment in total knee arthroplasty: Clin.Orthop.Relat Res., no. 259, p. 157-159.

Martin, A., M. Prenn, T. Spiegel, C. Sukopp, and S. A. von, 2004, [Relevance of wound drainage in total knee arthroplasty--a prospective comparative study]: Z.Orthop.Ihre Grenzgeb., v. 142, no. 1, p. 46-50

Martin, J. W., L. A. Whiteside, M. T. Milliano, and M. E. Reedy, 1992, Postoperative blood retrieval and transfusion in cementless total knee arthroplasty: J.Arthroplasty, v. 7, no. 2, p. 205-210.

Mauerhan, D. R., D. Nussman, J. G. Mokris, and W. B. Beaver, 1993, Effect of postoperative reinfusion systems on hemoglobin levels in primary total hip and total knee arthroplasties. A prospective randomized study: J.Arthroplasty, v. 8, no. 5, p. 523-527.

Mengal, B., J. Aebi, A. Rodriguez, and R. Lemaire, 2001, [A prospective randomized study of wound drainage versus non-drainage in primary total hip or knee arthroplasty]: Rev.Chir Orthop.Reparatrice Appar.Mot., v. 87, no. 1, p. 29-39.

Minnema, B., M. Vearncombe, A. Augustin, J. Gollish, and A. E. Simor, 2004, Risk factors for surgical-site infection following primary total knee arthroplasty: Infect.Control Hosp.Epidemiol., v. 25, no. 6, p. 477-480.

Munoz, M., A. Cobos, A. Campos, D. Ariza, E. Munoz, and A. Gomez, 2006, Post-operative unwashed shed blood transfusion does not modify the cellular immune response to surgery for total knee replacement: Acta Anaesthesiol.Scand., v. 50, no. 4, p. 443-450.

Munoz, M., D. Ariza, M. J. Garceran, A. Gomez, and A. Campos, 2005a, Benefits of postoperative shed blood reinfusion in patients undergoing unilateral total knee replacement: Arch.Orthop.Trauma Surg., v. 125, no. 6, p. 385-389.

Munoz, M., A. Cobos, A. Campos, D. Ariza, E. Munoz, and A. Gomez, 2005b, Impact of postoperative shed blood transfusion, with or without leucocyte reduction, on acute-phase response to surgery for total knee replacement: Acta Anaesthesiol.Scand., v. 49, no. 8, p. 1182-1190.

Niskanen, R. O., O. L. Korkala, J. Haapala, H. O. Kuokkanen, J. P. Kaukonen, and S. A. Salo, 2000, Drainage is of no use in primary uncomplicated cemented hip and knee arthroplasty for osteoarthritis: a prospective randomized study: J.Arthroplasty, v. 15, no. 5, p. 567-569.

Noain, E., W. P. Rodriguez, J. J. Sanchez Villares, F. J. Artazcoz, M. J. Martinez de, and P. J. Lasanta, 2005, [Perioperative blood management in primary total knee arthroplasty]: An.Sist.Sanit.Navar., v. 28, no. 2, p. 189-196.

Okuyama, M., K. Ikeda, T. Shibata, Y. Tsukahara, M. Kitada, and T. Shimano, 2005, Preoperative iron supplementation and intraoperative transfusion during colorectal cancer surgery: Surg.Today., v. 35, no. 1, p. 36-40.

Ovadia, D., E. Luger, J. Bickels, A. Menachem, and S. Dekel, 1997, Efficacy of closed wound drainage after total joint arthroplasty. A prospective randomized study: J.Arthroplasty, v. 12, no. 3, p. 317-321.

Padala, P. R., E. Rouholamin, and R. L. Mehta, 2004, The role of drains and tourniquets in primary total knee replacement: a comparative study of TKR performed with drains and tourniquet versus no drains and adrenaline and saline infiltration: J.Knee.Surg., v. 17, no. 1, p. 24-27.

Parker, M. J., C. P. Roberts, and D. Hay, 2004, Closed suction drainage for hip and knee arthroplasty. A meta-analysis: J.Bone Joint Surg.Am., v. 86-A, no. 6, p. 1146-1152.

Pola, E., P. Papaleo, A. Santoliquido, G. Gasparini, L. Aulisa, and S. E. De, 2004, Clinical factors associated with an increased risk of perioperative blood transfusion in nonanemic patients undergoing total hip arthroplasty: J.Bone Joint Surg.Am., v. 86-A, no. 1, p. 57-61.

Porteous, A. J., and R. J. Bartlett, 2003, Post-operative drainage after cemented, hybrid and uncemented total knee replacement: Knee., v. 10, no. 4, p. 371-374.

Prasad, N., V. Padmanabhan, and A. Mullaji, 2005, Comparison between two methods of drain clamping after total knee arthroplasty: Arch.Orthop.Trauma Surg., v. 125, no. 6, p. 381-384.

Raut, V. V., M. H. Stone, and B. M. Wroblewski, 1993, Reduction of postoperative blood loss after press-fit condylar knee arthroplasty with use of a femoral intramedullary plug: J.Bone Joint Surg.Am., v. 75, no. 9, p. 1356-1357.

Reize, P., D. Endele, M. Rudert, and N. Wulker, 2006, [Postoperative autologous transfusion from blood drainage after total hip joint arthroplasty--how much value is really there?]: Z.Orthop.Ihre Grenzgeb., v. 144, no. 4, p. 400-404.

Rosencher, N., H. E. Kerkkamp, G. Macheras, L. M. Munuera, G. Menichella, D. M. Barton, S. Cremers, and I. L. Abraham, 2003, Orthopedic Surgery Transfusion Hemoglobin European Overview (OSTHEO) study: blood management in elective knee and hip arthroplasty in Europe: Transfusion., v. 43, no. 4, p. 459-469.

Rowe, S. M., T. R. Yoon, Y. S. Kim, and G. H. Lee, 1993, Hemovac drainage after hip arthroplasty: Int.Orthop., v. 17, no. 4, p. 238-240.

Roy, N., M. Smith, M. Anwar, and C. Elsworth, 2006, Delayed release of drain in total knee replacement reduces blood loss. A prospective randomised study: Acta Orthop.Belg., v. 72, no. 1, p. 34-38.

Saleh, K., M. Olson, S. Resig, B. Bershadsky, M. Kuskowski, T. Gioe, H. Robinson, R. Schmidt, and E. McElfresh, 2002, Predictors of wound infection in hip and knee joint replacement: results from a 20 year surveillance program: J.Orthop.Res., v. 20, no. 3, p. 506-515.

Schmitt, S., and F. Weyand, 1997, [Correlation between postoperative duration of Redon drainage and wound healing. A study of 150 patients with total endoprosthetic hip replacement]: Unfallchirurgie, v. 23, no. 5, p. 205-209.

Sehat, K. R., R. Evans, and J. H. Newman, 2000, How much blood is really lost in total knee arthroplasty?. Correct blood loss management should take hidden loss into account: Knee., v. 7, no. 3, p. 151-155.

Senthil, K. G., O. A. Von Arx, and J. L. Pozo, 2005, Rate of blood loss over 48 hours following total knee replacement: Knee., v. 12, no. 4, p. 307-309.

Seyfert, C., K. Schulz, and G. Pap, 2002, [The influence of the drain suction in knee arthroplasty]: Zentralbl.Chir, v. 127, no. 10, p. 886-889.

Shander, A., K. Knight, R. Thurer, J. Adamson, and R. Spence, 2004, Prevalence and outcomes of anemia in surgery: a systematic review of the literature: Am.J.Med., v. 116 Suppl 7A:58S-69S., p. 58S-69S.

Shen, P. C., I. M. Jou, Y. T. Lin, K. A. Lai, C. Y. Yang, and T. C. Chern, 2005, Comparison between 4-hour clamping drainage and nonclamping drainage after total knee arthroplasty: J.Arthroplasty, v. 20, no. 7, p. 909-913.

Simpson, M. B., K. P. Murphy, H. G. Chambers, and A. L. Bucknell, 1994, The effect of postoperative wound drainage reinfusion in reducing the need for blood transfusions in elective total joint arthroplasty; a prospective, randomized study: Orthopedics, v. 17, no. 2, p. 133-137.

Sinardi, D., A. Marino, S. Chillemi, M. Irrera, G. Labruto, and E. Mondello, 2005, Composition of the blood sampled from surgical drainage after joint arthroplasty: quality of return: Transfusion, v. 45, no. 2, p. 202-207.

Slagis, S. V., J. B. Benjamin, R. G. Volz, and G. F. Giordano, 1991, Postoperative blood salvage in total hip and knee arthroplasty. A randomised controlled trial: J.Bone Joint Surg.Br., v. 73, no. 4, p. 591-594.

Strumper, D., E. W. Weber, S. Gielen-Wijffels, D. R. Van, S. Bulstra, R. Slappendel, M. E. Durieux, and M. A. Marcus, 2004, Clinical efficacy of postoperative autologous transfusion of filtered shed blood in hip and knee arthroplasty: Transfusion, v. 44, no. 11, p. 1567-1571.

Thomas, D., K. Wareham, D. Cohen, and H. Hutchings, 2001, Autologous blood transfusion in total knee replacement surgery: Br.J.Anaesth., v. 86, no. 5, p. 669-673.

Trammell, T. R., D. Fisher, F. R. Brueckmann, and N. Haines, 1991, Closed-wound drainage systems. The Solcotrans Plus versus the Stryker-CBC ConstaVAC: Orthop.Rev., v. 20, no. 6, p. 536-542.

Tsumara, N., S. Yoshiya, T. Chin, R. Shiba, K. Kohso, and M. Doita, 2006, A prospective comparison of clamping the drain or post-operative salvage of blood in reducing blood loss after total knee arthroplasty: J.Bone Joint Surg.Br., v. 88, no. 1, p. 49-53.

Turajane T, Larbpaiboonpong V, Kongtharvonskul J, and Maungsiri S, 2009, Results of computer assisted mini-incision subvastus approach for total knee arthroplasty.: J Med Assoc Thai, v. 92, no. s6, p. s51-s58.

Umlas, J., R. R. Foster, S. A. Dalal, S. M. O'Leary, L. Garcia, and M. S. Kruskall, 1994, Red cell loss following orthopedic surgery: the case against postoperative blood salvage: Transfusion, v. 34, no. 5, p. 402-406.

Walmsley, P. J., M. B. Kelly, R. M. Hill, and I. Brenkel, 2005, A prospective, randomised, controlled trial of the use of drains in total hip arthroplasty: J.Bone Joint Surg.Br., v. 87, no. 10, p. 1397-1401.

Weinrauch, P., 2005, Diagnostic value of routine drain tip culture in primary joint arthroplasty: ANZ.J.Surg., v. 75, no. 10, p. 887-888.

Widman, J., H. Jacobsson, S. A. Larsson, and J. Isacson, 2002, No effect of drains on the postoperative hematoma volume in hip replacement surgery: a randomized study using scintigraphy: Acta Orthop.Scand., v. 73, no. 6, p. 625-629.

Willemen, D., J. Paul, S. H. White, and D. W. Crook, 1991, Closed suction drainage following knee arthroplasty. Effectiveness and risks: Clin.Orthop.Relat Res., no. 264, p. 232-234.

Woda, R., and J. E. Tetzlaff, 1992, Upper airway oedema following autologous blood transfusion from a wound drainage system: Can.J.Anaesth., v. 39, no. 3, p. 290-292.

Wojan, M., R. Scholz, G. von Salis-Soglio, M. Schmidt, and A. Wild, 2005, [Retransfusion of unwashed drainage blood after total hip and knee arthroplasty]: Biomed.Tech.(Berl), v. 50, no. 11, p. 355-360.

Wollinsky, K. H., M. Oethinger, M. Buchele, P. Kluger, W. Puhl, and H. H. Mehrkens, 1997, Autotransfusion--bacterial contamination during hip arthroplasty and efficacy of cefuroxime prophylaxis. A randomized controlled study of 40 patients: Acta Orthop.Scand., v. 68, no. 3, p. 225-230.

Xenakis, T. A., K. N. Malizos, Z. Dailiana, T. Koukoubis, E. Zervou, C. Golegou, and P. N. Soucacos, 1997, Blood salvage after total hip and total knee arthroplasty: Acta Orthop.Scand.Suppl, v. 275, p. 135-138.

Zamora-Navas, P., F. Collado-Torres, and l. T.-S. de, 1999, Closed suction drainage after knee arthroplasty. A prospective study of the effectiveness of the operation and of bacterial contamination: Acta Orthop.Belg., v. 65, no. 1, p. 44-47.

Zufferey, P., F. Merquiol, S. Laporte, H. Decousus, P. Mismetti, C. Auboyer, C. M. Samama, and S. Molliex, 2006, Do antifibrinolytics reduce allogeneic blood transfusion in orthopedic surgery?: Anesthesiology., v. 105, no. 5, p. 1034-1046.

8

Acoustic Emission Studies in Hip Arthroplasty – Peak Stress Impact *In Vitro* Cemented Prosthesis

N. Gueiral and E. Nogueira
CIETI - Centre of Innovation in Engineering and Industrial Technology,
ISEP - School of Engineering, Polytechnic of Porto
Portugal

1. Introduction

Engineering has a very important role in the development of non-destructive monitoring of orthopaedical systems allowing the evaluation of its integrity.
Sir John Charnley revolutionized the field of joint arthroplasty in the 1960s with the development of the total hip replacement. He replaced the diseased hip joint with a steel femoral component and a plastic acetabular socket cup combination, both fixed into the bone using a self-curing acrylic cement, polymethylmethacrylate (PMMA) (Browne et al, 2005). That way, he has restored some of the most problematic joints in the human body.
The placement of the metal implant in the channel open in the femoral bone without using cement or by mechanical attack, called a non cemented arthroplasty, came into use in an effort to solve the problem.
A study about prostheses reviews, between 1979 and 2005, show that's were higher in non-cemented prosthesis, leading to studies on new forms of interface bone/metal. The growth of cemented arthroplasties has been observed since 2005.
By Ramos (Ramos et al, 2005), cemented arthroplasty is one of the most successful surgical techniques in orthopaedics. However, the cemented prosthesis has a tendency to fray during the time of their life due to stress and fatigue of the cement material leading to it cracking.
The growing importance of different Total Hip Arthroplasty (THA) studies is due to increased life expectancy of the population and its social and clinical relevance. Interdisciplinary THA studies such as: biomechanics (Bergmann et al, 2001; Fonseca et al, 2010; Nabais, 2006; Ramos et al, 2005; Stolk et al, 2006; Teixeira et al, 2008; Vieira, 2004); finite element analysis (Bachtar et al, 2006; Nizam Ahmad et al, 2006; Ridzwan et al, 2006) and acoustic emission monitoring (Browne et al, 2005; Cristofolini et al, 2003; Davies et al, 1996; Franke et al, 2004; Gueiral, 2008; Qi et al, 2005; Qi, 2000; Rowland et al, 2004) have been published.
Research has been done to improve the performance of artificial implants, addressing factors such as geometry, materials, cements, and other surgical techniques that directly or indirectly, might influence the performance and success of cemented arthroplasty.
Although the lifetime of a THA is between 10 and 15 years, there are factors that lead to loss of prosthesis such as the separation of the femoral prosthesis due to the splitting of connection between the implant/cement and cement/bone. The human body responds through its immune system causing inflammation and pain in osseous structure, which in most cases leads to the replacement of the prosthesis.

One the mechanisms of failure in total hip arthroplasty cemented prosthesis is the cement fatigue. So it becomes relevant to perform the monitoring integrity of these structure types (Gueiral, 2008).
It's important to have a technical solution capably reliable to indicate the time to have a replacement surgery. In this context the Acoustic Emission (AE) has a major role because it allows to determine and analyze cracks, microcracks and defects which can lead to delamination of cement and/or rupture of the connection implant/bone (Browne et al, 2005). The monitoring of the structural integrity of cement and interfaces (implant and bone) by detection of acoustic emission waves, represents a significant advance in the assessment and inspection of the performance of cemented prosthesis, in relation to usual practice, which is the patient operation for prosthesis inspection.
It is in this context that fits the presented work on the AE acquisition and signal processing obtained *in vitro* fatigue testing in the femoral component, being of great importance to identify the location of the sources that originates it.
AE is certainly the most promissory method for orthopaedic diagnostic not only *in vivo* but also *in vitro*. This diagnostic preferably should include non-destructive methods without intrusion or radiation for the patient (Franke et al, 2004). AE studies have been done since 1990 in THA with different issues of evaluation of fixation parameters of prostheses, cement fatigue and others. The first studies *in vitro* of the prostheses metal/cement interface integrity with acoustic emission and ultrasound have been done in 1996 (Davies et al, 1996). Acrylics and synthetic cement studies appear in 2000 (Qi, 2000).
The results of different THA biomechanical simulation studies identified areas in an implant-cement and cement-bone that are subjected to greater stresses and strains (Fonseca et al, 2010; Nabais, 2006; Prendergast et al, 1989; Stolk et al, 2004). The AE technique is important to observe the impact of stress and strain, translated into microcracks, in the aforementioned areas in cemented hip prostheses as in interfaces implant-cement and cement-bone. So, AE monitoring better allows to understand the orthopaedic construction mechanisms and in focusing other mechanisms that were not detected by conventional ways.
According to Browne (Browne et al, 2005), signals of AE allows to study the fatigue behaviour of the cement that holds the implant to the bone in orthopaedic implants. With the fatigue test the mechanisms leading to the failure of an hip prosthesis are characterized.
The second part of this work characterizes the Acoustic Emission phenomena, considering the origin and propagation, parameters and detection of AE signals as well as modelling studies. The third part, describes the methods of AE sources location, in particular the 3D methods which are needed to study the hip arthroplasty *in vitro*. The fourth part describes *in vitro* experimental tests of femoral components with cemented prostheses. The last part contains the conclusions and final remarks.

2. Acoustic emission

2.1 AE origin and propagation

Acoustic Emission belongs to the class of phenomena where transient elastic waves arising in the material are generated by the rapid release of small amounts of energy of the material (ASTM E1316, 2007).
These elastic waves are developed from an epicentre, commonly called AE source, and propagated indefinitely in all directions throughout the material and according to their characteristics will be attenuated until the total loss. We can liken the phenomenon to an earthquake, with due consideration of materials and proportions.

Acoustic emission wave propagation out of the source it generated over the structure is always a complex mechanical puzzle. Waves of different types propagate at different velocities and with different oscillation directions. Moreover, passing through a medium, waves undergo multiple changes due to attenuation, dispersion, diffraction, scattering, reflection from boundaries, interaction with reflections and other (Muravin, 2009).
The attenuation refers to the decrease in AE amplitude as a stress wave propagates along a structure due to energy loss mechanisms, from dispersion, diffraction or scattering.
The AE wave dispersion is caused by the frequency dependence of the speed of waves. Sound waves are composed of different frequencies hence for different frequency spectrums there are distint wave' speeds.
The spreading or bending of waves passing through an aperture or around the edge of a barrier is called difraction.
Scattering is the dispersion, deflection of waves when encounter a discontinuity in the material such as holes, sharp edges, cracks inclusions, etc.
Depending on the properties of each material, the response to the phenomenon will be different for external requests, such efforts, torsions, distensions and contractions.
One base theory to AE propagation is called Modal Acoustic Emission (MAE). It begins with the assumption that the AE waves are mechanical in nature, treating them as such. The general theory of wave propagation in solid media, says that AE waves propagate through a structure in a variety of modes with dispersion and attenuation characteristics. The separation of these modes in sensors can make possible to extract accurate information about the source that produces the wave. According to Jiao (Jiao et al, 2004) AE signals are in fact dispersive elastic waves.
The AE sources are usually manufacturing defects, minor cuts resulting from a defective welding, delamination, displacements, cracks, crevices and others. These AE sources only produce AE signals when subjected to new stresses, taking into account the Kaiser and/or Felicity effect. Thus, a possible source in the existing AE first time it is placed under the inspection sensors AE does not give any response because the source is asleep, i.e., need of higher efforts to generate new AE signals.
The number of AE sources in a particular structure depends largely on type of material that constitutes the structure. If the material is glass, ceramic or metal, the number of AE sources is low due to the crystalline structure of the material and the signal is well defined with relatively high amplitudes. If the material is concrete or composite it will increase the number of AE sources. On concrete, usually due to the porosity of the mortar there are a lot of AE sources whereas in composites these increase exponentially because just a short blow of the composite filament is enough to generate a new AE source. However, the amplitude is much lower compared with the AE sources in ceramic or glass.

2.2 AE signals: parameters and detection

Generally there are two types of AE signals which are represented in figure 1. One of them, a continuous signal is a qualitative description of the sustained signal produced by time-overlapping signals, figure 1a). The other one, a burst signal is a qualitative description of the discrete signal's related to individual emission events occurring within the material, figure 1b).
Each type of signal is related to the material under study/stretched. Porous materials or composites produce continuous AE signals. Ceramic or metallic materials produce signals AE burst.

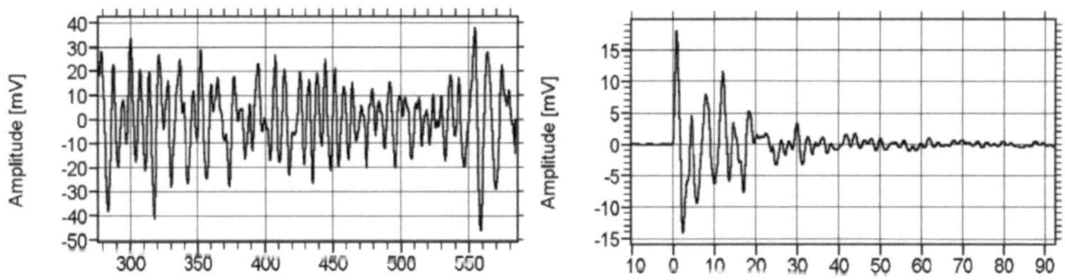

(a) Continuous signal. (b) Burst signal

Fig. 1. "AE Testing Fundamentals, Equipment, Applications" , H. Vallen

The electrical signal identified as an AE signal is generated by fracture phenomena. Therefore characteristics of AE parameters have been studied to infer fracture or physical phenomena. Signal parameters most widely used are explained from definitions (ISO 12716 2001):

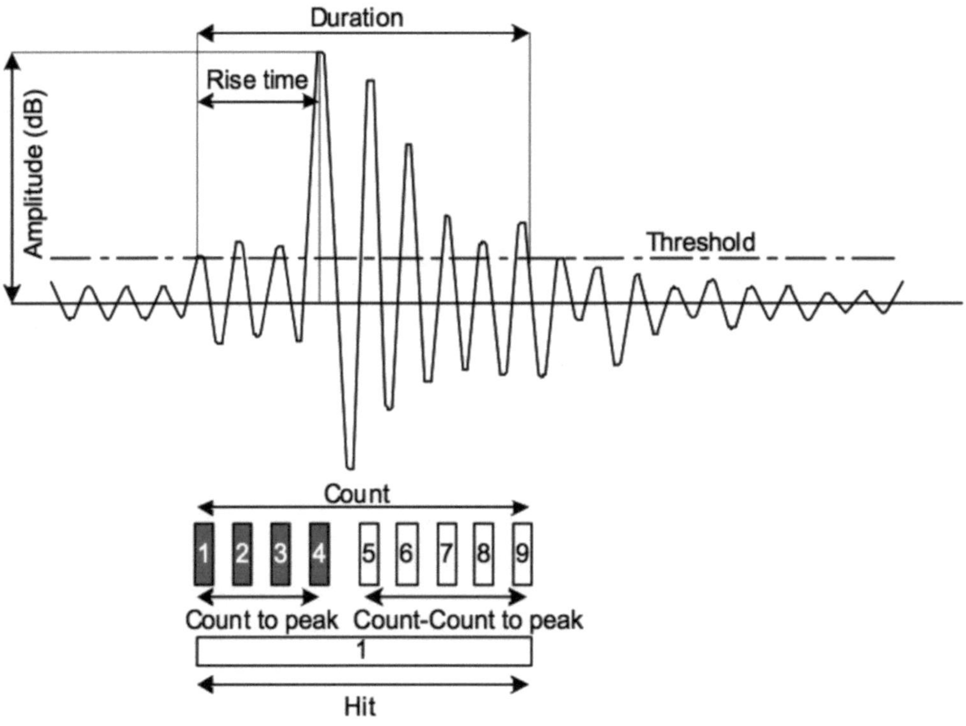

Fig. 2. Conventional AE signal features (Shiotani, 2008)

- *Hit:* a signal that exceeds the threshold and causes a system channel to accumulate data. It is frequently used to show the AE activity with counted number for a period (rate) or accumulated numbers. In figure 2, one waveform correspond one "hit".
- *Count/ring-down count/emission count:* the number of times within the duration, where one signal (waveform) exceeds a present threshold. In figure 2, nine counts are observed. "Count" is also employed to quantify the AE activity as well as "hit". It is noted

that "counts" depend strongly on the employed threshold and the operating frequency. Sometimes, counts between the triggering time over the threshold and the peak amplitude is referred to as "Counts to Peak", which is equal to four in figure 2.

- *Amplitude:* a peak voltage of the signal waveform is usually assigned. Amplitudes are expressed on a decibel scale instead of linear scale where $1\mu V$ at the sensor is defined as 0dB AE. The amplitude is closely related to the magnitude of source event. As mentioned the AE signals are detected on the basis of the voltage threshold, the amplitude is also important parameter to determine the system's detectability. Generally the detected amplitude shall be understood as the value does not represent the emission-source but the sensor response after losing the energy due to propagation. The magnitude of amplitude in each signal has been often analyzed in relation with frequency distribution.
- *Duration:* a time interval between the triggered time of one AE signal (waveform) and the time of disappearance is assigned. The duration, which depends on source magnitude and noise filtering is expressed generally in microseconds.
- *Rise time:* a time interval between the triggering time of AE signal and the time of the peak amplitude is assigned. The rise time is closely related to the source-time function, and applied to classify the type of fracture or eliminate noise signals.
- *Energy:* definitions of energies are different in AE system suppliers, but it is generally defined as a measured area under the rectified signal envelope. The energy is preferred to interpret the magnitude of source event over counts because it is sensitive to the amplitude as well as the duration, and less dependent on the voltage threshold and operating frequencies.

Before addressing specifically the process of detecting AE sources, it is of particular importance to observe the concepts and specifics of the AE system detection.
AE waves are detected by sensors, which convert dynamic motions at the surface of a material into electrical signals. Because AE signals are weak, they are normally amplified. The signal-to-noise ratio of equipments shall be low, and the amplifiers often provide more than 1000 times gain. Normally is set 100 times or so. The band-pass filter is successfully employed to eliminate the noises. In engineering materials, the band width from several kHz to several 100 kHz or 1 MHz is recommended in the measurement (Ohtsu, 2008).
AE signals emerge rapidly and randomly. As a result, the discrimination of AE signals from running waves is the first step for analyzing AE activity. To this end, the voltage threshold of AE wave, which is equivalent to a voltage level on an electronic comparator, is set. Then, the signals which exceed the voltage threshold are identified as AE signals (Shiotani, 2008).
The main purpose of AE sensors is to detect stress waves motion that cause a local dynamic material displacement and convert this displacement to an electrical signal. AE sensors are typically piezoelectric sensors with elements maid of special ceramic elements like lead zirconate titanate (PZT). Mechanical strain of a piezo element generates an electric signal. Besides PZT sensors, new types of sensors are under development. Other types of sensors include between others capacitive transducers and laser interferometers. Typical frequency range in AE applications varies between 20 kHz and 1 MHz. Sensors may have internally installed a preamplifier (integral sensors).
Selection of a specific sensor depends on the application and type of flaws to be revealed. There are two qualitative types of sensor according to their frequency response: ressonant and wideband sensors. Thickness of piezoelectric element defines the ressonance frequency of sensor. Diameter defines the area over which the sensor averages surface motion.

Another important property of AE sensors includes Curie Point, the temperature under which piezoelectric element loses permanently its piezoelectric properties. Curie temperature varies for different ceramics from 120 to $400C^o$. There are ceramics with over $1200C^o$ Curie temperature (Muravin, 2009).

2.3 AE process modelling

To understand the signals obtained by AE sensors it is necessary to model mathematically the whole AE process. The ability to accurately model acoustic emission process offers significant potential to improve the interpretation of AE data.

Applications of such models include the determination of optimal placement of sensors in an AE test, the scaling of AE results from laboratory coupons to structures of practical interest, the calibration of transducers, identify source mechanisms and insight into inversion of AE data to eliminate extraneous noise.

Several models of acoustic emission process, taking into account the application and the materials, are referred following. Source modelling (Hora, 2010); physicomathematical model of generation of AE (Belikov, 2008; 2010); crack grouth finite element modelling in plate structures (Wilcox et al, 2007); micromechanical model of microcrack formation in heterogeneous materials (Nosov et al, 2003) and AE waveforms modelling in thin plates (Prosser et al, 1998).

In the following text a more detailed description of these studies which are the best suited to the AE process of THA is made in *in vitro* system which consists of a femoral component with multiple layers of different materials (glass fiber reinforced - cortical bone, polyurethane foam - trabecular bone, cement and metal implant).

Hora (Hora, 2010) presented an acoustic emission source modelling by means of finite element method system COMSOL Multi-physics. Growth of cracks is an important AE source, and the study of the waves that they generate has played a major role in the understanding of the inner structure of the materials and the nature of the AE source. Energy release during growth of crack can be simulated by the concentrated force or concentrated force moment.

The kinds of the acoustic emission sources used in this paper, were the spatially concentrated force and concentrated dipole. The simplest problem corresponds to a spatially concentrated force (or point source) directed along one of the coordinate axes. The starting point is the scalar wave equation with a source term, which is first solved for an impulsive source, in which case the solution is known as Green's function for the problem. Then the Helmholtz decomposition theorem is used to reduce the solution of the elastic wave equation to the solution of two simpler ones.

This study aims to choose the best model of concentrated force and dipole. These models will be used to calculate the surface displacements in real steel constructions for the purpose of comparing that with surface displacements obtained by non destructive testing.

Belikov (Belikov, 2008) presented a physicomathematical model of generation of AE that is based on a system of average equations of heat and mass transfer in heterogeneous media (HM). The equation (1) describes the propagation of longitudinal and transverse waves in an HM consisting of a certain finite number of phases (Belikov, 2008; 2010). In the following expression ν represents the frequency that corresponds to vibrations of the interphase surface between two phases.

$$\nu = \sqrt{\frac{\Delta\tilde{\alpha}\Omega}{\rho\tilde{L}}} \quad (1)$$

$\Delta\tilde{\alpha}$ is the average difference of the elastic stresses at the interface between arbitrary two phases of the HM. Ω is the specific internal surface that corresponds to the internal surface S which separates the two phases, $\tilde{L}$ is the vibration amplitude of the interphase surface that corresponds to the contact between the two phases and ρ is the HM density.
The results of solving the direct problem, that is, constructing the AF spectrum using the relation of the AE frequency to the structural characteristics of a medium, allow to solve the inverse problem. This make the reconstruction of the characteristics of a damaged solid, including primarily the crack size distribution function using the observed amplitude - frequency spectrum of the acoustic emission. This algorithm was proposed by Belikov (Belikov, 2010).
A micromechanical model of acoustic emission of heterogeneous materials is presented by Nosov (Nosov et al, 2003). The model describes acoustic emission at the stage of delocalized microcrack formation that precedes crack formation or crack pop-in, relates fracture and elastic radiation parameters, shows directions for experimental studies and approaches to the development and modification of diagnostic methods.
Forecasting the fracture of structural materials is based on monitoring the damage kinetics. Of all non-destructive testing methods, this kind of observation can be carried out most successfully by the acoustic emission method. In this case, the time dependences and absolute values of the number of detected pulses, the type and parameters of the frequency spectrum of AE signals, the amplitude distributions of signals, the time intervals between pulses, etc., are used as data sources. The results of AE observations are generally interpreted in terms of crack growth mechanics, which does not allow micromechanical aspects of fracture and elastic radiation to be taken sufficiently into account and hence does not allow improvement in forecast accuracy.
The fine fracture relies on the statements of the kinetic failure theory, the micromechanics of fracture of solids, and the model that takes into consideration the number of AE pulses recorded at time t is directly proportional to the concentration of microcracks in a material. The acoustic emission coefficient (AEC) makes that direct proportion. Considering the stochastic nature of elastic radiation, the acoustic emission coefficient can be understood as the probability that the parameters of elastic waves coming from the AE source fall in the ranges of AE signal frequencies, amplitudes, and time intervals between the signals recorded by the measuring equipment.
The instability of AEC values during AE measurements breaks the similarity of fracture and elastic radiation processes, leading to errors in the evaluation of informative forecasting parameters and to a decrease in the forecast accuracy. This circumstance should be taken into account when processing primary AE data.
Wilcox (Wilcox et al, 2007) presented a modelling of the acoustic emission process in the crack growth in plate structures. The modelling framework referred as Quantification of Acoustic Emission Forward (*QAE-Forward*), is a forward model of the AE process from source to detection. The goal is to be able to simulate the time-domain signal that is received from a transducer when an AE even occurs anywhere in a structure.
This model was based on a modular linear system's architecture using frequency-domain transfer functions and was implemented within MATLAB. This modular architecture of *QAE-Forward* enables the source, propagation and detection of AE signals to be separated. The overall model for the frequency spectrum, $H(\omega)$, of a received time-domain signal, excluding noise terms, can be expressed as a single equation (2):

$$H(\omega) = \sum \left[E(\omega)P(\omega)BA(\omega)R_X(\omega)\prod R_C(\omega)\prod T_C(\omega)\right] \quad (2)$$

in which $E(\omega)$ is the modal excitability at the source, $P(\omega)$ is the delay due to propagation, $A(\omega)$ is attenuation, B is beam spreading, $R_X(\omega)$ is the sensitivity of the receiver, $\prod R_C(\omega)$ is the product of reflections coefficients of all features at which the ray is reflected and $\prod T_C(\omega)$ is the product of transmission coefficients of all features that the ray acoustic has traversed. The final received time-domain signal is the inverse Fourier transform of $H(\omega)$.

Such a model has a great importance for the development of AE-based Structural Health Monitoring (SHM) applications, because it can be used to optimize the spatial distribution of the sensors taking into account the sensitivity desired, to perform probability detection and false responses received by the sensors and to support cases based on the use of AE in a complex structures.

Prosser (Prosser et al, 1998) presented a study in which a comparison was made between two approaches to predict acoustic emission waveforms in thin plates. The geometries of many practical structures of interest for AE monitoring, though, are neither infinite in lateral extent, nor composed of thick plates or large components where propagation of bulk waves is dominant. Thin plates, pipes, shells, rods, and beams are common. In such geometries, the distance from the receiver to the AE source is often many times the specimen thickness and the wave propagation is dominated by guided modes.

A normal mode solution method for Mindlin plate theory (MPT) was used to predict the response of the flexural plate mode to a point source, step-function load, applied on the plate surface. The second approach used a dynamic finite element method (DFEM) to model the problem using equations of motion based on exact linear elasticity. This research has led to improved accuracy in the locating the sources of emission, better ability to discriminate and eliminate extraneous noise signals and enhanced identification of AE sources.

3. AE sources location

The main purpose of using an AE test is the detection, location and classification of the active source. The location of the source has been seen such as one of the benefits of using AE technique in different problems, in particular 3D methods which are needed to study the hip arthroplasty *in vitro*.

The location type depends on the geometry of the structure to be tested. If the structure's geometry is a little flat surface it is possible to locate a zone with one sensor. For pipes (cilindrical geometry) it is necessary two sensors to detect a plan and to detect a point source in a 3D structure geometry is necessary to use three or more sensors.

There is a variety of different location methods for different structural geometries and applications. One work about acoustic emission source location in dispersive media uses a non-iterative method with time-of-arrival (TOA) of several events received in an array of sensors arbitrary positioning in the 3D space (Lympertos et al, 2007). Complications arise, due to the dispersive, modal nature of ultrasound in most real structures and inhomogeneities in the wave propagation medium. The modal nature of the waves is countered by ensuring that the fastest mode is used at all times, but the inhomogeneities in the structure are less simple to overcome.

Moreover in composites materials, the wave speed along the fibre directions is faster than that perpendicular to the fibres due to the differing fibre and matrix material properties. In metallic engineering structures, where one would expect the wave speed to be constant in all directions, the geometry of the structure, thickness changes, holes, lugs, grease nipples, bearings and welds are only some of the features that dismiss the assumption that the wave propagation path from source to sensor is simple. In order to overcome this, Baxter

(Baxter et al, 2007) proposed the 'Delta T' method for locating AE events based on a set of artificial training data, generated by Hsu-Nielsen pencil lead fractures. Hensman in the paper "Locating acoustic emission source in complex structures using Gaussian processes" (Hensman et al, 2010) makes an extend to the work of Baxter.
Most of the location methods are based on evaluation of time difference between wave arrivals to different sensors. In the procedure of locating AE sources is essential to determine the arrival times of AE waves at different sensors (Jiao et al, 2004). In cases when time of arrivals is difficult or impractical to detect, other methods are applied. These include cross correlation methods for location of continuous acoustic emission signals or different zone location methods based on effect of signal parameters attenuation with a distance (Muravin, 2009).
In the procedure of locating AE sources, there are two typical options, a more traditional one based on the parameters of the signal and another that uses the Wavelet Transform (WT). Different authors demonstrated, that it is possible to extract accurately the arrival times of AE signals with the results of WT (Grosse et al, 2002; Hamstad, 2004; Hamstad et al, 2003; 2002; Jeong et al, 2000; Jiao et al, 2004).
More important information is possible to obtain from peak stress. Every peak stress corresponds to a larger number of AE events and a consequent larger release of acoustic energy. So it is possible to verify the existence of AE sources through energy studies. In study of Qi (Qi et al, 2005), the average energy for the crack follows the expression (3) where v represents the voltage AE (in nV) and t time:

$$Energy = U = \int |v| dt \tag{3}$$

The energy U is measured in eu (1eu = 1nV.s). In order to have a better understanding of the mechanism of defect-induced microcrack formation, the value of the slope of the energy-time (ET) relationship allows to divide fatigue process into three phases: initiation phase (ET > 0.6 - 0.8); transient phase (0.3 < ET< 0.8); and stable phase (ET < 0.3).
Based on the acoustic signal energy levels obtained, it is possible categorize microcracks into two types: type I and type II. A type I microcrack is a crack whose location is well defined because the AE signals from it are captured by four or more sensors. A type II microcrack is defined as one whose location is unknown because its energy/amplitude is so low that majority of the sensors are unable to capture it.
According Axinte (Axinte et al, 2005) methods to locate AE sources to three and two dimensions are based on triangulation sensors placed on different planes of the structure analysis such as shown in figure 3. In the figure 3 sensor S_1's position is considered the origin of axis system. That $x_1 = 0, y_1 = 0, z_1 = 0$ so $S_1(0,0,0)$. The intersection of three spherical surfaces centered on each of the sensors results in the point P whose coordinates define the location of source. Radius r is the distance between P and the sensor used as a reference system of axes. The radius of the spherical surface for each sensor is the sum of ray r with the path difference between that sensor and reference.
In the femoral component according to Gueiral (Gueiral, 2008; Gueiral et al, 2009) the calculus of source location was made by an analogy between the system used by Axinte (Axinte et al, 2005).
To quantify the failure mechanisms related to the loosening of cemented hip joint replacements were used techniques capable of monitoring nondestructively the initiation and progression of failure during *in vitro* fatigue tests.

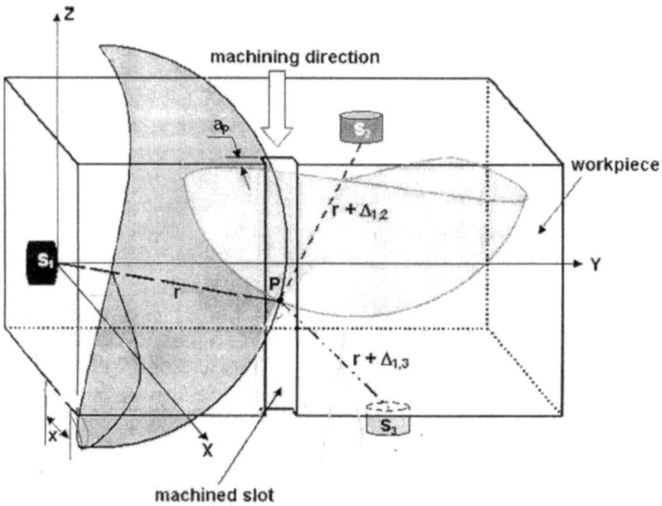

Fig. 3. Axis system and placement sensors (Axinte et al, 2005)

4. *In vitro* experimental tests of femoral component with cemented prostheses

A third generation in composite material, long left model 3306, femoral component by Sawbones was used in the study presented in the following text. The cement to fix the implant was CMW3 (polymethylmethacrylate with gentamicin) that is the most usual in cemented prosthesis.

The position of the femural component in the fatigue test to reflect the load on the THA to a certain amount of daily human activity was placed under the "femur coordinate system" defined by Bergmann (Bergmann et al, 2001).

The fatigue equipment was a pressure machine constructed according to the standards by an investigation group of Biomechanical Engineering which is part of the Mechanical Department of Aveiro University, Portugal. In the fatigue test the placement of the prosthesis in the testing machine follows the ISO 7206 standard (Qi, 2000; Ramos et al, 2005). The femur position was 9° in sagittal plan and 11° in frontal plan and was done by a base that supported the femoral component in the fatigue machine. The prosthesis fatigue test employed was done in accordance with (Ramos et al, 2005) being considered as the most severe by other authors (Cristofolini et al, 2003; Stolk et al, 2006). The sinusoidal charge cycles had a frequency of 2.5 Hz and 450 N in median amplitude. It was done between 900 N (minimum amplitude) and 1800 N (maximum amplitude). The femoral component under test had been constructed (prostheses collocated) about 3 years ago and it has been already used in a charge of 1 million of cycles and it does not present any visible crack. The test lasted 247343 s which corresponds to 618433 sinusoidal cycles.

Four sensors by Physical Acoustic Corporation (PAC) and Digital Wave Corporation (DAC) were mounted by a cylindrical distribution, as shown by Qi (Qi et al, 2005). The coordinates of the placement of sensors are presented in figure 4. To acquire the signals AE were used the AMSY5, Acoustic Emission System by Vallen.

The interface between sensors and femoral component was made by special synthetic silicon for polymers with excellent properties for the conduction of sound waves. Good collocation and attenuation (verified by Hsu Nielsen principle) essays were implemented to warranty a

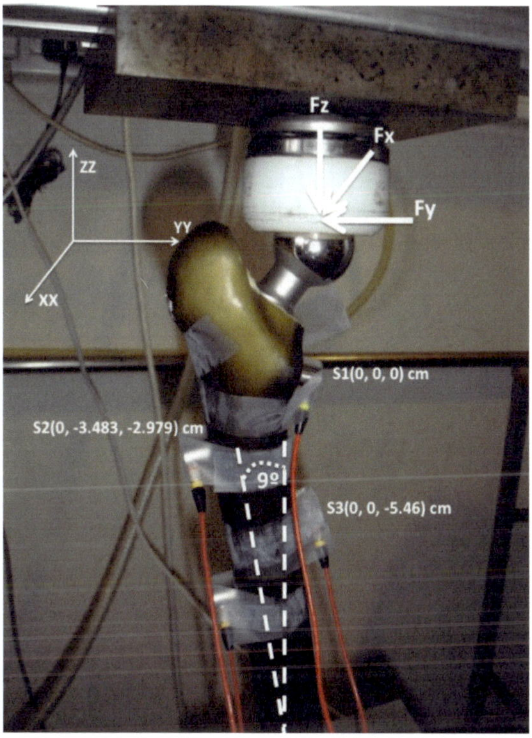

Fig. 4. Schematic placement of sensors and system of forces applied (Gueiral, 2008).

good signal AE acquisition. Usually tape-glue was used to sustain the sensors attached to femoral component.

During the process charge, sensor number 4 has been removed because it does not obtain any signal. After the charge we obtained three sets of AE events, the first appeared close to 7500 s (approximately two hours in fatigue), the second set of events appeared above 20000 s (approximately five and half hours in fatigue) and the third set of events appeared close to 55000 s (approximately fifteen hours in fatigue). Table 1 shows the acoustic energy during the component femural load process, that allows to conclude which of the events and which sensors have a peak stress, so an higher energy release. Analyzing the energy values in table 1,

Events	Sensor	Energy(eu)
1 (7500 s)	1	141×10^1
	2	331×10^2
	3	738×10^1
2 (20000 s)	1	155×10^1
	2	336×10^2
	3	814×10^1
3 (55000 s)	1	604×10^1
	2	127×10^3
	3	307×10^2

Table 1. Acoustic Energy

conclude that the femoral component was subject to maximum peak stress around the 55000 s, the third set of events. The sensor further "punished" is the sensor number two, because it presents a higher acoustic energy released as well as a larger amplitude measured by the sensor as we determine in the following analysis by WT.
To process the AE signal the WT software of Vallen was used to calculate the waves arrival times. That way, one could analyze all transients of acoustic emission signals and obtained really important information not possible with another analysis (Gueiral et al, 2009). Table 2 shows the obtained values for the wavelet coeffcient and arrival times to every set of events and to every sensors. The amplitude values have a permissible maximum error of 0.05 mV

Events	Sensor	Amplitude(mV)	WT Coefficients	Arrival Time (μs)
	1	1.7	0.00210	11.5
1	2	7.0	0.00825	23.5
	3	3.5	0.00394	60.0
	1	1.7	0.00226	11.0
2	2	6.5	0.00842	24.0
	3	3.6	0.00401	60.0
	1	3.6	0.00426	13.5
3	2	13.0	0.01452	26.0
	3	6.5	0.00755	59.5

Table 2. Wavelet Transform data (Gueiral, 2008)

and 0.5 s for the arrival time. Observing the values in table 2 it is visible that the three sets of events happened at different hours of the charge cycle, but the arrival time is similar in every set of events. This analysis makes the possibility that a crack has occurred (source AE) in the femoral component. Another fact observed is that the amplitude rises from the second to the third set, this probably means that the crack spread from inside to the surface of the femoral component.
The amplitude in sensor S_2 is greater than in sensor S_1 and S_3, which indicates that the position of sensor S_2 is near the crack (source AE). The smallest arrival time is in S_1. So considering the above and the results according to Gueiral (Gueiral et al, 2009) shows that the most probable zone where it happened the crack is between S_1 and S_2.
Making restrictions in sensors positions (Gueiral et al, 2009) according to Axinte (Axinte et al, 2005) the AE sources location methods was made by iterative calculus and the real coordinates of AE source is presented in table 3. The sensor S_1 was considered the origin of axis system (figure 4). The femoral component was cut into sections to realize complementary diagnostic by liquid penetrant test and by optical microscopy (200x). The crack was located in the marked zone shown in figure 5a)-b) [with a crack zoom c)].
The finite element analysis in the field of orthopaedics has earned a privileged position in the use of numerical computational techniques applied to the evaluation of stresses and displacements in structural components. Some application of the finite element method in the field of orthotics make analysis of the mechanical behavior of bone and joints, as well as

Events	X(cm)	Y(cm)	Z(cm)
1(7500s)	-0.601	- 2.556	0.972
2(20000s)	-0.821	- 2.473	1.025
3(55000s)	-0.697	- 2.611	0.732

Table 3. Coordinates of the location of the source EA (Gueiral, 2008)

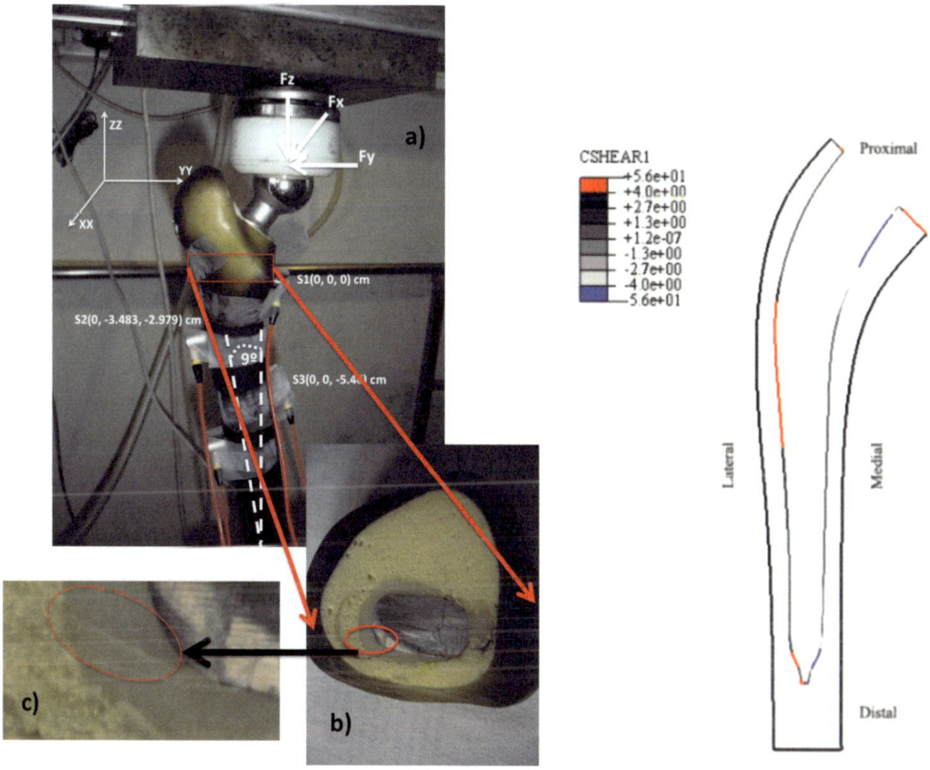

(a) Crack location in femural component (Gueiral, 2008) (b) Maximum shear stresses (Nabais, 2006)

Fig. 5. AE source location versus finite elements simulation

modelling of bone-implant failure. The displacement of the implant-cement interface and the failure of the implant-bone interface results in an increase of tensions in the cement mantle (Nabais, 2006).

According Nabais (Nabais, 2006), the maximum shear stress simulated by finite elements method are showed in the figure 5b). As one can see is really possible that the AE source detected in this study is located in the region of high stress concentration, figure 5b, when the femoral component is subjected to a fatigue test.

5. Conclusion

The monitoring of acoustic emission in evaluation structures integrity has the advantage to be done when the process is in charge, this does not happen in other non-destructives tests. That advantage is very important when one work with organic structures or organic substitution like in the study developed.

The signals obtained by the sensors system have the typical profile of a burst AE which means a good amplitude, duration and sufficient number of crossing the threshold.

The analysis of the acoustic emission results indicate the location coordinates of a crack in the structure, which coincides with the crack image observed in the optical microscope.

The surface metal prostheses have to be well polished because it may be the cause of cracking. As was observed in the microscopic images, in the local of the beginning AE crack formation, the metal implant had a sharp ridge.
In future work, given the constitution of the femoral component (different materials in thin layers) methods more stringent to locate sources should be used, not forgetting the fact that given the type of materials in question, the answer has a little number of AE events.

6. References

Axinte, D. A.; Natarajan, D. R. & Gindy, N. N. Z. (2005). An approach to use an array of three acoustic emission sensors to locate uneven events in machining - Part1: method and validation. *School of Mechanical - Materials an Manufacturing Engineering*, University of Nottingham, UK.

ASTM E1316-07 (2007). Standard Termninology for Nondestructive Examinations. *ASTM International.*

Bachtar, F.; Chen, X. & Hisada, T. (2006). Finite element contact analysis of the hip joint. *Med Bio Eng Comput* , Vol. 44: pages (643Ð651).

Baxter, M. B.; Pullin, R.; Holford, K. M. & Evans, S. L. (2007). Delta T source location for acoustic emission. *Mechanical Systems and Signal Processing,* Vol. 21: pages (1512-1520).

Belikov, V. T. (2008). Modeling of Acoustic-Emission Processes in a Solid. *Russian Journal of Nondestructive Testing*, Vol. 44, No.6: pages (429-435).

Belikov, V. T. (2010). Reconstruction of structural charateristics os a damage solid from Amplitude-Frequency spectrum of acoustic emission. *Russian Journal of Nondestructive Testing*, Vol. 46, No.1: pages (42-48).

Bergmann, G.; Deuretzbacher, G.; Heller, M.; Graichen, F.; Rohlmann, A.; Strauss, J. & Duda, G. N. (2001). Hip Contact forces and gait patterns from routine activities. *Journal of Biomechanics*, Vol. 34: pages (859-871).

Browne, M.; Taylor, A. & Roque, A. (2005). The Acoustic Emission Technique in orthopaedics - a review. *J. Strain Analysis,* Vol. 40, No.1-IMechE: pages (59-79).

Cristofolini, L.; Teutonivo, A. S.; Monti, L. ; Cappello, A. & Toni, A. (2003). Comparative in vitro study on the long term perfomance of cemented hip stems: validation of protocol to discriminate between good and bad designs. *JBiomech* , Vol. 36: pages (1603-1615).

Davies, J. P.; Tse, M. K. & Harris, W. H. (1996). Monitoring the integrity of the cement-metal interface of total joint components in vitro using acoustic emission and ultrasound. *Journal of Arthroplasty* , Vol. 11: pages (594-601).

Fonseca, E. M. M.; Mendes, C. S. & Noronha, J. K. (2010). Comparative study of the influence of different prosthetic materials in human femur. *8th National Congress of Experimental Mechanics*, Bragança, Portugal.

Franke, R. P.; Dorner, P.; Schwalbe H., & Ziegler, B. (2004). Acoustic Emission Measurement System for the orthopaedical Diagnostics of the Human Femur and Knee Joint. *DGZfP-Proceedings*, EWGAE.

Gueiral, N. (2008), Evaluation of Structural Integrity of Cemented Prosthesis by Acoustic Emission. *Master thesis in Electrotecnic and Computers Engineering*, ISEP - School of Engineering, Polytechnic of Porto, Portugal.

Gueiral, N.; Ramos, A. & Nogueira, E. (2009). Crack detection by Wavelet-based acoustic emission test - in vitro cemented implant. *Journal Materials Science Forum*, Vol. THERMEC 2009, 638 - 642: pages (558-563).

Grosse, C. U.; Motz, M.; Kroplin, B. H. & Reinhardt, H. W. (2002). Signal conditioning in acoustic emission analysis using wavelets. *Institute of Construction Materials and Statics and Dynamics of Aerospace Structures* , University of Stuttgart, Germany.

Hamstad, M. A. (2004). Electronic Noise Effects on Fundamental Lamb-Mode Acoustic Emission Signal - Arrival Times Determined Using Wavelet Transform Results. *DGZfP-Proceedings BB 90-CD Lecture 62* , EWGAE.

Hamstad, M. A.; Downs, K. S. & O'Gallagher, A. (2003). Practical Aspects of Acoustic Emission Source Location by a Wavelet Transform. *Journal of Acoustic Emission* , Vol. 21: pages (70-94), A1-A7.

Hamstad, M. A.; O'Gallagher, A. & Gary, J. (2002). Examination of the Application of a Wavelet Transform to Acoustic Emission Signals: Part 2 - Source Location. *Journal of Acoustic Emission* , Vol. 20: pages (62-81).

Hensman, J.; Mills, R.; Pierce, S. G.; Worden, K. & Eaton, M. (2010). Locating acoustic emission sources in complex structures using Gaussian processes. *Mechanical Systems and Signal Processing*, Vol. 24: pages (211-223).

Hora, P. & Cervena, O. (2010). Acoustic emission source modeling. *Applied and Computational Mechanics*, Vol. 4: pages(25-36).

Jeong, H. & Jang, Y. S. (2000). Wavelet analysis of plate wave propagation in composite laminates. *Division of Mechanical Engineering* , Wonkwang University, South Korea.

Jiao, J.; Wu, B.; Fei, R.; Wang, X. & He, C. (2004). Application of wavelet transform on modal acoustic emission source location in thin plates with one sensor. *College of Mechanical Engineering and Applied Electronics Technology - Beijing*, University of Technology, China.

Lympertos, E. F. & Dermatas, E. S. (2007). Acoustic emission source location in dispersive media. *Signal Processing*, Vol. 87: pages (3218-3225).

Muravin, B. (2009). Acoustic Emission Science and Technology. *Journal of Building and Infrastructure Engineering of the Israeli Association of Engineers and Architects*, Israel.

Nabais, C. (2006). Numerical Analysis of Interface Bone - Cement in Hip Arthroplasty. *Master thesis in Biomedical Engineering*, Faculty of Engineering, University of Porto, Portugal.

Nizam Ahmad, M.; Shuib, S.; Hassan, A. Y.; Shokri, A. A.; Ridzwan, M. I. Z. & Ibrahim, M. (2007). Application of multi criteria optimization method in implant design to reduce stress shielding. *Journal of Applied Sciences* , Vol. 7(3): pages (349-355).

Nosov, V. V. & Burakov, I. N. (2003). A Micromechanical Model of Acoustic Emission of Heterogeneous Materials. *Russian Journal of Nondestructive Testing* , Vol. 40, No. 2: pages (113-119).

Ohtsu, M.(2008). History and Fundamentals. in book: Acoustic Emission Testing, Springer-Verlag Berlin Heidelberg , ISBN 978-3-540-69895-1, pages (11 18).

Prendergast, P. J.; Monaghan, J. & Taylor, D. (1989). Materials selection in the artificial hip joint using finite element stress analysis. *Clinical Materials* Vol.4: pages (361-376).

Prosser, W. H.; Hamstad, M. A.; Gary, J. & O'Gallagher, A. (1998). Finite Element and Plate Theory Modeling of Acoustic Emission Waveforms. *Journal of Nondestructive Evaluation*, USA.

Qi, G.; Li, J.; Mouchon, W. P. & Lewis, G. (2005). Defect-induced fatigue microcrack formation in cement mantle. *Medical Acoustic Research Laboratory - Department of Mechanical Engineering*, University of Memphis, Tennessee, USA.

Qi, G. (2000). Attenuation of acoustic emission body waves in acrylic bone cement and synthetic bone using wavelet time-scale analysis. *Journal of Biomedical Materials Research - Part A*, Vol. 52 Issue1: pages (148Ð156).

Ramos, A.; Fonseca, F. & Simões, J. A. (2005). Fatigue cracks and shifts in Cemented Hip Prostheses: in vitro study. *Department of Mechanical Engineering*, University of Aveiro, Portugal.

Ridzwan, M. I. Z.; Shuib, S.; Hassan, A.Y.; Shokri, A. A. & Ibrahim, M. (2006). Optimization in implant topology to reduce stress shielding problem. *Journal of Applied Sciences*, Vol. 6(13): pages (2768-2773).

Rowland, C.; Browne, M. & Taylor, A. (2004). Dynamic health monitoring of metal hip prostheses using Acoustic Emission. *DGZfP-Proceedings*, EWGAE.

Shiotani, T. (2008). Parameter Analysis. *in book: Acoustic Emission Testing*, Springer-Verlag Berlin Heidelberg , ISBN 978-3-540-69895-1, pages (41-51).

Stolk, J.; Verdonschot, N. & Huiskes, R. (2002). Stair Climbing is more detrimental to the cement in hip replacement than Walking. *Clin Orthop Rel Res 405* : pages (294-305).

Stolk, J.; Verdonschot, N.; Murphy, B. P.; Prendergast, P. J. & Huiskes, R. (2004). Finite element simulation of anisotropic damage accumulation and creep in acrylic bone cement. *Engineering Fracture Mechanics*, Vol 71: pages (513-528).

Teixeira, C.; Fonseca, E. & Barreira, L. (2008). Resistance variation of the femoral neck by age, using a nonlinear finite element. *School of Health*, Polytechnic Institute of Bragança, Portugal.

Vieira, A. F. (2005). Project of a Femoral Component of Hip Prosthesis articulate in Composite Materials. *Master thesis in Biomedical Engineering*, Faculty of Engineering, University of Porto, Portugal.

Wilcox, P. D.; Lee, C. K.; Scholey, J. J.; Wisnom, M. R.; Friswell, M. I. & Drinkwater, B.W. (2007). Quantification of acoustic emission from crack growth in plate structures. *Department of Mechanical Engineering*, University of Bristol, UK.

Part 2

Materials

9

Titanium as a Biomaterial for Implants

Carlos Oldani and Alejandro Dominguez
Department of Materials and Technology, Faculty of Exact, Physical and Natural Sciences, Universidad Nacional de Córdoba
Argentina

1. Introduction

An ideal biomaterial is expected to exhibit properties such as a very high biocompatibility, that is, no adverse tissue response. Also, it must have a density as low as that of bone, high mechanical strength and fatigue resistance, low elastic modulus and good wear resistance. It is very difficult to combine all these properties in only one material.

Some metals are used as biomaterials due to their excellent mechanical properties and good biocompatibility. Since the metallic bonds in these materials are essentially non-directional, the position of the metals ions can be altered without destroying the crystal structure, resulting in a plastically deformable solid. This is also an advantage when thinking about the device manufacture technology.

The principal disadvantage of metals is its corrosion tendency in an in-vivo environment. Most metals can only be tolerated by the human body in small amounts even as metallic ions. The consequences of corrosion are the disintegration of the material implant, which will weaken the implant and the harmful effect of corrosion products on the surrounding tissues and organs.

Some metals are used as passive substitutes for hard tissue replacement such as total hip and knee joints, for fracture healing aids as bone plates and screws, spinal fixation devices and dental implants. Some metallic alloys are used for more active roles, as actuators such as vascular stents, and orthodontic archwires.

Metallic biomaterials can be conveniently grouped in the following categories:

- Stainless steel
- Cobalt base alloys
- Titanium base alloys
- Specialty metallic alloys

Examples of ASTM standards for some of these metallic biomaterials are shown in Table 1.

The first metal alloy developed specifically for human use was the "vanadium steel" but it was no longer used in implants because its corrosion resistance is inadequate *in vivo*. Later in the 1950s, 18-8sMo with very low carbon content (known as 316L) stainless steel was introduced and is actually widely used for implant fabrication. This alloy has a very good resistance to chloride solutions and poor sensitization.

The castable CoCrMo alloy has been used for many decades in dentistry and, relatively recently, in making artificial joints. The wrought CoNiCrMo alloy is relatively new, now used for making the stems of prostheses for heavily loaded joints such as the knee and hip. Both alloys have excellent corrosion resistance.

Attempts to use titanium for implant fabrication dates to the late 1930s. It was found that titanium was tolerated as was stainless steels and cobalt alloys. Titanium's lightness and good mechano-chemical properties are salient features for implant application.
Titanium was found the only metal biomaterial to osseointegrate (Van Noort, 1987). Also, there were even assumptions on a possible bioactive behaviour (Li et al., 1994) due to the slow growth of hydrated titanium oxide on the surface of the titanium implant that leads to the incorporation of calcium and phosphorous.

Material designation	Common name	ASTM Standard
Stainless Steel Fe-18Cr-14Ni-2.5Mo	316L Stainless Steel	ASTM F 138
Cobalt base alloys Co-28Cr-6Mo Co-35Ni-20Cr-10Mo	Cast CoCrMo Wrought CoNiCrMo	ASTM F 75 ASTM F 572
Titanium base alloys Ti CP (grade 1 to 4) Ti-6Al-4V ELI	Commercially pure Ti Ti6Al4V	ASTM F 67 ASTM F 136
Specialty metallic alloys Ta Ni-45Ti	Unalloyed Tantalum Nitinol	ASTM F 560 ASTM F 2063

Table 1. Examples of metallic biomaterials (An introduction to biomaterials , 2006)

2. Titanium base alloys developments

2.1 Commercially pure titanium

Commercially pure titanium (Ti CP) and extra low interstitial Ti-6Al-4V (ELI) are the two most common titanium base implant biomaterials. These materials are classified as biologically inert biomaterials. As such, they remain essentially unchanged when implanted into human bodies. The human body is able to recognize these materials as foreign and tries to isolate them by encasing it in fibrous tissues. However, they do not promote any adverse reactions and are tolerated well by the human tissues.
These metals do not induce allergic reactions such as has been observed with some stainless steels, which have induced nickel hypersensitivity in surrounding tissues.
Titanium is very light with a density of 4.5 g/cm^3. The Ti CP is 98.9 - 99.6 % Ti, being the oxygen content (and other interstitial elements such as C and N) the main element influencing significantly its yield, tensile and fatigue strengths (Table 2). Interstitial elements strengthen the metal through interstitial solid solution strengthening mechanism, with nitrogen having approximately twice the hardening effect (per atom) of either carbon or oxygen.
Pure Ti is an allotropic metal having hexagonal α–phase (HCP) below 882 °C and transforming to a cubic β–phase (BCC) over that temperature. As its typical microstructure is a single alpha phase, cold work is also an applied strengthening mechanism.
Its very good biocompatibility is due the formation of an oxide film (TiO_2) over its surface. This oxide is a strong and stable layer that grows spontaneously in contact with air and prevents the diffusion of the oxygen from the environment providing corrosion resistance.

It is a biomaterial with a high superficial energy and after implantation it provides a favourable body reaction that leads to direct apposition of minerals on the bone-titanium interface and titanium osseointegration (Acero et al., 1999).

Element	Grade 1	Grade 2	Grade 3	Grade 4	Ti6Al4V[a]
N máx	0.03	0.03	0.05	0.05	0,05
C máx	0.10	0.10	0.10	0.10	0,08
H máx	0.015	0.015	0.015	0.015	0,0125
Fe máx	0.20	0.30	0.30	0.50	0,25
O máx	0.18	0.25	0.35	0.40	0,13
Ti	Balance	Balance	Balance	Balance	

[a] Aluminium 6%, Vanadium 4%

Table 2. Chemical composition of Ti CP (ASTM F 67) and Ti6Al4V alloy (ASTM F 136)

2.2 Ti6Al4V alloy

Ti6Al4V alloy is widely used to manufacture implants and its chemical composition is given in Table 2. The addition of alloying elements to titanium enables it to have a wide range of properties because aluminium tends to stabilize the α-phase and vanadium tends to stabilize the β-phase, lowering the temperature of the transformation from α to β. The alpha phase promotes good weldability, excellent strength characteristics and oxidation resistance. The addition of controlled amounts of vanadium as a β-stabilizer causes the higher strength of beta-phase to persist below the transformation temperature which results in a two-phase system. The β-phase can precipitate by an ageing heat treatment. This microstructure produce local strain fields capable of absorbing deformation energy. Cracks are arrested or deterred at the particles. The mechanical properties of the Ti CP and the Ti6Al4V are given in Table 3.

Property	Grade 1	Grade 2	Grade 3	Grade 4	Ti6Al4V
Tensile strength (MPa)	240	345	450	550	860
Yield strength (MPa)	170	275	380	485	795
Elongation (%)	24	20	18	15	10

Table 3. Mechanical properties of Ti CP (ASTM F 67) and Ti6Al4V alloy (ASTM F 136)

The modulus of elasticity of these materials is about 110 GPa. This is much lower than stainless steels and Co-base alloys modulus (210 and 240 GPa, respectively (Dadvinson & Gergette, 1986). When compared by specific strength (strength/density) the titanium alloys exceed any other implant materials.

Titanium and titanium alloys, nevertheless, have poor shear strength, making them less desirable for bone screws, plates and similar applications. They also tend to gall or seize in sliding contact with itself or another metal.

2.3 Low modulus titanium alloys

The Ti6Al4V alloy has some disadvantages: its elastic modulus, although low, is 4 to 6 times that of cortical bone and has low wear resistance that is a problem in articulations surfaces.

Also, V can cause potential citotoxicity and adverse tissue reactions (Steinemann, 1980), and Al ions from the alloy might cause long-term Alzheimer diseases (Rao et al., 1996).
Briefly, a biocompatible titanium base alloy suitable for bone implant should meet at least the following requirements (Mehta, 2008):

- Potentially toxic elements, such as vanadium, cooper and tin, should be avoided completely
- Elements that may have potential toxicological problems, such as chromium, nickel and aluminium, should be used only in minimum, acceptable amounts
- The alloy should have high corrosion resistance
- The alloy should have, at least, the following desirable mechanical properties: low modulus, high strength and good smooth and notched fatigue strength
- The alloy should have good workability and ductility.

Consequently, the recent trend in research and development of titanium for biomedical applications is to develop alloys composed of non-toxic and non-allergenic elements with excellent mechanical properties (low modulus-high strength) and workability (Niinomi, 1999).
The first generation of design orthopaedic alloys try to replace the V and Al alloys with other non toxic components such as Nb, Fe and Mo (for the V) and Ta, Hf and Zr (for the Al).
Subsequent developments in orthopaedic Ti-base alloys have been motivated by the requirement of low elastic modulus. The stiffness of titanium and its alloys is still largely greater than that of cortical bone, although it is less than that of Co-Cr type alloys and stainless steels used for biomedical applications. This difference of rigidity produced the stress-shielding phenomenon. Stress shielding occurs because of the mismatch between the stiffness of the bone, which has a Young modulus of 7–25 GPa (Currey, 1998), and that of the metal implant stem.
Various methods of solving this problem have been considered, including changing the size and shape of the stem to reduce the differences in the structural stiffness of the implant and the surrounding bone and changing the implant material from steel to commercially pure titanium or Ti alloys with low modulus (Sarmiento et al., 1979).
Metastable β-Ti alloys were developed for this purpose, with low elastic modulus. In Table 4 it could be observed some old and new Ti-base alloys develop specifically for biomedical purpose (Guilemot et al., 2004).
Low modulus alloys are nowadays desired because the moduli of alloys are required to be much more similar to that of bone. These new alloys have an elastic modulus ranging 55-85 GPa, so it could be minimized the stress shielding phenomena because it is more proximally to the bone modulus. However, they are still greater than that of cortical bone.

1. Titanium CP (ASTM F 67)	10. **Ti-12Mo-6Zr-2Fe** (ASTM F1813- low modulus)
2. Ti-6Al-4V ELI (ASTM F 136)	11. **Ti-15Mo** (low modulus)
3. Ti-6Al-4V (ASTM F 1108)	12. Ti-16Nb-10Hf (low modulus)
4. **Ti-6Al-7Nb** (ASTM F 1295)	13. Ti-15Mo-5Zr-3Al (low modulus)
5. Ti-5Al-2.5Fe (ISO 5832)	14. Ti-15Mo-2.8Nb-0.2Si-0.26O (low modulus)
6. Ti-5Al-3Mo-4Zr	15. Ti-35Nb-7Zr-5Ta (low modulus)
7. Ti-15Sn-4Nb-2Ta-0.2Pd	16. Ti-29Nb-13Ta-4.6Zr (low modulus)
8. Ti-15Zr-4Nb-2Ta-0.2Pd	
9. **Ti-13Nb-13Zr** (low modulus)	

Table 4. Ti alloys developed for biomedical applications (in bold) and for other uses

3. Problems and solutions

Bulk titanium alloys used in implants present three main problems:
- High cost because the amount of processing energy and melting and casting difficulties
- Higher elastic modulus compared to bone
- Although the inert behaviour of Ti is a good property, its bone attachment is difficult because it do not react with the human tissues

3.1 The processing

A great problem of these new alloys is its fabrication processes because most beta titanium alloys contain considerable amounts of refractory elements with high melting temperatures. This results in heavily weight, difficult melting and solidification processing, low plastic deformability and high materials costs.

The various refractory materials employed in casting are attacked by titanium with such severity that sounds castings, possessing good mechanical properties are difficult to obtain. So, conventional methods are not practical with titanium.

The molten metal and the hot casting are susceptible to atmospheric contamination. Because Ti is very reactive with oxygen and other atmospheric gases, the melting and casting processes implies high temperature fusion and casting under vacuum or protective neutral atmospheres. Another casting problem is the maintenance of good flow over severe changes of dimensions or direction within the mold.

Powder metallurgy (P/M) is an alternative method of fabrication in which metal powders are utilized by compacting and sintering to form useful products. This method is employed primarily to produce simple shapes with good dimensional stability, to form shapes with material of extremely high melting temperatures and to produce parts not feasible by other means.

Production of cast titanium today takes 16 times more energy per tonne than the production of steel. Instead of conventional melting, milling and machining, P/M techniques implies powders that remain in solid form during the entire procedure. This saves a tremendous amount of processing energy with a reduction of over 50% (Mehta, 2008).

3.2 The elastic modulus

As was said, the elastic moduli and strength of titanium and its alloys are much higher than those of human bones, which may result in stress shielding and the failure of implants. People have tried to develop new types of titanium alloys, such as β-Ti alloys, to reduce the modulus of the implants to the level approaching human bones. On the other hand, the mechanical properties of porous titanium can be adjusted by pore fraction and morphology, and the stress shielding effect will be reduced. Porous titanium with porosity in a wide range can be prepared with powder metallurgy methods (Zhiguang et al., 2009), from which other kinds of powders as second phase in green bodies would be removed during subsequent heat treatment.

3.3 The inert behaviour

Despite the great progress achieved in orthopaedic biomaterials, fixation of implants to the bone host remains a problem. As titanium has an inert behaviour, the body tries to encapsulate the Ti-based implant. However, titanium does not bond directly to bone resulting in micro-movements and, eventually loosening of the implant. Undesirable

movements at the implant-tissue interface results in failure cracks of the implant. As osseointegration starts with the cellular stage and continues with the nucleation of mineral and the structuring of the new vital bone, the overall required time is varying in a broad range. A proposed solution for a better control of osseointegration is the bioactive fixation.
One approach to improving implant lifetime is to coat the metal surface with a bioactive material that can promote the formation and adhesion of hydroxyapatite ($Ca_{10} (PO_4)_6(OH)_2$), the inorganic component of natural bone.
The application of bioactive coatings to titanium-based alloys enhance the adhesion of Ti-based implants to the existing bone, resulting in significantly better implant lifetimes than can be achieved with materials in use today (Katti, 2004). Typically, several silicates glasses or hydroxyapatite (HA) are used as bioactive coatings. Some properties of hydroxyapatite are shown in Table 5.

Hardness (Mohs)	5
Density (g/cm^3)	3.1
Elastic Modulus (GPa)	100
Ultimate Tension Stress (MPa)	100
Compression Stress (MPa)	> 50 (good)
Toughness K_{IC} ($MPa\ m^{1/2}$)	1
Solubility	It has the less solubility in body fluids media, so it is impossible to have Ca^{2+} or PO_4^{3+} ions in water (PH=7)

Table 5. Hydroxyapatite properties

An ideal bioactive coating would bond tightly both to the bone and the metal. Two problems arise when attempting to coat metals with ceramics. For one side, the thermal expansion coefficients of the ceramic and metal are usually different, and as a result, large thermal stresses are generated during processing. These stresses lead to cracks at the interface and compromise coating adhesion. In addition, chemical reactions between the ceramic and metal can weaken the metal in the vicinity of the interface, reducing the strength of the coated system. This problem is particularly important when coating Ti alloys, due to their high reactivity with most oxide materials. However, bioactive ceramics coatings on Ti implants further improves the biocompatibility of these implants.

4. Titanium-Hydroxyapatite composite

Biocomposite materials have been developed in order to combine bioactivity of ceramics and mechanical properties of metals. Hydroxyapatite (HA) is known for its weakness and brittles (see Table 5) but has an excellent biocompatibility and is a bioactive material. When HA is added to titanium, an improvement of the biomaterial chemical properties occurs. New developments try to aggregate hydroxyapatite as a second phase to the Ti alloy, with powder metallurgy techniques (P/M). In this composite material, particles of HA are incorporated in a porous titanium matrix providing points of good bone reaction. These solutions allow improved adhesion strength of the load bearing metallic component to the bone, resulting in shorter healing periods as well as predictable behaviour of the implant for longer periods of time.

Although this benefits, there are some problems in the manufacture of the composite material and some doubts about its biocompatibility.
One processing problem is that, as Ti is stable in vacuum or reducing atmospheres and HA is stable only in oxidizing atmospheres (Weng et al., 1994), sintering of this type of composites is difficult. Also, there are some reports indicating intense HA decomposition at temperatures lower than the decomposition temperatures of the monolithic powders, due the interaction with the Ti powder (Yang et al., 2004), which declines its bioactivity and mechanical properties According to literature the Ca titanates $CaTiO_3$ and $CaTi_2O_5$ are formed through reactions between HA and TiO_2 in vacuum, both when the titanium oxide was intentionally added or when it resulted from the oxidation of metallic Ti in Ti-HA composites (Yang et al., 2004).
Another problem of porous metals is its fatigue behaviour. The porosity of most implants is usually determined to compromise between maintaining the mechanical strength of the implant while still providing adequate pore size for tissue ingrowth. Although optimum pore size required for implant fixation remains undefined, the consensus is that in order to optimize mineralised bone ingrowth, pore sizes between 100 and 400 μm are necessary (Cameron et al., 1976). A major concern with the use of porous implants in highly loaded applications is the effect the porous matrix might have on fatigue strength. Ti alloys experienced drastic reductions in fatigue strength till one-third that of the solid alloy equivalent shape (Wolfrth & Ducheyne, 1994). Stress intensification due to these pores are major sources of weakness in the fatigue strength. This is sometimes referred to as the nocth effect. To achieve a functionally strong implant, porous implant design needs to account for these losses in metal strength.
Nevertheless titanium-hydroxyapatite porous structures are promising biomaterials to be used as replacement implants.

5. Finite element analysis

As an artificial hip joints need to be designed to withstand the loads that they are expected to bear without fracture or fatigue, stress analysis is therefore required to ensure that all components of the device operate below the fatigue limit. For simple calculations, simple analytical calculations usually suffice. Unfortunately, analytical solutions are limited to linear problems and simple geometries governed by simple boundary conditions.
Implants as a hip joint involve some combinations of material or geometry non-linearity, complex geometry and mixed boundary conditions. Applying analytical methods to such a problem would require so many assumptions and simplifications. An alternative is the use of approximate or numerical methods. The most popular numerical method for solving problems in continuum mechanics is the finite element method (FEM), also referred to as finite element analysis (FEA).
FEA uses a complex system of points called nodes which make a grid called a mesh. The complex structure is divided into a large number of smaller parts, or elements, with interconnecting nodes, each with geometry much simpler than that of the whole structure. This mesh is programmed to contain the material and structural properties which define how the structure will react to certain loading conditions. Nodes are assigned at a certain density throughout the material depending on the anticipated stress levels of a particular area. Regions expected to receive large amounts of stress usually will have a higher node density than those which experience little or no stress.

The behaviour of the unknown variable within the element and the shape of the element are represented by simple functions that are linked by parameters that are shared between the elements at the nodes. Using boundary conditions, a large system of equations results and they are solved simultaneously using interactive means.
The essential steps in the FEM follow:

i. Discretization of the region of interest by the subdivision of the region (continuum) in small elements,
ii. Definition of the unknown variables (stress, strain and displacement) in each element within the continuum,
iii. Formulation in each element of the equations that define the behaviour of the unknown variables (stress-strain or strain-displacement relationships) in the form of matrices. These element matrices are assembled into a global system of equations for the entire discretized domain,
iv. Solving of the global system of equations by interactive means.

Following are presented some examples of the application of FEM in the estimation of fatigue life in a hip implant made in different materials. The materials implant analysed were: 316L stainless steel, Ti6Al4V, Ti-35Nb-7Zr-5Ta (low modulus β-Ti alloy) and sintered porous Ti.

5.1 Mechanical behaviour of hip implant

Currently, total hip arthroplasty (THA) is a common technique used in cases of reconstruction when the functionality of the natural hip joint and the leg is impaired. Despite great progress in biomaterials, fixation of the prosthesis to the bone remains a problem because the commercial metallic THA implants are five to six times stiffer than bone. The difference in elastic modulus between the bone and the implant material has been identified as the major cause of implant loosening from stress shielding.
The regenerative and remodelling processes in bone are directly triggered by loading, i.e. bone subjected to loading or stress regenerates and bone not subjected to loading results in atrophy. Thus, the effect of a much stiffer bone implant is to reduce the loading on bone resulting in the phenomenon called as stress shielding (Katti, 2004).
A stem of a lower stiffness material (e.g. a titanium alloy) will transfer more of the load to the femur proximally, reducing stress shielding, however, this is achieved at the expense of higher load transfer stresses at the cement interfaces with the bone and implant and the risk of cement failure (Gross & Abel, 2001). A goal to reach would be a low stress shielding and low interface shear stresses in this type of implant, but nowadays there are no means to reach that goal, so, the existing designs are based in a compromise between them.
There are many issues related to implants and prostheses, but in general the magnitude and direction of the load change and are not accurately known, and are patient dependant in any case. The average load on a hip joint is estimated to be up to three times body weight and the peak load during other activities such as jumping can be as high as 10 times body weight. Besides, hip joints may undertake cyclic loading as high as 10^6 cycles annually. This led the setting of different standards for testing mechanical strength.

5.2 Simulation of the mechanical behaviour of uncemented femoral stem of a hip prosthesis

For the present study we considered two conditions. The first of them corresponds to the layout and loads used in the fatigue test established in the Standard IRAM 9422-3

Determination of fatigue properties of the femoral stem components without the application of torsion. The second condition corresponds to the implant attached to bone under the action of an arbitrary load. This last condition analysed the distribution of stresses and strains that produces the implant on the femur.
The proposed stem design was thought to minimise stress shielding.

5.2.1 Methods

Three materials were considered in the simulation: a low carbon stainless steel 316L in semi hard condition, a typical Ti-6Al-4V titanium alloy and a low modulus beta-Ti alloy, Ti-35Nb-7Zr-5Ta. The mechanical properties of these materials are given in Table 6.
For the stem support for fatigue testing, the material of the support was assumed to have an elastic modulus E of 2.7 GPa and a Poisson ratio of 0.3.
To characterize the mechanical behaviour of the bone, all materials were considered as isotropic. The cortical and cancellous bones were assumed to have an elastic modulus of 16,200 MPa and 380 MPa, respectively and to have a Poisson ratio of 0.3

5.2.2 Finite element models

For fatigue testing, we performed three finite element models in which, in each case, it was changed the material properties of the implant. The models accounted for stem, the test stand and also a piece to apply the load. Full 3D model were considered, with solid tetrahedral and hexahedral elements.

Material	Young's modulus (GPa)	Tensile strength (MPa)	Yield strength (Mpa)	Poisson ratio
316L	196	861	620	0.3
Ti6Al4V	115	860	795	0.33
Ti35Nb7Zr5Ta	55	596	547	0.33

Table 6. Mechanical properties of implant materials considered in the simulation

Because the stem consists of two parts and a fastener, frictional contact was modelled at the interface. The remaining interactions were assumed as tied. A total of 106,195 elements and 26,192 nodes were used in the analyses. The meshed finite element model is shown in Figure 1.
For implant attached to bone finite elements models were realized, in which the hip implant and the femur were represented. Four nodes solid elements were used in the models, to realize 4 finite elements models. Three of them were developed with the implant and an additional model was analyzed without the implant. This was considered as a control solution for evaluation of stress shielding.
One of the meshed finite element model is shown in Figure 2.
For those models with implant, the implant was completely fastened to the bone through an interaction in which "slave" nodes are tied to the master surface of the bone. So the degrees of freedom in the exterior side of the implant associates to the degrees of freedom of the bone surface in contact to it.

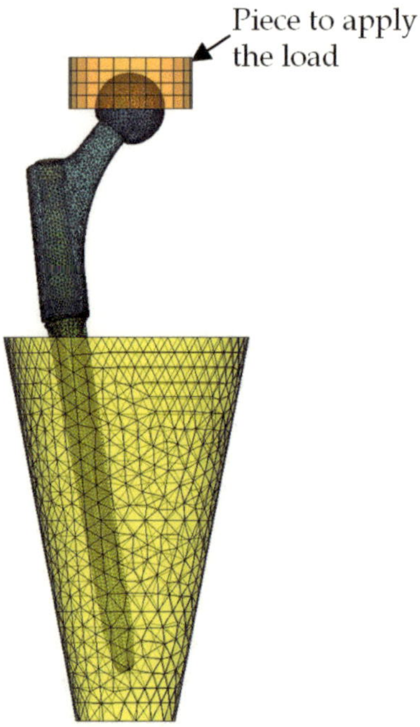

Fig. 1. Fatigue testing. The 3D finite element model developed in the analysis

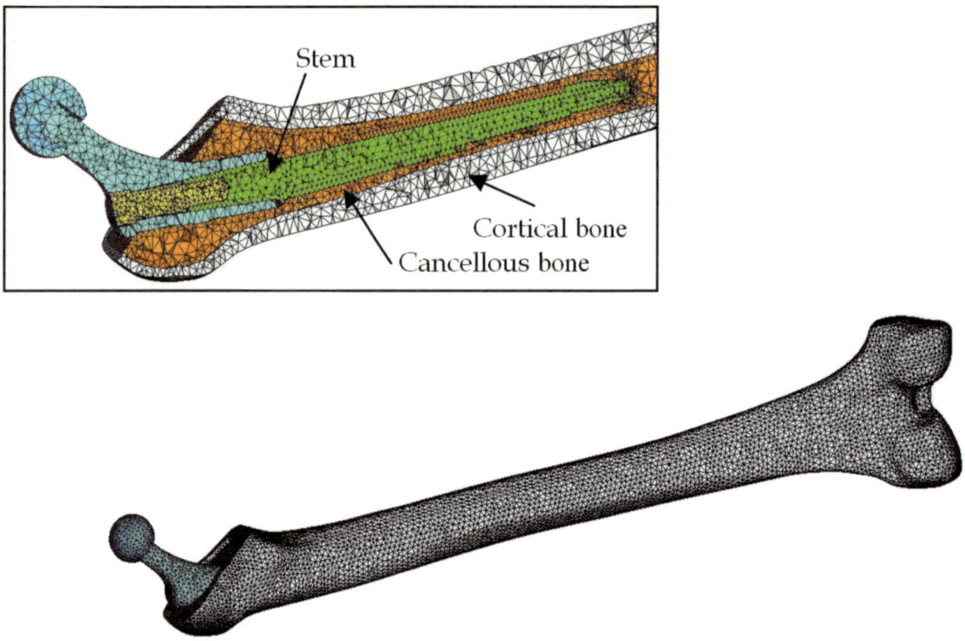

Fig. 2. Implant attached to bone. Finite element model developed in the analysis

All the models were created, analyzed and afterwards the results were processed using Abaqus 6.4.5.

5.2.3 Loads

In all cases for fatigue testing, the applied load was the load specified in the standard, of 2300 N. The load was applied on the upper surface of the piece that applys the load.
For implant attached to bone the applied load was an arbitrary load of 1000 N in the acetabular component of the prosthesis. Besides the pre-tensioning bolt load was simulated.

5.2.4 Results

a. Fatigue testing:

Due to the assembly load between the stem components, high levels of compressive contact stress were obtained. Therefore, and to wean the study of the influence of these stresses, we considered in the analysis the stress components S33, which would be responsible for a possible material fatigue. The simulation results obtained for the three models using different materials are given in Table 7.
Figure 3 shows the S33 stress distribution in the implant made of beta titanium alloy.

Material	Implant maximum flexural stress S33 (MPa)	Vertical displacement in the head of the implant (mm)
316L	+379 -602 (*)	- 0.57
Ti6Al4V	+397 -624 (*)	- 0.94
Ti35Nb7Zr5Ta	+455 -580 (*)	- 1.87

(*) The indicated compression component was mainly due to the contact stresses.

Table 7. Simulation results for the three models

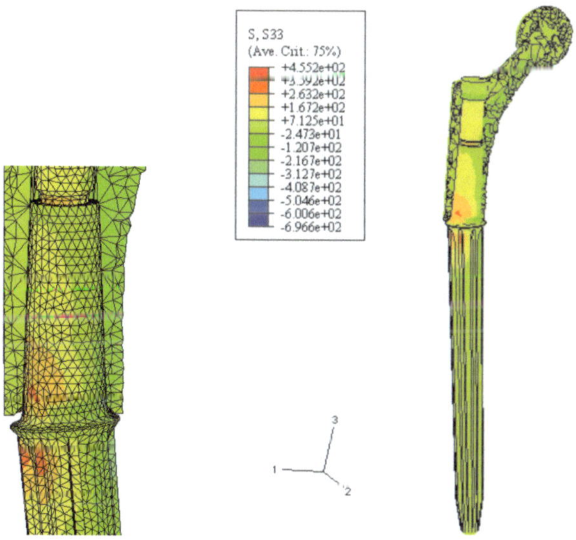

Fig. 3. S33 stress distribution (MPa)

Whereas the applied load varies between zero and 2300 N, the minimum stresses are related to those produced by the preload of the bolt connecting both parts of the implant, and the maximum stresses are due to the load of 2300 N.

Using the mechanical properties of the materials, were drawn Goodman diagrams and plotted the points corresponding to the applied loading (Figures 4 and 5). From them, it could be seen that the implants have unlimited duration of life with the geometry, loads and properties considered. However, it can be seen in the diagram for the stainless steel implant that the point representing working conditions is located near the boundary of the safe zone.

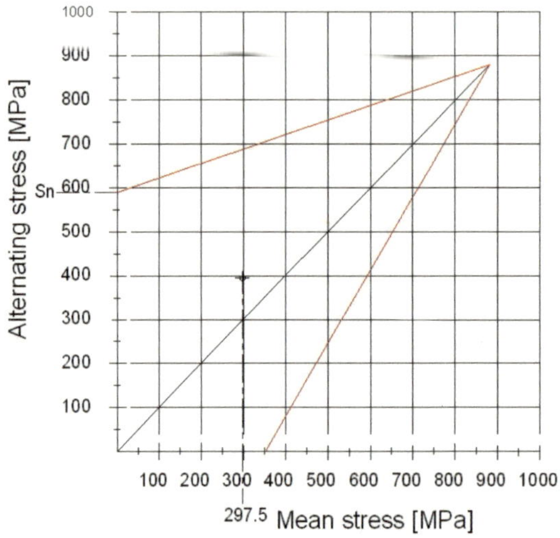

Fig. 4. Goodman's diagram. Ti6Al4V

It should be noted that the environment in which the implant should work would influence the final fatigue behaviour.

b. Implant fixed to bone:

In Figure 6 the S33 stress is shown for the bone, from the analysis of the stemmed Ti35Nb7Zr5Ta implant. Comparing whit the model without the implant, in the stemmed ones it was observed a change in the stress pattern, because the stem shielded the bone from

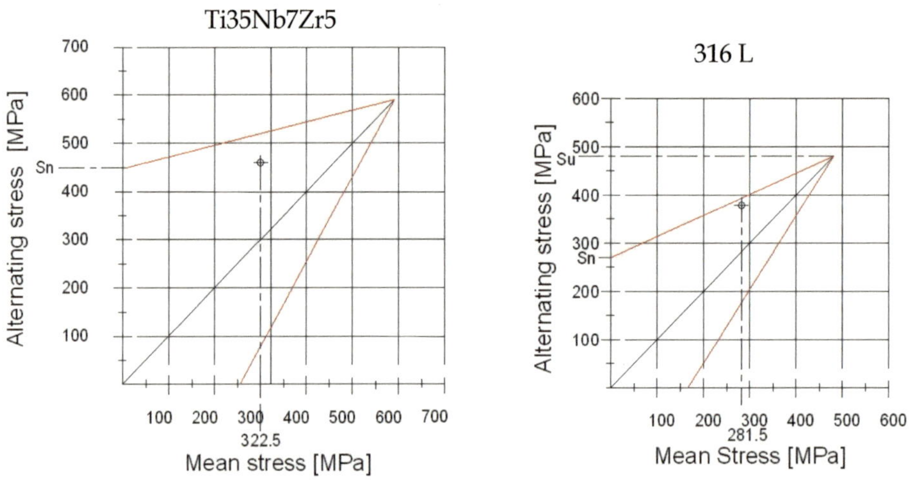

Fig. 5. Goodman's diagram. 316L and Ti35Nb7Zr5Ta

the loads. Comparing the stemmed models, from the point of view of stress and displacements that were produced in the bone, with the titanium Ti35Nb7Zr5Ta implant, the behaviour of the whole bone-implant is nearer to the natural bone, and the effect of stress shielding was the smaller.

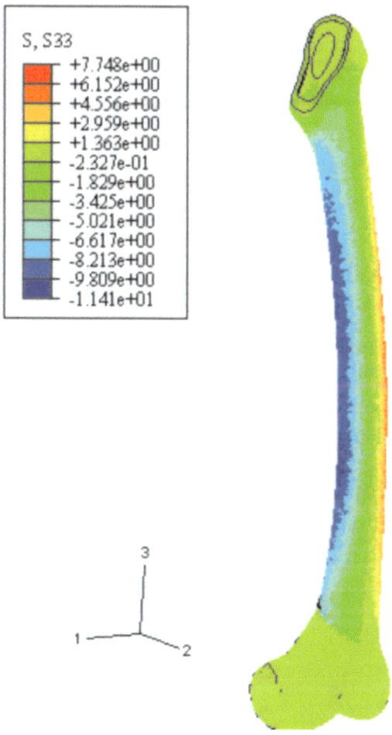

Fig. 6. S33 Stress in the bone, stemmed Ti35Nb7Zr5Ta implant model

5.3 Fully porous material in hip implants

It is well known that porosity decreases the Young's modulus of a material, thus it could be thought as a means to reduce stress shielding. It is difficult to get the properties for FEA analysis but it could be used some approach to represent the Young's modulus of a material with a given fraction of porosity. However, the effect the porosity on fatigue strength discourage using fully porous material in joint arthroplasty implants because porous metal alone does not provide sufficient mechanical strength to sustain the physiological loads (Ryan et al., 2006).

6. References

Acero, J.; Calderón, J.; Salmeron, J.; Verdaguer, J. & Consejo, C. (1999). The behaviour of titanium as a biomaterial: microscopy study of plates and surrounding tissues in facial osteosynthesis. *Journal of Cranio-maxillofacial Surgery*, Vol.27, No.2, (April 1999), pp. 117-123

Cameron, H.; Pilliar, R. & Macnab, I. (1976). The rate of bone ingrowth into porous metal. *Journal of Biomedical Materials Research*, Vol.10, No.2, (March 1976), pp. 295-302, ISSN 00219304

Currey, J. (1998). Mechanical properties of vertebrate hard tissues. *Proceedings of the Institution of Mechanical Engineers, Part H: Journal of Engineering in Medicine*, Vol.212, No.6, (1998), pp. 399-411, ISSN 09544119

Dadvinson, A. & Gergette, F. (1986). State of the art in materials for orthopedic prosthetic devices. *Proceedings of Implant Manufacturing and Materials Technology, Soc. Manufact. Eng.*, Em87-122, pp. 122-126

Gross, S. & Abel, E. (2001). A finite element analysis of hollow stemmed hip prostheses as a means of reducing stress shielding of the femur. *Journal of Biomechanics,* Vol.34, No.8, (2001), pp. 995-1003, ISSN 00219290

Guelcher, S & Hollinger, J. (Ed(s).). (2006). *An introduction to biomaterials*. CRC Press, ISBN 9780849322822

Guilemot, F.; Prima, F.; Latta, L. ; Bareille, R. ; Gordin, D. ;Gloriant, T. ; Porté-Durrieu, M. , Ansel, D. & Baquey, Ch. (2004). Design of new titanium alloys for orthopaedic applications. *Medical and Biological Engineering and Computing,* Vol.42, No.1, (January 2004), pp. 137-141, ISSN 01400118

Katti, K. (2004). Biomaterials in total joint replacement. *Colloids and Surfaces B: Biointerfaces,* Vol.39, No.3, (December 2004), pp. 133-142, ISSN 09277765

Li, P.; Kangasniemi, I. & De Groot, K. (1994). Hydroxyapatite Induction by a Gel-Derived Titania on a Titanium Substrate. *Journal of the Ceramic Society,* Vol.77, No.5, (May 1994), pp. 1307-1312

Mehta, R. (01 Jul 2008). Powder metallurgy processing for low-cost titanium, In: *Materials World Magazine,* Available from:
http://www.iom3.org/news/powder-metallugy-processing-low-cost-titanium

Niinomi, M. (1999). Recent titanium R&D for biomedical applications in Japan. *JOM Journal of the Minerals, Metals and Materials Society,* Vol.51, No.6, (June 1999), pp. 32-34, ISSN 10474838

Rao, S.; Ushida, T.; Tateishi, T.; Okazaki, Y. & Asao, S. (1996). Effect of Ti, Al, and V ions on the relative growth rate of fibroblasts (L929) and osteoblasts (MC3T3-E1) cells. *Bio-Medical Materials and Engineering,* Vol.6, No.2, (1996), pp. 79-86, ISSN 09592989

Ryan, G.; Pandit, A. & Panagiotis, D. (2006). Fabrication methods of porous metals for use in orthopaedic applications. *Biomaterials,* Vol.27, No.13, (May 2006), pp. 2651-2670, ISSN 01429612

Sarmiento, A.; Zych, G.; Latta, L. & Tarr, R. (1979). Clinical experiences with a titanium alloy total hip prosthesis. *Clinical Orthopaedics and Related Research,* Vol.144, (October 1979), pp. 166-173, ISSN 0009921X

Steinemann, S. (1980). Corrosion of surgical implants—in vivo and in vitro tests, In: *Evaluation of biomaterials*. Winter, G.; Leray, J. & de Groot, K., Wiley, ISBN 471276588, New York

Van Noort, R. (1987). Titanium: the implant material for today, *Journal of Material Science,* Vol.22, (1987), pp. 3801-3811

Weng, J.; Liu, X.; Zhang, X. & Ji, X. (1994). Thermal decomposition of hydroxyapatite structure induced by titanium and its dioxide. *Journal of Material Science Letters,* Vol.13, No.3, (January 1994), pp. 159-161, ISSN 02618028

Wolfrth, D. & Ducheyne, P. (1994). Effect of a change in interfacial geometry on the fatigue strength of porous-coated Ti-6A1-4V. *Journal of Biomedical Materials Research,* Vol.28, No.4, (April 1994), pp. 417-425, ISSN 00219304

Yang, Y.; Kim, K.; Agrawal, C. & Ong, J. (2004). Interaction of hydroxyapatite-titanium at elevated temperature in vacuum environment. *Biomaterials,* Vol.25, No.15, (July 2004), pp. 2927-2932, ISSN 01429612

Zhiguang, L.; Yumei, Z.; Huan, S.; Lijuan, X.; Yuyong, C. & Woo, K. (2009). Porous Ti/HA biocomposites for biomaterials applications. *Materials Science Forum,* Vol.614, (March, 2009), pp. 73-78

10

The Bearing Surfaces in Total Hip Arthroplasty – Options, Material Characteristics and Selection

Hamid Reza Seyyed Hosseinzadeh, Alireza Eajazi and Ali Sina Shahi
Shahid Beheshti Medical University Tehran
Iran

1. Introduction

During total hip arthroplasty, both the femoral and acetabular bearing surfaces are surgically replaced with metallic, polymeric, and/or ceramic components. Throughout the twentieth century, many different combinations of these materials have been proposed and examined as bearing surfaces for total hip arthroplasty. Metal-on-metal total hip replacements were first implanted by Wiles in the 1930s and later developed in the 1950s and 1960s by pioneering surgeons like McKee and Ring. In 1958, Charnley introduced a ''low-friction arthroplasty'' based on the principle of a metallic femoral component articulating against a polymeric acetabular component, and in 1970, Boutin developed the first ceramic-on-ceramic total hip replacement. Charnley's hard-on-soft bearing concept eventually dominated the hard-on-hard bearing alternatives. Today the most widely accepted bearing couple (i.e., combination of bearing materials for the hip joint) consists of a femoral head made from cobalt chromium molybdenum (cobalt chrome or CoCr) alloy articulating against a polymeric component fabricated from ultrahigh molecular weight polyethylene (UHMWPE). The use of the CoCr/UHMWPE bearing couple has proved consistent results in total hip arthroplasties around the world for the past four decades. (Older 2002)
In 1998, an estimated 700,000 UHMWPE hip components were implanted worldwide. Based on the report of major orthopaedic manufacturers, at most 200,000 metal-on-metal or ceramic-on-ceramic components have been implanted in patients worldwide between 1988 and 2000, corresponding to less than 10% of total hip replacements during the same time period. Therefore, the overwhelming majority (over 90%) of total hip arthroplasties currently in service throughout the world includes an UHMWPE or a modified UHMWPE component and is based upon Charnley's original concept of hard-on-soft bearing. Despite the worldwide acceptance of total hip arthroplasty, wear of the UHMWPE component is a major obstacle limiting the longevity of these reconstructions. It is well established that particulate debris generated from the hard-on-soft articulating surfaces initiates a cascade of adverse tissue response leading to osteolysis and in certain cases loosening of the components. Extending the longevity of total joint replacements using alternative bearing technologies with improved wear behavior has been the subject of ongoing research in the orthopaedic community. Since the 1970s, researchers have attempted to improve the tribological characteristics of UHMWPE by modifying the polymer's structure, with the ultimate goal of improving the in vivo wear performance of hip bearings. In the 1970s,

carbon fiber-reinforced UHMWPE with a potentially improved wear resistance was clinically introduced. In the 1980s, a high-pressure recrystallized form of UHMWPE was clinically introduced for its improved creep resistance. In the late 1990s, many researchers confirmed that crosslinking of UHMWPE can substantially improve the wear performance of the polyethylene in hip joint simulators. Based on these in vitro analyses, a number of radiation cross-linked materials have been clinically introduced in the late 1990s.

2. Tribology of articulating surfaces

According to the ASM International handbook, tribology is defined as the science and technology of interacting surfaces in relative motion and all practices related thereto. It includes the study of wear, friction, and lubrication. Total joint replacements have bearing surfaces that must transmit normal joint loads and motions. Low friction has been an important design objective for prosthetic joints for two reasons. First, if large shear forces due to friction are applied to the articulating surfaces, the risk of loosening may be increased. Second, the addition of frictional shear increases the stresses associated with surface damage due to contact, which can result in the release of wear debris to the surrounding tissue that also increases the risk of loosening.

2.1 Friction

Friction arises from the interaction between moving solids in contact and hinders (sliding friction) or prevents (static friction) motion. The friction force is proportional to the normal load applied to the surface and the coefficient of friction. The coefficient of friction is determined, in part, by the bearing surface material. There are two coefficients of friction, static and dynamic. It requires a greater force to initiate sliding than to maintain it, so the latter is generally considered to be 70% of the former. The contact area also determines the frictional force. The true contact area for many bearing surfaces is far less than the apparent contact area, somewhere in the region of 1%.(Fig.1)

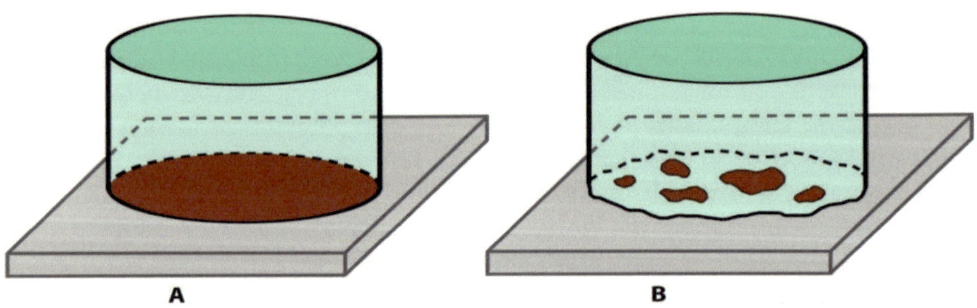

Fig. 1. Apparent (A) and Real (B) area of contact

This is due to the marked irregularity of the surfaces (asperities) at microscopic level. Only very small peaks from each surface contact each other.

The friction force is defined as the force acting tangentially to the interface resisting motion, when, under the action of an external force, one body moves or tends to move relative to another. The friction force F may be associated with sliding motion or with pure rolling motion of the bodies.

The coefficient of friction μ is a dimensionless number, defined as the ratio F/N between the friction force F and the normal force N acting to press the two bodies together. The kinetic coefficient of friction μ_k is the coefficient of friction under conditions of macroscopic relative motion between the two bodies, while the static coefficient of friction μ_s is the coefficient of friction corresponding to the maximum friction force that must be overcome to initiate macroscopic motion between the two bodies. F is approximately linearly proportional to N over quite large ranges of N. The equation

$$F = \mu N \tag{1}$$

is sometimes called "Amontons Law". The value of μ can be expected to depend significantly on the precise composition, topography and history of the surfaces in contact, the environment to which they are exposed, and the precise details of the loading conditions. Although tables of coefficients of friction have been published, they should not be regarded as anything more than general indications of relative values under the specific conditions of measurement. The coefficient of friction usually lies in the range from 0 to 1, although there is no fundamental reason why it need do so.

In order to initiate sliding, the bonds between the contact points need to be broken, thus explaining the higher force required to initiate movement with respect to maintaining it. The friction begins by cyclic elastic or plastic deformation of contact spots of the real contact area. Then it is transformed into elastic or plastic deformation energy within interlocking surface asperities and/or leads to crack initiation and propagation. This deformation may be responsible for the generation of particles. This (progressive) loss of particulate debris from the surface of a solid body due to mechanical action has been defined as wear. The adhesion of the surface atoms and molecules of body and counterbody contributes to friction. The probability of adhesion depends on mechanical properties and the tendency of atoms and molecules to react chemically. Both the deformation and adhesion contributions to friction can be distinctly lowered by means of surface modifications or coatings as well as by lubrication. At least 90% of the introduced energy is dissipated into heat, leading to an increase of the temperature within the contact zone. Depending on local normal forces and the relative velocity, the average as well as the flash temperatures may rise. Although the average temperature is primarily governed by the normal force, the flash temperature depends mostly on the relative velocity and lasts for only a few nanoseconds or milliseconds. The remaining 10% is dissipated by storing mechanical energy within lattice defects generated by cyclic elastic and plastic deformation, phase transformation or chemical reaction of body, counterbody, interfacial medium, and environment. Friction also results in the transfer of force from the articulating areas to the fixed interfaces.

2.2 Lubrication

Friction can be reduced by lubrication. The principal idea behind lubrication is to interpose a material between two contacting solids to minimize interaction between them. For example, wetting of the surfaces reduces adhesion. The extent of fluid film formation plays an important role in the wear process of artificial joints in vivo. The effectiveness of a lubricant film can be defined by the specific film thickness which is dependent on the viscosity of the lubricant, the relative velocity between body and counterbody, the pressure across the interface, and the roughness of the mating surfaces.

Sommerfield number is the determiner of the thickness of the lubrication fluid and depends on a number of factors:

- Viscosity
- Sliding velocity (velocity at which the fluid is forced into gaps)
- Applied pressure

$$\text{Sommerfield number} \propto \text{Fluid viscosity x Sliding velocity/Applied pressure} \quad (2)$$

The higher the value, the thicker the lubrication film.(Howcroft 2008)
The wettability of the materials also plays a part. This is essentially describes how hydrophobic or hydrophilic they are. The ceramics are the most wettable of the currently used bearings.
The lambda ratio (λ) refers to the ratio of fluid-film thickness to the surfaces roughness. Lambda values greater than 3 imply that the fluid-film thickness is greater than the height of asperities on the articular surface and represent fluid-film lubrication. Lambda values between 1 and 3 represent mixed film lubrication, and values less than 1 represent boundary lubrication.
Lubrication between the bearing surfaces of hip implants and its effect on friction generated during articulation is commonly illustrated by a Stribeck diagram. (Fig.2)

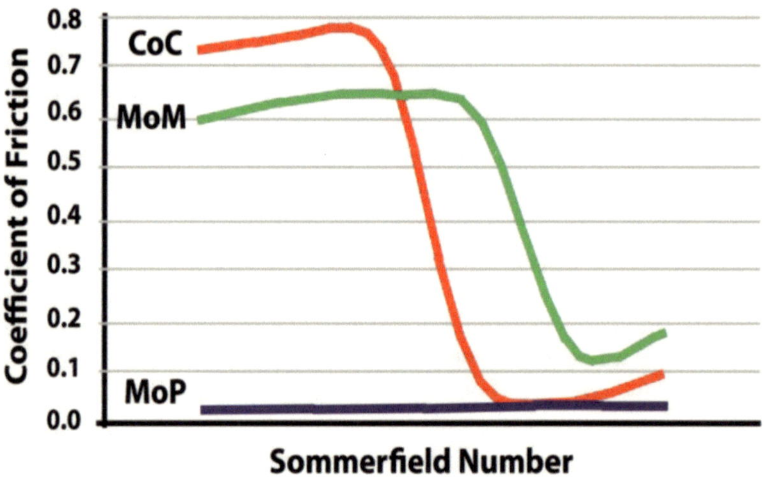

Fig. 2. The Stribeck diagram of different bearing combination materials

The Stribeck curve is traditionally depicted in three phases. When the thickness of the fluid film is less than or equal to the average surface roughness of the articulating surfaces, boundary lubrication (BL) is achieved. In this phase, the asperities of the articulating surfaces are in contact at all times. It is not ideal and is more likely to occur in rough bearing surfaces, or as a result of third body formation or protein deposition. It is improved with better manufacture tolerances of the bearing surfaces. The longer implants remain in situ the more likely they are to develop this type of lubrication. As the thickness of the fluid film increases, the articulating surfaces become separated from each other. There is a transition stage called mixed lubrication (ML), where there is a combination of fluid film and boundary lubrication. The coefficient of friction continues decreasing until full fluid film lubrication (FFL) is generated, where the articulating surfaces are separated by the lubricant. It is also called hydrodynamic lubrication and is divided into two groups depending on whether the two surfaces are conforming or not. Native joints are conforming (hydrodynamic lubrication) unlike artificial joints that deform elastically (elastohydrodynamic lubrication). Elastohydrodynamic (EHD) lubrication occurs when the pressure in the fluid film is sufficiently high to deform the asperities of the solid surfaces. Thus, even if the thickness of the fluid film is less than the heights of the asperities of body and counterbody, a total separation may be still achieved. Under realistic loads and in the presence of synovial fluid, metal-on-polyethylene hip joints articulate in the mixed film or boundary lubrication regime. Hard-on-hard bearings primarily work in the elastohydrodynamic and mixed film lubrication regime; however, with increasing femoral head size (>28 mm), a shift toward full fluid film (hydrodynamic) lubrication can be observed as well. (Smith 2001b; Dowson 2006)

2.3 Wear and wear mechanisms

Wear can be defined as damage to a solid surface, generally involving progressive loss of material, due to relative motion between that surface and a contacting substance or substances. Materials in contact are subjected to relative motion in many different applications. The creep and plastic deformation are not forms of wear per se because they do not produce wear debris but dimensional changes of the contacting surfaces. Also, corrosion is not directly related to wear because it can take place without any mechanical activation at all.(Buford 2004)

2.3.1 Types of wear

It is important, especially when describing wear, to distinguish clearly between the nature of the relative motion responsible for the wear and the physical mechanisms by which the material is removed or displaced in wear. The wear mechanisms in bearing surfaces are as follows:

2.3.1.1 Adhesive wear

The bonds that form between to surfaces need to be broken to allow movement. If the bonds are the weakest point then they will break. But sometimes one of the materials is weaker than the bonds so it breaks preferentially. Thus a layer of the weaker material lines the stronger material, changing the interface at which movement takes place. During mechanical action, these microjunctions are torn off, and fragments may become particles or be transferred from body to counterbody and vice versa, bringing about surface damage in the form of flakes and pitting. If the generated flakes and particles are bigger than the clearance of the bearing, they may act as abrasive particles or even block the joint.(Howcroft 2008)

2.3.1.2 Abrasive wear

When material is removed from a surface by hard asperities on the counterface or hard particles (third body) trapped between the two contact surfaces, abrasive wear occurs.(Howcroft 2008) (Fig.3)

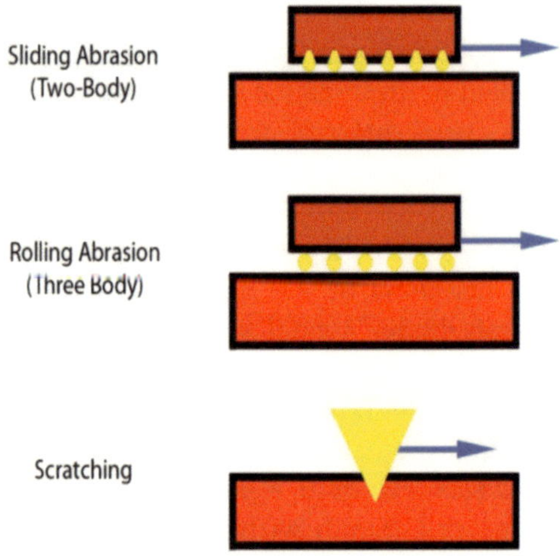

Fig. 3. Examples of abrasive wear

2.3.1.3 Corrosive wear

This type of wear occurs by the combination of mechanical wear and chemical reaction. (Howcroft 2008)

2.3.1.4 Surface fatigue wear

Fatigue acts during repeated sliding or rolling over the same wear track. The repeated loading and unloading can induce the initiation and propagation of microcracks parallel and orthogonal to the surfaces for mechanical or material-related reasons. As a result, shallow pits and filaments (delaminations) are generated.

2.3.2 Wear mode

The wear mode defines the general mechanical conditions under which the bearing is functioning when wear occurs. Wear modes are defined by two sets of criteria: first by the macroscopic structure of the tribosystem and the kinematic interaction of its elements and second by the combination of acting wear mechanisms. It should be noted that the wear mode is not a steady-state condition and can change from one form to another. For example, particulate debris generated by two-body abrasion may function as an interfacial medium and turn the problem into a particle-related (third-body) phenomenon. Depending on the circumstances, this may reduce or increase the wear rate. Mode 1 wear results from the motion of two primary bearing surfaces one against each other, as intended. Mode 2 refers to the condition of a primary bearing surface moving against a secondary surface, which is not intended. Usually, this mode of wear occurs after excessive wear in mode 1. Mode 3 refers to the condition of the primary surfaces moving against each other, but with third-body particles interposed. In mode 3, the contaminant particles directly abrade one or both of the primary bearing surfaces. This is known as three-body abrasion or three-body wear. The primary bearing surfaces may be transiently or permanently roughened by this interaction, leading to a higher mode 1 wear rate. Mode 4 wear refers to two secondary (nonprimary) surfaces rubbing together. Examples of mode 4 wear include wear due to metal-cement or bone-cement interface motion or from relative motion of a porous coating, or other metallic surface, against bone; relative motion of the superior surface of a modular

PE component against the metal support, so-called back-side wear; and fretting and corrosion of modular taper connections and extra-articular sources.(Jacobs 2006) (Fig.4)

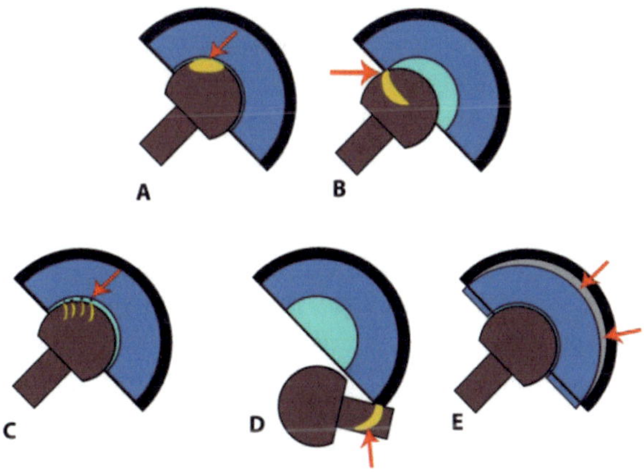

Fig. 4. The modes of wear for a total hip arthroplasty: **A:** Mode 1 or normal wear, **B:** Mode 2 or subluxation wear, **C:** Mode 3 or third body abrasive wear, **D and E:** Mode 4

Particles produced by mode 4 wear can migrate to the primary bearing surfaces, inducing third-body wear (mode 3). Wear particles are a function of the type of wear. A smooth, highly polished femoral head wearing against PE in the absence of third bodies generates very small wear particles with comparatively little variation in size and shape.

2.4 Material properties

Materials used in the manufacturing of femoral heads for metal-on-polyethylene (MOP) total hip replacement (THR) include the metal alloys, stainless steel, cobalt-chromium, and titanium alloy as well as ceramic materials, aluminum oxide, and zirconium oxide. Properties to consider when evaluating materials for bearings in THR include corrosion resistance, strength, ductility, hardness, and frictional characteristics. Frictional characteristics are a result of material properties such as wettability (related to surface energy), manufacturing variables such as surface finish, and operating conditions such as lubrication. The degree of resistance is proportional to the load. Because both chemical and mechanical interactions may occur, frictional forces depend on both the material composition and the roughness of the opposed surfaces. Lubricating conditions can change the nature of the interface between the moving surfaces and decrease friction. As described earlier, the coefficients of friction depend upon the nature and amount of lubricant present, as well as the speed of relative motion and the applied load.

2.5 Surface roughness

A thorough surface roughness evaluation should include a visual comparison of the actual tracings and representative photomicrographs (scanning electron microscope) of the surface. The surface roughness of currently available femoral heads ranges from an average height (R_a) of less than 0.03 µm to about 0.10 µm and maximum height ranging from less than 0.10 to about 0.40 µm. The surface roughness of a femoral bearing can change over time in vivo. In the presence of hard third bodies, as can occur in vivo, surface abrasions (scratches) result

in an increased surface roughness, and the wear rate of polyethylene (PE) can increase. Conversely, in "clean" operating conditions with little or no hard third bodies, motion against PE may result in polishing of the metal surface and a lower surface roughness. This suggests that differences in the initial surface roughness of a femoral head may not be as important in the long run as the in vivo operating conditions. The susceptibility to scratching is a function of the hardness of the material. The decreased hardness of titanium alloy results in decreased abrasion resistance. Although the initial surface roughness of a titanium alloy femoral head may be equivalent to that of other bearing materials, there is greater potential for surface roughness to increase in vivo. In an environment with few or no hard third bodies, the wear performance of titanium alloy against PE can be comparable to the other metals, but the performance of titanium alloy against PE is affected to a greater degree by the presence of hard third bodies. The abrasion resistance of cobalt-chromium alloy is considered superior to that of titanium alloy and stainless steel.(Fisher 2004)
The abrasive particles are mainly released from modular interfaces, metal backing, and/or porous coating. Increased femoral head surface roughness may dramatically accelerate two-body abrasive wear of PE. Experimental studies indicate that a threefold increase in femoral roughness can cause at least a tenfold increase in the wear rate of PE. Specific increases in wear rate are dependent on the nature of the damage to the femoral head. Ceramics are harder and therefore more resistant to damage by third-body particles than metal counterfaces. For this reason, the increased hardness of ceramic materials is considered advantageous. The pattern of damage by a hard third body in metals and ceramics differs.(Raimondi 2008) (Fig.5)

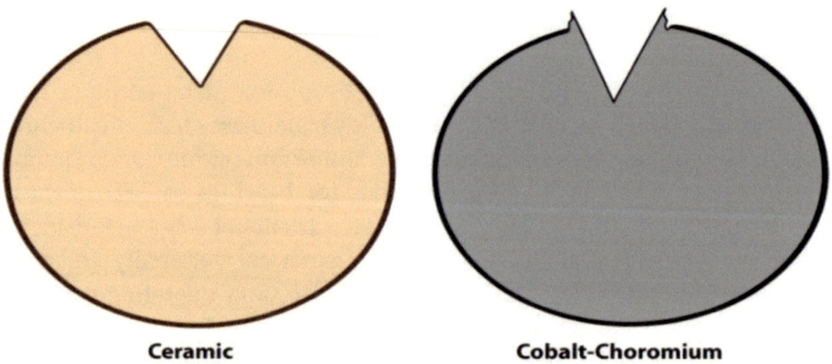

Fig. 5. Scratch profiles of metal and ceramic femoral heads

2.6 Frictional torque

The frictional torque of the Charnley prosthesis with a load of 890 N has been reported between 0.4 to 1.2 Nm. Under similar conditions, the frictional torque of a 28-mm prosthesis, a 43-mm prosthesis, and a 51-mm prosthesis averaged 1.3, 2.7, and 3.2 Nm, respectively. These values are 20 to 100 times smaller than the reported static torques to failure for cemented acetabular components. The coefficient of friction for the MOM bearing of the McKee-Farrar hip is roughly two to three times greater than that for the Charnley. The larger diameter of the McKee-Farrar (about 40 mm) amplifies this difference, and the result is a frictional torque that is up to 10 times greater than that in the Charnley. This value is still an order of magnitude less than the static torque-to-failure of an acutely implanted cemented acetabular component and lower than that reported for surface replacement components. Contrary to theoretical considerations, frictional torque has not been demonstrated to be important in the initiation of aseptic loosening of either femoral or acetabular components. Accumulating evidence indicates that PE wear particles have a greater effect on the durability of implant fixation than frictional torque. From this perspective, the success of the Charnley low-friction arthroplasty is primarily a function of the low volumetric wear of the 22-mm bearing, not low frictional torque. Higher bearing surface friction and frictional torques can be tolerated if the release of wear particles to periprosthetic tissues is sufficiently low. Within the range of frictional torques generated by implants used to date, wear is a more important factor in survivorship than frictional torque. Large-diameter bearings can be successful if the wear rate is low. This is an important consideration as alternatives to PE bearings are being investigated.

2.7 Stresses caused by contact

When contact occurs between metal and polyethylene components, both surfaces deform, but the deformation of the metal component is negligible and the metal component behaves like a rigid indenter. Thus, when an artificial joint is loaded, the polyethylene is squeezed between the rigid metal component and the supporting material (bone, cement, or metal backing), and in the region of contact, the articulating surface of the polyethylene is forced to conform to the shape of the metal surface. The resulting deformation causes compressive, tensile, and shear stresses in the polyethylene. The magnitude of the stress depends on the magnitude of the joint load. These loads are large (3-5 times body weight) and in combination with the relative motion of the articulating surfaces, cause damage that increases with time of implantation (number of cycles of loading) and patient weight (magnitude). This provides strong evidence that surface damage in total joint replacements is the result of fatigue processes. The stresses associated with damage to the articulating surfaces occur both at the surface and within the polyethylene component. Two types of stresses can be applied to the surface: normal compressive stresses (contact stresses), and tangential shear stresses due to friction. Metal and polyethylene were originally chosen for bearing surface materials to produce low-friction total joint replacements. The stresses acting on the surface produce normal and shear stresses within the polyethylene. At the surface, the largest compressive stresses are the contact stresses that act perpendicular to the surface. They decrease nonlinearly with depth through the thickness of the polyethylene. Joint contact also produces compressive and tensile stresses within the polyethylene component that act tangent to the articulating surface. Tangential compressive stresses occur because the polyethylene under the center of the contact area expands radially as the component is compressed. This expansion is resisted by the surrounding material, and tangential compressive stresses are produced. Tangential tensile stresses near the articulating surface occur because the surface must stretch as the polyethylene conforms to the shape of the metal component when the joint is loaded. The stretching occurs near the edge of the contact area. The resulting tensile stresses are largest at the surface of the component. Surface damage is most likely due to combinations of stress components. The maximum shear stress occurs at the surface for conforming joints like hip joints. Although artificial joints produce a range of particle sizes, conforming joints such as hip replacements produce a number of smaller particles greater than the number of larger particles produced by nonconforming total knee replacements.

2.8 Reducing surface damage

By minimizing the stresses associated with the types of damage that can occur or by increasing the strength of the polyethylene, the risk of surface damage can be decreased. We know that abrasive wear which occurs in hip joints can be minimized by a reduction in contact stress. Interestingly, both the range of the maximum principal stress and the maximum shear stress generally decrease when contact stress is decreased. Therefore, one can reduce the risk of abrasive wear and pitting and delamination by reducing the contact stress. The overall design goal is to choose the geometry of the articulating surfaces and material properties of the polyethylene that minimize contact stress.

2.8.1 Minimizing contact stress

Contact stresses in acetabular components are affected by changes in loading, conformity of the articulating surfaces, thickness of the polyethylene, and stiffness of the material. Contact stresses increase with increasing load. If the same prosthesis (same conformity, thickness, and material) is used in patients with different weights, the stresses will be higher in the heavier patients. The stresses are not directly proportional to the load. As the load between the contacting surfaces increases, the contact area also gets larger. The contact stresses, of course, are not uniform over the contact area. The metal component of a total joint replacement is a rigid indenter. The contact stress will be greatest where the surface displacement of the polyethylene is greatest. Consequently, the displacement of the polyethylene surface in a direction normal to the surface will be determined by the shapes of the two contacting surfaces. For example, if the indenter and the polyethylene are both spherical, as they are in an ideal total hip replacement, then the maximum displacement of the polyethylene will occur at the center of contact. Therefore, the maximum contact stress will occur at the center of the contact area, and the minimum contact stress (zero) will occur at the edge of contact. Furthermore, the shape of the contact area in this ideal case will be circular. If the surfaces are not spherical because of either design or manufacturing variations, then the maximum contact stress may not be at the center of the contact area. The acetabular surface has ripples in it. As a result, when the femoral head is pressed into the polyethylene, the largest displacement normal to the surface of the polyethylene component will be at the apexes of the ripples. Therefore, the greatest contact stresses will also occur at these points. The stress in the valleys in the contact area will be small, because the deformation (difference between the dashed and solid lines) will be small at these points. Surface waviness can be caused by normal variations in manufacturing processes. Changes in conformity, thickness, and material properties cause changes in the contact area. In general, changes that decrease the contact area will increase the stresses, because the same load must be distributed over a smaller region. The contact area decreases when the conformity between the articulating surfaces decreases, when the thickness of the material decreases, and when the stiffness of the material increases. The effects of changes in thickness and elastic modulus on contact stresses may be understood as follows. Conceptually, the polyethylene may be considered to be supporting the metal indenter by a collection of parallel rods that are aligned along the direction of loading. Each rod supports a portion, δP, of the total load P. The stiffness of a rod under axial load is given by

$$K_{rod} = \delta P/\Delta = EA/L \tag{3}$$

where Δ is the displacement of the rod, E is the elastic modulus of the rod material, A is the cross-sectional area of the rod, and L is the length of the rod, which corresponds to the thickness of the polyethylene component. It can be seen from this equation that the structural stiffness of the rod increases as the length of the rod decreases. In a similar way, the structural stiffness of polyethylene components increases with decreasing thickness. When the stiffness of the component increases, the indenter does not displace as much, the contact area decreases, and the contact stresses increase. The rod analogy further shows that structural stiffness also increases when the elastic modulus of the rod material increases. Similarly, the structural stiffness of a polyethylene component increases when the elastic modulus of the polyethylene increases, leading to a decrease in contact area and an increase in contact stress. The contact stresses for acetabular components are within the elastic limit of the polyethylene. For perfectly conforming spherical contact, it can be shown that the contact stresses are independent of cup thickness and modulus. This is consistent with observations of in vivo head penetration rates, which are constant with time after an initial wearing-in period. On the basis of contact stress alone, larger head sizes would be preferred. But it has been shown that wear at a point is proportional to pressure times sliding distance. Consequently, there is a trade-off between the relative sliding of the contacting surfaces and the contact stress, both of which are a function of diameter. The maximum shear stress in polyethylene acetabular components occurs very close to the articulating surface and this fact has not yet been directly linked to the wear seen in these components.(Teoh 2002)

2.9 Particle debris

The generation of particulate debris is a central focus of attention in the arthroplasty literature. The biologic response to wear debris is currently heralded as the single most important factor limiting the long-term durability of contemporary total hip and total knee replacement arthroplasty.

2.9.1 Types of particles

Current data suggest that tissues adjacent to a failed joint prosthesis contain billions of particles per gram of tissue. A wide variety of particle types have been retrieved from periprosthetic tissues at the time of autopsy or revision, as well as from joint simulators. In general, these particles types may be classified as metallic, polymeric, and ceramic. The majority of reports on periprosthetic metal debris pertain to Co-Cr and titanium. Metallic particles are characteristically gray to black, and although they may appear weakly birefringent under polarized microscopy, the appearance of birefringence is an optical artifact because the particles are actually opaque. The metal particles are generally smaller than polymer particles but larger than ceramic particles.

Submicrometer metallic particles have been described as globular or irregularly shaped as well as elongated with sharp corners. Larger Co-Cr particles, in the 1- to 5-μm size range, have been described more often as needle, rod, or splinter shaped. Even larger Co-Cr particles, from 5 μm to over 1 mm, have been described as irregularly shaped or globular. These particles tend to be extracellular and may actually represent aggregates or clusters of smaller particles. The majority of titanium particles likewise range from under a micrometer to less than 5 μm in size and have been described as blackish-gray material and fine powder. Occasional titanium particles from 5 μm up to 1 mm in size have been reported. (Malviya 2010)

The most common polymer particles encountered in association with joint prostheses are PMMA and UHMWPE particles. PMMA, unlike UHMWPE, is normally not birefringent. There are several potential sources of PMMA particles, including intraoperative debris, fatigue failure of cement and fretting of bone-cement and prosthesis-cement interfaces. In addition, unconsolidated or poorly mixed PMMA may release 25- to 35-μm "prepolymerized spheres". Certain elements of tissue processing for light microscopy dissolve PMMA and therefore it may be represented by histologic voids, ranging from less than 1 μm to greater than 1 mm in size. The particles or voids are irregularly shaped and have been described as multifaceted or resembling slivers of glass. Barium sulfate or zirconium oxide which have been added to most PMMA since the 1970s to permit visualization of the cement on radiographs has been reported in tissue voids left by PMMA. UHMWPE debris is translucent and strongly birefringent under polarized light microscopy. The particles from the femoral area of aseptically loose femoral components are predominantly spherical or globular in shape, ranging from 0.1 to 1 μm with a mean of 0.5 μm. Over 90% of these particles are less than 1 μm in size. The spherical particles are also associated with fibrillar attachments either singly or forming aggregates of fine particles. The fibrils ranged from 0.3 to 1.0 μm wide to 10 to 25 μm in length. Debris over 100 μm in length have been described as shredded fibers and flattened UHMWPE rolled in the articulation and resembling cigars. There has been great recent interest in the use of highly cross-linked UHMWPE in total joint arthroplasty as a means of decreasing the wear rates of the polyethylene bearing surfaces. It is known that the mechanical properties of UHMWPE are directly related to its molecular weight, crystalline ultrastructure, chemical structure and thermal history. The increased intramolecular cross-links of highly cross-linked UHMWPE are thought to better resist deformation and wear. The wear particles from highly cross-linked polyethylene are smaller (often in the submicrometer and nanometer range) than those from conventional UHMWPE. Controversy exists regarding the ability of these submicrometer particles to generate the inflammatory response that ultimately results in osteolysis. It is well known that particle morphology can strongly influence biological response. The elongated particles of UHMWPE were more biologically active than globular particles.(Gul 2003)

A resurgence of interest in ceramic articulating surfaces has been driven by various reports of their excellent wear characteristics. Still, ceramic wear debris is reported and particles are most commonly 1 to 5 μm in size. In a study of tissue retrieved at the time of revision, Hatton et al. found a bimodal distribution of sizes of ceramic wear debris. Using low resolution electron microscope, ceramic particles between 0.05 and 3.2 μm were found. Using high resolution electron microscope, particles between 5 and 90 nm were visualized. It was theorized that the larger particles were generated from microseparation and impaction of the ceramic surfaces and that the smaller particles were generated from normal articulation of the bearing surfaces.(Hatton 2002b) While often thought of as inert, ceramic wear debris may be able to generate a biologic response that leads to osteolysis. Many studies have shown that ceramic particles can incite inflammatory and cytotoxic effects. Hatton et al. demonstrated that tissues from around ceramic-ceramic hips had areas rich in macrophages, large amounts of neutrophils and lymphocytes, and areas with up to 60% necrosis. The control group, tissue from Charnley metal-on-poly hips, showed the presence of giant cells and a dense macrophage infiltrate, but there was less than 30% necrosis. There were significantly more neutrophils in the ceramic-ceramic tissues and significantly more macrophages and giant cells in the metal-on-poly group.(Hatton 2002b; Hannouche 2005)

In certain clinical settings, relatively large numbers of particles of corrosion products have also been identified. Chromium-orthophosphate-hydrate-rich particles were noted at the modular prosthetic head-neck junction, in the UHMWPE liner, and in the pseudocapsule around the prosthesis. In fact, in certain cases, chromium orthophosphate was second only to UHMWPE in number of intracellular particles found in periprosthetic tissues. The vast majority of chromium orthophosphate particles are less than 5 μm, and they are described as noncrystalline, translucent, and colorless. In addition to particles arising from the prosthesis or cement, certain anomalous particles have also been described. Silica has been reported in interfacial membranes, most likely a remnant of the catalyst used in UHMWPE manufacturing or a remnant of the sandblasting of metal prosthetic components. These are likely sources of trace amounts of aluminum as well. Furthermore, iron- and nickel-containing particles (stainless steel) were likely contaminants from surgical instruments. Calcium- and phosphorous-rich particles were noted and, judging from the ratio of their concentrations, were probably from bone mineral. Thus, bone particles are also present in the periprosthetic milieu.(Jacob 2006)

2.10 Osteolysis

Osteolysis is a significant cause of aseptic loosening and is the biggest cause of revision surgery. It is due to resorption of bone, which is seen more commonly around the acetabulum than the femur. There is a link between wear and corrosive debris formation and osteolysis and is seen more commonly in patients with high wear of their implants. It is often seen as lucency around the implants on radiographs taken years after the original procedure, but can be underestimated on plain films. The primary cellular mediator is the macrophage. In the presence of debris it produces a number of cytokines and inflammatory mediators (IL-1, IL-6, IL-10, TNF-α and prostaglandins). These initiate increased osteoclast activity and also increase osteoclastic differentiation, whilst the debris particles actually have a detrimental effect on osteoblastic bone formation. (Howcroft 2008) Within osteolytic areas other cell lineages may be found including fibroblasts and lymphocytes. Both of these contribute to the ongoing osteoclastic activity and periprosthetic bone resorption.(Archibeck 2000) It is now becoming evident that the size of the wear particles is of equal importance to their number. Nanometer particulate wear debris does not appear to affect the osteoblasts significantly, and coupled with a lower wear rate longer implant survival could be predicted. As the bearing surfaces clearly have an effect on implant survival, it is important to consider the different pairings and look at the relative merits of each. (Harris 2001)

2.11 Clicking and squeaking

With the aid of fluoroscopy, articular surfaces separation during the hip motion has been observed. During this hip separation there is a loss of contact area, leaving only edge contact. Although separation has been well documented, it has not been correlated to clinical complications nor has a more in-depth understanding of the cause and effect been developed. Glaser et al studied the correlation between hip separation and sound production in different bearing surfaces.(Glaser 2008) In their study, among all analyzed subjects, the patients with a metal-on-polyethylene articulating surface experienced the highest magnitude of separation. The ceramic-on-polyethylene group had, on average, relatively low separation values, and these subjects demonstrated much less jerky motion. The maximum separation for the metal-on-metal polyethylene sandwich subjects was 1.5

mm. Interestingly, in the metal-on-metal group with large femoral heads (52 mm), all patients experienced very high separation values after heel-strike in the first 30% of stance phase, which decreased to a no-separation condition during midstance. In the metal-on-metal group with small-size femoral heads (38 mm), the trend was similar to the other bearings with small femoral heads.(Komistek 2002) For all patients, the sound signals were examined and compared with the kinematic findings. Interestingly, there was a distinct correlation of a high-frequency sound occurring at the time when the femoral head slid back into the acetabular component. As the femoral component impacted the acetabular cup, the sound sensor revealed a high-frequency sound, representing impact conditions. A thud-like "clicking" sound was detected for the subject having a metal-on-polyethylene bearing. Similar, but much more accentuated, was the sound recorded for the subjects with a ceramic-on-polyethylene prosthesis. Clear and rich "clicking," combined with some crepitus, was observed for the subjects having a metal-on-metal polyethylene sandwich total hip arthroplasty. The subjects with a metal-on-metal total hip prosthesis experienced a sound similar to a "rusty door hinge". Ceramic-on-ceramic total hip arthroplasty subjects experienced a "squeaking" sound of variable degree, which was present throughout the entire gait cycle. The ceramic-on-ceramic articulations were considered to be the noisiest.(Rodriguez 2008) In all patients with separation, a knocking sound was observed when the femoral head contacted the acetabulum.(Glaser 2008)

Mismatched ceramic couples, acetabular component malposition and impingement have been proposed as factors in the development of squeaking. However, not all mismatched and malpositioned components lead to squeaking. (Restrepo 2008) Additionally, squeaking has been observed in properly matched and positioned implants and when no evidence of neck-to-rim impingement is present. Audible squeaking of a hip replacement remains a still unexplained phenomenon. The sliding motion within the acetabular cup could lead to the induction of vibrational propagation across the interface of the femoral head and acetabular cup, possibly leading to audible interactions. It is also hypothesized that the "squeaking" sound, which mainly occurs in ceramic-on-ceramic total hip prostheses, may be due to separation of the femoral head. This movement of the femoral head from the acetabular component and the impact conditions generated from sliding back can be a source for the acoustic emission observed in total hip prostheses. (Jarrett 2009)

3. Alternate bearing surfaces

During total hip arthroplasty, both the femoral and acetabular bearing surfaces are surgically replaced with metallic, polymeric, and/or ceramic components.(Fig.6) Throughout the twentieth century, many different combinations of these materials have been explored as candidate bearing surfaces for total hip arthroplasty. Today the most widely accepted bearing couple (i.e., combination of bearing materials for the hip joint) consists of a femoral head fabricated from cobalt chromium molybdenum (CoCr) alloy articulating against a polymeric component fabricated from ultrahigh molecular weight polyethylene (UHMWPE). The use of the CoCr/UHMWPE bearing couple has provided consistent results in total hip arthroplasties around the world for the past four decades. In 1998, an estimated 1.4 million UHMWPE components were implanted worldwide, with approximately half of these bearings being implanted in the hip. At most 200,000 metal-on-metal or ceramic-on-ceramic components have been implanted in patients worldwide between 1988 and 2000, corresponding to less than 10% of total hip replacements during the same time period. Despite the recognized success and worldwide acceptance of total hip arthroplasty, wear of the UHMWPE component is a major obstacle limiting the longevity of these reconstructions.

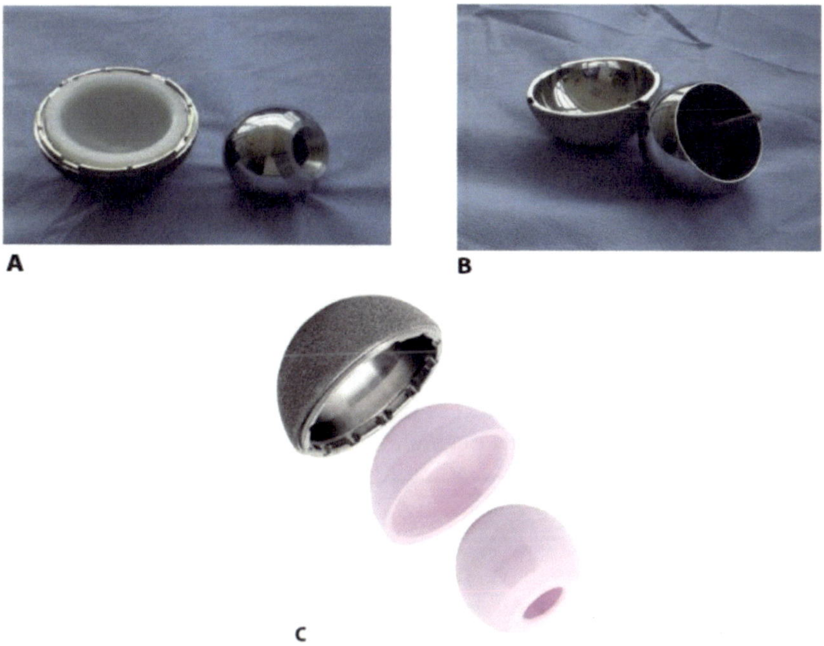

Fig. 6. Different current bearing surface options; A, metal-on-polyethylene, B, metal-on-metal, and C, ceramic-on-ceramic

3.1 Materials bearing against polyethylene

3.1.1 Metal-on-polyethylene bearings

The metals used in conjunction with polyethylene principally have included stainless steel, cobalt-chromium alloy (in the vast majority), and titanium alloy. In some cases, the metal components have been surface hardened; for example, by nitriding or ion-implanting. In general, the wear rate of polyethylene against stainless steel has been comparable to that against cobalt chrome alloy in laboratory tests and in clinical use. In contrast, although the wear rate of polyethylene against titanium alloy under clean conditions appears to be comparable to that with the other metals, the greater vulnerability of titanium alloy to abrasion by entrapped third-body particles can cause severe, runaway wear. Hardening of the surface of the titanium alloy by techniques such as gas nitriding, solution nitriding, or ion implanting can markedly improve its resistance to abrasion by third-body particles, and good 10-year results have been reported for titanium nitride-hardened TiAlNb alloy balls used with polyethylene cups. Nevertheless, if a hardened surface eventually is penetrated, severe wear of the underlying alloy still can be triggered. Consequently, even hardened titanium alloys have seen limited clinical use as bearing surfaces. The vast majority of metal-on-polyethylene bearings used in hip prostheses have involved cobalt-chrome alloy femoral balls, including cast or forged alloys, and the wear rate of this combination now forms the clinical baseline against which potentially improved bearing combinations are evaluated. As noted above, the average wear rate of the polyethylene against cobalt-chrome alloy is typically reported to be in the range of 0.1 to 0.2 mm/yr. However, it should be noted that this average includes those implants that have accelerated wear rates due to excessive third-body damage to the bearing surfaces, radiation-induced oxidative degradation of the polyethylene, or other causes. Thus, the inherent wear rate of a polyethylene cup with a cobalt-chrome alloy ball under clean conditions is probably somewhat below the clinical average wear rate, possibly as low as 0.05 mm/yr. Ion implanting and other surface hardening techniques also have been applied to cobalt-chromium alloy. Laboratory tests of hardened cobalt-chromium alloy have been reported to both markedly reduce wear and to increase wear of the opposing polyethylene, and clinical results are not yet sufficient to resolve this contradiction. Whereas it seems likely that surface hardening of cobalt-chrome may improve its resistance to moderate amounts of third-body abrasion, the uncertainty of the advantage in general has limited its clinical application.(Kim 2005)

3.1.2 Ceramic-on-polyethylene bearings

Alumina and zirconia femoral balls have been used widely as bearing surfaces against polyethylene cups, and most clinical studies have shown substantially lower polyethylene wear rates than with metal balls, with the wear ratios ranging from 0.75 to as low as 0.25 with alumina balls. A comparable advantage has been reported with zirconia against polyethylene.(Urban 2001) Unacceptably high rates of polyethylene wear, lysis, and loosening with an early type of zirconia ball were reported in a study. Similarly, although the majority of the laboratory tests have indicated lower wear of polyethylene with alumina or zirconia than with metal, in one hip simulator study slightly greater polyethylene wear was reported with alumina balls, but less with zirconia balls.(Yoshitomi 2009) The greater hardness of ceramic balls renders them more resistant than metal balls to scratching by entrapped abrasive contaminants that can, in turn, accelerate the wear of the opposing polyethylene cup (wear mode 3). The differences in the relative wear rates in the various clinical studies might reflect differences in the amount of third-body contamination, with those studies having relatively little such contamination showing comparable polyethylene wear rates for ceramic or metal balls. Nevertheless, contamination by metal particles may be detrimental even with a ceramic ball, because the particles can adhere to the surface of the ceramic, effectively roughening it and, thereby, increasing abrasion of the polyethylene. Metal also can be transferred to the ceramic by contact against metallic components or instruments during surgery.(Garvin 2009) Regardless of the bearing material used, care must be taken to minimize the formation of abrasive contaminants in vivo, for example, by avoiding those porous coatings that are prone to shed particles. (Clarke 2000)

3.2 Polyethylenes

3.2.1 Chemical structure and molecular weight

Polyethylene is a polymer of ethylene and consists of a carbon backbone chain with pendant hydrogen atoms. It is the simplest of polymer molecules chemically, but as the length of the polymer chain increases, so too does the complexity of the material. UHMWPE, used in orthopedic hip and knee applications since 1962, has a molecular weight ranging from 2 to 6 million daltons. By virtue of its molecular weight, UHMWPE has the desirable attributes of wear and impact resistance, together with ductility and toughness. These attributes make UHMWPE highly suitable as a bearing material. There has been some confusion in the historical arthroplasty literature, in which what is now considered UHMWPE was historically referred to as high-density polyethylene (HDPE) or polythene. Today, high-density polyethylene refers to a material with a molecular weight of 100 to 250,000 daltons and is suitable for milk jugs, not artificial joints. In a hip simulator, HDPE has a wear rate that is four times higher than that of UHMWPE.

The ultra-high molecular weight polyethylenes (UHMWPEs) that were used for acetabular cups implanted during the past 30 years were fabricated from raw powder (also called resin). The powder is converted to solid form using one of three distinct methods. In the extrusion process, the polyethylene powder is driven by a ram through a heated nozzle, fusing the flakes into a continuous bar, typically several inches in diameter. The components are machined from the bar stock. In bulk compression molding, the powder is placed in a large mold and heated under pressure to fuse it into a block or sheet from which the final components are machined. In net-shape molding, the powder is placed in a metal mold having the desired shape of the implant and then fused under heat and pressure, such that little or no final machining is required. The final step in any fabrication process was sterilization.

3.2.2 Crystallinity

Crystallinity is an important attribute of all polyethylenes, including cross-linked polyethylene. The molecular chains in polyethylene have a natural tendency (driven by thermodynamics) to preferentially fold up against themselves whenever possible, hindered by the considerable crowding and thermal jostling presented by adjacent molecules. Regions of the polymer with folded chains are referred to as crystallites, whereas the regions with randomly oriented polymer chains are referred to as the amorphous regions. In polyethylene, the crystallites have a particular "lamella" shape. If we were to dissolve away the amorphous regions, the crystalline lamellae in polyethylene would look something like twisted, interconnected sheets. The molecular chains are oriented perpendicular to the plane of the lamella and may emerge to connect with adjacent lamellae.(Fig.7)

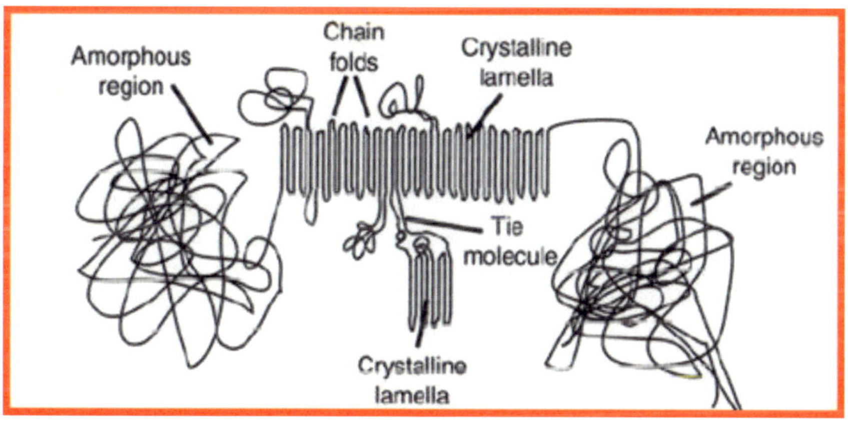

Fig. 7. Schematic crystalline structure of polyethylene

These connective polymer chains (not shown) are referred to as tie molecules. In particular, it is thought that tie molecules contribute greatly to the inherent wear resistance of polyethylene. The elastic modulus and yield stress of polyethylene will increase in direct relation to the number of crystals present. Many of the processing steps for clinical polyethylenes are tailored specifically to optimize the crystalline structure and thereby tune its material properties. Polyethylene typically has a crystalline content of about 50%. The thermal processing alters the basic organization of molecular chains in polyethylene by modifying the size and shape of the crystals.

3.2.3 Cross-linking

Cross-linking is the foundation of all modern polyethylene total hip bearings. Cross linking is defined as the joining of two independent polymer molecules by a chemical covalent bond. Only radiation cross-linking has been commercialized by orthopedic device manufacturers. The first step involves irradiation of the polyethylene molecule. Next, irradiation produces a hydrogen radical, leaving a so-called "free" radical on the polyethylene molecule. Actually, the radical on the polymer chain has extremely limited mobility and is hindered by the adjacent molecule. For cross-linking to occur, free radicals must be present on adjacent polyethylene molecules, and the molecules must be mobile. Free radical recombination takes place primarily in the amorphous phase of the polymer, where the molecules are in close enough proximity to allow the formation of the interchain carbon-carbon bond that constitutes the cross-link. When the adjacent radicals react, a covalent bond, or cross-link, is formed between the two polyethylene molecules. In the crystalline phase, because of the increased distance between the molecules, crosslinking is not favored. As a result, the free radicals generated in the crystalline regions are postulated not to take part in the crosslinking reactions and become trapped. These residual free radicals are the known precursors of oxidation-induced embrittlement secondary to gamma sterilization. (Muratoglu 2001)

The extent of cross-linking in polyethylene is proportional to the absorbed dose of radiation. Historically, polyethylene bearings were gamma sterilized at a dose of 25 to 40 kGy. This dose resulted in the formation of some cross-links. Saturation of cross-linking was achieved only at approximately 100 kGy of absorbed dose. Today, cross-linked polyethylenes are processed with a total dose ranging from 50 to 105 kGy. In general, increasing the dose provides a proportional improvement in wear resistance, with diminished benefits observed above 100 kGy. (Geedink 2009)

3.2.4 Thermal processing: Annealing and remelting

In the production of a highly cross-linked UHMWPE, the material is subjected to a thermal treatment step to reduce the level of free radicals via further cross-linking reactions. At higher temperatures the polymer molecules have increased mobility, thereby increasing the probability of free radicals on adjacent chains to react and form cross-links.(Fig.8) For the thermal treatment to be effective at eliminating all free radicals, it must be conducted above the melting temperature of the material at 150°C. Heating above the melting temperature destroys the crystalline regions of the material, thus making the free radicals that were in the crystals available for cross-linking. The disadvantage of melting is the reduction in polymer crystal size and in mechanical properties (e.g., material yield and ultimate strength) that ensues when the material returns to room temperature. A compromise solution is to heat the material to 130°C to 135°C, just below the melting temperature. This solution preserves the original crystal structure, retains mechanical properties, and makes more free radicals available for cross-linking than would be available without thermal treatment. Some free radicals are retained in the crystal domains, but the number is substantially reduced by the elevated temperature. When thermal treatment is conducted below the melt transition of 135°C, it is referred to as annealing, and above the melt transition, it is called remelting.

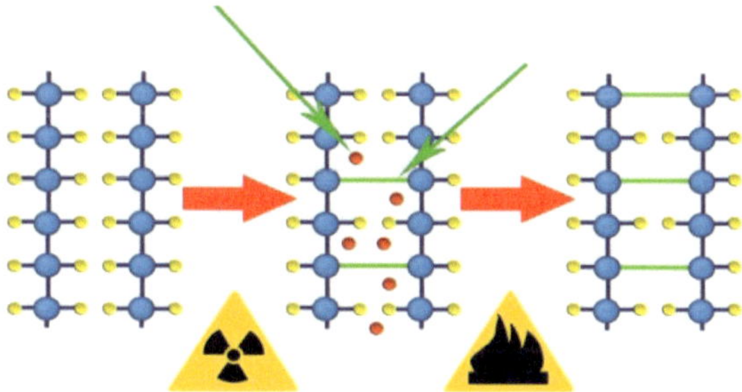

Fig. 8. Diagrammatic representation of the manufacturing process of highly cross-linked polyethylene; the effects of radiation and heat treatment

3.2.5 The effect of crosslinking on mechanical properties of polyethylene

The changes in the mechanical properties of the radiation- and heat-treated polyethylene are primarily dominated by changes in the crosslink density and crystallinity. Under multiaxial loading conditions, it is more difficult to separate effects of crystallinity and cross-linking, since both appear to influence the large-strain mechanical behavior in a more complex, synergistic manner. The crystallinity of polyethylene is a function of the radiation dose level and thermal treatment history. Irradiation generates smaller chains with increased mobility, leading to recrystallization and a slight increase in the crystallinity of the polymer. The changes in the crystallinity during the postirradiation thermal treatment depend on temperature. If the thermal treatment is carried out below the melting transition (<135°C), the chain mobility increases, which, in turn, increases the crystallinity of the polymer. When the thermal treatment is performed at temperatures above the melting transition (>135°C), during cool-down to room temperature, the crystallization of the polymer takes place in the presence of the crosslinks. This leads to a decrease in the crystallinity of the polymer. The radiation dose level used in the irradiation step determines the crosslink density. The crosslink density of the polyethylene limits the ultimate elongation that can be achieved during plastic deformation prior to failure. Therefore, at higher radiation dose levels, the cross-linked polymer exhibits reduced ultimate tensile strength and elongation at break under uniaxial tension. As a result, the work to failure also decreases. As the crosslinking reduces the chain mobility, it also inhibits the active energy-absorbing mechanisms. Therefore, at high uniaxial deformation rates, such as impact loading, the energy absorption before failure decreases, leading to a decrease in the toughness.(Baker 2003) Another important variable that affects the mechanical properties of the radiation- and heat-treated polyethylene is the irradiation temperature. When the polymer is irradiated at an elevated temperature (90°C < T < 135°C) the effect of the crosslink density on the large strain mechanical properties decreases significantly. This may be explained by a nonstatistical distribution of the crosslinks resulting at increased irradiation temperatures. As a result, the low crosslink-density matrix controls the large-strain mechanical properties.(Dumbleton 2006) The polyethylenes irradiated at increased temperatures have been reported to exhibit better large-strain mechanical properties than those irradiated at room temperature with identical radiation dose levels.(Affatato 2005)

3.2.6 Conventional polyethylene surfaces

Although ultra-high-molecular-weight polyethylene (UHMWPE) has low friction and dampening properties, it has one major disadvantage, which is adhesive and abrasive wear. The UHMWPE particles produced from cyclical loading are thought to play a major role in particle-induced osteolysis and secondary implant failure and loosening. Osteolysis results from the intrusion of polyethylene debris between the implant surface and bone, inducing a macrophage response. Polyethylene also can fail as a result of third-body wear secondary to polyethylene degradation. A polyethylene wear rate of 0.10 mm per year is the threshold for the development of osteolysis. In addition, conventional polyethylene thickness should not decrease below 6 to 8 mm, or accelerated wear polyethylene failure and osteolysis will develop.(Lundberga 2006)

3.2.7 Highly cross-linked polyethylene surfaces

Highly cross-linked polyethylene was introduced to reduce the polyethylene wear rate in THA.(McKellop 1999) It is well documented that young age, male gender, and high activity level increase the risk of wear, osteolysis, and mechanical failure. However, these different factors that influence wear rate in conventional polyethylene have no significant influence when using highly cross-linked polyethylene.(Rohrl 2007) In vitro studies on highly cross-linked polyethylene have shown that wear can be reduced by 42% to 100% compared with that of conventional polyethylene, and, multiple in vivo studies support many of these in vitro results. The annual linear wear for highly cross-linked polyethylene has been reported to be 45% that of the conventional liner at 5 years after implantation. This wear rate is well below the threshold for lysis. Long-term results (10 to 20 years) of highly cross-linked polyethylene support that the low wear rates reported approach that of MOM and ceramic-on-ceramic bearings.(Digas 2007; Atienza 2008)

3.2.8 Sterilization techniques

Today, polyethylenes are sterilized by different techniques with regard to the fact that sterilization process can affect the physical properties of polyethylene. Some brands of the polyethylene components are now sterilized without irradiation, using either ethylene oxide or gas plasma, in order to minimize the oxidative degradation. Because these methods do not generate free radicals in the polyethylene, they completely avoid the potential for immediate and long-term oxidative degradation of the mechanical properties and wear resistance. However, because ethylene oxide or gas-plasma do not induce cross-linking, these polyethylenes do not take advantage of improving the wear resistance following cross-linking.(Digas 2003) Other brands of polyethylenes are still sterilized with gamma radiation, but for doing so, the polyethylene components are sealed in some type of low-oxygen atmosphere, including vacuum, inert gas, or with an oxygen scavenger. In addition, one manufacturer anneals the polyethylene acetabular cups after sterilization by heating them in the nitrogen packaging at 37° to 50°C (well below the melt temperature of 135°C to avoid distorting the components) for about 6 days to reduce the level of residual free radicals that were induced by the gamma radiation. These modifications in sterilization techniques can markedly reduce but not necessarily eliminate the oxidation that would otherwise occur during gamma sterilization and subsequent shelf-storage, and the remaining free radicals may induce some oxidation during long-term use in vivo. The moderate level of cross-linking that was present in the vast majority of UHMWPE components implanted over the past three decades was an unintentional byproduct of the 2.5 to 4 Mrads of gamma radiation used to sterilize the components. The improvement in wear resistance in these polyethylenes relative to non-cross-linked polyethylene ranges from about 30% to 50%, compared to the 85% or more reduction achieved with intentionally elevated cross-linking doses. A number of laboratory wear simulations have demonstrated that the wear rate of UHMWPE cups decreases markedly with an increasing level of radiation-induced cross-linking. The greatest reduction per Mrad occurs as the dose increased from zero to about 8 Mrads, with progressively less improvement at higher doses and no additional benefit after 15 to 20 Mrads. While this dose-wear relationship was the basis for the recent development of a variety of intentionally-cross-linked polyethylenes, the developers have arrived at very different opinions regarding the appropriate dose and other processing parameters for optimizing the clinical performance of a polyethylene implant.

3.2.9 Optimum method for cross-linking

In addition to the optimum method of cross-linking, the optimum amount of cross-linking to use is also a subject of current debate. Because increasing the level of crosslinking causes a progressively greater reduction in some mechanical properties, such as ultimate strength, ductility, fracture toughness, and fatigue strength, one extreme is to avoid cross-linking altogether (for example, by simply sterilizing with ethylene oxide or gas plasma). This avoidance is to retain the maximum values of strength, elongation, and fracture toughness, despite the fact that it results in substantially higher wear of the polyethylene. Among those who advocate crosslinking, the particular dose used represents that manufacturer's approach to balancing reduced wear against the need to maintain other mechanical properties well above that needed for acceptable clinical performance. Those using the high levels of cross-linking (9.5 to 11 Mrads), about 3 to 4 times the typical dose used historically to sterilize polyethylene components, maintain that these high levels are justified to obtain the additional 5% to 10% improvement in wear over that provided by a moderate dose, despite the corresponding reduction in other physical properties. In contrast, advocates of a moderate cross-linking dose, such as 5 Mrads, maintain that the corresponding reduction in wear to 85% below that of a noncross-linked polyethylene will be sufficient to avoid an osteolytic reaction in even the most active patients, without unnecessarily reducing other physical properties. Clearly, it is not desirable to use a dose that will result in mechanical failure of the polyethylene components.(Moore 2008; Bradford 2004)

3.3 Metal-on-metal bearings

The first widely used total hip replacements featured cobalt-chromium alloy bearing against itself, primarily the McKee-Farrar (Howmedica, Limerick, Ireland) design, along with the Mueller (Sulzer AG, Winterthur, Switzerland), Ring (Downs, Ltd, Mitchham, England) and others. Because of a relatively high rate of early failure, the first-generation metal-on-metal hips were largely supplanted by the Charnley prosthesis, which featured a stainless steel ball and a polyethylene socket. Disregarding the early failures, the long-term survivorship of the early metal-on-metal designs has been comparable to that of the metal-on-polyethylene Charnley. In particular, the steady-state wear rates have been on the order of a few micrometers per year compared with the average of 100 to 200/µm of polyethylene wear per year typically reported for metal-on-polyethylene hips. In view of the growing awareness of the problem of extensive osteolysis caused by polyethylene wear debris, a number of second-generation metal-on-metal implants have been developed, including conventional total hips and surface replacements. The first to be widely used clinically was the Metasul (Sulzer AG, Winterthur, Switzerland) hip. Hip simulator studies and clinical retrievals of modern metal-on-metal bearings also typically have shown steady-state wear rates on the order of a few micrometers per million cycles (with one million cycles being the equivalent of about 1 year's use in a patient of average activity). It is also apparent that metal-on-metal implants have the ability to self-heal, that is, to polish-out isolated surface scratches caused by third-body particles or subluxation damage. The overall clinical performance of second-generation metal-on-metal hips to date has been comparable to that of conventional metal-on-polyethylene hips. Clinical and laboratory wear studies have indicated that metal-on-metal implants often exhibit 10 to 20 times greater wear-in during the initial 1 to 2 years of clinical use, or one to two million cycles in a hip simulator. In addition, some first-generation and second-generation metal-on-metal hips have exhibited extensive surface micropitting, possibly due to a fatigue-corrosion mechanism associated with the smaller carbides.

3.3.1 Tribology

The principle constituents of alloys for MOM bearings are cobalt, chromium, and molybdenum, but they can be differentiated as being either high carbon (0.20% to 0.25%) or low carbon (0.05% to 0.08%), with the former usually demonstrating lower in vitro wear rates. MOM hip bearings produce wear particles by some combination of the four classic mechanisms of adhesion, abrasion, corrosion, and surface fatigue, with an emphasis on abrasion and surface fatigue.(Wimmer 2003) Wear in metal-on-metal total hip arthroplasty implants is known to consist of two distinct phases. A relatively high-wear running-in phase, which lasts for between 0.5 and 2 x 10^6 cycles, is followed by a steady-state phase, during which the wear rate is constant and much lower. This decrease in wear has been demonstrated to be secondary to the so-called self-polishing effect of metal-on-metal bearing surfaces. Opposing metallic bearing surfaces are thought to run-in in the contact zone as surface asperities are polished or removed, improving the initial surface finish, with a commensurate reduction in the wear rate as the lubricating fluid film becomes more coherent. Metal-on-metal total hip arthroplasty implants can operate in the mild mixed-lubrication regime in which much of the applied load is supported by elastohydrodynamic films. Correct tribological design leads to remarkably low steady-state wear rates. Promotion of the most effective elastohydrodynamic films calls for the largest possible head diameters and the smallest clearances that can be reasonably adopted consistent with fine surface finishes, good sphericity, polar contact, and minimal structural elastic deformation of the cup on its foundations.(Udofia 2003) With current manufacturing techniques, a surface roughness of 5 to 15 nm is typically achieved. This results in improved sphericity and surface finish. The presence of depressions or holes (rather than scratches) with smooth (rather than sharp) edges seems to improve the lubrication and wettability properties. The wear of metal-on-metal bearings is affected by various design parameters, such as the clearance or surface roughness. The predictive role of the λ ratio in the evaluation of wear behavior of metal-on-metal total hip replacements has also been well documented. In an in

vitro study, Affatato et al. demonstrated that femoral heads of 36 mm in diameter work in the mixed-lubrication regime ($\lambda > 1$) and 28-mm diameter heads were associated with a λ ratio of <1, thus showing their aptitude to work in the boundary-lubrication regime, with substantially higher volume depletion due to wear. With the 32-mm heads, the λ ratio varied in a range around 1, suggesting the possibility of their operating in the mixed-lubrication regime.(Affatato 2008) Hip-joint-simulator tests on metal-on-metal total hip replacements have shown a transition from boundary to mixed lubrication as the diameter of the femoral head increased. An increase in diameter up to 54 mm resulted in a marked reduction in wear rates, which was attributable to growing support from the fluid-film action in a mixed-lubrication regime. Reducing the clearance between the femoral and acetabular components also reduces the amount of wear debris. Significant reduction in the wear debris associated with large-diameter (54-mm) heads has been noted when clearances were reduced. When clearances are designed, cup flexibility needs to be taken into account so that the minimum clearance is always more than the maximum flexibility of the cup.
Thick (8 to 12-mm) chromium nitride (CrN) and chromium carbon nitride (CrCN) coating leads to twenty-two-fold lower wear rates as compared with those associated with standard metal-on-metal couples. Also, CrN wear particles were found to be less cytotoxic than standard metal-on-metal bearings when co-cultured with macrophage and fibroblast cells. The substantially lower ion concentration released by these surface-engineered components along with the reduced wear volumes and the reduced cytotoxicity per unit volume of wear points to the potential for clinical application of this technology. However, there is concern about the durability of this coating.(Williams 2004)

3.3.2 Materials and design considerations

The interplay of material(s), macrogeometry (diameter and clearance), microgeometry (surface topography), and lubrication influences the wear of MOM-bearing THRs to a far greater degree than MOP-bearing ones. Alloys of cobalt (Co) and chromium (Cr) have been preferred for MOM bearings in THR because of their hardness. High chromium content provides good corrosion resistance. Cast Co-Cr-Mo alloy, which was used to manufacture the majority of first-generation MOM hips, has a relatively high carbon content of 0.2% to 0.3% and contains primarily Cr and Mo carbides, which result in asperities on the polished surface. The macrogeometry of a MOM bearing can be described in terms of the diameter(s) of the ball and the socket and the clearance of the resultant bearing couple. Clearance is the size of the gap between the surfaces at the equator of the bearing. For hemispherical bearings, clearance is a function of the difference in the diameters of the surfaces of the ball and socket. A ball and socket of exactly equal diameter mated together would have zero clearance and a maximal contact area for that size bearing. Contact area can be increased by increasing the size (diameter) of the bearing surfaces and/or by decreasing the clearance. Conversely, for a given diameter, increasing clearance decreases contact area. Contact stresses are a function of material properties and are inversely proportional to contact area. Clearance also influences lubrication, as the size of the gap has implications for the amount and type of lubrication. Smaller clearances encourage fluid film lubrication. Large clearances lead to a reduced contact area, loss of effective lubrication, and more rapid wear.(Reiker 2005) However, too little clearance may lead to equatorial contact, very high frictional forces, high torque, and loosening of the implant.(Chan 1996)

The limitations of current mass production manufacturing set the lower limit of clearance at about 20 µm. Wear rate, particularly during the initial run-in, increases rapidly with clearances above about 150 µm. In addition to the contact area, another important variable is where the contact occurs. Given bearings of equivalent diameters, equatorial contact is associated with higher frictional torques than the same contact area in a more polar location. Equatorial bearing may have been a factor associated with failure of some early MOM THRs, and this is supported by retrieval studies. Consequently, relatively polar contact is preferred.(Dowson 2004; Isaac 2006) (Fig.9)

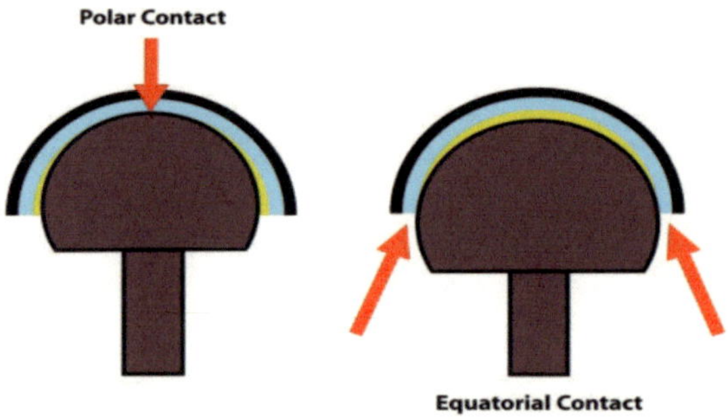

Fig. 9. Too much reduction in the "clearance" can result in conversion a polar contact to an equatorial contact resulting in the articulation seizing

3.3.3 Lubrication

The lubricating fluid and conditions are important variables which influence friction and wear. The synovial fluid of normal, osteoarthritic, and rheumatoid joints has been characterized to some degree. The fluid is thixotropic; viscosity is a function of the shear strain rate, or velocity of motion, for practical purposes. Less is known about the fluid formed around total joint arthroplasties, but the composition and rheology are likely variable. A favorable film thickness to surface roughness ratio (λ ratio) is desirable in order to maintain low friction between the articulating surfaces. Mixed-film lubrication appears to be the operative mechanism in most MOM hip joints. For a given load and surface velocity, fluid film thickness is dependent on the properties of the fluid but can be influenced by the properties of the bearing materials, the macrogeometry of the bearing (which is a function of diameter and clearance), and the surface microtopography (surface finish). (Affatato 2008) Within the apparent contact area, the surfaces make actual contact only at the tips of asperities, and a lubricant film can influence wear significantly. As wear proceeds, the contact area at the asperity tips increases, and such "running-in" can produce a more favorable microgeometry for lubricant films to separate the surfaces and reduce wear. Fluid-film lubrication is encouraged by making the femoral head as large as practically possible and the clearance as small as practically possible. For MOM bearings, in distinction from PE bearings, larger diameters can actually produce lower wear rates for similar manufacturing parameters.(Smith 2001a; Chan 1999)

3.3.4 Composition and microstructure of CoCr alloys

CoCr alloys consist of a primary cobalt alloy matrix phase and a secondary metal carbide phase. In the cobalt-based matrix, chromium enhances the mechanical properties of the alloy and promotes the formation of a passive oxide layer, whereas molybdenum is included in the alloy for corrosion resistance. The size and distribution of the carbide phase contributes to the hardness and mechanical behavior of the alloy. The properties of CoCr alloys depend upon their processing history—whether fabricated by investment casting or by a thermomechanical forming process. During an investment casting process, a wax replica of the prosthesis is first fabricated and coated with a silicate slurry. The replica and slurry are raised above the melting point of the wax (100–150°C) and burned away in a furnace, leaving only the slurry mold with an interior cavity having the dimensions of the replica. The cavity is then filled with molten alloy and, after cooling, the mold is broken to remove the cast implant. Mechanical forming, on the other hand, can be accomplished by a wide range of thermomechanical manufacturing methods, including rolling, forging, swaging, and drawing, all of which lead to a wrought CoCr alloy. Both cast and wrought CoCr alloys are subjected to annealing heat treatments for optimization of microstructure and mechanical properties. Historically, the first-generation metal-on-metal components were fabricated by casting(Hernandez-Rodriguez 2005), whereas contemporary second-generation metal-on-metal implants are manufactured from wrought CoCr alloys. (Barnes 2008)

Wrought CoCr alloys have significantly enhanced hardness, yield strength, and ultimate properties as compared with cast alloys, resulting from their more uniform carbide microstructure. All CoCr alloys used in orthopaedics contain trace constituents of carbon (0.35%), nitrogen (max 0.25%), nickel (max 1%), iron (max 0.75%), silicon (max 1.0%), and manganese (max 1.0%). Cast CoCr alloys may also contain tungsten (max 0.20%), phosphorus (max 0.020%), sulfur (max 0.010%), aluminum (max 0.30%), and boron (max 0.01%). Of these secondary constituents, the effect of carbon content on CoCr alloys has been examined most closely by researchers in the orthopaedic community because of the link between carbon content, carbide formation, and properties of the bearing surface. CoCr alloys may be further classified as either low-carbon (<0.05%) or high-carbon (>0.20%). The majority of contemporary metal-on-metal bearings are fabricated from a high-carbon CoCr alloy. In contemporary hip simulator studies, high- and low-carbon CoCr alloys have exhibited comparable wear mechanisms and wear rates. (Isaac 2006)

3.3.4.1 Metal ions

Ion levels have been measured in whole blood, serum, and erythrocytes. Metal ions from hip implant materials include the following: titanium; vanadium; chromium; cobalt; and molybdenum. In reports of metal ion concentrations in urine, for maximal accuracy and to minimize the effect of variations in the level of hydration that may occur throughout the day, a 24-hour urine collection should be performed. Healthy controls have been demonstrated to have a mean serum cobalt level of 0.24 mg/L (median, 0.23 mg/L; range, 0.08 to 0.50 mg/L) and a mean serum chromium level of 0.28 mg/L (median, 0.29 mg/L; range, 0.06 to 0.93 mg/L). Currently there are two methods for measuring trace metals: inductively coupled plasma mass spectroscopy (ICP-MS) and graphite furnace atomic absorption spectrophotometry (GFAAS), with the former method being favored because of higher sensitivity to detect low levels of metal ions, allowing multielement determinations.(Engh 2009) Numerous studies have reported an increase in the levels of metal ions in serum, urine, and blood of patients with MOM implants. However, serum/plasma levels of cobalt and chromium ions appeared to be higher than those in red blood cells, suggesting that serum may reflect better the true ion levels when using blood to assess systemic ion levels.(Daniel 2007; Antoniou 2008) In a study looking specifically at the serum cobalt concentrations in patients during the first 5 years after an MOM THA, Brodner and colleagues showed a moderate concentration of 1 μg/L at 1 year and 0.7 μg/L at 5 years. They did not find any significant difference in the levels from 3 to 12 months and the subsequent measurements and, therefore, concluded that the serum cobalt concentrations did not reflect the higher run-in wear of MM implants.(Brodner 2003) In modern MM surface arthroplasty, Skipor and colleagues reported elevations in serum chromium that were 22-fold, 23-fold, and 21-fold higher at 3, 6, and 12 months postoperatively, respectively, than preoperatively. The corresponding serum cobalt levels were eightfold, sevenfold, and sixfold higher than preoperative levels, and the authors reported that the values seen with the current generation of surface arthroplasties were in the same range as those observed in association with conventional MOM THA.(Skipor 2002) Comparison of serum cobalt and chromium ion levels in patients with a MOM compared with a MOPE bearing and a MOM compared with a ceramic-ceramic bearing showed that there were always higher ion levels in the patients with the MOM bearings. In a study analyzing the whole blood cobalt and chromium ion levels in 68 patients, Hart and colleagues reported a decrease in cytotoxic $CD8^+$ T-lymphocytes, which are involved in the defense against intracellular pathogens and cancerous cells.(Hart 2009) Of interest, Back and colleagues noted a significant decrease in the cobalt levels at 2 years compared with the levels at 6 months, as well as a decrease in the chromium levels at 2 years compared with the levels at 9 months. When looking at the effects of the size of the femoral head and the orientation of the acetabular component on the overall concentrations of metal ions in the whole blood of patients with MOM resurfacings, Langton et al. reported higher ion concentrations in patients with smaller components and when the inclination angle was greater than 45 degrees and the anteversion angle exceeded 20 degrees.(Langton 2008)

Wear particles from MOM bearings are nanometers in linear dimension, which is substantially smaller than PE wear particles. Light microscopic analysis of tissue obtained from around MOM joints showed particles with variable and irregular shape. The size of metal particles reported by scanning electron microscopy studies ranges from 0.1 to 5 μm. The studies have suggested that large metallic particles observed with light microscopy were agglomerates of the smaller particles. Transmission electron microscopy has demonstrated wear particles from Co-Cr-Mo bearings to be round to oval in shape with irregular boundaries. Most of the particles are smaller than 50 nm (range 6 nm to 1 μm). Additional analysis of these retrieved wear particles indicates that the particles have several different elemental compositions. There are Co-Cr-Mo particles, but there is an even greater number of chromium oxide particles. It has been hypothesized that the Co-Cr-Mo particles are produced by the wear of the carbides on the bearing surfaces and the prosthesis matrix, and that the chromium oxide particles come from the passivation layer on the implant surface and possibly from oxidized chromium carbides. There is little known about the rates of metallic particle production in vivo, lymphatic transport of metallic particles from the joint, and systemic dissemination. Utilizing information on volumetric wear rate and average particle size, it has been estimated that 6.7×10^{12} to 2.5×10^{14} metal particles are produced per year, which is 13 to 500 times the number of PE particles produced per year by a typical MOP joint. The aggregate surface area of these metal wear particles is substantial. (Malviya 2010)

It is important to recognize that in modern THR prostheses there may be several sources of metal particle and ion generation.(Savarino 2006) Systemic dissemination of soluble and particulate corrosion products from modular junctions has been described, including the presence of metallic particles in the lymph nodes, liver, and spleen. In modular total hips with a MOP bearing, with no or mild corrosion at the modular head and neck junction, serum and urine levels of Co averaged 0.94 ppb (range <0.54 to 1.65) and 0.92 ppb (range <0.3 to 1.14), respectively, and urine Cr levels averaged 1.0 ppb (range 0.54 to 1.92). With moderate or severe corrosion at the modular head and neck junction, the serum and urine levels of Co averaged 1.06 ppb (range 0.8 to 1.4) and 0.87 ppb (range <0.3 to 1.3), respectively, and the average urine Cr levels were 1.59 ppb (range 0.6 to 3.0).(Jacobs 1998) The levels of metal ions in serum and urine are further elevated in patients with MOM bearings. It appears that the ion levels are higher in the short term and decrease over time. This is consistent with a conditioning phase or running-in of the bearing. The ion levels in subjects with Co-Cr alloy MOM THRs that had been in situ for an average of 24 years have been reported. The average serum Co level was 0.9 ppb (range <0.3 to 2.0). The average serum Cr level was 1.28 ppb (range 0.21 to 2.56), and the average urine Cr level was 1.22 ppb (range 0.26 to 2.59).(Bitsch 2007) The longer-term serum and urine ion levels produced by MOM bearings are not much higher than those produced by the modular junctions of femoral components. Unfortunately, the toxicological importance of these trace metal elevations has not been established, and available data do not answer questions regarding the risks of ion hypersensitivity, toxicity, and carcinogenesis. Since wear of a MOM bearing cannot generally be measured on a radiograph, serum and urine metal ion concentrations may be useful indicators of patient activity and the tribological performance of these bearings.(MacDonald 2004) The distribution and histological effects of wear particles from a McKee-Farrar THR with an in vivo use of nearly 30 years has been described. Clinically, the implant was functioning well. Serum and urine levels of chromium and serum levels of cobalt, obtained 25 years after implantation and while the patient was healthy and active, were found to be 1.02 ppb, 0.51 ppb, and 0.66 ppb, respectively. Sections from multiple samples of the lymph nodes, spleen, liver, and kidney were examined with light microscopy. This tissue analysis did not reveal any evidence of end-organ damage or accumulation of metal particles. It appears that a patient with normal renal function is capable of clearing cobalt and chromium ions from his or her system. Potential additional sources of ions include the acetabular morse taper connection.(Brodner 2003)

3.3.4.2 Biological response

Although the periprosthetic tissue reactions surrounding MOM THA demonstrate some histological characteristics similar to those typically seen around MOPE THAs, they have been reported to be less intense with fewer histiocytes present in the tissues. It is still uncertain whether this difference can be attributed to variations in particle concentration, size, shape, or composition. The wear particles produced by MOM implants in vitro and in vivo are in the nanometer size range, mostly round to oval but with the presence of some needle-shaped particles as well, mainly depending on the number of cycles (for in vitro particles) and the implantation time (for in vivo particles). In addition, most of the particles contain Chromium (Cr) and Oxygen (O) but no Cobalt (Co) and are therefore most likely chromium oxides. Therefore, in addition to focusing on CoCrMo particles, attention to the effects of chromium oxide particles should be addressed in future in vitro and in vivo biologic studies. Finally, because of their nanometer size, those particles have a high surface

area and are subject to corrosion, releasing metal ions into the surrounding areas, and therefore the biologic response to metal ions also need to be considered.
The large aggregate surface area of metal wear particles may have both local and systemic effects. Surface area has been identified as a variable affecting the macrophage response to panicles. However, the local tissue reaction around MOM prosthesis, indicated by the number of histiocytes, is about one grade lower than that around MOP prostheses. A number of hypotheses have been proposed to explain this discrepancy. Since metal particles are considerably smaller than PE particles, histiocytes are able to store a larger number of metal particles, and therefore, the total number of histiocytes required to store the metal particles is lower. Very small particles may enter macrophages by pinocytosis instead of phagocytosis, which may alter the cellular response to the particles. It is also recognized that Co-Cr particles have greater potential for cytotoxicity than PE particles, and the cell may be incapable of the same inflammatory response. There may be a difference in the relative proportion of metal wear particles that are retained locally versus systemically distributed compared to PE wear particles. Dissolution of metal particles results in elevation of the cobalt and chromium ion concentrations in erythrocytes, serum, and urine. The metal particles have shown a dose-response effect. Low to moderate concentrations of metal particles stimulate the release of cytokines, such as interleukin-1 (IL-1), interleukin-6 (IL-6), tumor necrosis factor-α, and prostaglandin E1, that can lead to periprosthetic osteolysis and aseptic loosening. At higher concentrations, however, Co-Cr particles have been found to be cytotoxic, altering the phagocytic activity of macrophages and leading to cell death.(Kwon 2009; Huber 2010)
Although the volume of reactive periprosthetic inflammatory tissue associated with MOM bearings is less than with MOP, osteolysis can occur in hips with MOM bearings. The incidence of osteolysis associated with MOM bearings has not been well established but appears to be comparatively low.(Bharma 2006)

3.3.4.3 Inflammatory versus immunological responses

Because metal ions remain a major cause for concern in the widespread clinical use of MOM implants, in vitro studies have also been conducted on the effects of these metal ions. Co^{2+} and Cr^{3+} have been demonstrated to induce tumor necrosis factor (TNF)-α secretion. Petit and colleagues examined the effect of Co^{2+} and Cr^{3+} ions on protein oxidation in human U937 macrophages and showed that both Co^{2+} and Cr^{3+} ions induced a time- and dose-dependent protein oxidation, reaching 6.5 and 2.9 times the control levels after 72 hours, respectively.(Bagchi 2002) A histological study of tissues surrounding MOPE and MOM THAs by Campbell and colleagues showed that fewer macrophages were present in the tissues surrounding MOM THAs than in the tissues surrounding MOPE THAs. Catelas and colleagues demonstrated that tissues surrounding failed MOM THAs with low to moderate quantities of metal particles could induce the production of potentially osteolytic cytokines. In addition to the potential for wear products to induce osteolysis through inflammatory response as observed surrounding conventional MOPE implants, a concern has emerged regarding the possibility of specific immunological responses. These immunological responses could be due to the release of metal ions that act as antigens and stimulate an allergic (hypersensitivity) reaction when they form organometallic complexes with proteins. Hypersensitivity reactions can be mediated by antibodies (type I, II, or III) or can be cell-mediated (type IV, i.e., delayed type hypersensitivity). Type IV reactions to metal ions involve the activation and clonal expansion of metal-ion-specific major histocompatibility complex (MHC) class II restricted CD4+ T-lymphocytes by professional antigen-presenting cells (APCS). However, in addition to conventional peptide antigens, T cells can also react directly with metal ions. Regardless of the mechanisms, the consequences are that metal ions-sensitized CD4+ T-lymphocytes would elaborate cytokines, including interferon γ, that will attract and activate more macrophages, leading to the release of additional osteolytic cytokines and possibly causing a T-cell-mediated periprosthetic osteolysis.(Hallab 2001; Whittingham 2008) In a review study, Gawkrodger concluded that although early MOM displayed high incidences of hypersensitivity, no conclusion could be drawn about the new generation of MOM implants.(Gawkrodger 2003) Finally, it is still unclear if the loosening of the implants can be linked to an increased reactivity of the lymphocytes to metal particles or ions. When comparing tissues surrounding MOPE and MOM THAs, Campbell and colleagues showed more lymphocytes in the MOM THAs.(Campbell 2005) Although this infiltration of lymphocytes could be indicative of a delayed-type hypersensitivity response to the metal wear products and the development of a typical immunological response, Willert and colleagues also reported the presence of plasma cells, B-lymphocytes, and massive fibrin exudation, which are not characteristic of a type IV delayed-type hypersensitivity reaction. These authors described this reaction as an aseptic lymphocyte-dominated vasculitis-associated lesion (ALVAL) or as a lymphocyte-dominated immunologic (LYDIA) answer. Pandit et al. reported the presence of pseudotumors surrounding MOM surface replacements. These pseudotumors were characterized by an extensive necrosis of dense connective tissue, a focaly heavy macrophage and lymphocytic infiltration as well as the presence of plasma cells and eosinophils in some cases. The observed reaction was somewhat similar to ALVAL reaction reported by Willert et al. but with possibly a more diffuse lymphocyte infiltrate and the presence of extensive connective tissue necrosis.(Willert 2005) However, the specificity of such pseudotumors to MOM implants remains to be determined.(Pandit 2008) The potential adverse effects of MOM wear particles are mainly due to their local and systemic distribution and their capacity for releasing corrosion products, especially if they are in situ for several decades. Systemic dissemination of soluble and particulate corrosion products has been described, including the presence of metallic particles in the liver and spleen and raises questions about potential genotoxicity.(Urban 2000)

3.3.4.4 Local and systemic effects

Metal wear debris may cause DNA damage through the action of metal particles and/or through the action of metal ions by a chemical effect. Cobalt-chromium particles may exert a purely particulate effect that damages DNA by inducing free-radical formation in a way similar to the actions of nonmetallic particles. Alternatively, the cobalt-chromium particle might produce a chemical effect as a result of the release of cobalt and/or chromium ions. Cr^{3+} and Cr^{6+} cause DNA-strand breaks. Co^{2+} itself causes DNA-strand breaks, but in addition it inhibits DNA repair, therefore potentially augmenting the damage caused by chromium. Metal ions and wear debris may lead to genomic instability, similar to that induced by ionizing radiation, and this may increase the probability of DNA damage or mutation during normal cellular function.(Cobb 2006)

Temporary increases in the incidence of hematopoietic cancers at different follow-up points were observed in some cohorts. A study by Visuri et al. demonstrated a 3.77-fold increase in the rate of hematopoietic cancer following metal-on-metal total hip arthroplasty compared with the rate following metal-on-polyethylene total hip

arthroplasty, but this difference was not significant.(Visuri 2006) Recent evidence from studies of patients who have undergone metal-on-metal hip resurfacing has shown raised circulating levels of cobalt and chromium ions to be associated with T-cell lymphopenia, with the lymphocyte counts of these patients differing from those of control subjects with a total hip arthroplasty that did not produce metal wear debris. The effect was consistent only for CD_8^+ T-cell lymphocytes.(Hart 2006, 2009)
Another concern regarding increased metal-ion levels following metal-on-metal total hip arthroplasty is that the ions may cross the placental barrier. Initially, it was thought that the placenta was an effective barrier to metal ions, but a subsequent study showed that the placenta actually exerts a modulatory effect on the rate of metal ion transfer. The transfer rate at low maternal metal-ion levels is higher than that at higher maternal levels. The transplacental transfer rate was in excess of 95% in the controls for both metals, but only 29% for chromium and 60% for cobalt in study patients, suggesting that the placenta exerts a modulatory effect on the rate of metal ion transfer.(Ziaee 2007) On the basis of these findings and the lack of comprehensive knowledge regarding the potential effects of metal ions on fetal development, metal-on-metal total hip arthroplasty probably should not be performed in women of child-bearing age until additional information is available.(Brodner 2004)

3.3.4.5 Cancer risk

Co and Cr wear particles have been shown to induce carcinoma in animal models, giving rise to the concern that such alloys could have the same effect in human tissues if present in sufficient amounts for a sufficient length of time. The first well-documented case of cancer associated with total joint replacement was in a patient who developed a malignant fibrous histiocytoma 3.5 years after a MOM THR performed in December 1969. There have been, at least, 24 additional cases reported in the English literature of malignancy occurring in association with a total hip or knee prostheses. Of the 25 reported cases of cancer following a total joint replacement, 21 involved sarcomas.(Gillespie 1988) The risk of cancer after MOM THR has been assessed specifically in only one epidemiological study. In that study, the relative risk of cancer was reported to be 0.95, suggesting that there is no apparent increased risk of cancer development after MOM total hip arthroplasty. In addition, the risk of sarcoma after MOM THR was found to be 0.00. However, the same study found the relative risk of hematopoietic cancer to be 1.59 following MOM THR and 3.77 for leukemia when MOM implants were compared with MOP implants. From an epidemiological perspective, these data are limited because of the small number of patients who underwent MOM THR. Furthermore, the majority of patients in these reports have less than 10 years of follow-up. The latency of known carcinogens, such as tobacco, asbestos, and ionizing radiation, is several decades. Longer follow-up of large patient groups is needed to better assess the risk of cancer with any implant system.(Tharani 2001) Since the goal of more wear resistant bearings is to reduce the need for reoperation, theoretical risks should be weighed against the risks of revision THR. In the Medicare population, the 90-day mortality following revision THR is 2.6%, which is significantly and substantially higher than that of primary total hip and directly related to the revision procedure. Rigorous long-term studies are needed to assess the relative risk to benefit ratios for total hip bearings.

3.4 Ceramic bearings

Ceramic bearings, made of alumina, have demonstrated the lowest in vivo wear rates to date of any bearing combination. The same principles of friction and lubrication reported for

MOM bearings apply to ceramic-on-ceramic (COC) bearings. However, ceramics have two important properties that make them an outstanding material regarding friction and wear. Ceramics are hydrophilic, permitting a better wettability of the surface. This ensures that the synovial fluid-film is uniformly distributed over the whole bearing surface area. Secondly, ceramic has a greater hardness than metal and can be polished to a much lower surface roughness. Although the better wettability results in a slightly thinner fluid-film than with MOM bearings it is compensated by the reduced size of the asperities on the surface. Overall, this results in a favorable higher λ ratio and in a reduced coefficient of friction. This bearing combination is the most likely to achieve true fluid-film lubrication. However, because of the hardness of ceramics, the wear characteristics are sensitive to design, manufacturing, and implantation variables. Rapid wear has also been observed, generally associated with suboptimal positioning of the implants. COC bearings currently in clinical use are made of alumina. Developments in the production process (sintering) have improved the quality of the material. Modern alumina ceramics have a low porosity, low grain size, high density, and high purity. Thus, its hardness, fracture toughness, and burst strength increased. The alumina on alumina bearing is considered the standard ceramic on ceramic articulation.(D'Antonio 2009) Alumina ceramic bearings have been in clinical use for more than three decades, and significant basic science and clinical research support their use. The small amount of ceramic particulate debris that is generated has been noted to be much less biologically reactive than metal or polyethylene particles. Most important, the incidence of osteolysis associated with use of ceramic on ceramic bearings appears to be minimal or nonexistent. (Bierbaum 2002)

3.4.1 Mechanical properties

Alumina ceramics are classified as hard, stiff, and brittle materials. Because alumina ceramics are highly oxidized, they are biologically inert and resistant to further oxidation. The hardness of alumina creates a product with significant resistance to surface damage, and ceramics are much harder than other materials routinely used in orthopedic surgery. The hardness of alumina makes it very abrasive and wear resistant. In addition, the hardness of alumina increases its resistance to scratching, and it is much less likely to scratch than titanium or cobalt chromium alloys. In fact, the only material capable of scratching alumina is diamond. Clinically, this is important because alumina can resist third-body wear and is not scratched by retained cement particles or bone. Although alumina has poor bending characteristics, it is extremely strong in compression. This lack of bending strength has currently limited its use in total hip arthroplasty to the femoral head and cup liner. Because alumina is very stiff, it does not deform under high loads. Therefore very precise production techniques are needed in order to ensure proper fit of the head within the socket. Polyethylene will mold around a femoral head if there is an initial, small incongruity, which is not true with ceramics, and poor manufacturing can lead to high wear rates. The lack of ceramic deformation makes the contact areas between the head and socket smaller as compared with metal on polyethylene articulations. In order to maximize the contact surface area, clearance must be optimized. Alumina is more than 300 times stiffer than cancellous bone and almost 200 times stiffer than polymethlymethracrylate. Because of this significant modulus mismatch, cemented ceramic components have been found to be associated with higher cement fracture and loosening rates than all-polyethylene components. Alumina is very brittle and under compression will deform linearly until fracture. No plastic deformation occurs before fracture. By definition, its fracture toughness is considered to be its resistance to fracture. The initial flaws in the material determine the risk of ceramic fracture, and flaws are related to the purity and density of the ceramic. A combination of improvements, including improved processing with smaller grain sizes, fewer impurities, laser etching, and proof testing, have led to a lower incidence of material fracture. The burst strength of alumina components improved from 38 kilonewtons in 1977 to 98 kilonewtons in 1998. (Tateiwa 2008)

3.4.2 Alumina and zirconia

Medical-grade alumina is consolidated from a high-purity (>99%) alumina powder through a hot isostatic pressing step. Modifications to the sintering process over the past three decades have resulted in increased density, hardness, and strength of medical-grade alumina. Modifications to the sintering also led to a decrease in the average grain size from 4.5 μm to about 1.8 μm, with a narrower grain size distribution. The improved regulation of the grain size did not lead to any noticeable changes in the fracture toughness of alumina. While alumina remains the most widely used ceramic in the total hip, zirconia is also utilized as a replacement for alumina femoral heads, but only for applications where the counterface is UHMWPE. Zirconia is stronger than alumina; therefore it can withstand higher stresses, which may be induced when smaller and thinner implants are used. During deformation, pure zirconia undergoes a crystalline-phase transformation from monoclinic to tetragonal, with the former occupying more space. This transformation adversely affects the mechanical properties of pure zirconia, leading to internal stresses within the deformation zone ahead of propagating cracks. Zirconia can be stabilized with the addition of either magnesium oxide (MgO) or yttrium oxide (Y_2O_3) to avoid the detrimental effects of deformation-induced phase transformation.(De Aza 2002)
Alumina was the first ceramic to be widely used in hip arthroplasty, following its introduction in 1970. Aluminium oxide (Al_20_3) can be highly polished to produce a very low coefficient of friction and is also highly resistant to abrasion. It has a more stable structure than the more recently developed Zirconia so the properties are more predictable. Improved manufacturing techniques have resulted in smaller grain size and smoother finish helping to reduce the fracture risk that was encountered when using earlier generations. (D'Antonio 2009)
Zirconium oxide (ZrO_2)(Zirconia) was introduced in 1985 as an alternative to alumina. Its superior mechanical strength was attractive with a theoretical reduction in fracture risk. It also allowed smaller femoral head sizes whilst maintaining excellent wear characteristics when coupled with UHMWPE. Clinical trials have shown that UHMWPE wear when coupled with a zirconia femoral head is at least as good as that with a Co-Cr femoral head and in many cases is much better.(Affatato 2001) However Zirconia undergoes phase transformation. The strongest tetragonal phase is also the most unstable, so, for medical purposes, a stabilizer, Yttrium oxide, is used. In vivo studies have shown that phase transformation still occurs at the bearing surface secondary to temperature and pressure changes which transforms zirconia to the more stable monoclinic phase. This results in a 3% increase in volume producing surface roughness. Hence it performs poorly when articulating against itself and can also result in accelerated polyethylene wear bearing on UHMWPE. As a result it has fallen out of favour.(Fernandez-Fairen 2007)

3.4.3 Tribologic properties

In vitro wear studies have proved that alumina on alumina is a very low friction couple, and wear is significantly reduced. The outstanding tribologic properties of the alumina articulation are due to its low surface roughness (secondary to small grain size), hardness, enhanced wettability, and fluid film lubrication. It has been shown that there are two wear phases during in vitro testing. The "run-in" phase is the first phase and involves the first million or so cycles. Volumetric wear rates for alumina against alumina bearings during this run-in phase measure 0.1 to 0.2 mm^3 per million cycles. The second phase is called the "steady-state" phase. During this period, volumetric wear rates decrease to less than 0.02 mm^3 per million cycles. Compared with metal on polyethylene couples, during both the run-in and steady-state phases, wear is reduced up to 5000 fold. Under certain clinical conditions, accelerated wear can occur with alumina on alumina couples. One phenomenon called "stripe wear" occurs when accelerated wear is present over a discrete area. Stripe wear may be associated with separation of the ball from the socket such as during the swing phase of gait or when the ball is levered out of the socket by impingement. In vitro testing under the conditions of separation of the femoral head from the socket leads to increased volumetric wear. It was noted that wear as high as 1.24 mm^3 per million cycles could occur with separation and stripe wear results. A bimodal distribution of particle size was also noted in this study, with nanometer-sized particles (1 to 35 nm) probably associated with polishing of the articulation and micrometer-sized particles (0.05 to 10 μm) that likely originated from stripe wear and transgranular fracture of the alumina ceramic. Numerous retrieval studies of ceramic bearings have been performed, and the results are interesting. One study examined retrieved alumina components associated with aseptic loosening of the socket at a mean of 11 years after implementation. Components were classified into three groups: (1) low wear with no visible signs of material loss; (2) stripe wear with a visible oblong worn area on the femoral head and a penetration rate below 10 μm/year; and (3) severe wear with visible loss of material on both components and maximum penetration higher than 150 μm.(Fig.10 and 11) Evaluation of these 11 components revealed massive, severe wear on two devices. The remaining nine components had liner wear rates less than 15 μm/year. The authors concluded that two different types of wear are associated with ceramic on ceramic couples-one that is limited and has negligible effect on long-term performance of the implant, and a second type that catastrophically leads to rapid destruction of the bearing surface. Published wear rates examining clinical performance of the alumina on alumina bearing surface have reported wear to range from 0.3 μm/year to 5.0 mm/year. These variations may be related to implanted material and design issues or surgical and patient factors. However, it is important to note that most catastrophic wear

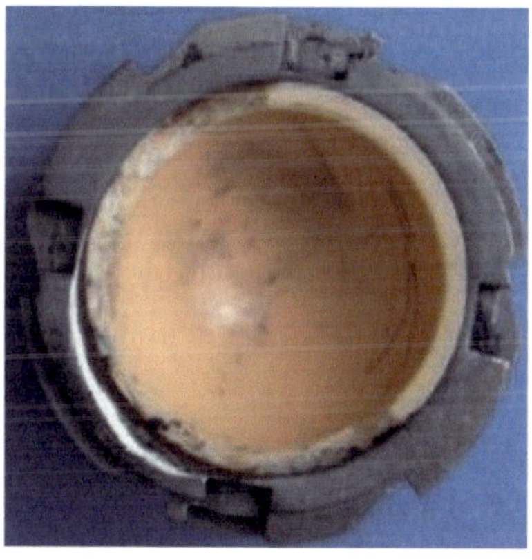

Fig. 10. Acetabular liner showing gross damage to the liner

has been reported with products produced before 1990. In recent years, wear rates below 15 μm/year have been consistently reported. Many investigators believe that severe wear is related to clinically exceptional circumstances and that with properly implanted bearing surfaces, catastrophic wear is essentially nonexistent.(Capello 2008)

3.4.4 Microseparation and wear particles

Ceramic materials may have better biocompatibility than metal alloys, but the relative size, shape, number, reactivity, and local versus systemic distribution of the wear particles have not been fully determined. Hatton et al. investigated the tissues from ten noncemented COC THAs undergoing revision surgery. The tissues from the femoral and acetabular regions demonstrated the presence of intracellular particle agglomerates and mixed pathology, with areas that had no obvious pathology and areas that were relatively rich in macrophages, and over half of the tissues had 60% of necrosis. A bimodal size range of ceramic wear debris was observed, with particles as small as 5 to 90 nm (mean 24 nm) and as large as 0.05 to 3.2 μm (mean 430 nm).(Hatton 2002a) These two types of ceramic wear debris are generated by two different wear mechanisms in vivo, with very small wear particles being generated under normal articulating conditions and larger particles being generated under microseparation conditions. After total hip arthroplasty, the femoral head and the acetabular insert can separate up to 2 mm during the swing phase of a normal gait cycle. When a load is applied at heel strike in the stance phase, the femoral head moves vertically to relocate in the cup. With the geometry of a typical COC prosthesis, separations of only 2 mm will allow the femoral head to contact the rim acetabular liner, resulting in changes in the wear performance of the bearing couple (stripe wear). (Stewart 2001, 2003)

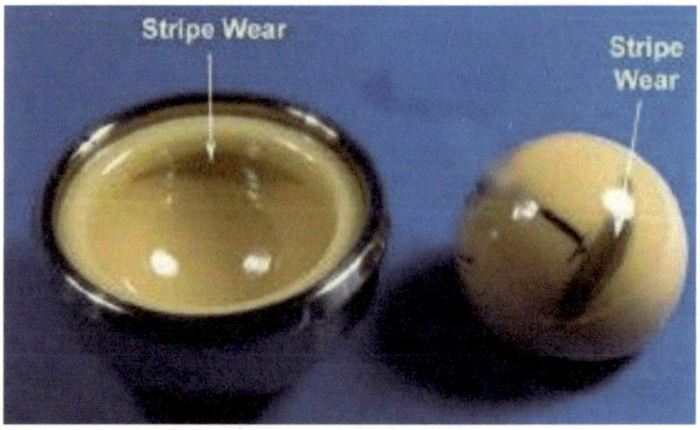

Fig. 11. A ceramic head and acetabular liner from a patient with "squeaking" hip with evidence of impingement and "stripe wear.

It is hoped that improvements in the manufacturing of ceramics and ceramic components will minimize or eliminate mechanical problems such as fracture and accelerated wear.

3.4.5 Wear debris and tissue response

It has been shown, in vitro and in vivo, that alumina wear debris is biologically inert and well tolerated. Alumina particles induce very little cellular response and formation of granulomatous tissue. The small nature of most alumina on alumina wear particles and the low volume of particles generated leads to a low level of bioactivity. Giant cells have not been observed in contact with alumina wear debris. Lerouge and colleagues compared 12 periprosthetic membranes obtained during revision for aseptic component loosening with an alumina on alumina couple. These were compared with a series of membranes obtained from revisions of a metal on polyethylene bearing. In the alumina on alumina group, the cellular reaction, which was generally mild, was determined to be in response to the zirconia ceramic particles used in the cement as an opacifying agent. No cellular reaction to the alumina particles was noted.(Lerouge 1997) This contrasted with the significant cellular activity noted in the metal on polyethylene group with reaction to the polyethylene debris. Osteolysis associated with alumina on alumina total hip arthroplasty has been infrequently reported. In one study, when an implant made with large-grain-size ceramics, low density, and high porosity was used, large production of debris resulted and osteolysis occurred. Tissue obtained from failed hips with an alumina on alumina couple was shown to have significantly lower prostaglandin E_2 (PGE_2) levels compared with tissue obtained from hips with metal on polyethylene articulation. Both alumina and polyethylene debris stimulate cellular release of tumor necrosis factor (TNF)-α. However, polyethylene particles cause more release of TNF-α, and in fact the stimulation may be 8 to 10 times greater. Of importance, alumina particles induce macrophage apoptosis, which leads to decreased macrophage activity. This induced apoptosis explains the decreased levels of TNF-α associated with alumina and may also account for the paucity of ceramic-related osteolysis. Ceramic debris may not be bio-inert as initially assumed, because osteolysis has been described in some patients with a COC bearing.(Nam 2007) Some studies describe inflammatory and cytotoxic reactions on the cellular level, but the relationship to material, size, and particle number remains uncertain. It seems that there is less inflammatory reaction compared to MOM or MOP bearings in well-functioning prostheses. In contrast with polyethylene or metallic particles, foreign body reactions are routinely observed. Ion toxicity is not an issue with ceramics.(Mehmood 2008)

3.4.6 Ceramic-on-metal articulation

In a simulator study, Firkins et al demonstrated superior wear for alumina ceramic-on-metal articulations. Femoral heads 28 mm in diameter made of medical-grade alumina were articulated against acetabular cups manufactured from medical-grade, high-carbon-wrought cobalt-chromium alloy. The implants were tested for 5 million cycles. Wear and surface analyses were performed every 1 million cycles. The results were compared with metal-on-metal articulations that used medical-grade, low-carbon, cobalt-chromium alloy femoral heads against medical-grade, high-carbon, cobalt-chromium alloy sockets. The metal-on-metal bearings initially showed high bedding-in and subsequently developed a steady-state volumetric wear rate of 1.23 mm3 per 1 million cycles. No bedding-in period was observed with the ceramic-on-metal, and a volumetric wear rate of 0.01 mm3 per 1 million cycles was reported. This represents more than a 100-fold decrease in wear with the ceramic-on-metal articulation. Surface analysis of the ceramic head showed no signs of wear or change in surface roughness. Metal particles from both articulations were of nanometer size (6 to 30 nm). In addition, the ceramic-on-metal articulations produced slightly smaller particles although they were far fewer in number. (Firkins 2001) Clinical studies are currently under way to assess the performance of these bearings. The potential advantage of this novel ceramic-on-metal bearing is lower wear and the generation of significantly fewer metal particles compared with currently available metal-on-metal bearing surfaces. This bearing combination allows for the use of large femoral heads, similar to metal-on-metal bearings. With larger ceramic heads, the fracture risk is reduced, and an increased number of femoral head options are available to the surgeon. Potential disadvantages of this new bearing articulation include the risk of a ceramic femoral head fracture and its as-yet unknown clinical performance.(D'Antonio 2009)

3.4.7 Ceramic advantages

The potential advantages of using a ceramic on ceramic articulation for total hip arthroplasty can be quickly summarized as decreased wear and elimination of osteolysis. Osteolysis from wear debris is commonly viewed as the major obstacle blocking the development of a "lifetime" hip replacement. The need to eliminate wear and osteolysis has been magnified by the extension of indications for total hip arthroplasty to younger, more active, healthier patients with long life expectancies. The potential for decreased wear is derived from the tribologic properties inherent to alumina. Alumina can be highly polished. Alumina bearings are also very hard, and this characteristic increases their resistance to scratching. The hardness minimizes third-body wear from entrapped bone, polymethylmethacrylate, or metal debris derived from surgical instruments or component fretting. Alumina has ionic properties and therefore, in combination with body fluids, has better wettability than chrome cobalt. The fluid film that develops on ceramic surfaces decreases frictional drag and adhesive wear. Wear rates for modern ceramic on ceramic articulations have been shown to be as low as 4 µm/year. This low wear rate coupled with less alumina bioreactivity minimizes the likelihood of osteolysis. With currently used implant designs, osteolysis has not been reported with follow-up as long as 18.5 years.

3.4.8 Ceramic concerns

One significant drawback of ceramic materials is their inherently lower strength and toughness under tension and bending, which are the loading modes that favor the initiation and propagation of cracks. One such adverse loading arises from the mismatch at the taper junction between the metal stem and ceramic head. To prevent this from leading to early fracture, the tolerances at the taper are matched and may be manufacturer-specific. The surgical placement of the components may also predispose the ceramic components to high stresses and initiate fracture. For instance, a third body (bone cement or bone fragment) left in the taper interface or impingement of the femoral component on the rim of the ceramic acetabular liner secondary to malpositioning of the components could also initiate ceramic fracture.(Barrack 2004)

3.4.8.1 Fracture (Fig.12)

Improved material processing, smaller grain sizes, fewer impurities, laser etching, and proof testing have greatly diminished the risk of catastrophic in vivo fracture. The risk of ceramic fracture is estimated to have decreased nearly 100-fold in the last two decades. In 1990 the incidence of fracture was approximately 0.8%, and today is likely between 0.004% and 0.010%. Nonetheless, this complication is devastating and still occurs.(Min 2007) Even with proof testing, it is unlikely that failure by fracture will be eliminated. Although theoretically proof testing eliminates weaker components, flawed products that are likely to fail are not always eliminated. Proof testing theoretically is designed to be stringent enough to remove components with manufacturing flaws that are likely to clinically fail. However, the test must be nondestructive and not cause damage to the tested part. No proof test currently available is 100% effective. So, it must be remembered that production errors can and still do occur. In 1998 a manufacturing change resulted in a high fracture rate of ceramic balls.

About one in three components clinically failed, and this was despite negative proof testing of all fractured devices. The production of ceramics is far more demanding than the manufacture of metal and polyethylene components, and the incidence of catastrophic failure for ceramics will always be higher than with other materials. Ceramic component fracture may occur secondary to poor surgical technique. Improper component insertion predisposes the implant to fracture. Impaction of the femoral head on the trunnion should be performed only after ensuring it is concentrically placed. Placing the head nonconcentrically on the trunnion or not cleaning and drying it properly leads to stress concentrations in the femoral head.(Poggie 2007) In addition, placing a ceramic head on a damaged trunnion also leads to stress concentration and a significantly reduced burst strength with the potential for fracture.(Anwar 2009) It is also possible to nonconcentrically place the ceramic liner in the metal acetabular shell. However, the adverse effects and long-term consequences of this error have not been reported. Ceramic component fracture is a double-edged sword. After fracture the patient is confronted with immediate debilitating pain and the need for emergency revision surgery. However, secondarily, revision of a fractured ceramic component carries the risk of a less than optimal outcome. Because of trunnion damage, revision with a ceramic head is usually not possible. Ceramic fracture debris embedded in the soft tissue can cause third-body wear and premature failure owing to accelerated wear if a metal and polyethylene articulation is used for the revision. During revision of fractured ceramic components, it is now recommended to perform meticulous synovectomy and debridement to remove as much fracture debris as possible and revise the femoral head with a metallic alloy, such as CoCr, to avoid further catastrophic failure. Another option on the femoral side is to revise the femoral stem and use a ceramic femoral head.(Ha 2007; D'Antonio 2009)

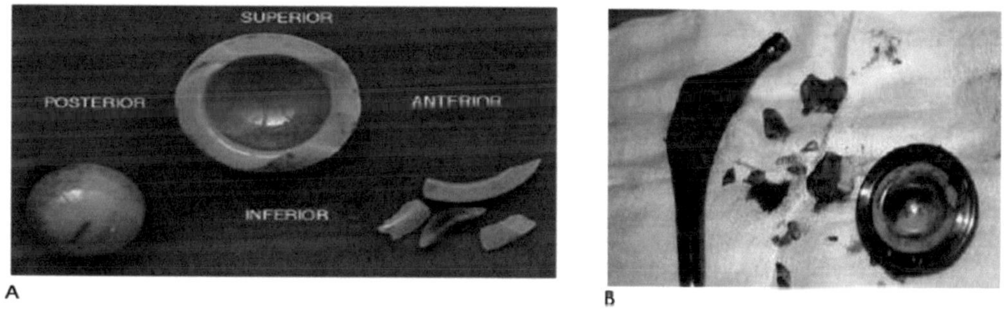

Fig. 12. Retrieved Ceramic-on-Ceramic implants showing fractured acetabular liner (A) and femoral head (B)

3.4.8.2 Stripe wear

Separation of the ball from the socket in patients with a hip arthroplasty may occur during the swing phase of gait or with impingement of the trunnion on the acetabular rim levering the ball from the socket. When this separation occurs, the contact area of the femoral head on the acetabular liner becomes small and stripe wear can result.(Fig.15) Stripe wear is concerning because volumetric wear associated with this phenomenon is high. In one study, stripe wear produced volumetric wear that averaged 1.24 mm^3 per million cycles. Equally concerning, a bimodal array of nanometer- and micrometer-sized particles was created with an enhanced profile of bioreactivity. Separation of the ceramic on ceramic hip articulation is most likely to occur in individuals with tissue laxity or excellent range of motion. Also, patients with vigorous lifestyles and those who perform activities that require placing the hip through a provocative range of motion may be prone to impingement and stripe wear.(Walter 2004) For patients with these risk factors, other articulation choices should be considered. Of course, malpositioned components, as with any articulation, increase the risk of impingement. (Park 2006)

3.4.8.3 Motion-related noise

Hard on hard bearings can produce noise that can be disconcerting and annoying enough that revision surgery is requested by the patient. Specifically, with alumina on alumina bearings patients may describe this noise as "squeaking."(Keurentjes 2008) Ranawat and his colleagues reported that 10 of 159 ceramic on ceramic articulations squeaked and that the phenomenon was self-reported by the patient. The squeaking usually occurred in midrange of motion and was generally considered a significant issue of concern for the patient. In a study on patients with COC THAs who had squeaking, ideal cup position was described as 25 degrees ±10 degrees of anteversion and 45 degrees ±10 degrees of inclination. Clearly, these data suggest that squeaking is related to cup position.(Ranawat 2007; Walter 2007) However, conversely, Parvizi and associates reviewed the incidence of squeaking after 1056 ceramic on ceramic total hip arthroplasties. Thirty-three patients reported squeaking. The patients who had a noisy hip were matched against a control group, and cup position for both groups was carefully determined using computed tomography. There was no significant difference in acetabular position between the two groups.(Restrepo 2008) Retrieval of revised noisy ceramic bearings has so far been inconclusive. Noisy retrieved bearings frequently have a small zone of stripe wear and metallic staining, possibly associated with the head subluxing and making contact with the protective metal rim around the ceramic or the acetabular shell. (Taylor 2007) The management of squeaking begins with informed consent. The occurrence of noise in an otherwise well-functioning arthroplasty is very disconcerting to the patient. The patient's perception that the articulation is malfunctioning can prompt litigation which could involve the surgeon. Reassurance is appropriate because there is no evidence at this time that the noise reflects that the articulation is deteriorating. Certainly the patient should avoid provocative activities because this recommendation seems logical. There is empirical evidence that squeaking is related to a "dry" joint, and oral hydration or injection of viscosupplements can alleviate the noise. If a patient presents with a squeaking ceramic hip, first ceramic breakage must be excluded with a computed tomography scan because a broken ceramic insert can cause squeaking and it may not be obvious on plain radiographs. The computed tomography scan also provides an accurate measure of the acetabular component anteversion. If the noise itself is infrequent, and occurs only with a specific activity, then revision surgery may not be necessary. If the noise itself is troubling, if there is gross component malposition, if there is impingement, or if the patient has symptoms of pain, revision surgery should be recommended. The cup and stem need to be carefully inspected to be sure they are correctly positioned and well fixed. Because the trunnion may be damaged, revision to a metal ball and polyethylene socket is best, as metal on metal articulations have also been reported to occasionally make noise. Using a metal on metal articulation, if it also squeaks, would not likely be acceptable to the patient.(Walter 2008)

3.4.8.4 Other ceramic concerns

The number of femoral head size and neck length options available to the surgeon when using ceramic articulations is limited. In general, for each acetabular component there is only one size liner diameter and paired head girth available. In addition, collared heads are not manufactured, and this significantly reduces the neck length options available. Also, offset and lipped acetabular liners are not produced because they would lead to impingement and chipping. These limitations have caused some experts to speculate that instability and dislocations will be more common when ceramic on ceramic bearings are used. However, clinically this has not proved to be a problem. Impingement of the femoral component trunnion on the ceramic liner edge is also an area of concern. This impingement can lead to chipping of the ceramic liner or notching of the femoral component. A protective metal rim has been added to the ceramic shell liner. Of course, impingement can still occur; however, this protective rim does seem to prevent ceramic damage. Nonetheless, impingement with the protective rim may still cause femoral neck notching and generate metallic debris. The consequences of this type of impingement are unknown; however, the generation of metallosis may theoretically contribute to the problem of noise and squeaking.

3.4.9 Delta ceramic-on-alumina ceramic articulation in primary THA

The newest generation of Ceramic-on-Ceramic bearings incorporate nanosized, yttria-stabilized tetragonal zirconia particles producing an alumina matrix composite. This new bearing surface provided high survivorship.

The newest generation of ceramics, incorporating zirconia into the alumina matrix (marketed as Biolox delta by CeramTec, Plochingen, Germany). Nanosized, yttria-stabilized tetragonal zirconia particles improve the mechanical properties by preventing the initiation and propagation of cracks. Oxide additives produce platelet-like crystals that dissipate energy by deflecting cracks. The addition of chromium oxide further increases the strength and toughness by composite hardening. The final product is a mixture of roughly 75% aluminum oxide, 25% zirconia, and less than 1% chromium oxide and strontium oxide. The result is a composite ceramic with improved mechanical properties and reduced wear as shown on scanning electron microscopy (SEM) and a predicted longer lifespan. These improved mechanical properties reduce overall wear rates of 28-mm heads in a hip simulator wear test from 1.84 mm^3 per million cycle to 0.16 mm^3 per million cycle, comparing alumina-on-alumina versus alumina matrix composite-on-alumina matrix composite, respectively. (Lombardi 2010; Hamilton 2010)

3.4.10 Other advances

There are some laboratory and very short-term clinical data to support the use of ceramic femoral heads articulating with metal acetabular components. These appear to produce less stripe wear with edge loading than metal-on-metal implants. It also appears that there is a reduction in metal ions in the patients at 6 months. Though there have been reports of early catastrophic failure if this pairing is reversed and a metal head is articulated with a ceramic acetabular component.

3.4.10.1 Fabrication and testing of silicon nitride bearings in total hip arthroplasty

A concern with ceramic femoral heads is brittle catastrophic failure in vivo. Improvements in the quality and manufacturing of Al_2O_3 have not eliminated this risk. In the past, zirconia

femoral heads were introduced as a stronger alternative to Al_2O_3, but zirconia can undergo phase transformation and weakening, leading to unpredictable outcomes in vivo. Another strategy to reduce polyethylene wear is to modify the surface of zirconium alloy femoral heads. This avoids brittle failure, but the wear reduction, surface hardness, and scratch resistance of oxidized zirconium are less favorable than Al_2O_3, and oxidized zirconium cannot be used in ceramic-ceramic articulations. An alternative ceramic material was fabricated from silicon nitride (Si_3N_4) powder. Mechanical testing showed high-flexural strength, fracture toughness, Weibull modulus, and resistance to hydrothermal degradation. The Si_3N_4 cups produced low wear rates when tested with either CoCr or Si_3N_4 femoral heads. The Si_3N_4 showed a near 100% theoretical material density (3.20 g/cm^3) and a uniform microstructure of fine, elongated grains (average grain width, 1.5 μm). The flexural strength was 923 ± 70 MPa, with a Weibull modulus of 19, and a fracture toughness of 10 ± 1 MPa.m$^{1/2}$.
The Si_3N_4-Si_3N_4 and Si_3N_4-CoCr bearings produced wear volumes of 0.2 mm^3 and 0.18 mm^3, respectively, at 1 million cycles. These data were extrapolated to 10 million cycle wear because previous hip simulator studies have shown that hard-on-hard bearing wear follows a characteristic biphasic pattern with higher wear in the early, run-in period to about 0.5 million cycles, followed by a lower, steady state linear wear pattern that can be extrapolated to predict long-term wear. A consistent wear rate, that is, the gradient of the linear regression trend is considered more significant than the actual magnitude of wear at any point in time. Accordingly, we calculated the volumetric wear rate from the slope of the linear regression curve during steady state wear; thus, at 10 million cycles, the predicted wear for Si_3N_4-Si_3N_4 and Si_3N_4-CoCr bearings was calculated to be 0.65 mm^3 and 0.47 mm^3, respectively. For THA bearings of the same diameter, the clinical wear volume of CoCr-polyethylene THA is 62 mm^3, and the experimental wear volumes of CoCr-CoCr and Al_2O_3-Al_2O_3 measured in other hip simulators are 6.5mm^3 and between 0.35 and 0.6 mm^3, respectively. After wear testing, Si_3N_4 surfaces remained smooth and glossy, without scratches or damage.
Modern Si_3N_4 is used in aerospace bearings and in high-temperature applications such as diesel engines. The Si_3N_4-Si_3N_4 pairings have a friction coefficient of 0.001 compared to 0.08 for Al_2O_3-Al_2O_3. The CoCr-Si_3N_4 articulations produced low wear rates in this study because of the favorable material hardness, tensile strength, fracture toughness, and lubricity of Si_3N_4 and the close match in elastic modulii between the bearing materials. Because Si_3N_4 has a higher fracture toughness than Al_2O_3, it is more resistant to the initiation and propagation of microcracks that can lead to brittle failure. The fracture toughness and strength of Si_3N_4 also result in superior damage resistance, that is, the ability of the material to retain strength after contact damage. Practically, this means that Si_3N_4 can withstand high loads even if contact stress-related damage were to occur.
It has been postulated that hard bearings in THA could produce a greater number of smaller-sized wear particles, thereby increasing the exposed surface area of bioreactivity in vivo. Wear particles were characterized in this study, and those findings have been reported separately. Because wear between dissimilar mating surfaces originates from the softer, sacrificial material, Si_3N_4-CoCr couplings should generate predominantly CoCr metal particles. Assuming so, the volume of metal wear from Si_3N_4-CoCr calculated in this study was an order of magnitude lower than the wear of retrieved CoCr-CoCr THA bearings. Furthermore, particle size analysis has shown a mean equivalent circular diameter (ECD) of Si_3N_4 wear particles of 0.7 ± 0.6 μm in this study. This figure is comparable to ultrahigh-

molecular-weight polyethylene (mean ECD, approximately 0.4 ± 0.2 μm) and Al_2O_3 (mean ECD, approximately 0.4 ± 0.4 μm) particles obtained from clinical retrievals. Furthermore, the morphology of Si_3N_4 wear particles in this study was similar to Al_2O_3 particles produced under similar testing conditions. For the same size and concentration, ceramic particles may be less bioreactive than those of polyethylene. Previous biocompatibility tests have shown that Si_3N_4 does not elicit adverse in vivo reactions; specifically, exposure to Si_3N_4 does not produce acute or chronic toxicity, mutagenicity, allergenicity, carcinogenicity, or localized tissue toxicity.(Bal 2009)

4. New horizons in bearing surfaces

Metal on polyethylene, metal on metal, and ceramic on ceramic bearings will continue as the dominant bearing materials for total hip arthroplasty because of their excellent track record, resistance to damage, and ease of manufacture and use. Clinically, most bearing combinations consist of cobalt-chromium (CoCr) alloy or ceramic femoral heads articulating against highly cross-linked ultra-high-molecular weight polyethylene acetabular inserts. Alumina on alumina ceramic and CoCr on CoCr articulations are used in younger and more active patients. Each bearing combination has advantages and potential disadvantages. Second-generation HXPE materials are now available. Ceramic composite materials with high fracture toughness are under clinical investigation, as are ceramic on CoCr articulations. Outside this main area of bearing development, research efforts have been under way for some 20 years with two quite different classes of materials. The two classes of materials are carbon fiber polymeric composites and elastomeric materials.

4.1 Carbon fiber polymeric composites

Carbon fiber ultra-high-molecular weight polyethylene (UHMWPE) composites were introduced in the early 1980s as tibial bearings.(Fruh 1998) However, the clinical performance was poor with many revisions. Load can be transferred only by compressive forces between the fibers and matrix, resulting in an inefficient reinforcement. Carbon fiber-reinforced epoxy composites (CFRP) were introduced in Europe in the late 1980s as acetabular components with alumina femoral heads. Simulator studies reported a wear rate of 1 to 3 μm per million cycles. Canine hips with CFRP cups were implanted in six dogs for up to 5.5 years with no adverse consequences. A clinical study began in 1989, and 101 patients received cups of CFRP. In cases of revision, there were few particles in the tissue and the biologic response was benign. The wear of retrieved components was 6.1 to 6.3 μm/year. These wear rates are comparable to those seen with HXPE materials. Epoxy resins are thermoset materials and cannot be shaped other than by machining once they have "set" via chemical reaction. Many thermoplastic composites can be shaped by combinations of heat and pressure and "set" thereafter. Polyether ether ketone (PEEK) is a thermoplastic high performance polymer that is attractive as a composite matrix owing to its strength, toughness, stability, and biocompatibility.(Wang 1999)

4.2 Compliant bearings

There has long been interest in developing bearing materials that exhibit friction and wear behavior similar to that of articular cartilage. Cartilage is an example of a compliant bearing that has a low modulus but is capable of large deformation without failure. The friction coefficient between cartilage surfaces in a synovial joint is less than 0.01. This low friction is achieved via three lubrication mechanisms: elastohydrodynamic (EHD) lubrication, μEHD, and squeeze-film lubrication. Elastic deformation of the articular surfaces under load assists in allowing joint fluid to separate the surfaces, avoiding solid-solid contact with consequent wear. μEHD has a similar effect confined to the surface asperities (roughness) of the cartilage. EHD and μEHD predominate during the stance phase of walking, when pressure is generated in the synovial fluid by an entraining motion between the joint surfaces. Squeeze-film action predominates during heel strike, as the two cartilage surfaces move toward each other, squeezing the joint fluid from between the surfaces. Deformation of the articular cartilage assists in retention of the synovial fluid film. Healthy cartilage has a thickness of 2 to 4 mm at the femoral head and acetabulum. The modulus of elasticity is 10 to 50 MPa with a Poisson ratio of 0.42 to 0.47. The surface roughness is about 2 μm. Polyurethanes are synthetic polymers having properties comparable to those of articular cartilage. There have been extensive studies to determine the suitability of polyurethanes as bearing surfaces. The intent is to have a bearing in which the surfaces are separated by the pressure developed in the joint fluid as well as by the deformation of the articular surfaces, resulting in low friction and low wear. This is a different approach from that of using UHMWPE, CoCr, or alumina bearings that operate under mixed lubrication conditions with higher friction and a degree of solid to solid contact.(Scholes 2000)

5. References

Affatato S, et al. (2005). Wear behaviour of crosslinked PE assessed in vitro under severe conditions. *Biomaterials*, 26, 2005: 3259–3267

Affatato S, et al. (2008). Predictive role of the lambda ratio in the evaluation of metal-on-metal total hip replacement. *Proc Inst Mech Eng*, 222, 2008: 617-628

Antoniou J, et al. (2008). Metal ion levels in the blood of patients after hip resurfacing: a comparison between twenty-eight and thirty-six-millimeter-head metal-on-metal prostheses.*J Bone Joint Surg Am*, 90 (Suppl 3), 2008: 142-148

Anwar I, et al. (2009). Delayed catastrophic failure of a ceramic head in hybrid total hip arthroplasty. *J Arthroplasty*, 24, 2009: 158–162

Archibeck MJ, et al. (2000). The basic science of periprosthetic osteolysis. *J Bone Joint Surg Am*, 82, 2000: 1478-1489

Atienza C Jr, Maloney WJ. (2008). Highly cross-linked polyethylene bearing surfaces in total hip arthroplasty. *J Surg Orthop Adv*, 17, 2008: 27-33

Bagchi D, et al. (2002). Cytotoxicity and oxidative mechanisms of different forms of chromium. *Toxicology*. 180, 2002: 5-22.

Baker D, et al. (2003). The effects of degree of crosslinking on the fatigue crack initiation and propagation resistance of orthopedic grade polyethylene. *J Biomed Mater Res*, 66, 2003: 146

Bal BS, et al. (2009). Fabrication and Testing of Silicon Nitride Bearings in Total Hip Arthroplasty. *J Arthroplasty*, 24, 1, 2009: 110-116

Barnes CL, et al. (2008). Wear Performance of Large-Diameter Differential-Hardness Hip Bearings. *J Arthroplasty*, 23(6), Suppl. 1, 2008: 56-60

Barrack RL, et al. (2004). Concerns about ceramics in THA. *Clin Orthop Relat Res*, 429, 2004: 73–79

Beaul´e PE, et al. (2001). Osteolysis in a cementless, second generation metal-on-metal hip replacement. *Clin Orthop Relat Res*, 386, 2001: 159-165

Bhamra MS, Case CP. (2006). Biological effects of metal-on-metal hip replacements. *Proc Inst Mech Eng, 220,* 2006: 379-84

Bierbaum BE, et al. (2002). Ceramic-on-ceramic bearings in total hip arthroplasty. *Clin Orthop Relat Res*, 405, 2002: 158-63

Bitsch RG, et al. (2007). Ion Production and Excretion in a Patient with a Metal-on-Metal Bearing Hip Prosthesis. A Case Report. *J Bone Joint Surg Am*, 89, 2007: 2758-2763

Bozic KJ, et al. (2009). The Epidemiology of Bearing Surface Usage in Total Hip Arthroplasty in the United States. *J Bone Joint Surg Am*, 91, 2009: 1614-1620

Bradford L, et al. (2004). Early failure due to osteolysis in highly cross-linked ultrahigh molecular weight polyethylene: a case report. *J Bone Joint Surg Am*, 86A, 2004: 1051

Brodner W, et al. (2003). Serum cobalt levels after metal-on-metal total hip arthroplasty. *J Bone Joint Surg Am*, 85, 2003: 2168-2173

Brodner W, et al. (2004). Does the placenta inhibit the passage of chromium and cobalt after metal-on-metal total hip arthroplasty? *J Arthroplasty*, 19 (Suppl), 2004: 102-106

Buford A, Goswami T. (2004). Review of wear mechanisms in hip implants. *Mat Des*, 25, 2004: 385–393

Campbell PA, et al. (2005). An unusual lymphocytic perivascular infiltration in tissues around contemporary metal-on-metal joint replacements. *J Bone Joint Surg Am*, 87, 2005: 18-27

Capello WN, et al. (2008). Ceramic-on-ceramic total hip arthroplasty: update. *J Arthroplasty*, 23, 2008: 39–43

Catelas I, et al. (2006). Wear particles from metal-on-metal total hip replacements: effects of implant design and implantation time. *Proc Inst Mech Eng*, 220, 2006: 195–208

Chan FW, et al. (1996). Engineering issues and wear performance of metal on metal hip implants. *Clin Orthop Relat Res*, 333, 1996: 96-107

Chan FW, et al. (1999). Wear and lubrication of metal-on-metal hip implants. *Clin Orthop Relat Res*, 369, 1999: 10-24

Clarke IC, Gustafson A. (2000). Clinical and hip simulator comparisons of ceramic-on-polyethylene and metal-on-polyethylene wear. *Clin Orthop Relat Res*, 379, 2000: 34–40

Cobb AG, Schmalzreid TP. (2006). The clinical significance of metal ion release from cobalt-chromium metal-on-metal hip joint arthroplasty. *Proc Inst Mech Eng*, 220, 2006: 385-398

D'Antonio J, et al. (2009). Ceramic Materials as Bearing Surfaces for THA. *J Am Acad Orthop Surg*, 17, 2009: 63-68

Daniel J, et al. (2006). The effect of the diameter of metal-on-metal bearings on systemic exposure to cobalt and chromium. *J Bone Joint Surg Br*, 88, 2006: 443-448

Daniel J, et al. (2007). The validity of serum as a surrogate measure of systemic metal ion exposure in hip arthroplasty. *J Bone Joint Surg [Br]*, 89B, 2007 : 736-741

De Aza AH, et al. (2002). Crack growth resistance of alumina, zirconia and zirconia toughened alumina ceramics for joint prostheses. *Biomaterials*, 23, 2002: 937–945

Digas G, et al. (2003). Increase in early polyethylene wear after sterilization with ethylene oxide: radiostereometric analyses of 201 total hips. *Acta Orthop Scand*, 74, 2003: 531-541

Digas G, et al. (2007). 5-year experience of highly cross-linked polyethylene in cemented and uncemented sockets. Two randomized studies using radiostereometric analysis. *Acta Orthop*, 78(6), 2007: 746-754

Dowson D, et al. (2004). A hip joint simulator study of the performance of metal-on-metal joints. Part II: design. *J Arthroplasty*, 19 (Suppl 3), 2004: 124-130

Dowson D, Jin ZM. (2006). Metal-on-metal hip joint tribology. *Proc Inst Mech Eng*, 220, 2006: 107-118

Dumbleton JH, et al. (2006). The basis for a second-generation highly cross-linked UHMWPE. *Clin Orthop*, 453, 2006: 265-271

Engh CA, et al. (2009). Metal Ion Levels After Metal-on-Metal Total Hip Arthroplasty: A Randomized Trial. *Clin Orthop Relat Res*, 467, 2009: 101–111

Fernandez-Fairen *M, et al.*(2007). Aging of Retrieved Zirconia Femoral Heads. *Clin Orthop Relat Res*, 462, 2007, 122–129

Firkins PJ, et al. (2001) A novel low wearing differential hardness, ceramic-on-metal hip joint prosthesis. *J Biomech*, 34, 2001: 1291-1298

Fisher J, et al. (2004). Wear of surface engineered metal-on-metal hip prostheses. *J Mater Sci Mater Med*, 15, 2004: 225-235

Fruh HJ, Willmann G. (1998). Tribological investigations of the wear couple alumina-CFRP for total hip replacement. *Biomaterials*, 19, 1998: 1145-1150

Garvin KL, et al. (2009). Wear Analysis in THA Utilizing Oxidized Zirconium and Crosslinked Polyethylene. *Clin Orthop Relat Res*, 467, 2009: 141–145

Gawkrodger DJ. (2003) Metal sensitivities and orthopedic implants revisited: the potential of metal allergy with the new metal-on-metal joint prostheses. *Br J Dermatol*, 148, 2003: 1089

Geerdink CH, et al. (2009). Cross-linked Compared with Historical Polyethylene in THA An 8-year Clinical Study. *Clin Orthop Relat Res*, 476, 2009: 979–984

Gillespie WJ, et al. (1988). The incidence of cancer following total hip replacement. *J Bone Joint Surg Br*, 70, 1988: 539-542

Glaser D, et al. (2008). Clicking and Squeaking: In Vivo Correlation of Sound and Separation for Different Bearing Surfaces. *J Bone Joint Surg Am*, 90, 2008: 112-120

Greenbaum ES, et al. (2004). Effect of lipid absorption on wear and compressive properties of unirradiated and highly crosslinked UHMWPE: an in vitro experimental model. *Biomaterials*, 25, 2004: 4479–4484

Gul RM, et al. (2003). Effect of consolidation on adhesive and abrasive wear of UHMWPE. *Biomaterials*, 24, 2003: 3193–3199

Ha YC, et al. (2007). Ceramic liner fracture after cementless alumina-on-alumina total hip arthroplasty. *Clin Orthop Relat Res*, 458, 2007: 106–110

Hallab N, et al. (2001). Metal sensitivity in patients with orthopaedic implants. *J Bone Joint Surg Am*, 83, 2001: 428-36

Hamilton WG, et al. (2010). THA with Delta Ceramic on Ceramic; Results of a Multicenter Investigational Device Exemption Trial. *Clin Orthop Relat Res*, 468, 2010: 358–366

Hannouche D, et al. (2003). Fractures of ceramic bearings: history and present status. *Clin Orthop Relat Res*, 417, 2003: 19–26

Hannouche D, et al. (2005). Ceramics in total hip replacement. *Clin Orthop Relat Res*, 430, 2005: 62-71

Harris WH. (2001). Wear and periprosthetic osteolysis: the problem. *Clin Orthop Relat Res*, 393, 2001: 66-70

Hart AJ, et al. (2006). The association between metal ions from hip resurfacing and reduced T-cell counts. *J Bone Joint Surg Br*, 88, 2006: 449-454

Hart AJ, et al. (2009). Circulating levels of cobalt and chromium from metal-on-metal hip replacement are associated with CD_8T-cell lymphopenia. *J Bone Joint Surg Br*, 91, 2009: 835-842

Hatton A, et al. (2002a). Alumina-alumina artificial hip joints: Part I. A histological analysis and characterisation of wear debris by laser capture microdissection of tissues retrieved at revision. *Biomaterials*, 23, 2002: 3429

Hatton A, et al. (2002b). Alumina-alumina artificial hip joints. Part II: characterisation of the wear debris from in vitro hip joint simulations. *Biomaterials*, 23, 2002: 3441–3448

Hern´andez-Rodr´ıguez MAL, et al. (2005). Wear of cast metal–metal pairs for total replacement hip prostheses. *Wear*, 259, 2005: 958–963

Howcroft D, et al. (2008). Bearing surfaces in the young patient: out with the old and in with the new? *Current Orthopaedics*, 22, 2008: 177-184

Huber M, et al. (2010). Postmortem Study of Femoral Osteolysis Associated with Metal-on-Metal Articulation in Total Hip Replacement; An Analysis of Nine Cases. *J Bone Joint Surg Am*, 92, 2010: 1720-1731

Isaac GH, et al. (2006). Metal-on-metal bearings surfaces: materials, manufacture, design, optimization, and alternatives. *Proc Inst Mech Eng*, 220, 2006: 119-133

Jacobs JJ, et al. (1998). Metal release in patients who have had a primary total hip arthroplasty. A prospective, controlled, longitudinal study. *J Bone Joint Surg Am*, 80, 1998: 1447-1458

Jacobs JJ, et al. (2006). Wear Particles. *J Bone Joint Surg Am*, 88, 2006: 99-102

Jarrett CA, et al. (2009). The squeaking hip: an underreported phenomenon of ceramic-on-ceramic total hip arthroplasty. *J Bone Joint Surg Am*, 91, 2009: 1344-1349

Keurentjes JC, et al. (2008). High incidence of squeaking in THAs with alumina ceramic-on-ceramic bearings. *Clin Orthop Relat Res*, 466, 2008: 1438–1443

Kim YH. (2005). Comparison of polyethylene wear associated with cobalt-chromium and zirconia heads after total hip replacement. A prospective, randomized study. *J Bone Joint Surg Am*, 87(8), 2005: 1769-1776

Komistek RD, et al. (2002). In vivo comparison of hip separation after metal-on-metal or metal-on-polyethylene total hip arthroplasty. *J Bone Joint Surg Am*, 84, 2002: 1836-1841

Kwon YM, et al. (2009). Dose-dependent cytotoxicity of clinically relevant cobalt nanoparticles and ions on macrophages in vitro. *Biomed Mater*, 4, 2009: 18-25

Lerouge S, et al. (1997). Ceramic-ceramic and metal-polyethylene total hip replacements comparison of pseudomembranes after loosening. *J Bone Joint Surg Br*, 79B, 1997: 135

Lombardi AV, et al. (2010). Delta Ceramic-on-Alumina Ceramic Articulation in Primary THA; Prospective, Randomized FDA-IDE Study and Retrieval Analysis. *Clin Orthop Relat Res*, 468, 2010: 367–374

Lundberga JH, et al. (2006). Problematic sites of third body embedment in polyethylene for total hip wear acceleration. *Journal of Biomechanics*, 39, 2006: 1208–1212

MacDonald SJ. (2004). Can a safe level for metal ions in patients with metal-on-metal total hip arthroplasties be determined? *J Arthroplasty*, 19 (Suppl 3), 2004: 71-77

Malviya A et al. (2010). Metal-on-Metal total hip arthroplasty. *J Bone Joint Surg Am*, 92, 2010: 1675-1683

McKellop H, et al. (1999). Development of an extremely wear-resistant ultrahigh molecular weight polyethylene for total hip replacements. *J Orthop Res*, 17, 1999: 157–167

Mehmood S, et al. (2008). Review of ceramic-on-ceramic total hip arthroplasty. *J Surg Ortho Adv*, 17, 2008: 45–50

Min BW, et al. (2007). The Delayed Fracture of a Ceramic Insert With Modern Ceramic Total Hip Replacement. *J Arthroplasty*, 22(1), 2007: 136-139

Moore KD, et al. (2008). Early failure of a cross-linked polyethylene acetabular liner. A case report. *J Bone Joint Surg Am*, 90, 2008: 2499–2504

Muratoglu OK, et al. (2001). A novel method of cross-linking ultra–high-molecular-weight polyethylene to improve wear, reduce oxidation, and retain mechanical properties. *J Arthroplasty*, 16, 2001: 149

Nam KW, et al. (2007). Alumina-Debris-Induced Osteolysis in Contemporary Alumina-on-Alumina Total Hip Arthroplasty A Case Report. *J Bone Joint Surg Am*, 89, 2007: 2499-2503

Older J. (2002). Charnley low-friction arthroplasty: a worldwide retrospective review at 15 to 20 years. *J Arthroplasty*, 17, 2002: 675-680

Park YS, et al. (2006). Ceramic failure after total hip arthroplasty with an alumina-on-alumina bearing. *J Bone Joint Surg Am*, 88, 2006: 780–787

Poggie RA, et al. (2007). Failure analysis of a ceramic bearing acetabular component. *J Bone Joint Surg Am*, 89, 2007: 367–375

Raimondi MT, et al. (2001). Quantitative evaluation of the prosthetic head damage induced by microscopic third-body particles in total hip replacement. *J Biomed Mater Res*, 58(4), 2001: 436–448

Ranawat AS, Ranawat CS. (2007). The squeaking hip: a cause for concern—agrees. *Orthopedics*, 30, 2007: 738–743

Restrepo C,et al. (2008). The noisy ceramic hip: is component malpositioning the cause? *J Arthroplasty*, 23, 2008: 643–649

Rieker CB, et al. (2005). Influence of the clearance on in-vitro tribology of large diameter metal-on-metal articulations pertaining to resurfacing hip implants. *Orthop Clin North Am*, 36, 2005: 135-142

Rodrı´guez JA, et al. (2008). Squeaking in total hip replacement: a cause for concern. *Orthopedics*, 31, 2008: 877–878

Ro¨hrl SM, et al. (2007). Very low wear of non-remelted highly-linked polyethylene cups. An RSA study lasting up to 6 years. *Acta Orthop*, 78(6), 2007: 739-745

Savarino L, et al. (2006). Differences in ion release after ceramic-on-ceramic and metal-on-metal total hip replacement. Medium-term follow-up. *J Bone Joint Surg Br*, 88, 2006: 472-476

Scholes SC, Unsworth A. (2000). Comparison of friction and lubrication of different hip prostheses. *Proc Inst Mech Eng*, 214, 2000: 49-57

Scholes SC, et al. (2006b). Compliant layer acetabular cups: Friction testing of a range of materials and designs for a new generation of prosthesis that mimics the natural joint. *Proc Inst Mech Eng*, 220, 2006: 583-596

Skipor AK, et al. (2002). Serum and urine metal levels in patients with metal-on-metal surface arthroplasty. *J Mater Sci Mater Med, 13,* 2002:1227-1234

Smith SL, et al. (2001a). The effect of femoral head diameter upon lubrication and wear of metal-on-metal total hip replacements. *Proc Inst Mech Eng*, 215, 2001: 161-170

Smith SL, et al. (2001b). The lubrication of metal-on-metal total hip joints: a slide down the Stribeck curve. *Proc Inst Mech Eng*, 215, 2001: 483-493

Stewart TD, et al. (2001). Long-term wear of HIPed alumina on alumina bearings for THR under microseparation conditions. *J Mater Sci*, 12, 2001: 1053–1056

Stewart TD, et al. (2003). Long-term wear of ceramic matrix composite materials for hip prostheses under severe swing phase microseparation. *J Biomed Mater Res*, 66, 2003: 567–573

Tateiwa T, et al. (2008). Ceramic total hip arthroplasty in the United States: safety and risk issues revisited. *Am J Orthop*, 37, 2008: 26–31

Taylor S, et al. (2007). The role of stripe wear causing acoustic emissions from alumina ceramic-on-ceramic bearings. *J Arthroplasty*, 22(7 Suppl. 3), 2007: 47-51

Teoh SH, et al. (2002). An elasto-plastic finite element model for polyethylene wear in total hip arthroplasty. *Biomechanics*, 35, 2002: 323–330

Tharani R, et al. (2001). The risk of cancer following total hip or knee arthroplasty. *J Bone Joint Surg Am*, 83, 2001: 774-780

Udofia IJ, Jin ZM (2003). Elastohydrodynamic lubrication analysis of metal-on-metal hip resurfacing prostheses. *J. Biomech*, 36, 2003: 537–544

Urban RM, et al. (2000). Dissemination of wear particles to liver, spleen, and abdominal lymph nodes of patients with hip or knee replacement. *J Bone Joint Surg Am*, 82, 2000: 457-477

Urban JA, et al. (2001). Ceramic-on-polyethylene bearing surfaces in total hip arthroplasty: seventeen to twenty-one year results. *J Bone Joint Surg Am*, 83, 2001: 1688–1694

Walter WL, et al. (2004). Edge loading in third generation alumina ceramic-on-ceramic bearings: stripe wear. *J Arthroplasty*, 19, 2004: 402–413

Walter WL, et al. (2007). Squeaking in ceramic-on-ceramic hips: the importance of acetabular component orientation. *J Arthroplasty*, 22, 2007: 496–503

Walter WL, et al. (2008). Squeaking hips. *J Bone Joint Surg Am*, 90 (Suppl 4), 2008: 102–111

Wang A, et al. (1999) Suitability and limitations of carbon fiber reinforced PEEK composite as bearing surfaces for total joint replacement. *Wear*, 229, 1999: 724-727

Whittingham-Jones PM, et al. (2008). Immune Responses in Patients with Metal-on-Metal Hip Articulations: A Long-term Follow-up. *J Arthroplasty*, 23(8), 2008: 1212-1218

Williams S, et al. (2004). Comparative wear under different conditions of surface-engineered metal-on-metal bearings for total hip arthroplasty. *J Arthroplasty*, 19 (Suppl 3), 2004: 112-117

Wimmer MA, et al. (2003). Tribochemical reaction on metal-on-metal hip joint bearings: a comparison between in-vitro and in-vivo results. *Wear*, 255, 2003: 1007–1024

Yoshitomi H, et al. (2009). Manufacturers Affect Clinical Results of THA with Zirconia Heads A Systematic Review. *Clin Orthop Relat Res*, 467, 2009: 2349–2355

Ziaee H, et al. (2007). Transplacental transfer of cobalt and chromium in patients with metal-on-metal hip arthroplasty: a controlled study. *J Bone Joint Surg Br*, 89, 2007: 301-305

11

The Use of PEEK in Spine Arthroplasty

T. Brown[1], Qi-Bin Bao[1] and Hansen A. Yuan[2]
[1]*Pioneer Surgical*
[2]*SUNY Upstate, New York*
USA

1. Introduction

Cervical and lumbar disc arthroplasty are one component in the continuum of treatment for symptomatic degenerative disc disease (DDD) that is unresponsive to conservative care. In the lumbar spine, this may be accomplished via nucleus replacement or total disc replacement, and in the cervical spine by total disc replacement. The goal of both lumbar disc arthroplasty treatments are the same; relieving discogenic back pain through removing the pain source and restoring or maintaining motion segment function. For cervical arthroplasty, the goal is to relieve radicular pain as a result of nerve root compression, and/or myelopathy as a result of spinal cord compression, in addition to preserving motion. From a design standpoint, nucleus replacement technology consists of elastomers and non-elastomers, both preformed and *in-situ* cured, and can incorporate articulation similar to total disc replacements, with the intent of replicating to various extents the natural nucleus and preserving most of the annulus, thereby relying on a biomechanically intact annulus to share the compressive load. Also, most artificial nucleus devices are not fixed to the vertebral endplates, and therefore allow small, relative motion between their external surfaces and the vertebral endplates. In contrast, the majority of total disc replacement technology consists of articulating designs and material combinations that have been developed based upon the wealth of scientific and clinical information produced by the success of total joint arthroplasty. An artificial disc is designed to replace the entire disc tissue by excising almost all the disc materials, and therefore removing all the natural constraints in the anterior column. In addition, all artificial discs have a superior plate and an inferior plate, which are fixed to the two adjacent vertebrae. These represent key design differences between the two technologies.

A key challenge for a disc arthroplasty device is selecting the proper material(s) for the various components that consitute its design. Unlike total joint replacement, a candidate for disc arthroplasty is on average 40 years of age with a target indication of 18 to 60 years (Zigler et al., 2007; Murrey et al., 2009). As a consequence, these devices are expected to last much longer than those of total joint recipients, whose average age is 70 years (Bergen, 2011, Garellick et al., 2010). Therefore, there are stringent requirements for long term implantable materials, and this will significantly limit the selection of materials available. Biocompatibility and biodurability, otherwise known as the abilities of a material to maintain its physical and chemcial integrity under *in vivo* applications without eliciting an aggressive host immune response for a given application, are essential for permanent medical implants. Since a central tenet of all arthroplasty devices is the preservation of motion, it is therefore expected that these devices will produce wear particulate, and the subsequent potential biologic activity needs to be evaluated. This is in addition to exhibiting sufficient strength and fatigue performance over the expected lifetime of the device within the *in vivo* environment. Subsequently, disc arthroplasty devices should be introduced into clinical use only after a successful preclinical evaluation of their mechanical and biological properties within the scope of their intended use, as failure can lead to a technically challenging revision, increased economic burden and more importantly, a significant risk to the patient (Devin et al., 2008, Cavanaugh et al., 2009, Francois et al., 2007, Guyer et al. 2011, Lucina & Thorpe, 2004, Punt et al., 2009).

Initially, much of the preclinical testing of candidate materials is not conducted on the device but rather the material itself. Logical progression then leads to testing of the device itself, since the design of the device will also affect a given materials performance. These tests should include bench top testing such as static and fatigue assessments, wear testing, and evaluation in human cadaver and animal models. The wear, mechanical durability and potential resultant biologic activity of disc arthroplasty devices are a key component that needs to be addressed prior to clinical use. This can be assessed to a large extent by the appropriate wear tests for articulating devices and fatigue tests in the case of devices that utilize elastomers for the basis of their motion. However, in the absence of significant implant retrievals, the appropriate tests to perform in assessing a respective devices' durability properties becomes critical. Device fatigue and wear may decrease the devices' lifespan for its intended application. In addition, the wear particulate generated may result in a particle mediated inflammatory response potentially leading to osteolysis or delayed type hypersensitivity. Evaluation of the particulate generated can allow for assessment of potential biologic reactivity. Successful animal models can act as a final spring board for initiation of clinical studies by evaluation of the mechanical behavior and elicited histopathological response of the device component materials following long-term implantation. Analyses can based upon gross necropsy, MRI radiography, plain X-ray, microradiography, multi-directional flexibility testing and biocompatibility assays (local and systemic histology). The overall successful completion and evaluation of these studies allows for advancement to the clinical stage.

Traditionally metal alloys, ceramics and polymers have been the materials of choice for arthroplasty applications. Ceramics are noted for their high wear resistance and strength, and metal alloys, such as titanium (Ti) and cobalt chrome (CoCr) for their high strength, fracture toughness and hardness; properties that are necessary for long term implantable materials. Polymers are a more compliant material, with low-friction properties ideal for articulating surfaces which produce relatively inert wear debris. These materials and combinations thereof have a long clinical history in total joint arthroplasty. Therefore, material combinations such as metal on UHMWPE and metal on metal are typically used for articulating disc replacements based upon the established scientific and clinical history of these bearing couples in total joint arthroplasty. Poly-ether-ether-ketone (PEEK) is a linear, aromatic thermoplastic with proven biocompatibility and biostability. It can be repeatedly steam and gamma sterilized with no detrimental effects on its bulk material properties. It is an exceptionally strong engineering thermoplastic that retains its mechanical properties even at very high temperatures (Rae, 2007). The material is tough and abrasion resistant with high-impact strength and excellent flexural and tensile properties. It has a low coefficient of friction and resists attack by a wide range of organic and inorganic chemicals and solvents. To this end, PEEK is widely used in the lumbar spine for both fusion

(Rousseau et al., 2007) and non-fusion applications (Balsano, 2011; Senegas, 2002) due to its excellent mechanical strength, biostability, biocompatibility and radiolucency (Kurtz & Devine, 2007), and has replaced to a significant extent the use of metallic cages. It is also commonly used in the cervical spine in the form of interbody cages for fusion. Therefore, it potentially has most of the material characteristics deemed to be required for use as material in spine arthroplasty applications. However, unlike traditional polymers and metals, common materials used in the spine arthroplasty arena, the use of PEEK represents a new material for disc arthroplasty applications in the cervical and lumbar spine, and as such, its use as a material for this technology has largely gone unexplored.

PEEK has recently been used in the form of a nucleus replacment device and in the form of a cervical total disc replacement. Both devices utilize a ball and socket articulation for motion. As part of evaluating the safety and effectiveness profile of both devices, several preclinical tests were successfully performed to satisfy FDA and the Essential Requirements of the Medical Device Directive (MDD) for CE mark requirements prior to clinical use. Each device is CE marked and currently in clinical use. Worldwide clinical results as measured by validated measures such as Oswestry Disability Index (ODI), Visual Analog Scale (VAS), along with patient satisfaction, suggest that both devices can relieve the symptoms of their respective degenerative processes, with no adverse events occurring as a direct result of the device not performing as expected from a biomaterial perspective. The methodology, results and interpretation of these preclinical studies that have allowed for advancement to the clinical stage will be discussed, along with the clinical results in light of both devices' clinical performance.

2. Preclinical studies and results

2.1 PEEK cervical total disc replacement device

The cervical arthroplasty device incorporates a unique, Ti cam blade fixation system that can be described as a rotating shaft with blades for primary fixation (Figure 1). Given that PEEK is a relatively bio-inert material, bone apposition does not readily occur onto the material. Therefore, a plasma-sprayed hydroxyapatite (HA) coating was added to the outer endplates. The design objectives are to achieve secure, long term fixation within the disc space, exhibit the necessary strength and durability for the lifetime of the patient for its intended use, and restore or maintain the range of motion (ROM) at the operative level while simultaneously not adversely affect the biomechanics at the adjacent levels.

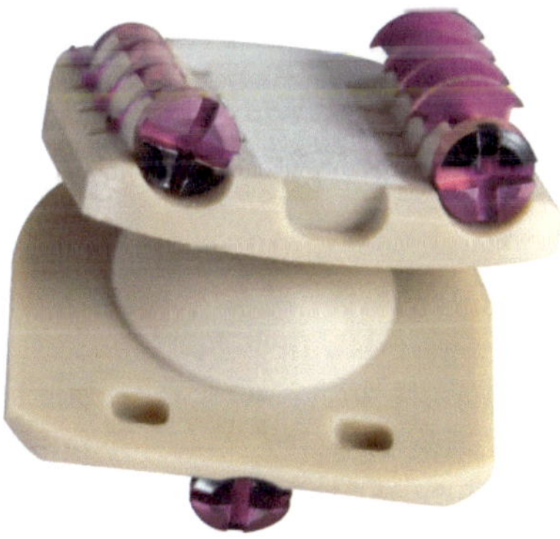

Fig. 1. PEEK cervical arthroplasty device.

2.1.1 Axial static and fatigue strength

To determine the static and fatigue strength of the device, the smallest footprint (12x14 mm) and height (5 mm) was utilized. Testing was performed on an MTS 858 Mini-Bionix II test frame with the devices mounted on steel fixtures. A comparison was made between HA coated devices and uncoated devices to determine if the coating had an adverse effect on the static and fatigue strength of the device. A sample size of 6 was used for the static test with a displacement rate of 2 mm/min. The acceptance criteria was an offset yield load of greater than 1200 N for the axial static testing. For the fatigue tests, a sample size of 2 was used with a starting fatigue load of 75% of the static offset yield load of the uncoated devices, with R=10 at 10 Hz.

For the axial static testing, the results showed that the mean load at offset yield was calculated to be 7,631 ± 171 N at a displacement of 0.50 ± 0.01 mm for the uncoated devices and 9640 ± 251 N at a displacement of 0.70 ± 0.02 mm for the coated devices, which was significantly greater (t-test, $p<0.001$). The primary mode of failure in the tested constructs was fracture of the PEEK. For the axial fatigue testing, the uncoated and coated samples reached 10 million cycles at a load of 5723 N (R=10). No evidence of failure, such as fatigue cracks or gross deformation, was seen during the inspections or after test. When the coated devices were tested at a load of 7230 N, implant fracture occurred at 867,966 cycles.

The literature suggests that the maximum compressive load on the cervical spine during the performance of physical tasks is 1.2 kN [Moroney, 1988] and that the elastic limit of single motion segments could be as high as 1.23 kN, with a predicted ultimate compressive strength of 2.40 kN [Przybyla, 2007]. The results showed that the loads reached were significantly above the expected *in vivo* loads of the cervical spine, and that the HA coating did not negatively affect the axial compressive static or fatigue performance.

2.1.2 Shear static and fatigue strength

To determine the shear static and fatigue strength of the device, the smallest footprint (12x14 mm) and height (5 mm) was utilized. Testing was performed on an MTS 858 Mini-Bionix II test frame with the devices mounted on steel fixtures. According to the literature, the total ROM for flexion/extension of the cervical spine is greatest at the C_4-C_5 level, and appears to be slightly more than 20° when measured *in vivo* using computer assisted tracking software [Reitman, 2004]. The literature also shows that the amount of mean flexion is only slightly higher than the mean extension [Panjabi, 2001]. Therefore, the shear test was conducted at 10° for both flexion and extension. A comparison was made between HA coated devices and uncoated devices to determine if the coating had an adverse effect on the shear static and fatigue strength of the device. A sample size of 6 was used for the static tests with a displacement rate of 2 mm/min. The acceptance criteria was an offset yield load of greater than 135 N [Moroney, 1988] for the shear static testing and for the fatigue tests, a sample size of 2 was used with a run out load greater than 135 N [Moroney, 1988] with R=10 at 10 Hz.

For the shear static testing at 10° flexion, the mean load at offset yield was calculated to be 4774 ± 372 N at a displacement of 0.44 ± 0.01 mm. For the shear static testing at 10° extension static shear, the mean load at offset yield was calculated to be 6788 ± 412 N at a displacement of 0.53 ± 0.02 mm. The primary mode of failure was fracture of the PEEK (Figure 2). Since the results of the static compressive shear strength resulted in a lower offset yield load in flexion (4744 N) versus extension (6788 N), the fatigue test was run at 10° flexion as a worst case scenario. The results of the fatigue testing at 1600 N showed the devices reached 10 million cycles without experiencing any visible plastic deformation or fracture. For the coated devices, since the shear static loading was significantly higher than the acceptance criteria and the coating was shown to not have a detrimental effect on the axial static properties of the device, only shear fatigue testing was performed. The results were the same as the coated devices, 1600 N of compressive shear to 10 million cycles without experiencing any visible plastic deformation or fracture. Therefore, it was concluded that shear fatigue loads can be withstood far beyond those that would be expected *in vivo*.

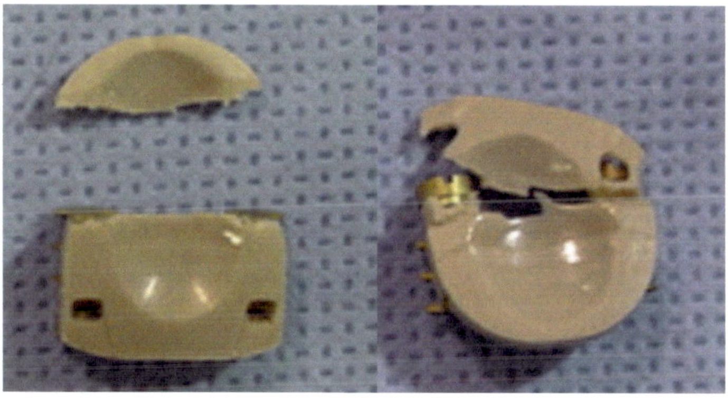

Fig. 2. PEEK cervical arthroplasty device after static compressive shear testing to failure. Left - tested under 10° flexion, right - tested under 10° extension.

2.1.3 Fixation strength

The fixation strength of the device was assessed by determining its pull out strength using a synthetic vertebral model. The largest (17x17 mm) and smallest footprints (12x14 mm) of 8 mm height were utilized. To avoid the variability produced by human cadaveric tissue, including bone mineral density and endplate geometries, a synthetic fixation medium of ASTM grade 15 polyurethane foam was selected for use. The fixation pull out test model consisted of compressing the device between two polyurethane blocks to 60 lbs, and then performing a uniaxial tensile load to failure test, thereby forcibly removing the implant. The test was conducted on an MTS 858 Mini-Bionix II test frame with appropriate fixturing. The displacement rate was 2.5 mm/sec. The implant was placed between the blocks in accordance with the surgical technique. A minimum of ten pullout tests were performed for each implant size. This data was then compared to eight previously tested cervical disc arthroplasty devices used clinically in cervical reconstruction that utilize press fit, keel or screw fixation using the same test protocol and laboratory [Cunningham, 2010]. Therefore, the results of this testing provides for a standardized testing methodology to quantify the strength of fixation and resistance to migration.

In all pullout tests for the two implant sizes, there was no incidence of intrinsic device failure. Failure always occurred at the polyurethane block-implant interface. The cam blade fixation indicated the highest pullout strength, which was statistically different from nearly all other designs (Table 1). Prosthetic endplates containing toothed ridges and keel fixation ranked next in terms of fixation strength. Although intuition favored the coronal keel as affording an increased mechanical advantage over the toothed surface, there were no observed statistical differences in pullout strength between the two endplate designs ($p>0.05$). In fact, the toothed surfaces indicated a slightly higher failure load over the keel device, although not statistically different. Moreover, the utilization of toothed ridges

Experimental Group	Device Fixation Type	Endplate Surface Area (mm^2)	Failure Load (N)
PEEK cervical device (small)	Cam blade	168	386.3 ± 44.1*
PEEK cervical device (large)	Cam blade	289	566.2 ± 72.0**
PCM Low Profile	0.2 mm endplate serrations	300	257.4 ±28.5
PCM V-Teeth	0.2 mm endplate serrations with 1.0 mm toothed ridges	300	308.8 ± 15.3
PCM Modular Flange	Serration with (4) 4 mm x 15 mm screws	300	496.4 ± 40.0
PMC Fixed Flange	(4) 4 mm x 15 mm screws	300	528.0 ± 127.8
Prestige LP	2.3 mm height center keel with teeth	275	306.4 ± 31.3
Kineflex C	0.2 mm endplate serrations with 2.5 mm height center keel	250	286.9 ± 18.4
Anterior Cervical Plate with Interbody Cage	Serration with 4 screws	180	635.5 ± 112.6
Iliac Crest Autograft	N/A	235	161.6 ± 16.6

Table 1. Fixation strength of the PEEK cervical arthroplasty device as compared to other forms of fixation. * Fixation strength was significantly greater than all others with the exception of PCM Fixed Flange and Anterior Cervical Plate with Interbody Cage. **Fixation strength was significantly greater than all others with the exception of PCM Fixed and Modular Flange, Prestige LP and Anterior Cervical Plate with Interbody Cage. There were no statistical differences between endplate surface areas.

elevated beyond 1.0mm did not significantly improve fixation strength ($p>0.05$). Prosthetic endplates containing serrated edges (0.2mm) alone indicated the lowest fixation strength. These results indicate not only a high fixation strength but the ability of the PEEK housing for the cam blades to withstand the expected *in vivo* shear forces placed upon the device.

2.1.4 Wear testing and wear particulate characterization

Wear testing was performed on six devices of the smallest footprint (12x14 mm) and 5 mm height using an MTS Spine Wear Simulator. The test parameters consisted of ASTM F2423-05 recommended multidirectional motion and static load profiles from 0-10 million cycles followed by ISO 18192-1 recommended motion and dynamic load profiles from 10-20 million cycles. The test frequency was 2 Hz for motion and 4 Hz for load. The testing fluid consisted of newborn calf serum diluted with phosphate buffered saline (PBS) to a final protein content of 20 g/L. Ethylene-diamine tetraacetic acid (EDTA) was added to the serum at a concentration of 20 mM to bind the calcium ions present in the serum. EDTA is a known preservative, and together with the low protein content and PBS, the addition of sodium azide or other anti-bacterial agent was not used. The test fluid temperature was kept at 37 ± 3° C. Unloaded soak controls were used to account for moisture uptake. After 0.5 million cycles, the tests were stopped at 1 million cycles and at million-cycle intervals thereafter to clean, dry and gravimetrically assess the wear rates. The test fluid was subsequently collected and stored at -20° C. The average wear rates were determined using linear regression analysis with one-way-analysis-of-variance (ANOVA) used to determine if significant differences ($p < 0.05$) in the wear rates between methodologies were present. Complimentary to the wear testing, particle analysis was performed using light scanning electron microscopy (SEM). The proteinacious test serum containing PEEK wear debris underwent enzymatic digestion (5x Trypsin digestion and 1.5 mg/mL of Proteinase K per sample at 37° C for 24 hours) followed by a mild acid treatment (10% HCl at 37° C for 24 hours), meeting or exceeding similar protocols previously established to be equivalent for acid and base digestion (Niedzwiecki, 2001). The particles were then analyzed by SEM analysis and characterized according to their equivalent circle diameter (ECD), aspect ration (AR), roundness (R) and form factor (FF) in accordance with ASTM F 1877-05.

All implants maintained full functionality throughout each test duration. The results showed only a slight, non-significant variation in the wear rates over the course of 20 million cycles. The wear rate for the first 10 million cycles was approximately 0.26 ± 0.01 mm^3/million cycles. For the interval of 10 to 20 million cycles, the wear rate increased slightly, 0.32 ± 0.02 mm^3/million cycles. These wear rates are similar to other arthroplasty devices in clinical use (Figure 3). Although the wear rates were relatively consistent, the particle size was sensitive to the test method. The particle analysis revealed that the size (ECD) of the particulate was larger for the ISO testing methodology (2.56 μm) as compared to the ASTM methodology (1.67μm) (Figure 4). However the particle morphology, an equally important parameter influencing biological activity, was similar for both methods. The ASTM testing revealed a smaller particulate; however it may be unlikely that a static compressive load occurs in the cervical spine *in vivo*, since the literature suggests that a dynamic compressive load occurs due to muscle contraction during kinematic activities [Snijders, 1991].

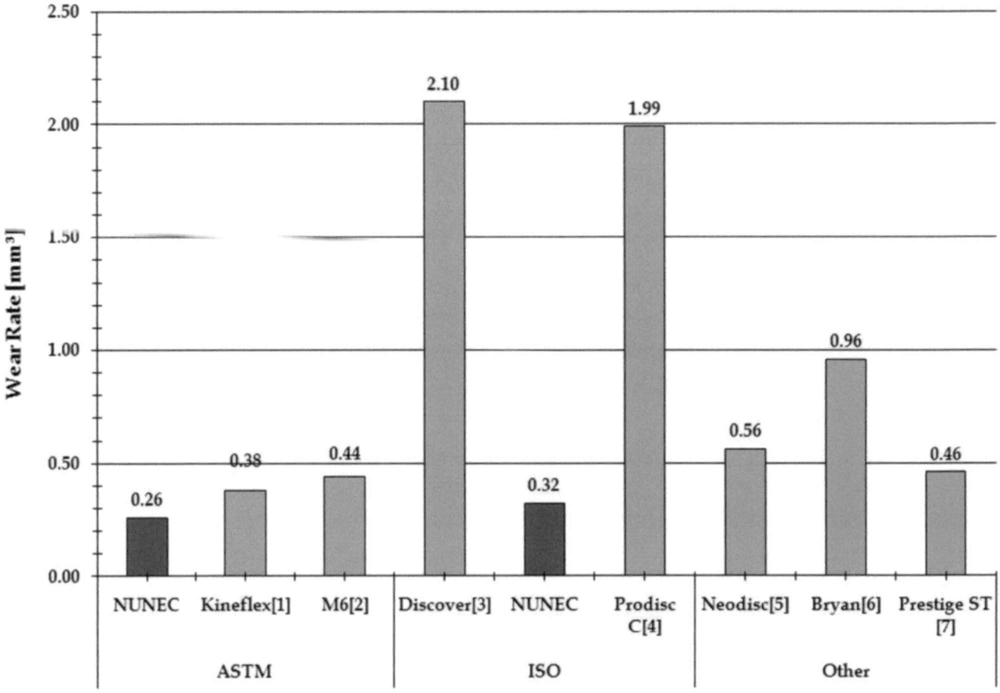

Fig. 3. Wear rate comparison of the PEEK cervical arthroplasty device to other devices in clinical use.

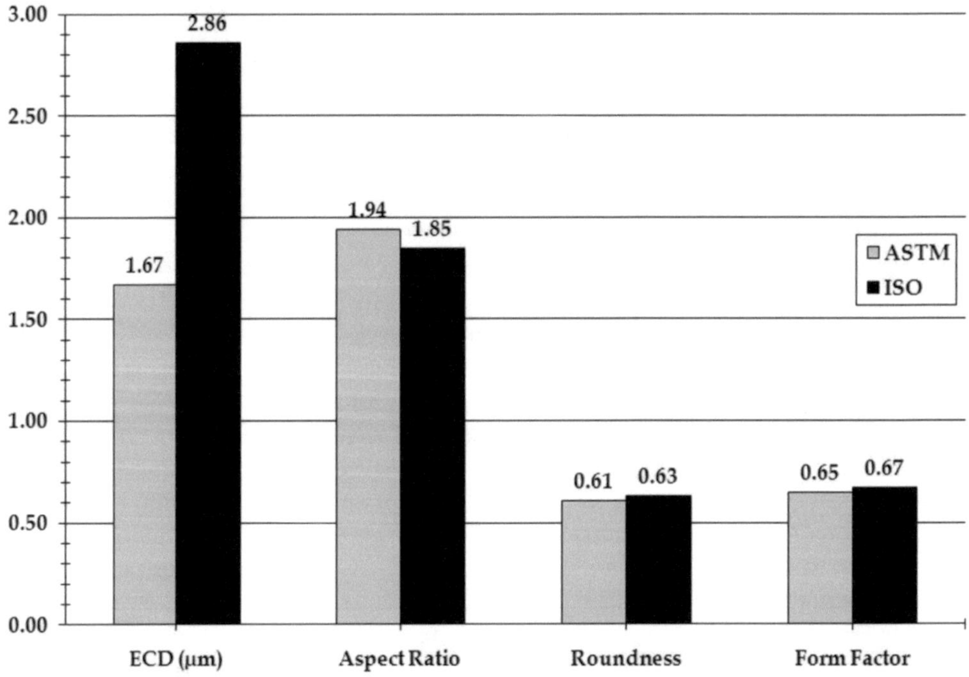

Fig. 4. SEM analysis of the PEEK particulate generated from the wear tests.

Methodology	Group 1- Normal Load	Group 2 - Artificially Aged	Group 3 – High Load
Environmental Condition			
Sterilization	30 kGy in air	200 kGy in air	30 kGy in air
Aging	N/A	Exposure to O_2 at 70° C for 40 days	N/A
Dynamic Compressive Load	225…1024 N	225…1024 N	200…2000 N
Motion	ISO - 6°/3° flexion/extension ±2° lateral bending and axial rotation to 10 million cycles	ISO - 6°/3° flexion/extension ±2° lateral bending and axial rotation to 10 million cycles	ISO - 6°/3° flexion/extension ±2° lateral bending and axial rotation to 10 million cycles
Test Frequency	Compressive Load 4 Hz Motion 2 Hz	Compressive Load 4 Hz Motion 2 Hz	Compressive Load 4 Hz Motion 2 Hz

Table 2. Summary of Testing Methodology for All Groups.

2.1.5 Hydroxyapatite coating and substrate effects

The HA coating is applied to the outer endplates of the device via the well known plasma spray process. The coating was characterized in accordance with FDA guidelines. Given that the device' material (PEEK) is being exposed to what is considered a high temperature process, a potential change in the materials biocompatibility profile and/or material properties could occur. Therefore, several tests were performed to ensure that the thermal and chemical signature of the PEEK substrate was not adversely affected. This consisted of Differential Scanning Calorimetry (DSC), Thermal Gravimetric Analysis (TGA) and Fourier Transform Infrared Spectroscopy (FTIR), the most common tools used to characterize polymers. This was then compared with the 20-year historical measurements of PEEK provided by the manufacturer (Invibio). Analyses were performed on bulk and surface samples.

For the DSC, TGA and FTIR analysis, six machined samples of HA coated PEEK that subsequently had the coating removed by a 10% phosphoric acid treatment were compared to machined PEEK samples that had not been coated. The DSC analysis showed similarity between all samples and to machined PEEK samples. Likewise, ATR-FTIR showed no appreciable difference in the tested samples. TGA analysis resulted in primary degradation of the samples starting at approximately 550°C and continuing until about 625°C, showing an initial degradation loss of 35%. There was a dramatic decrease in sample mass (65% of the initial mass down to 0% of the initial mass) of the samples between 625° C and 800° C. There was no appreciable difference in the samples, and the degradation response looked very similar to the machined PEEK samples. All observed values (mean, maximum and minimums) were within the 20 year historical ranges of PEEK as verified by Invibio. More importantly, from a biocompatibility standpoint, since there were no additional absorption peaks found in the regions that formerly had an HA coating, and the HA coating was readily removed with a mild solvent, it is highly unlikely that any covalent bonding occurred between the HA and the PEEK material. Furthermore, there was no measurable change in the molecular structure of the PEEK induced by adding the HA layer. Therefore, no chemical bonding was noted to occur, the surface properties and subsequently the biocompatibility profile of the PEEK substrate have not changed, and it can be concluded that only a mechanical bond exists between the PEEK and HA coating.

Biocompatibility tests in accordance with ISO 10993 parts 5, 10 and 11 were conducted at NAMSA. These tests were carried out on coated and an equal number of substrates having the coating removed with a mild solvent (phosphoric acid) in order to expose the underlying substrate. The control consisted of virgin PEEK:

ISO 10993, Part 5: Tests for Cytotoxicity-

HA coated PEEK and coated PEEK that had the coating removed, were prepared using single strength Miminum Essential Medium supplemented with 5% serum and 2% antibiotics (1X MEM). The test extracts were placed onto three separate monolayers of L-929 mouse fibroblast cells propagated in 5% CO_2. Three separate monolayers were prepared for the reagent control, negative control and for the posititve control. All monolayers were incubated at 37° C in the presence of 5% CO_2 for 48 hours at which point they were examined microscopically to determine any change in cell morphology. Under the conditions of this study, the 1X MEM test extract showed no evidence of causing cell lysis or toxicity. The reagent control, negative control and the positive control performed as anticitpated. Therefore the requirements of the study were met.

ISO 10993, Part 10: Test for Irritation and Delayed-Type Hypersensititivity-

A guinea pig (Hartley albino) maximization test was conducted to evaluate the potential for delayed dermal contact sensitization. HA coated PEEK and coated PEEK that had the coating removed, were extracted in 0.9% sodium chloride USP solution (SC) and sesame oil, NF (SO). Each extract was intradermally injected and occlusively patched to ten test guinea pigs per extract in an attempt to incude sensitization. Five additional guinea pigs served as a control. All sites were scored at 24 and 48 hours after patch removal. HA coated PEEK and coated PEEK that had the coating removed, were extracted in 0.9% sodium chloride USP solution (SC) and sesame oil, NF (SO). A 0.2 mL dose was injected by the intracutaneous route into five separate sites on the right side of the the back of two New Zealand white rabbits. Similarly, the corresponding control was injected on the left side of the back of each rabbit. Observations for erythema and edema were conducted at 24, 48 and 72 hours after injection. Under the conditions of this study, there was no evidence of the extracts causing delayed dermal contact sensitization in the guinea pigs or no erythema or edema from the extracts injected intracutaneously into the rabbits. The requirements of the study were met.

ISO 10993, Part 11: Tests for Systemic Toxicity-

HA coated PEEK and coated PEEK that had the coating removed, were extracted in 0.9% sodium chloride USP solution and sesame oil, NF. A single dose of the extract was injected into five mice per extract by either the intravenous or intraperitoneal route. Five mice served as a control. The animals were observed immediately and at 4, 24, 48 and 72 hours after injection. Under the conditions of this study, there was no mortality or evidence of systemic toxicity from the extracts, and therefore the requirements of the study were met.

2.1.6 Biomechanical analysis

Using an *in-vitro* human cadaveric model, the range of motion (ROM) of the device was evaluated at a single level, with data analysis based on the resulting operative and adjacent level multidirectional flexibility properties. A total of twelve fresh-frozen human cadaveric cervical spines (C_1T_3) were harvested en-bloc and utilized. Prior to biomechanical analysis, standard anteroposterior and lateral plain films were obtained to exclude specimens demonstrating intervertebral disc or osseous pathology. In preparation for biomechanical testing, the specimens were thawed to room temperature and cleaned of all residual musculature, with care taken to preserve all ligamentous attachments and facet joint capsules. The proximal (C_1C_3) and distal (T_1T_3) ends of the specimen were stabilized in metal tubing containers using four, four point compression screws. An optoelectronic motion measurement system (3020 Optotrak System) was used for kinematic analysis under a pure moment loading to evaluate the flexion/extension, lateral bending and axial rotational response after reconstruction of the C_4C_5 cervical level. A comparision was made between the intact, destabilized, reconstructed and fusion procedures.

Flexion/extension testing demonstrated the diskectomy condition as producing a five degree increase (10.5 to 15.6°) in operative level range of motion compared to the intact spine and was statistically greater than intact and anterior plate-cage groups ($p<0.05$). Implantation of the PEEK cervical artificial disc restored motion to near intact level (11.9°) which was not statistically different from the intact spine (10.5°) ($p > 0.05$). The final reconstruction using the anterior plate-cage decreased the mean range of motion to 8.71° at the operative level, which resulted in significantly less range of motion than the PEEK artificial disc (11.9°) ($p<0.05$) but not intact condition (10.5 dg) ($p>0.05$). The elevated mean range of motion value for this reconstruction is attributable to the segmental instability created by the diskectomy condition (ANOVA $F=3.72$, $p=0.018$). Biomechanical testing in lateral bending loading did not reveal any significant differences in range of motion when comparing the intact spine and three treatment groups ($p>0.05$). Diskectomy (7.63°), PEEK artificial disc (6.90°) or anterior plate-cage construct (6.77°) afforded a statistical change in flexibility compared to the native intact condition (7.10°). The high standard deviation in the range of motion account for the lack of statistical significance under this loading modality (ROM: ANOVA $F=0.58$, $p=0.633$). Biomechanical testing in axial rotation indicated no statistical differences in ROM between the intact spine, diskectomy, PEEK total disc replacement or anterior plate-cage group ($p>0.05$). The cervical disc replacement procedure (7.21°) resulted in a slight increase in operative level flexibility relative to the intact (6.05°) and diskectomy conditions (6.44°) ($p>0.05$). The trends under this biomechanical loading mode failed to reach statistical significance secondary to specimen variability and high standard deviations. (ROM: ANOVA $F=0.22$, $P=0.882$). Despite the use of the Panjabi Hybrid testing protocol, there were very minimal changes in adjacent level ROM when comparing the intact spine, diskectomy condition and two reconstruction groups ($p>0.05$). The only significant change was observed at the adjacent level in flexion extension loading condition. The normalized-to-intact ROM at C_6C_7 level in these two reconstruction conditions was significantly higher than that was detected in diskectomy condition ($p<0.05$). Similar to the operative level ROM, the trends under this biomechanical loading mode failed to reach statistical significance secondary to specimen variability and high standard deviations.

The greatest differences between the intact spine and three treatment groups were detected during flexion/extension loading. The fundamental trend in each loading condition demonstrated the diskectomy condition as producing, as expected, an increase in segmental motion. Reconstruction using the PEEK artificial disc restored motion to near intact levels. The final reconstruction using the anterior plate-cage construct reduced motion at the operative level. These reductions in segmental motion, however, were not as low as expected. These findings are attributable to the instability created by the diskectomy condition and follow patterns similar to previous biomechanical studies using anterior plate and interbody cages.

2.1.7 Pilot functional animal study

Using an *in-vivo* goat model, evaluation of implant osseointegration and biocompatibility properties of HA coated and uncoated devices was performed. These properties were radiographically and histologically evaluated at three months post-operatively. Mature female crossbred goats served as the experimental model in this pilot study as these animals are gentle, easy to care for and represent excellent models for cervical spine procedures. There were n = 4 animals for the HA coated and uncoated groups. Following the three month sacrifice, the operative cervical motion segments were sagittally sectioned along the geometric centerline of the implanted device using a Beuhler Isomet saw. Histologic preparation of all samples included dehydration in 100% ethanol, staining using the Villanueva Osteochrome Bone Stain, undecalcified solution processing and embedding in polymethyl-methacrylate (PMMA). Using the EXAKT Microgrinding Device, the embedded specimens were cut at 250 to 300 um thick, ground and polished to 75 um. Microradiographs were obtained of the slide-mounted specimens using Faxitron radiography. The slides were placed twelve inches from the beam and exposed for two minutes, using a technique of 45 kVp and 3mA while in direct contact with the single emulsion high-resolution graphics arts film. For all animals, the soft tissue organs and structures were resected, sectioned and prepared by a veterinarian pathologist. The specimens were fixed in a 10% formalin solution, underwent routine paraffin processing and slide preparation. Using thin-sectioning microtomy, the paraffin embedded sections were cut (3-5μm in thickness), slide mounted and stained using standard Hematoxylin and Eosin (H&E). The spinal cord and local tissue overlying the anterior aspect of the C_3-C_4 operative disc level were evaluated using routine H&E and Macrophage Staining Method (HAM-56). The use of this staining method highlights the presence of activated macrophages within the local tissues. Using plain and polarized light microscopy, histopathological readings of the slide-mounted tissue sections, activated macrophages, presence of wear debris as well as any signs of foreign body giant cells, granulomas inflammatory reactions, degenerative changes or autolysis could be discerned.

All operative cervical motion segments were examined for gross evidence of infection and local pathologic response at the time of necropsy. There was no apparent infection in any of the operative C_3-C_4 levels or adjacent motion segments. Based on gross examination at the time of necropsy, the local tissues from all animals were considered unremarkable and without evidence of ectopic bone formation or other significant histopathologic changes.

Histopathological interpretation of the slide-mounted undecalcified specimens indicated no evidence of significant pathological changes in tissues within or surrounding the specimens. For the HA coated group, there was good intercalation of cancellous bone with the Ti fixation cams and bone apposition to both endplates of the devce (Figure 5). For the

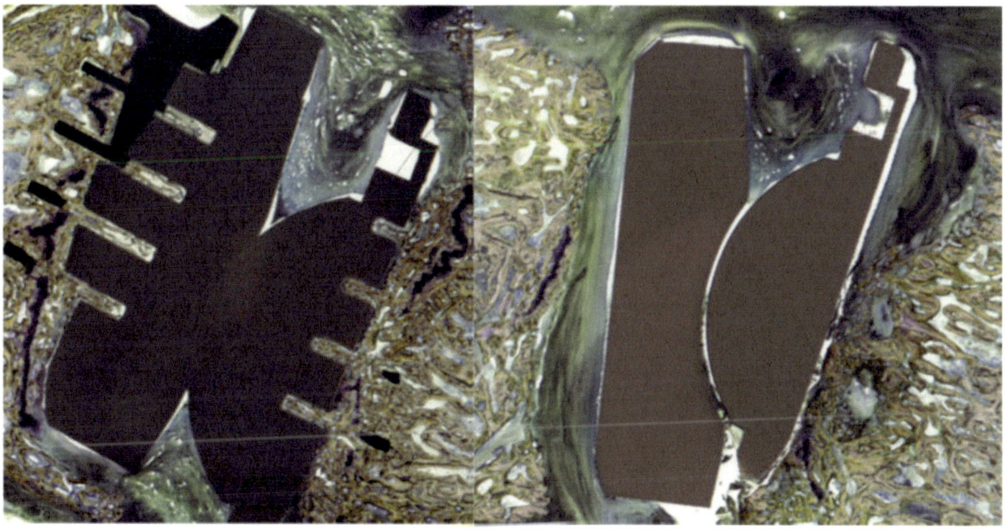

Fig. 5. Left - Good bone apposition to the HA coated devices was seen. Fibrous membranes are around the edges of both components where there is no coating applied, but there is no significant fibrosis at the bone/implant interface. Right – mostly fibrous tissue surrounded the uncoated devices. For all devices, no significant particles of debris were evident.

uncoated group, only focal bone ingrowth to the Ti cam's was noted, with no bone apposition to the PEEK, consistent with the relatively inertness of the material not allowing for bone apposition. For all groups, plain and polarized light microscopy of local tissues overlying the operative sites from experimental levels of both groups indicated a mild inflammatory reaction. The histiocytic infiltration responses were considered secondary to the surgical procedure and healing response. The spinal cord sections exhibited no significant pathological changes based on plain and polarized review. There was no evidence of giant cell reaction or other significant pathological changes, no debris associated with the device, aggresive inflammatory reactions, degenerative changes or autolysis noted.

2.2 PEEK nucleus replacement device

The PEEK nucleus replacement device is a two-piece implant comprised of a top and a bottom plate, with an inner ball and socket articulation (Figure 6). Since PEEK is radiolucent, tantalum (Ta) markers are used to facilitate the visualization of the device location when using radiographic methods. The articulation allows for rotational motions along all three major axes. The motion of the device in axial rotation is unconstrained, while the motions in flexion/extension and lateral bending are semi-constrained slightly beyond the physiological ROM. Similar to all nucleus replacement devices and unlike a total disc replacement, the device ranges of motion are largely dependent upon the constraints from the adjacent tissues, and is designed to restore or maintain the load sharing capabilities of the index disc.

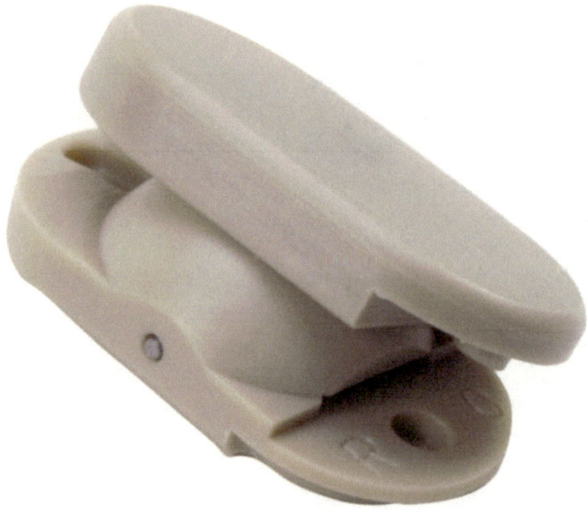

Fig. 6. PEEK nucleus replacement device.

2.2.1 Axial static and fatigue strength

To determine the static and fatigue strength of the device, the smallest footprint (11x20 mm) and height (8 mm) was utilized. These were considered the worst-case scenario for contact stress distribution. The specimens tested were representative of the smallest true contact stress area for all current designs. Testing was performed on an MTS 858 Mini-Bionix II test frame with steel fixturing. A sample size of 3 was used for the static tests with a displacement rate of 2 mm/min. The acceptance criteria was an offset yield load of greater than 2200 N (Lowe, 2004) for the axial static testing. For the fatigue tests, a sample size of 6 was used with a runout load criteria of 3000 N to 5 million cycles (FDA guidance), with R=10 at 10 Hz.

The results of the axial static testing showed that the mean offset yield was 10868 ± 413 N. The primary failure mode was excessive plastic deformation of the top component of the device. For the axial fatigue test, two specimens were tested at a peak compressive load of 9238 N with both failing within 200 cycles due to excessive plastic deformation of the top component, similar to the axial static testing. Two other specimens ran out to 10 million cycles at a peak compressive load of 8151 N. However, upon visual inspection, fatigue cracks emanating from the radiographic marker hole were discovered. Therefore, the load was dropped down to 7065 N for an addition two samples, with a successful outcome. This represented 85%, 75% and 65% of the mean offset yield compressive load, respectively. These results are thought to be well beyond those of the expected *in vivo* physiological loads, and therefore failure was not expected to occur in either static axial compression or dynmaic axial compression.

2.2.2 Shear fatigue strength

To determine the static and fatigue strength of the device, the smallest footprint (11x20 mm) and height (8 mm) was utilized. The specimens tested were also representative of the smallest true contact stress area for all current designs. Testing was performed on an MTS 858 Mini-Bionix II test frame with steel fixturing. A shear angle of 15° was selected based

upon a review of the relevant literature. Extreme flexion of the lumbar spine appears to be approximately 10° on average, with slightly more at the levels L_2L_3 to L_4L_5 and slightly less at L_1L_2 and L_5S_1 when measured *in vivo* (Pearcy, 1984). Therefore, a 15° angle was considered to be at the physiological extreme. Two specimens were used to characterize the shear fatigue strength of the device.
Given the compressive loads obtained during the axial testing, only shear fatigue testing was performed. The two test specimens were successfully tested to 10 million cycles at 6600 N. There is limited data on flexion fatigue testing of human cadaveric lumbar motion segments. The available data states that fatigue failure can occur on average at 263 ±646 cycles with 9 kg of cyclic loading (representing a peak load of 3150 N) at 6° of flexion (Gallagher, 2005). It was therefore thought that the device has adequate compressive-shear fatigue strength for its intended application.

2.2.3 Wear testing and wear particulate characterization

All implants used for wear testing were applicable to a clinical setting and were of the smallest height (8 mm) and footprint (11x20 mm) available. Three separate groups of six implants each were utilized in this wear study. Table 2 summarizes the test methodology. The peak compressive load of 1024 N was chosen based upon the physiological load sharing expected of nucleus replacement devices. The peak compressive load of 2000 N represents a worst case scenario in the event that the device must support the entire compressive load on the anterior column. Group 2 was exposed to 200 kGy of gamma radiation followed by simulated aging. The simulated aging process was similar to ASTM F2003-02, which was developed to measure accelerated aging of UHMWPE in air at 70° C and 5 atm of oxygen, except that the aging time was extended from 14 days to 40 days. All implants were pre-soaked in test fluid for at least 6 weeks. All groups were tested on a six-station spine wear simulator (EndoLab GmbH). The testing fluid consisted of newborn calf serum diluted with phosphate buffered saline (PBS) to a final protein content of 20 g/L. Ethylene-diamine tetraacetic acid (EDTA) was added to the serum at a concentration of 20 mM to bind the calcium ions present in the serum. EDTA is a known preservative, and together with the low protein content and PBS, the addition of sodium azide or other anti-bacterial agent was not used. The test fluid temperature was kept at 37 ± 3° C. Although not part of the test methodology, group 2 was temporarily stopped at 5 million cycles due to simulator availability whereupon the implants were immersed in saline at 37 ± 3° C for 33 weeks. Although unintended, this represented an additional test parameter. The test was subsequently resumed until 10 million cycles was reached. Unloaded soak controls were used for all groups to account for moisture uptake. Group 3 was tested at approximately double the compressive load. The tests were stopped at half million-cycle intervals to clean, dry and gravimetrically assess the wear rates. The average wear rates were determined using linear regression analysis with one-way-analysis-of-variance (ANOVA) used to determine if significant differences ($p < 0.05$) in the wear rates was present. The proteinacious test serum containing PEEK wear debris underwent enzymatic digestion (5x Trypsin digestion and 1.5 mg/mL of Proteinase K per sample at 37° C for 24 hours) followed by a mild acid treatment (10% HCl at 37° C for 24 hours), meeting or exceeding similar protocols previously established to be equivalent for acid and base digestion (Niedzwiecki, 2001). The particles were then analyzed by SEM analysis and characterized according to their equivalent circle diameter (ECD), aspect ration (AR), roundness (R) and form factor (FF) in accordance with ASTM F 1877-05.

All implants for each group maintained full functionality throughout each test duration with visual and light microscopy revealing no evidence of gross deformation, delamination or fatigue cracks. Since group 1 desplayed a wear-in period from 0-1.0 million cycle, the wear rates were calculated from 1 million cycles on for all groups. For group 1, the wear rate was calculated to be 0.41 ± 0.01 mm^3/million cycles. For group 2, the wear rate was calculated to be 0.52 ± 0.02mm^3/million cycles. For group 3, the wear rate was calculated to be 0.92 ± 0.01 mm^3/million cycles, which was significantly higher than groups 1 and 2. This increase in the wear rate was to be expected, given that the peak compressive load was increased from 1024 N to 2000 N. Overall, the wear rates are less than contempary lumbar total disc arthroplasty devices, which can range from 2.8 to 20.4 mm3/million cycles (Bushelow, 2007; Nechtow, 2006; Grupp, 2009) (Figure 7). The particle analysis conducted via SEM revealed that group 1 had the smallest particulate of 1.09 μm, followed by groups 2 and 3 at 1.71 μm and 1.86 μm respectively. Other than the aspect ratio for group 1, the morphology of the wear particulate appears to be similar for all the groups tested (Figure 8). Using standard nomenclature for describing particle morphology in accordance with ASTM F1877-05, the larger particulate tended to be mostly somewhat roughened or smooth flakes, with some shards and globular particles, along with a few fibrils. Any submicron particulate was smooth, with spheroidal granules.

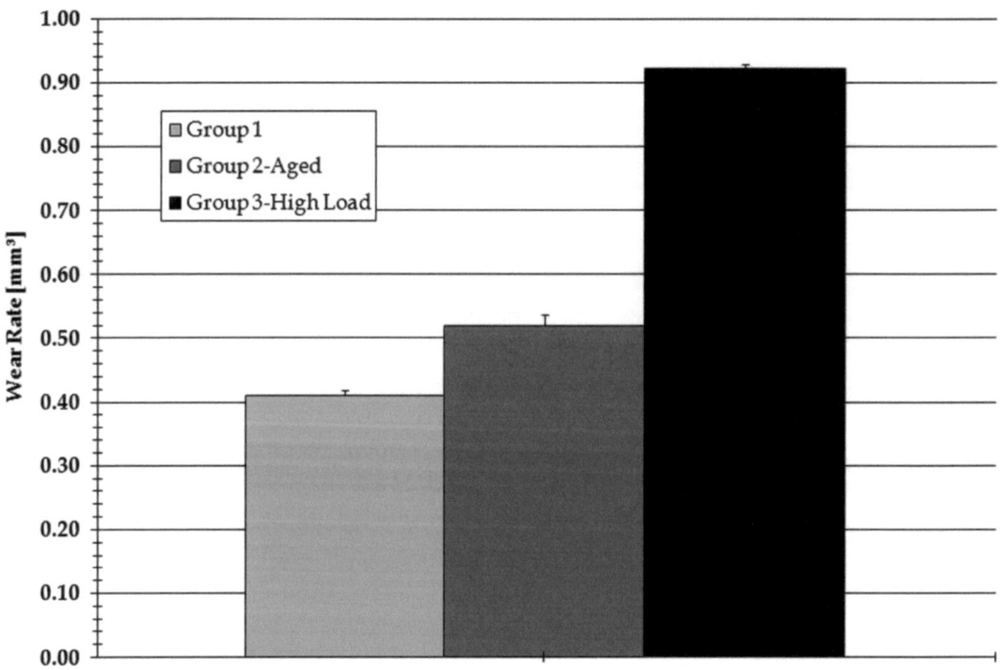

Fig. 7. Average wear rates for the PEEK nucleus replacement device.

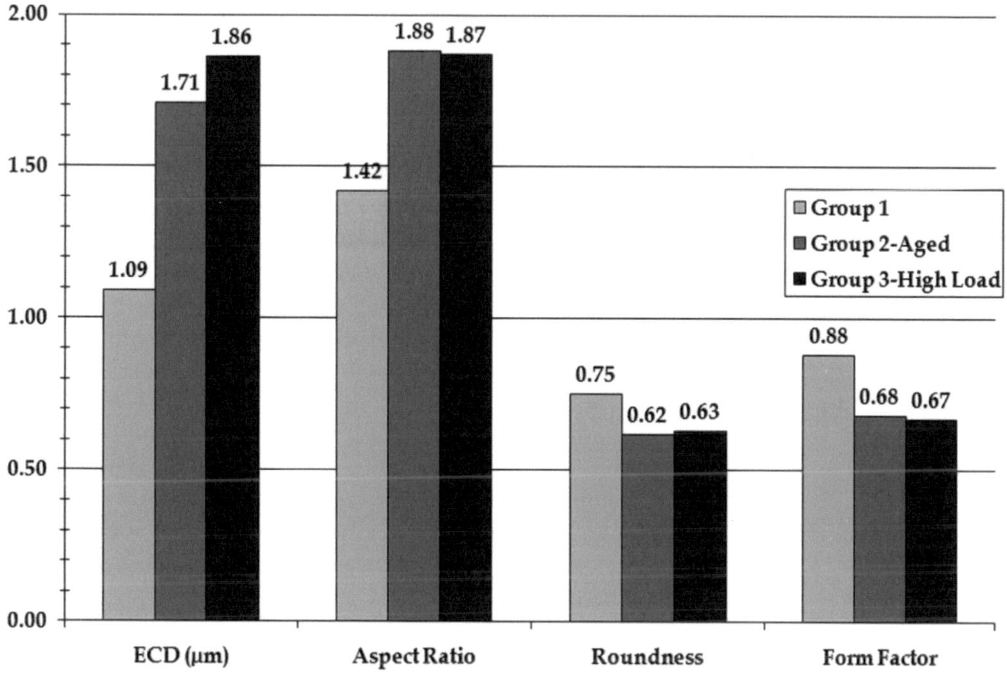

Fig. 8. SEM analysis of the PEEK particulate generated from the wear tests.

2.2.4 Biomechanical analyses

The first study sought to assess the restoration of disc height, the potential adverse effects of the device on the underlying vertebral endplate under physiological loading conditions and an initial assessment of the extrusion risk. A total of eight fresh-frozen human lumbar functional spinal units (L_2L_3 and L_4L_5) were harvested en-bloc and utilized in this investigation. Prior to biomechanical analysis, standard anterior/posterior and standard lateral plain films were obtained to exclude specimens demonstrating intervertebral disc or osseous pathology. Bone mineral density (BMD) scans (DEXA) were performed to exclude specimens demonstrating BMD's less than 0.9 g/cm^3. Each test specimen consisted of two contiguous functional spinal units (three vertebra and two intervertebral discs). One intervertebral disc served as a control and the other intervertebral disc was implanted with the device. To determine restoration of disc height, a 1200 N compressive load was applied. An annular incision followed by a box cut (6 mm x 10 mm) was created on the anatomic right, followed by a complete nucleotomy. A fatigue test was conducted under a left lateral bending moment ranging from 2.5 to 7.5 Nm (250 to 750 N compressive load offset 10 mm). The test was run at 2 Hz for 100,000 cycles. The left lateral bending mode represented a "worst case" scenario with regards to implant extrusion. Upon completion of the biomechanical analyses, each specimen was radiographed and examined for possible fractures and/or migration. Segments were then dissected transversely through the intervertebral discs. Both the intact and implanted discs were examined macroscopically for potential changes. Photographs of the disc were taken using a macro lens to document the condition of the endplates and the annulus. The L1 and L4 vertebrae were scanned on a mCT 80 (ScancoMedical AG, Bassersdorf, Switzerland) to examine the trabecular bone for potential fractures. The specimens were scanned with an x-ray energy of 70Kvp and current of 114 mA and at an isotropic voxel resolution of 74 microns (image matrix of 1024 x 1024). A total of 500 projections over 180 degrees were collected for each vertebra. An integration time of 700 ms/projection was used, which resulted in a scan-time of about 2.5 - 3 hours/specimen. A repeated measures ANOVA was used to examine differences in ROM between intact, discectomy, and implant conditions. Implant extrusion was assessed by direct observation made from the pre and post fatigue radiographs. Gross macroscopic fractures were determined from the dissection and radiographs for both the control and surgical levels. The microCT images were analyzed by a board certified radiologist (Medical Metrics, Inc. Houston, Texas, USA). The disc height of 2.2 ± 0.6 mm after discectomy significantly decreased ($p<0.05$) to 3.7 ± 1.1 mm for all specimens in comparison to the intact condition under 1.2 kN of compressive loading. Implantation of the nucleus device significantly increased ($p<0.05$) the disc height to 2.6 ± 0.7 mm compared to the discectomy condition. There was no significant difference between the intact and implanted conditions. There were no gross endplate fractures observed at the completion of 100,000 cycles of lateral bending. The evaluation of the microCT images noted no fractures in the endplates or vertebral bodies. There were slight migrations of the device towards the annulotomy, but no extrusions noted.

The second study performed was to quantify the ROM and destructive load to failure properties of the device. A total of eight fresh-frozen human lumbar functional spinal units (L_2L_3 and L_4L_5) were harvested en-bloc and utilized in this investigation. Prior to biomechanical analysis, standard anterior/posterior and lateral plain films were obtained to exclude specimens demonstrating intervertebral disc or osseous pathology. BMD scans using DEXA were performed to exclude specimens demonstrating BMD's less than 0.9 g/cm^3. To determine the multidirectional flexibility, six applied pure moments of ± 7 Nm (flexion and extension, left and right lateral bending, and left and right torsion) were applied to the superior end of the vertically oriented specimen while the caudal portion of the specimen remained fixed to a testing platform. Following the intact analysis, an annular incision followed by a box cut (10 mm x 10 mm) was created on the anatomic left, followed by a complete nucleotomy. After biomechanical testing of the destabilized condition, the nucleus device was implanted and the operative motion segment retested. As a final test, the reconstructed specimen was destructively evaluated under axial compression. Biomechanical data was normalized to the intact condition and expressed as mean ± one standard deviation, with a Repeated Measures Analysis of Variance (ANOVA) and Student-Newman-Keuls test to determine differences among individual groups ($p<0.05$).

Multidirectional flexibility testing indicated significant increases in the segmental range of motion and neutral zone secondary to the annulotomy/nucleotomy procedures after reconstruction of the operative segment. For both calculated parameters, the segmental rotation increased for the destabilized condition versus the intact and reconstructed specimens ($p<0.05$). Importantly, the neutral zone, an indicator of spinal stability of the reconstructed segment, returned to levels not statistically different from the intact condition. As a final test, the reconstructed specimens were destructively evaluated under axial compression. In all specimens except one, the observed failure mechanism was fracture of the vertebral body, without significant disruption of the vertebral endplate. The primary mode of fracture was through the vertebral bodies above and below the operative disc level. The mean failure load was 3340 ± 2029 N. This average fracture load is comparable to the compressive failure load for intact lumbar segment (Lowe, 2004).

2.2.5 Functional animal study

Evaluation of the mechanical behavior and elicited histopathological response following long-term implantation in a functional animal (baboon) model of the device was performed. Fourteen mature male baboons (Papio cynocephalus) were randomized into two post-operative time periods of six-months (n=7) and twelve-months (n=7). Each animal underwent a lateral transperitoneal surgical approach followed by complete nucleotomy at L_3-L_4 and L_5-L_6 levels. The inferior L_5-L_6 level was reconstructed using the nucleus replacement device while the adjacent level served as a control.

Analyses were based on gross necropsy, MRI radiography, plain X-ray, microradiography, and biocompatibility assays (local and systemic histology) performed at the six and twelve month post-operative time-points. resected, sectioned and prepared by a veterinarian pathologist. The specimens were fixed in a 10% formalin solution, underwent routine paraffin processing and slide mounting. Using thin-sectioning microtomy, the paraffin embedded sections were cut (3-5μm in thickness), slide mounted and stained using standard Hematoxylin and Eosin (H&E). The spinal cord sections, obtained from each operative disc level, were evaluated using routine H&E. The local tissues overlying the operative levels underwent the following immunocytochemistry analyses using standard immunocytochemistry techniques, including primary and secondary antibodies combined with the avidin-biotin complex (ABC) horseradish peroxidase. Immunohistochemical localization of intracellular and membrane bound macrophage expressing cytokines included IL-1, IL-2, IL-6 and Tumor Necrosis Factor-Alpha and beta (TNF-α,β). The Macrophage Staining Method (HAM-56) was used to highlight the presence of activated macrophages within the local tissues. Using plain and polarized light microscopy, histopathological readings of the slide-mounted tissues, activated macrophages, presence of wear debris as well as any signs of foreign body giant cells, granulomas inflammatory reactions, degenerative changes or autolysis could be discerned. Pathological assessment for all systemic and local tissues included, but was not limited to, the architecture of the tissues, presence of wear debris as well as any signs of foreign body giant cell / granulomas inflammatory reactions, degenerative changes or autolysis.

Multidirectional flexibility testing indicated no difference in axial rotation ($p>0.05$) for the six-month groups, comparing the intact spine to surgical motion segments. Flexion/extension and lateral bending exhibited reduced segmental motion for the nucleus replacement device and operative control levels at six months versus the non-operative intact spine ($p<0.05$). However, these findings were also noted in the operative control levels demonstrating the effect of surgical intervention itself on segmental stability. At twelve months, segmental motion was restored to the intact levels for the reconstructed levels ($p>0.05$). Histopathologic analysis of the nucleus replacement treatment exhibited increased densification of trabeculae along the endplate periphery, which corroborated with Modic Type I changes observed with MRI and radiographically. Evidence of implant subsidence was noted in 5/7 cases at six months and 7/7 cases at twelve months, which correlated with the absence of articular cartilage in some regions. A limitation of this study was the use of a single height nucleus replacement device for all treated discs. This resulted in difficulties in insertion and placement of the device and significant over distraction of the disc space. The difficulties in insertion and over distraction may have resulted in the use of more force for proper placement. This potentially induced endplate damage at the treated disc levels and led to abnormal high contact stress on the endplates, which may have been the precursor to the Modic changes and subsidence. Plain and polarized light microscopy of local tissues overlying the operative sites from both the experimental and control levels indicated a chronic inflammatory reaction, with evidence of fibrous connective replacement and infiltration of mononuclear cells. These observations were considered secondary to the surgical procedure and, importantly, occurred at both the control and experimental operative levels. There was no evidence of cellular apoptosis, giant cell reaction or other significant pathological changes. Analysis of the immunohistochemical antibody stains for the local tissues overlying the experimental and control levels were negative in each case. In the histological analyses, there was no detectable wear debris from the device and no evidence of an osteolytic response. There was no evidence of a pro-inflammatory cytokine reaction at any of the experimental or control levels.

3. Clinical summary

Worldwide clinical usage of both devices is ongoing. Currently, there have been no reported adverse events due to a material failure, such as device breakage, fatigue failure or an aggressive host immune response leading to a revision surgery to remove the device. Clinical results as measured by validated measures such as Oswestry Disability Index (ODI) and Visual Analog Scale (VAS), along with patient satisfaction, suggest that both devices can relieve the symptoms of their respective degenerative processes (Figures 9, 10). From a biomaterial perspective, no adverse events have occurred as a direct result of these devices not performing as expected. Based upon worldwide clinical success, and the success of a US pilot IDE study, the nucleus replacement device was granted approval by FDA to start a first of its kind IDE pivotal study in the US.

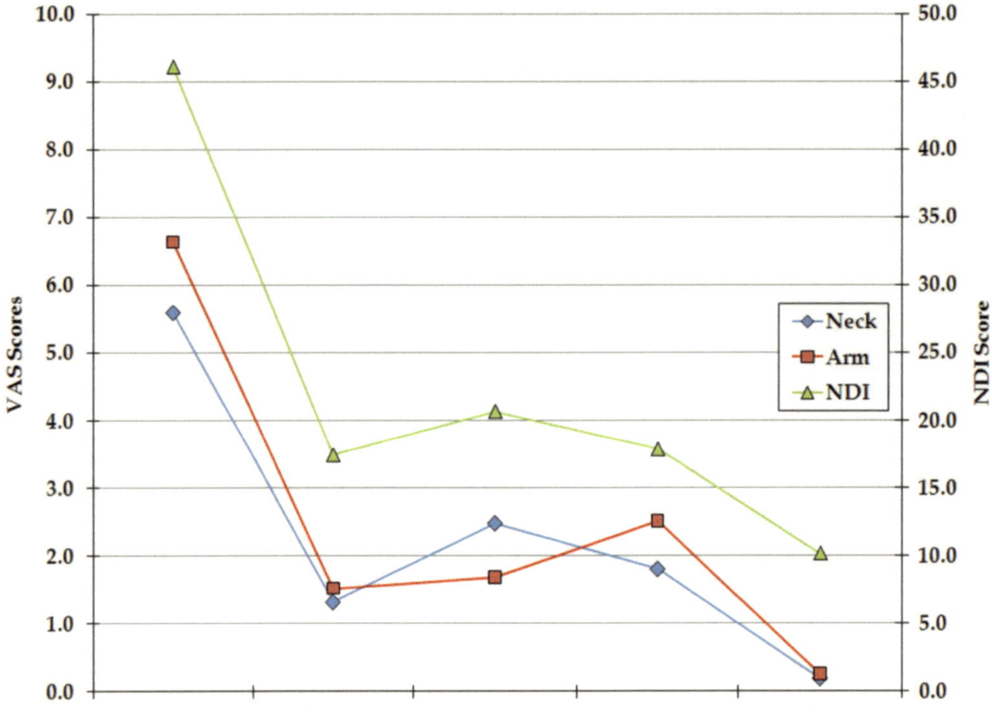

Fig. 9. ODI and VAS scores from the worldwide usage of the cervical arthroplasty device.

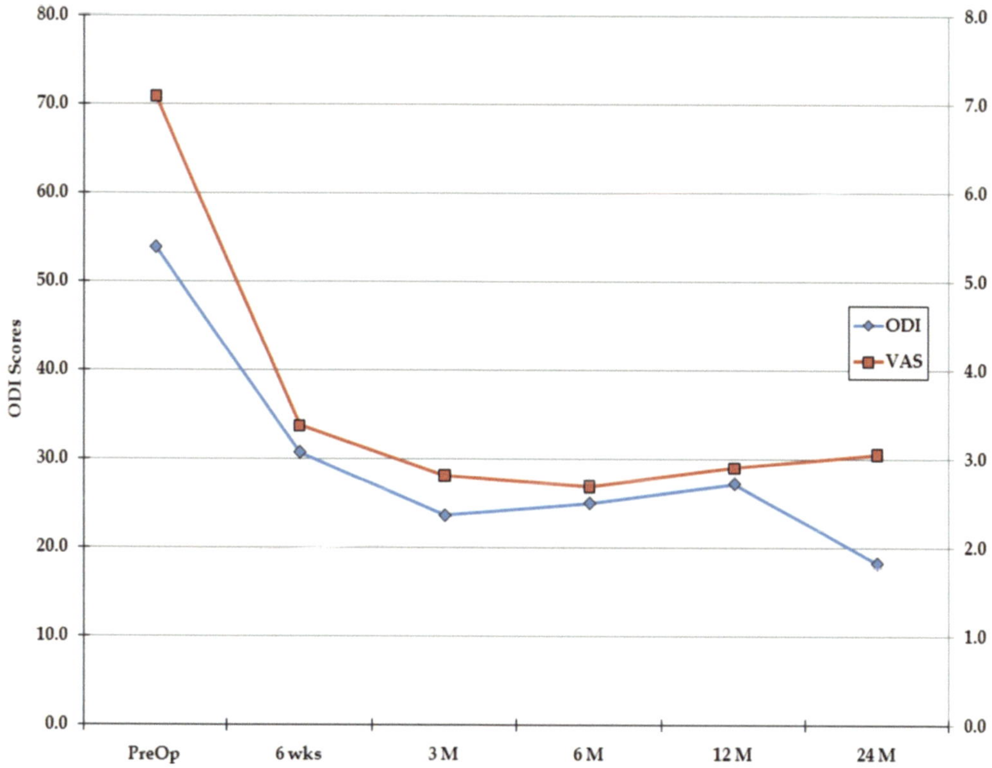

Fig. 10. ODI and VAS scores from the US IDE pilot study for the nucleus replacement device.

4. Conclusion

The concept of reconstruction of the lumbar and cervical disc is not new, as clinical experimentation goes back to the early 1950's. Since then, the scientific and clinical community has sought to improve upon the selection of available biomaterials for use in the disc arthroplasty arenas. The mainstay of these materials has been ceramics, metal alloys and polymers, in large part due to the history gained form their use in total joint reconstruction. Currently there is no universal material that is considered the ultimate biomaterial, and an in-depth knowledge of a given material is important in understanding and predicting its response when used in an application as demanding as an implantable biomaterial. Knowledge can be gained by not only performing the appropriate testing on the bulk properties of the material, but also proper preclinical testing of the constructed device. More importantly, adroit interpretation of these results is fundamental to the clinical success of the device (Fraser, 2004; Kurtz, 2009). The use of PEEK in spinal arthroplasty represents a new application of this material. Although the history of PEEK suggests that it has the necessary material properties to serve as a long-term implantable arthroplasty material, it's use in the form of any arthroplasty device has not been diligently explored. Therefore, a battery of preclinical testing was performed, and the interpretation of the results for both a cervical disc arthroplasty device and lumbar nucleus replacement device have allowed for successful advancement to the clinical usage. The results of these combined preclinical studies described can be used in an ongoing basis to further analyze the use of PEEK in arthroplasty applications. Long term clinical follow up is needed to further support the preclinical results.

5. Acknowledgment

The authors would like to acknowledge Nathaniel Ordway at SUNY Upstate New York for help with conducting the biomechanical studies, along with Bryan Cunningham of Union Memorial Hospital for help with conducting the biomechanical and animal studies. The authors would also like to acknowledge Dr. Nadim Hallab of Bioengineering Solutions for performing the particulate analyses, along with Markus W. Wimmer and Thorsten Schwenke at RUSH Medical Center for help in conducting the wear studies.

6. References

Balsano, M.; Zachos, A. & Ruggiu A. (2011). Nucelus desc arthroplasty with the NUBAC device: 2-year clinical experience. *Eur Spine J*, Vol. 20, Suppl 1 (May, 2011) pp. S36-40 ISSN 0940-6719

Bergen, H. (2011). The Norwegain Arthroplasty Register, In: Centre of Excellence of Joint Replacements, 07.07.2011, Available from http://nrlweb.ihelse.net/eng/Report_2010.pdf

Bushelow, M.; Walker, J. & Coppes J. Comparison of Wear Rates: Metal/UHWMPE and Metal-on-Metal Total Disc Arthroplasty. Trans 22nd (2007) NASS p32

Cavanaugh, D.; Nunely P. & Kerr J. (2009). Delayed Hyper-reactivity to Metal Ions After Cervical Disc Arthroplasty: A case report and literature review. *Spine*, Vol. 34, No. 7 (April, 2009) E262-265 ISSN 0362-2436

Cunningham, B.; Hu, N. & Zorn, C. Comparative fixation methods of cervial disc arthroplasty versus conventional methods of anterior cervical arthrodesis: serration, teeth, keels, or screws? *J Neurosurg Spine*, Vol. 12, No. 2 (February, 2010) pp. 214-220 ISSN 1547-5654

Devin, C.; Myers, T. & Kang J. (1889). Chronic failure of a lumbar total disc replacement with osteolysis. Report of a case with nineteen year follow up. *J Bone Joint Surg Am* Vol.90, No. 10 (October, 2008) pp. 2230-2234 ISSN 0021-9355

Francois, J.; Coessens, R. & Lauweryns P. (2007). Early removal of a Maverick disc prosthesis: surgical findings and morphological changes. *Acta Orthop Belg*, Vol. 73, No. 1(2007) pp. 122-27 ISSN 0001-6462

Fraser, R.; Ross, E. & Lowery G. (2004) AcroFlex design and results. *Spine J* Vol. 4, No. 6 Suppl (Nov-Dec, 2004) pp. 245S-51S 1529-9430

Gallagher, S.; Marras, W. & Davis, K. (2005) Torso Flexion Load and the Fatigue Failure of Human Lumbosacral Motion Segments. *Spine*, Vol. 30, No. 20 (October, 2005) pp. 2265-73, 2005 ISSN 0362-2436

Garellick, G; Darrholm J & Rogmark C. (2010). The Swedish Hip Arthroplasty Register, In: Swedish Hip Arthroplasty Register, Annual Report 2008, 07.07.2011, Available from https://www.jru.orthop.gu.se/

Grupp, T.; Yue, J. & Garcia R. (2008) Biotribological evaluation of artificial disc arthroplasty devices: influence of loading and kinematics patterns during in vitro wear simulation. *Eur Spine* J Vol. 18, No.1 (January, 2009) pp. 98-108 ISSN 0940-6719

Guyer, R.; Shellock, J & MacLennan, B. (2011). Early failure of metal-on-metal artificial disc prostheses associated with lymphocytic reaction: diagnosis and treatment experience in four cases. *Spine*, Vol. 36, No. 7, (April, 2001) E492-497 ISSN 0362-2436

Kurtz, S. & Devine J. (2007). PEEK biomaterials in trauma, orthropedic and spinal implants. *Biomaterials*, Vol. 28, No. 32, (November, 2007) pp. 4845-4869 ISSN 0142-9612

Kurtz, S. MacDonald, D. & Ianuzzi, A. (1976). The natural history of polyethylene oxidation in total disc replacment. *Spine*, Vol. 15, No. 34, (October, 2009) pp. 2369-2377 ISSN 0362-2436

Licina, P. & Thorpe P. (1948). Osteolysis and complications associated with artificial disc replacement. *J Bone Joint Surg*, Vol. 86-B, Suppl IV (2004) pp. 460-461 ISSN 0301-620X

Lowe, T.; Hashim, S. & Wilson, L. (1976). A biomechanical study of regional endplate strength and cage morphology as it relates to structural interbody support. *Spine*, Vol. 1, No. 29, (Novermber, 2004) pp. 2389-2394 ISSN 0362-2436

Moroney, S. Schultz, A. & Miller J. (1988). Analysis and measurement of neck loads. *J Ortho Res*, Vol. 6, No. 5, (September, 1988) pp. 713-720 ISSN 1554-527X

Murrey D.; Janssen M & Delamarter R. (2009). Results of the Prospective, Randomized, Controlled Multicenter Food and Drug Administration Investigational Device Exemption Study of the ProDisc-C Total Disc Replacement Versus Anterior Discectiomy and Fusion for the Treatment of 1-level Symptomatic Cervical Disc Disease. *The Spine Journal*, Vol.9, No. 4, (April, 2009) pp. 275-286 ISSN 1529-9430

Nechtow, W.; Hinter, M. & Bushelow M. IVD Replacement Mechanical Performance Depends Stronlgy on Input Parameters. Trans 52nd ORS (2006) p0118.

Niedzwiecki, S.; Klapperich, C, & Short J. (2001). Comparison of three joint simulator wear debris isolation techniques: acid digestion, base digestion, and enzyme cleavage. *J Biomed Mater Res* Vol. 56, No. 2, (August, 2001) pp. 245-249 ISSN 1549 3296

Pearcy, M.; Portek, I. & Shepherd J. (1976). Three-Dimensional X-ray Analysis of Normal Movement in the Lumbar Spine. *Spine*, Vol. 9, No. 3 (April, 1984) pp.294-297 ISSN 0362-2436

Panjabi, M.; Crisco, J. & Vasavada A. (2001) Mechanical Properties of the Human Cervical Spine as Shown by Three Dimensional Load Displacement Curves. *Spine*, Vol. 26, No. 24 (December, 2001) pp. 2692-2700 ISSN 0362-2436

Przybyla A.; Skrzypeic, D. & Pollintine, P. Strength of the cervical spine in compression and bending. *Spine*, Vol. 32, No. 15, (July, 2007), pp. 1612-1620 ISSN 0362-2436

Rae, P.; Brown, E. & Orler, E. (1960). The mechanical properties of poly(ether-ether-ketone) (PEEK) with emphasis on the large compressive strain response. *Polymer* Vol. 48, No. 2 (January, 2007) pp.598-615 ISSN 0032-3861

Reitman, C.; Mauro, K. & Nguyen. L. (2004). Intervertebral Motion Between Flexion and Extension in Asymptomatic Individuals. *Spine*, Vol. 29, No. 24 (December, 2004) pp. 2832-2843 ISSN 0362-2436

Senegas, J. (2002). Mechanical supplementation by non-rigid fixation in degenerative intervertebral lumbar segments: the Wallis system. *Eur Spine J* Vol. 11, Suppl 2 (October, 2002) pp. S164-169 ISSN 0940-6719

Snijders, C.; Hoek van Dijke, G. & Roosch E. (1991). A biomechanical model for the analysis of the cervical spine in static postures. *J Biomech*, Vol. 24, No. 9, (1991) pp. 783-792 ISSN 0021-9290

Zigler, J.; Delamarter R. & Linovitz R. (2007). Results of the Prosperctive, Randomized, Mulitcenter Food and Drug Administration Investigational Device Exemption Study of the ProDisc-L Total Disc Replacement Versus Circumferential Fusion for the Treatment of 1-Level Degernative Disc Disease. *Spine*, Vol. 32, No. 11, (May, 2007), pp. 1155-1162 ISSN 0362-2436

12

The Biology of Bone Grafts

Carlos Roberto Galia and Luis Fernando Moreira
Rio Grande do Sul Federal University, Porto Alegre, RS, Brazil School of Medicine, Post-Graduate Programme of Surgery and Hospital de Clinicas University Hospital Department of Surgery 1Division of Orthopaedics and 2Division of Surgical Oncology Brazil

1. Introduction

The use of bone transplants in orthopaedic procedures has become crucial to treat a great number of bone diseases including bone tumour operations, knee or total hip revision arthroplasty and even beyond the orthopaedic scope such as in craniomaxillofacial surgery.
Approximately 10% to 15% of the orthopaedic procedures carried out every year in the U.S.A. employ some kind of musculoskeletal transplant. Annually, about 650 thousand bone-based grafts are distributed by the American Tissue Banks, which clearly shows the importance of processing, controlling and storage of this type of material.
As opposed to other organs such as heart, liver or kidneys and most of the soft tissues, the bone can be processed by many ways, can be stored longer and has been implanted till recently without prior testing compatibility. Moreover, the grafts can be obtained from oneself, living or cadaver donors, or derived from other species or even from non organic biomaterials. However, the offer for grafts is far behind the demand. Despite the success rate of about 85% with the use of bone grafts in orthopaedic surgery, patient waiting list for these grafts keep growing day by day either in the public or private health service.
The homologous deep-frozen grafts have been frequently used, although availability is very limited and a certain risk of transmitting contagious diseases cannot be thoroughly ruled out. On the other hand, though homologous freeze-dried grafts have virtually eliminated the risk of transmissible diseases is still lacking availability and therefore, alternative biomaterials from synthetic or natural source have been considered and carefully studied. Among them, the use of freeze-dried grafts from bovine sources is a suitable alternative with many advantages over autologous or homologous deep-frozen ones due to their great physicochemical and structural resemblance to human bone and their practically endless availability. As a non specific xenograft however, it may possibly present adverse immunological and inflammatory reactions. Nevertheless, our physicochemical processing protocols have been developed in order to significantly minimise these problems, decreasing antigenicity and thus, turning the bovine freeze-dried bone an important biomaterial for large use in reconstructive surgery.
Up to date, it is necessary, an increased knowledge about some kinds of available grafts including biological and mechanical aspects, sources and a careful analysis of outcomes, since transplant of grafts in general is responsible for a remarkable improvement in people's quality of life and their social reinsertion. Moreover, bone implants are far from being a

novel issue and it is crucial that already in the XXI century, we have to know the reasons for its use and, over all matters, to clearly determine our results.
This chapter is intended to present a brief review of the history of bone grafts, indications for use, storage details and differences of processing techniques as well as to present the experience of our department with the use of freeze-dried bone from bovine origin in a thousand orthopaedic procedures.

2. History

The idea of transplanting tissues between individuals of the human species and even between individuals of distinct species is very ancient, dating to the early Christian era. Empirically, Cosmas and Damian, in the second century, were regarded as the pioneers of bone transplantation by having removed a leg of an individual due to an advanced tumour and soon deployed a new leg taken from a freshly killed Moro. However, it was Sir William MacEwan in 1880 who successfully reconstructed the humerus of a boy with the tibia obtained from another child. On the other hand, the first transplant between different species was conducted by the Dutch surgeon Job van Meekren in 1668. According to Godwin, he successfully transplanted part of the skull of a dog in a traumatic defect of the skull of a soldier. Deeply concerned of being excommunicated by the church for having undergone a non-Christian method of treatment, the soldier asked the surgeon to remove the graft, but due to time elapsed, this could not be completely removed since it was already fully integrated.
Is not well known when the first studies on bone grafts started. However, Ollier and Barth in the late 19th century, were the first to intensively investigate and report the biological properties of the tissue and concluded, though partially correct, that bone and periosteum remain viable when transplanted, contributing to new bone formation.
Assuming that the cells survive in the graft, even when removed from the donor, Albee in 1915, concluded in a classical work, the most suitable tissues for transplant are those originated from the connective tissue such as bone, fat and fascia. Ten years later, in 1925, Lexer published his experience with transplants and total joint replacement called "arthroplasty" to all surgical procedures performed in an attempt to restore joint movement.

3. Terminology

It is important to know the terminology frequently used when dealing with this kind of procedure in relation to (a) different types of graft; (b) distinction between grafts and transplants; (c) the process of new bone formation, and; (d) the use of consolidation and osteointegration, since these terms vary greatly in the literature and an attempt to standardized them has not been effective. The nomenclature most commonly used is as follows:

3.1 Types of grafts

Grafts received from oneself and reimplanted in oneself should be called autogenic, autogenous, autologous or autograft. The graft obtained from other individuals, but intended to a host of the same species, should be called allogeneic, allogenous, homologous, allograft or homograft, while grafts from donors to hosts of different species should be called xenogenic, xenogenous, xenologous, xenografts or interspecific.

a. Grafting and transplantation

A Brazilian Board Resolution on Biomaterials - BBRB No. 220 of December 27th, 2006 considers the term transplantation to describe the placement of bone graft during a surgical procedure, so the graft is the product and the use of this tissue is called a transplant.

b. Bone formation and osteointegration

In the process of bone formation and the biological events responsible for osteointegration the following terms are used: osteogenesis when bone growth is derived from osteoblasts transferred along with the graft; osteoinduction when the newly formed bone derives from the recruitment of mesenchymal cell receptors that differentiate into osteoblasts; osteoconduction when the ability of a material (usually inorganic) allows the new bone tissue from pre-existing bone, requiring the presence of osteoprogenitor (preosteoblast) cells or bone tissue.

c. consolidation and osteointegration

On the biological process occurring after transplantation it should be clear that the graft can consolidate and/or embedded (incorporate) into the host bone. Therefore, consolidation and incorporation processes are distinct and should be well understood respectively, as the union that occurs between the graft and host bone or reabsorption and cell recolonisation between graft and host bone resulting in a progressive replacement of one by another. Thus, the imaging methods for assessment of these features can only provide an idea of the evolution of this process, but precise assessment on the consolidation and incorporation can be only determined by histopathology.

4. Biological characteristics

Bone tissue basically consists of an organic matrix of collagen type I, containing low molecular weight proteoglycans and non-collagen proteins, a mineral part (mainly hydroxyapatite) and water, corresponding to 25%, 65% and 10% of the bone weight, respectively.

Despite the great power for repair, the bone does not always respond appropriately when affected by extensive osteolysis. Because of these situations, extremely frequent in orthopaedic surgery, especially in RTHAs, there is eagerness to search for high quality bone grafts and other biomaterials that can fill these gaps and restore availabilty.

Bone grafts can be of cortical, cancellous or cortico-cancellous types, depending on the site of origin and can be used in blocks, segments or morselised. These different types of bone grafts will provide distinct mechanical and biological responses. For instance, the cortical bone is less osteogenic than the spongy bone; showing however, a higher structural quality, for long periods and even in the absence of adequate integration. The greater osteogenic features of cancellous bone (Figures 1a, 1b and 1c) has been recognised for more than 40 years, which has stimulated its use in many situations, being crucial for use in RTHAs.

After the transplant of a spongy bone there is a sequence of histological events that starts with inflammatory response, macrophage invasion, neovascularization and differentiation of mesenchymal cells into osteoblasts that places an osteoid layer in a necrotic trabecular bone remainings. Viable nuclei are reabsorbed by osteoblasts and the matrix is eventually replaced by necrotic trabeculae of newly formed bone. All these events are probably mediated by inducing protein factors.

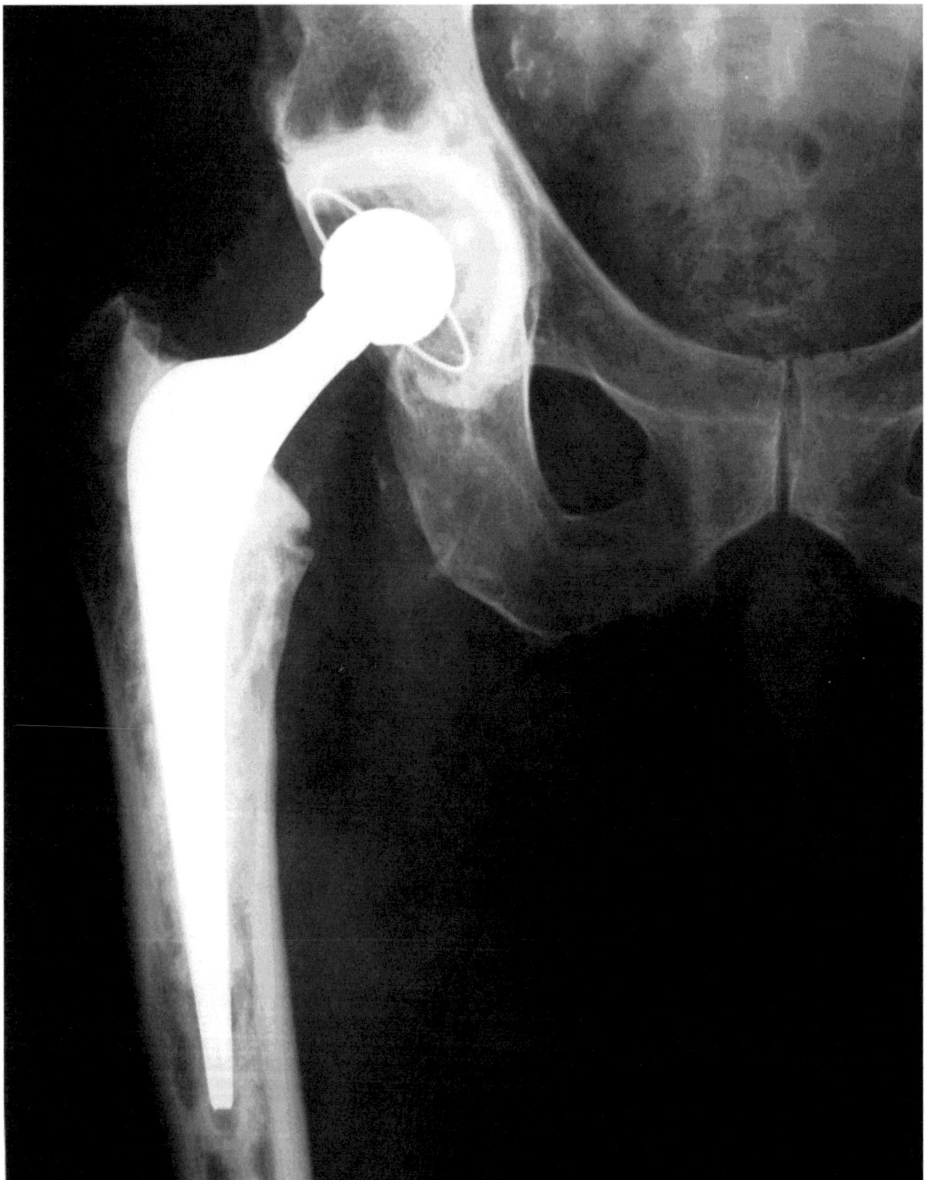

Fig. 1a. Revision as of right femoral component with bone graft and frozen morcelised impacted. 70 months of evolution.

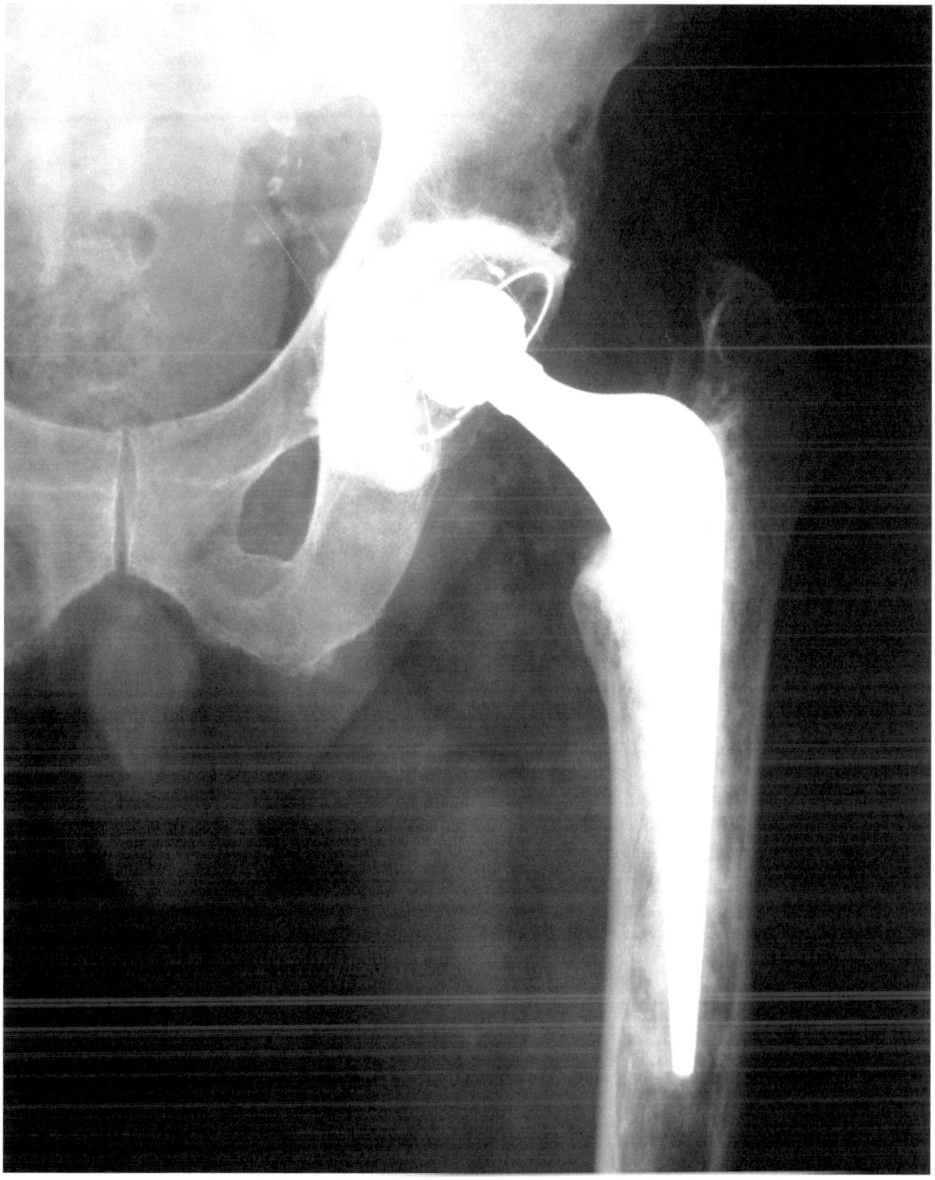

Fig. 1b. Revision of femoral component left with bone graft and bovine freeze-dried, morcelised impacted. 60 months of evolution.

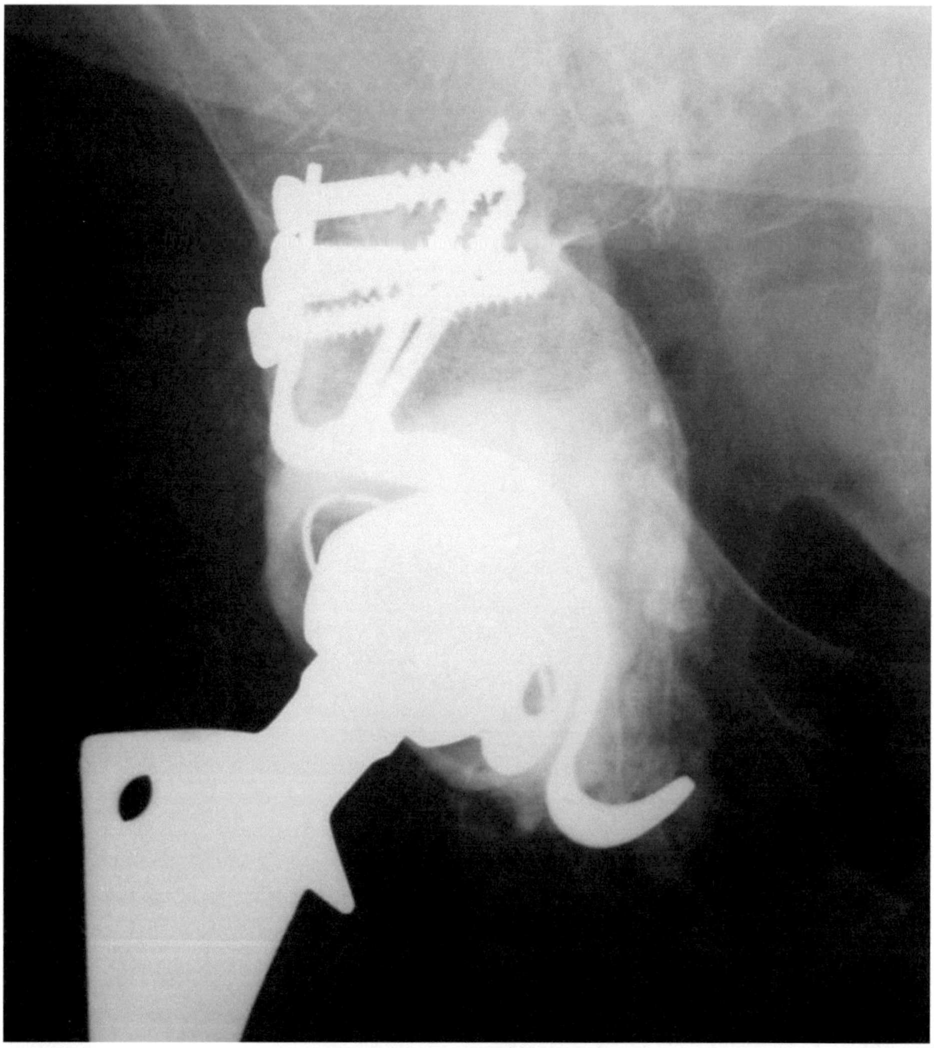

Fig. 1c. Revision of the acetabular component with lyophilized bovine bone graft and graft block frozen morcelised impacted. 82 months of evolution.

Histologic assessment was performed and described by Buma et al. in eight patients who underwent revision of the acetabular component after previous operation with impacted bone grafting technique. All but one, that has not even shown revascularization, samples revealed different stages of integration depending on the time elapsed following implantation. At 4 months, there was an established revascularization, osteoblasts replacing parts of the implant and presence of a small graft and new bone formation. Samples with a longer evolution showed the graft replaced with new bone. Another sample with 28 months in contact with the cement layer revealed viable bone presenting, however, a predominantly fibrous tissue interface5. Similar results on the femoral component were demonstrated in another study published by Ullmark and Obrant in 2002 and by Galia in acetabular biopsies in patients with traumatic dislocation of RTHA (Figures 2a and 2b) 3 years after the first revision procedure.

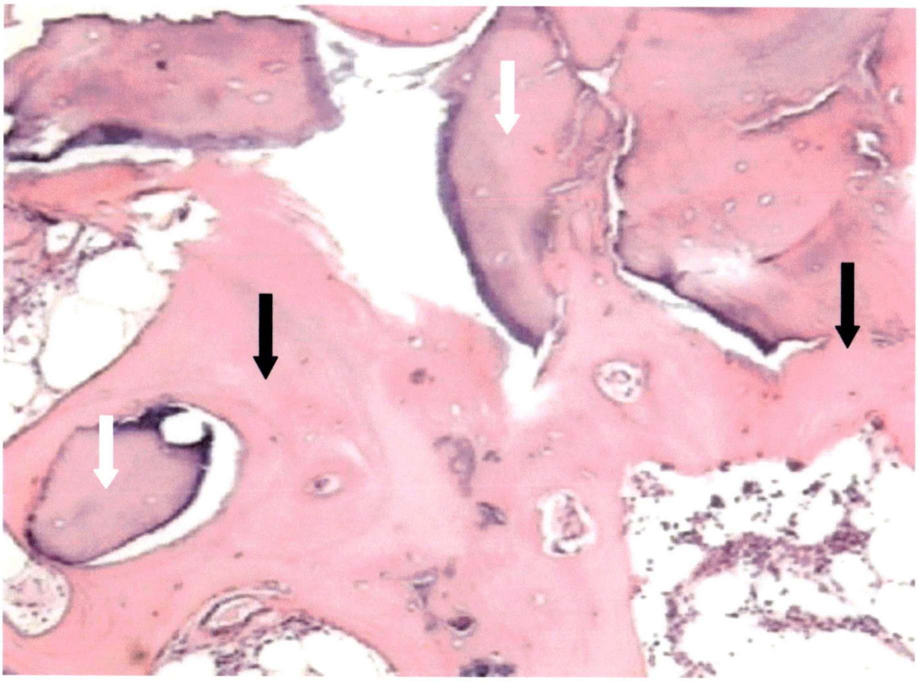

Fig. 2a. Biopsy bone grafting with bovinefreeze-dried three years after surgery. White arrow = graft; black arrow = new bone

In a classic study, Urist described ectopic bone formation after intramuscular implantation of demineralised bovine bone matrix in rabbits and rats. This discovery was crucial in the biomaterial and graft fields and supported the search for substances capable of inducing cell differentiation present in bone matrix. Subsequent investigations, led by Urist demonstrated that low molecular weight proteins could be extracted from demineralised bone matrix, having great osteogenic activity and being called bone morphogenetic proteins (BMPs), and belonging to a superfamily of proteins called transforming growth factors beta (TGF-ß) responsible for inducing growth. The superfamily of TGF-ß proteins regulates many biological processes including cell growth, differentiation and embryo formation. BMPs have been shown to be important regulators in the development and regeneration of skeletal tissue having the BMP2 and BMP7 the highest osteoinductive potential. Another important factor is the reaction triggered by antigenic grafts. The antigens present into the graft cells probably play a very important role on the outcomes of bone transplants. It seems clear that these reactions are not mediated by T or B lymphocytes, but by other cells in the bone marrow. In vitro evidences suggest that the granulocyte lineages in the bone marrow are responsible for triggering immune responses and removal of bone marrow cells therefore and can be directly related to a decrease in graft immune response.

Fresh, frozen and lyophilized bone grafts were experimentally compared in rabbits from the immunological point of view. The first two grafts caused serologically detectable immune response, while the third one, highly purified (free of fat and marrow cells) was not able to immunologically sensitize animals.

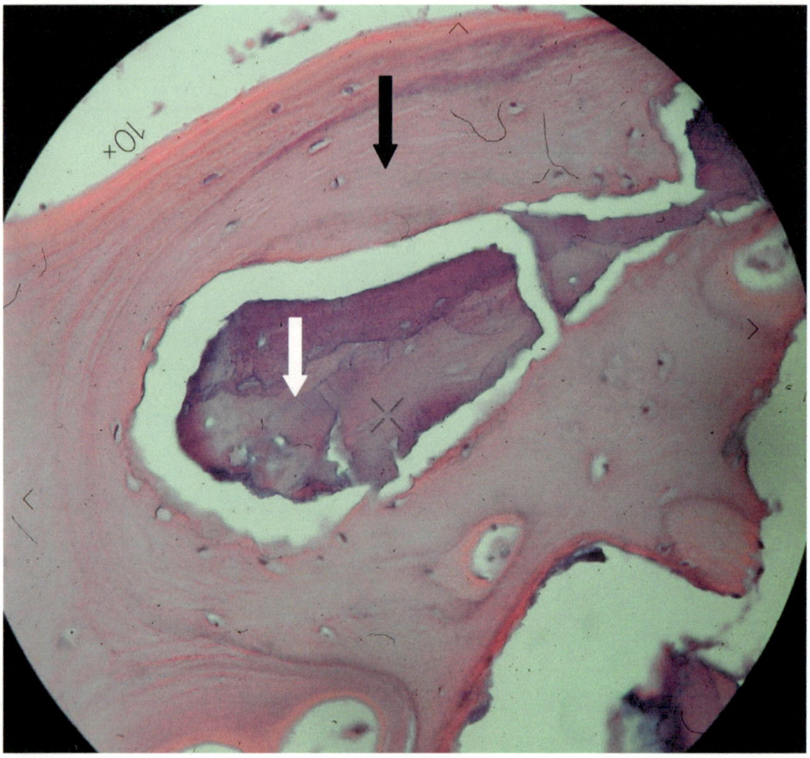

Fig. 2b. Biopsy of frozen human bone graft. 36 months of evolution. White arrow = graft; black arrow = new bone.

Although the freeze-dried grafts, whether human or bovine, are available in many medical centres worldwide, most work on RTHAs refers to the use of frozen bone grafts in blocks or cortical, but especially, most recently the spongy morcelised and impacted.

Tagil, in his PhD thesis published in 2000, attempted to explain the reasons for succeeding using the technique of frozen morcelised and impacted bone, once theoretically, the large volume of necrotic bone exposed to great mechanical stress tend to collapse, as in the vascular necrosis of the femoral head or knee. After detailed study, Tagil found out the following possibilities: (a) morcelised bone, as in a comminuted fracture, would produce extensive surface contact allowing access and release of biologically active substances; (b) impaction may improve osteoconductive properties of the graft leading to the release of BMPs and this way favouring osteointegration and; (c) the high elasticity may allow small deformations that would stimulate new bone formation. The importance of this study lays in the fact that it is essential, from a scientific standpoint, to know the pros and cons of a due technique and why results may be good or bad, to better use and indicate such a procedure more securely and confidentially.

5. Mechanical characteristics

In addition to the biological characteristics, the mechanical aspects are very relevant and can be decisive in the choice and obtained results using a due graft. Itoman and Nakamura, in

1991, studied the histological and biomechanical properties of different ways of bone graft processing in rats and noted that an increased stiffness of the bone after freezing at -80°C and lyophilising it. The freeze-dried demineralised bone has initially decreased its mechanical strength. However, after 16 weeks, a progressive increase in resistance of the grafts was observed and was likely related to its biological interaction, which might be an indicator of the osteoinductive properties of the graft. They also concluded that on the features of integration, as expected, the autologous bone showed the best results.

The physical properties of human and bovine trabecular bone are documented and their results are available, however, the range of dispersion is very wide. The Young's module, for example, in one study ranged from 70 to 673 MPa and compressive strength varied between 2.44 and 6.24 MPa. This dispersion occurred for both human and bovine bone and may be related to several factors such as donor age, bone density and methodology used in the study.

Cornu et al. in 2001, has demonstrated in vitro that the lyophilised morcelised and impacted bone is mechanically superior to the morcelised and impacted deep-frozen bone since, at least, has the same resistance after impaction, that is achieved however, more quickly and with fewer impacts, and the authors assumed as to the fact that lyophilised material was devoid of fat and bone marrow. Moreover, Macedo et al. in 1999, using an automated compression machine compared in vitro, the compressive strength of frozen and freeze-dried bovine bone rehydrated for an hour and found out that deep-frozen bovine bone grafts after defrosting, has similar compressive loads and deformation rate of the rehydrated lyophilised bovine bone.

6. Methods sterilization, infectious diseases and biosafety

Another extremely important issue is the study of methods of sterilization of frozen and freeze-dried grafts, since there still remains controversy and need for further studies. The currently available techniques have advantages and disadvantages regarding efficacy and maintenance of mechanical and biological properties. Significant deleterious effects on the use of cobalt 60 in the sterilisation of freeze-dried grafts have been reported, demonstrating that, even at low dosage, radiation is capable of destroying the morphogenetic properties, mainly in non-demineralised bone.

The effects of radiation on the biomechanics of the grafts are dose-dependent. Fidele et al. in 1995, studied the damage caused by the application of different doses of gamma radiation exposure on seven biomechanical parameters of frozen allogenic patellar bone-grafting. The sterilization dose accepted for inactivation of HIV, for example, is about 25 kGy. However, four out of the seven parameters measured were reduced after 20 kGy and after 30 kGy all parameters have shown significant reductions. Also, Zhang, Cornu and Delloye in 1997, in an experimental study in rats, compared the ability of graft osteoinduction after gamma radiation sterilisation (25 kGy), ethylene oxide (EO) at 55°C and 40°C or preservation in ethanol showing that the OE at 40°C and ethanol have not negatively affected the osteoinductive capacity, gamma radiation has decreased 40% and OE to 55°C had an almost completely loss of this potential. Some authors indicated that other factors in sterilisation need to be observed are the toxic residues from the OE that may remain in the graft and are released when in contact with liquids. Reference is also considered to the toxicity of gamma radiation when in contact with fat present in the graft, in addition to the mechanical change that the radiation may cause.

Another way to sterilise is to autoclave the bone, although it has also limitations. According to the recommendation of the European Community, aimed at inactivating prions (infectious proteins), tissues from bovine origin should be sterilised in an autoclave at 132°C for 1h, but the biomechanical effects of this method of sterilisation has proven to reduce in approximately 70%the mechanical resistance to compression of the graft. Moreover, many authors support the safety of non-sterilised bone grafts provided by banks that adopt appropriate methodology for donor selection and quality control and such control is so important that when applying these criteria, 20% to 30% of the harvested material will be discarded due to bacteriological or serological inadequate results. Despite this severe control, to name a few, in November 2001 there were two reported cases in the U.S., by Clostridium sordellii infection in surgical patients who received bone transplants. In March 2002, the Centre for Disease Control and Prevention (CDC, Atlanta) has received 26 reports from different locations of secondary bacterial infections in transplanted musculoskeletal tissues. In these events the CDC investigated donors and confirmed the presence of those bacteria in their tissues. Several other notifications have been done and are reported every year, which provides the need for even a more strict control, revision of adopted routines and, perhaps, searching for methods of sterilisation that may minimally interfere with quality of the graft.

Taylor in 2002, stated that prions, responsible for Creutzfeldt-Jakob disease in humans and bovine spongiform encephalitis, unlike bacteria and viruses, are resistant to procedures such as autoclaving or exposure to sodium hydroxide, but, the association of alkaline substances and heat even at 100°C for 1 minute appears to be effective to inactivate prions. In addition, when isolated used, sodium hypochlorite also demonstrated ability to deactivate prions.

Alike prions, potentially transmissible viral diseases such as hepatitis A, B or C, HIV and HTLV, and other more recently isolated viruses and certain types of tumour cells, should also be of concern, even with current knowledge and care from the point of view of serological or other diagnostic methods, which clearly demonstrates the importance of a wide discussion about sterilisation processes.

As published by Sugihara et al. in 1999, about 1% of tumour cells in 137 femoral heads subjected to histological examination in patients undergoing THA due to primary arthrosis and Palmer et al. also found high rates of histological abnormalities in 1146 patients with hip joint arthrosis, even suggesting that pathological examinations should be included as part of screening for donor tissues.

7. Processing and storage

Many ways of processing and storage bone tissue for clinical application have been proposed and used in Tissue Banks around the world. Among them, we highlight the deep-frozen (-80oC) and lyophilisation, which are the most widely used and accepted methods.

The ultralow freezing temperature is reached in freezers that go as low as -80oC with graphical systems constantly monitoring the temperature, having their own power generators and emergency alarms alerting when temperature increases. So, after rigorous screening of donors (living or dead), culture and serological tests for bacteria and fungi, and processing in a surgical environment the graft is subjected to freezing at-80C that allows its storage for up to 5 years. However, it is worth of note that low temperatures do not play any role in the sterilisation of the material, but decreases antigenicity indeed, allowing more useful handling of the graft.

Lyophilisation, as proposed and spread in 1951 by the USA Navy Tissue Bank24, is a technique by which dehydration of the water contained in a product is removed by sublimation, i.e., starting from a previously frozen material, placed under vacuum, the water goes directly from a solid state into mist30. Before that, however, the bone graft is washed, centrifuged, decellularised, chemically degreased and subjected to physical processes of cleaning and sterilisation preserving only the protein-mineral matrix, thus decreasing antigenicity23 (Figure 3).

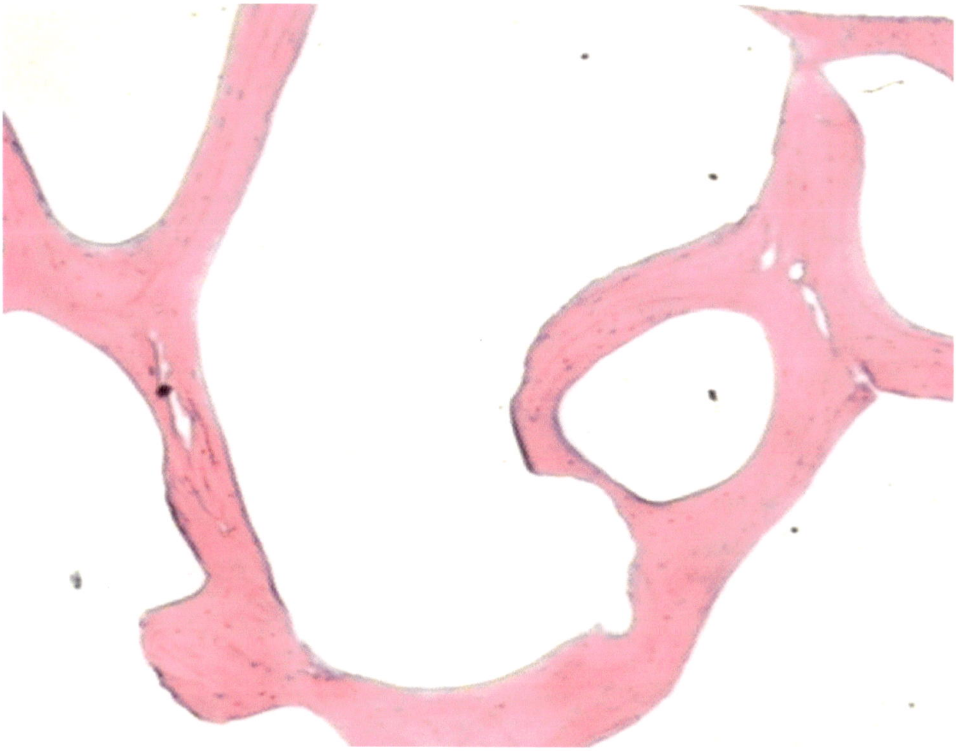

Fig. 3. Histological section of bone sample degreased, decellularized and freeze-dried. Note that the only remaining protein-mineral matrix.

Moreover, lyophilisation is a method of processing and storage of musculoskeletal tissues that allows not only the use of human bones, tendons and fascias (allogeneic), but also and mainly the bovine (xenogenic) ones, since by reducing antigenicity, provides biocompatibility, sterilisation and can be stored at room temperature.

Currently, in major health centres different types of bone grafts are available for reconstructive orthopaedic surgery: frozen and freeze-dried autologous, allogeneic and lyophilised xenogenic (bovine). The autologous graft, though not requiring processing, has been considered from the integration viewpoint, the preferred tissue for bone replacement. There is evidence that survival of osteoblasts and osteocytes from autologous graft are dependent on the quality of the receptor bed. Moreover, the amount of graft obtained is limited, surgical time is increased and complications, either systemic or local, of the intervention required to obtain the graft ranges from 21% to 49%.

The frozen allogeneic graft is the most widely used and accepted nowadays, but due to the reduced number of Tissue Banks in our country and the small number of donations is not always available to a wider use. Moreover, despite of all care and biosafety standards adopted by the banks there is still some risk of transmission of infectious diseases and tumours.

The lyophilised allogeneic graft, produced by the majority of U.S. tissue banks, is still not widespread among us, and few studies have reported the use of this graft in orthopaedic surgery and with a small number of cases and limited methods for assessing osteointegration, further studies are needed to better define its use (Figures 4a and 4b).

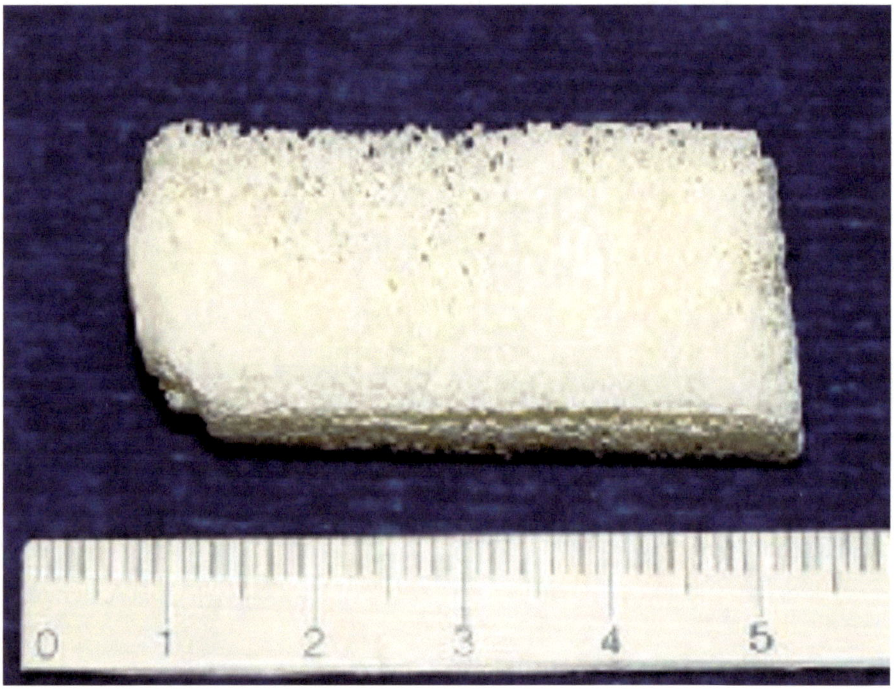

Fig. 4a. Sample of lyophilized bovine graft.

The xenogenic grafts, commonly used in dentistry, although controversial, are beginning to be used in orthopaedic surgeries, especially those of bovine origin, due to its easy preparation, availability and similarity. The bovine bone has chemical composition, porosity, size, shape and biological behaviour similar to its human counterpart as it can be clearly observed in Table 1. Besides those features, bovine graft provides structural support, osteoconduction and a high content of calcium and phosphorus, all of them essential factors for the newly formed bone tissue.

The most important issue, regardless of the type of graft chosen by the surgeon, is the guarantee that the graft has been processed and stored according to the standards of graft management as established by the Associations of Tissue Banks and the national and international health authorities.

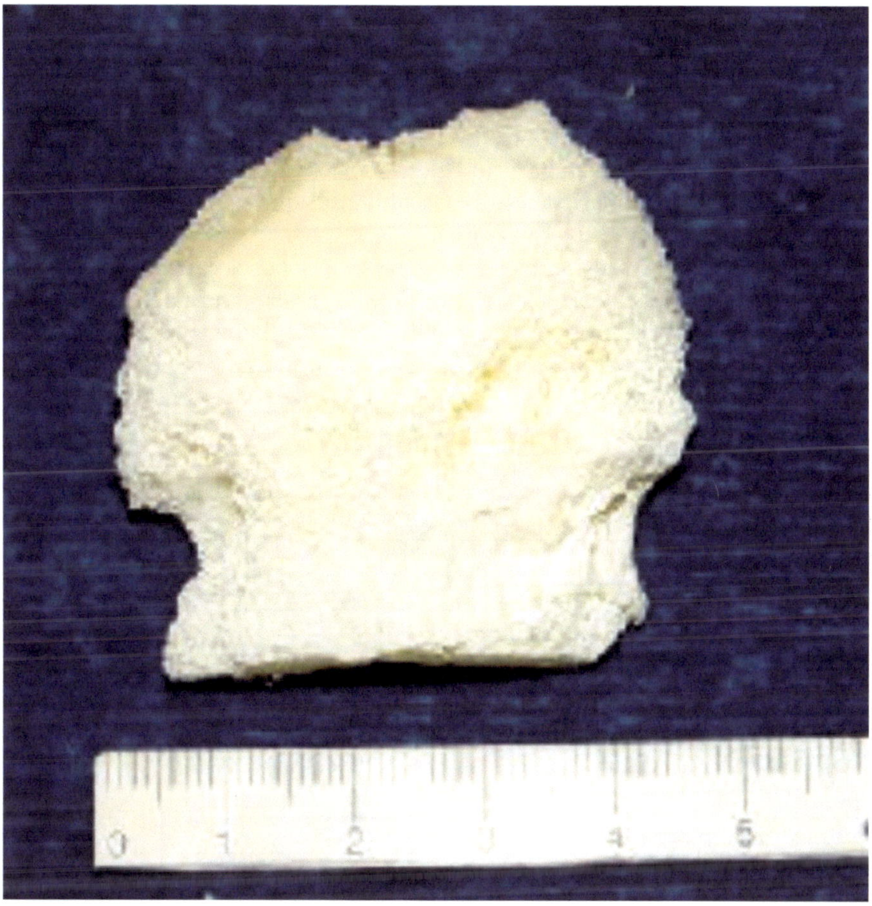

Fig. 4b. Sample graft ½ lyophilized human femoral head.

Readings	Human (%)	CI* 95%	Bovine (%)	CI* 95%
Water	7.93	-	7.75	-
Fat	0.06	0.1	0.1	0.1
Nitrogen	4.3	0.1	4.3	0.1
Proteins	27.5	0.2	27.2	0.2
Phosphorus	11.9	0.1	11.9	0.2
Total P_2O_5	27.1	0.2	27.2	0.7
Calcium	24.6	0.7	23.7	0.6
Ca/P	2.06	-	1.99	-
Total sodium	0.57	0.01	0.46	0.01
Ashes	64.8	0.6	64.3	0.1
Chlorides	1.3	0.06	1.3	0.2

*CI, Confidence Interval

Table 1. Physical and Chemical analysis of lyophilised bones HCPATB

8. Musculoskeletal tissue banks

Like in the USA, where the American Association of Tissue Banks (AATB) regulates and supervises the functioning of all in-country tissue banks since 1976, in Brazil the Ministry of Health, with the Norm No. 220 of December 27th, 2006, provides the technical regulations for the functioning of Musculoskeletal and Skin Tissue Banks of human origin. This regulation relates to the facility characteristics, screening of living donors or cadavers, equipment and human resources. These rules, although quite rigid, greatly increased the quality of processed tissues and the safety on its use.

In relation to screening, the decision to accept or reject a donor is carried out by the Medical Director of the Bank of Musculoskeletal Tissues (BMST) after rigorous tests and following a established protocol. As the protocols used by the Tissue Banks, one must consider the history, physical examination and laboratory tests of the donor.

Name:	**Medical record No.:**		
Date of Birth:	**Age (y):**	**Sex:**	**Race:**
Checking date:	**Collecting date:**		
DONOR PAST HISTORY			
• **CONDITIONS**		**YES**	**NO**
• Toxic substances or illegal drug abuses			
• **HAS THE DONOR HAD ANY BEHAVIOUR OR OTHER CONDITION BELOW IN THE PAST 12 MONTHS?**			
- Professional sex, illegal drugs or has any related person with this done so?			
- Multiple sexual partners?			
- Homosexual intercourse or sex with homosexual related persons?			
- Any unprotected sexual intercourse with known HIV, hepatitis B, C or other blood transmitted infection person?			
- Arrested or has been in a prison?			
- Submitted to acupuncture, tattooing, and permanent makeup or piercing?			
- A blood transfused or hemodialysed sexual partner?			
- Any malignant disease?			
- AIDS/HIV infection?			
- Any autoimmune disease?			
- Any neurological, degenerative or impairing disease?			
- Chronic kidney failure?			
- Past or active tuberculosis?			
- Sexually transmitted diseases?			
- Any osteometabolic diseases?			
- Any skin burns?			

-	Malaria or lived in an endemic area for malaria in the past 36 months?		
-	Creutzfeldt Jakob disease?		
-	Any undiagnosed situation or infection?		
-	Any human derived pituitary growth hormone treatment?		
-	Any duramater or corneal transplant?		
-	Chemotherapy or radiation therapy?		
-	Any orthopaedic surgery in the donor site?		
-	Any surgical procedure due to undefined situation?		
-	Any biopsy or suspicion of muscoskeletal tumour?		
-	Any non-obstructing jaundice or jaundice in any related person?		
-	Death by an unknown cause?		
-	Chronic use of steroids?		
-	Any diagnosed bacterial or fungal infection while in hospital?		
-	Vaccines:		
-	Unfit for 24h: toxoids or vaccines (diphteria, tetanus, cholera, typhus, paratyphus, influenza, pertussis, poliomyelitis Salk and serum non-derived B hepatitis)		
-	Unfit for 2 weeks: animal or virus attenuated vaccines (measles, parathyroid, yellow fever and Sabin poliomyelitis)		
-	Unfit for 1 month: rubeolla		
-	Unfit for 1 year: experimental vaccines, hepatitis B hyperimmune globulin, rabbis vaccine (prior animal bites), passive immunizations		
•	**CONDITIONS**	**YES**	**NO**
-	Any blood or blood product transfusion?		
-	Received any crystalloid solution resulting in hemodilution over 50% of the intravascular volume in the past 2h prior to blood sample analysis?		
-	Received any synthetic colloid solution resulting in hemodilution over 50% of the intravascular volume in the past 48h prior to blood sample analysis?		
-	Past history of accident or exposure to suspected or confirmed contaminated blood by HIV, hepatitis B or C?		
-	Hemophiliacs receiving blood or blood products from newly sexual partners within the past 12 months?		
-	Chronic hemodialysis?		
-	Mechanical ventilation over 72h?		
•	**AGE LIMITS FOR DONORS**		
	a. bone tissue:	below 18 and over 70 years	
	b. tendon tissue:	below 18 and over 55 years	
	c. osteochondral tissue:	below 18 and over 45 years	

• PHYSICAL EXAMINATION (CONDITIONS)	YES	NO
- Skin appearance of sexuallly transmitted or malignant diseases?		
- Tattoos, signs of piercing or definitive makeup?		
- Scars prior to the harvesting procedure?		
- Perineal or perianal skin appearance of sexually transmitted disease?		
- Needle punctures suggestive of intravenous drug abuse?		
- Jaundice?		
- Hepatomegaly?		
- Diffuse lymph node swelling/		
- Kaposi Sarcoma?		

• LAB PROFILE				
• EXAM	• RESULTADO	•	• EXAME	RESULTADO
• Hb/Ht	•	•	• WBC	
• ESR	•	•	• Glucose	
• Bilirubins	•	•	• Alcaline Phosphatase	
• GOT	•	•	• GPT	
• Coagulation	•	•	• Platelets	
• Urine analysis	•	•	• Urine culture	
• HbsAG	•	•	• Anti-HBc	
• Anti-HCV	•	•	• Anti-HIV 1+2	
• HTLV1/HTLV2	•	•	• Toxoplasmosis IgM/IgG	
• Chagas	•	•	• Epstein-Barr virus	
• CMV IgM/IgG	•	•	• HBV-PCR	
• HCV-PCR	•	•	• Lues PPR test	
• HIV-PCR	•	•	•	
• RADIOGRAPHIC EXAM				
Results:				
....				

Source: Bank of musculoskeletal tissues (BMST), Hospital São Vicente de Paulo - Passo Fundo BMST of the Hospital de Clinicas de Porto Alegre University Hospital (licensed, but awaiting accreditation by Ministry of Healthy Quality Control Committee - ANVISA)

Table 2. Screening protocol for muscoskeletal tissue donors.

9. Conclusion

There are many differences when comparing the types of graft, with variations as for the source, production methods, processing, uses (block or shredded) sterilisation, storage and cost of the process. Thus, it is essential the implementation of protocols for processing and quality control of all types of bone grafts. This measure will facilitate the monitoring and analysis of the results obtained in distinct surgical procedures, and shall provide grafting material of better quality, thoroughly tested and ready available.

Although there are reports of the use of bone grafts and transplants for many years, many mechanical and biological issues such as physical and chemical composition, incorporation, bone remodelling and immune responses are still incompletely assessed. These issues are still requiring more knowledge and further clinical and laboratory investigations to allow a more scientifically based choice of the graft and appropriate indication to surgical use on any particular situation.

There is no doubt on the importance of bone transplants in orthopaedic surgery, especially in hip procedures. Their results are well-known and, to some extent predictable when its use is carried out by experienced surgeons. It is also indubitable that bone tissue is a biologically privileged material, since several alternative bone grafts can be used quite well. It is undeniable, however, that we still knowing little about many aspects of the host-graft interaction and sometimes seems we are resigned with this situation, when in fact, many studies have yet to be carried out in several ways to attempt to answer questions that sometimes are underestimated, since "most of the time the graft works". For instance, why do 85% of the grafts theoretically integrate? Though it seems a good percentage, how about the other "not so lucky" 15% of the cases? Is it a matter of technique, immune response, mechanical effect or biological feature? Which is the best substitute for autologous grafts? The frozen allogeneic sterile or non-sterile or the freeze-dried irradiated or autoclaved graft? Should a method of definitive sterilisation be employed by the Tissue Banks?

These are just some of important yet unanswered issues that should be carefully investigated and analysed it best clinical responses, increased biosafety and lower complication rates as well as higher scientific basis to precisely and reliably analyse the grafts and surgical outcomes are to be sought.

10. References

American Association of Tissue Banks - AATB's. http://www.aatb.org [accessed Mar 29th, 2011]

Autograft, allograft, and xenograft [Lecture 17]. http://www.pharmacy.wisc.edu/courses/718-430/handouts/ tisgraft.pdf [accessed Feb 27th, 2011]

Barth H. Histologische untersuchungen uber knochen-transplantation. Beitr. Path. Anat. Allg. Path.;17: 65-142; 1895 (in German).

Buck BE, Malinin TI. Human bone and tissue allografts. Preparation and safety. Clin Orthop. Jun; (303):8-17; 1994.

Buma P, Lamerigts N, Schreurs BW, Gardeniers J, Versleyen D, Slooff TJ. Impacted graft incorporation after cemented acetabular revision. Histological evaluation in 8 patients. Acta Orthop Scand. Dec;67(6):536-40; 1996.

Cornu O, Bavadekar A, Godts B, Delloye C, Vantomme J, Banse X. Processed freeze-dried bone is more efficient than fresh frozen for impaction bone grafting. In: 47th Annual Meeting, Orthopaedic Research Society; Feb 25-28; San Francisco, California. 1081-81; 2001.

Czitrom AA, Axelrod T, Fernandes B. Antigen presenting cells and bone allotransplantation. Clin Orthop. Jul-Aug; (197):27-31; 1985.

de Roeck NJ, Drabu KJ. Impaction bone grafting using freeze-dried allograft in revision hip arthroplasty. J Arthroplasty. 2001 Feb, 16(2).201-6.

Fideler BM, Vangsness CT Jr, Lu B, Orlando C, Moore T. Gamma irradiation: effects on biomechanical properties of human bone-patellar tendon-bone allografts. Am J Sports Med. Sep-Oct; 23(5):643-6; 1995.

Finkemeier CG. Bone-grafting and bone-graft substitutes. J Bone Joint Surg Am. Mar; 84-A(3):454-64; 2002.

Fred II A. The fundamental principles involved in the use of the bone graft in surgery. Am J Med Sci. Mar; 149(3): 313-25; 1915.

Friedlaender GE, Strong DM, Sell KW. Studies on the antigenicity of bone. I. Freeze-dried and deep-frozen bone allografts in rabbits. J Bone Joint Surg Am. Sep; 58(6):854-8; 1976.

Galia, CR. Liophilised impacted bone grafts from human and bovine origin in TRHAs. Porto Alegre, 2004, 127p. Doctorate Thesis - Faculty of Medicine, Post-graduate Programme in Surgery. Rio Grande do Sul Federal University, 2004.

Garcia, VD. Tissue and organ transplants. 2 ed. São Paulo, SP, Brazil, 2006.

Gie GA, Linder L, Ling RS, Simon JP, Slooff TJ, Timperley AJ. Impacted cancellous allografts and cement for revision total hip arthroplasty. J Bone Joint Surg Br. Jan; 75(1):14-21; 1993.

Godwin L. Tissue banking and allograft transplantation Jun 2000. http://www.iscpubs.com/articles/abl/b0006god.pdf [accessed Nov 22nd, 2003]

Goldberg VM. Selection of bone grafts for revision total hip arthroplasty. Clin Orthop. Dec; (381):68-76; 2000.

Gonçalves HR. Methods of acetabular bone graft incorporation in THA with bone loss [dissertation]. São Paulo, SP, Brazil. Santa Casa de São Paulo Faculty of Medical Sciences 2003 (In Portuguese).

Heliotis M, Tsiridis EE. Fresh frozen bone in femoral impaction grafting: can developments in bone regeneration improve on this? Med Hypotheses. Dec; 57(6):675-8; 2001.

National Press. Brazil's official Press nº 185, 1, Section Sept 24th, 2002. Norm nº 1.686, Sept 20th, 2002. https://www.in.gov.br/imprimir.asp?id=1081142100&tela=imp. [accessed Apr 1st, 2011]

Invasive Streptococcus pyogenes after allograft implantation - Colorado, 2003. http://www.cdc.gov/mmwr/preview/mmwrhtml/mm5248a1.htm [accessed Jan 23rd, 2011]

Itoman M, Nakamura S. Experimental study on allogenic bone grafts. Int Orthop.;15(2):161-5; 1991.

Kakiuchi M, Ono K, Nishimura A, Shiokawa H. Preparation of bank bone using defatting, freeze-drying and sterilisation with ethylene oxide gas. Part 1. Experimental evaluation of its efficacy and safety. Int Orthop.;20(3):142-6; 1996.

Kreuz FP, Hyatt GW, Turner TC. et al: The preservation and clinical use of freeze-dried bone. J Bone Joint Surg (Am) 33:863-873, 1951.

Lexer E. Joint transplantations and arthoplasty. Surg Gynecol Obstet.;40: 782-809; 1925.

Li Zi-zuang, Lu Shi-bi, Wag Ji-fang. The study of repairing ability of freeze-dried bone allograft. Zhonghua Wai Ke Za Zhi Dec;32(12):765-7; 1994. (English abstract).

Lind M, Krarup N, Mikkelsen S, Horlyck E. Exchange impaction allografting for femoral revision hip arthroplasty: results in 87 cases after 3.6 years' follow-up. J Arthroplasty. Feb; 17(2):158-64; 2002.

Liu W. Reconstitution of osteoinductive bone xenograft: bioassay in mice. Zhonghua Yi Xue Za Zhi. Jul;71(7):378-80, 28, 1991(English abstract).

Lubboc. Maitrise orthopédique [accessed Jan 29th, 2011]:http://www.maitrise-orthop.com/gesto/lubboc.shtml (in French).

Luchese AC, Dec hechi ED. Lyophilisation process. In: XI Research and Bioethics Meeting 2003 (Oct 20th-22nd); Porto Alegre, RS, Brazil. www2.pucpr.br/educacao/pibic//evento/files/CE08.html. [accessed Mar 13th, 2011].

Macedo CAS, Galia CR, Silva ALB, César PC, Sanches PRS, Duarte LS et al. Compression resistance of deep-frozen and freeze-dried bone of bovine origin. Rev Bras Ortop. 34(9/10): 529- 33; 1999 (in Portuguese).

Moreau MF, Gallois Y, Basle MF, Chappard D. Gamma irradiation of human bone allografts alters medullary lipids and releases toxic compounds for osteoblast-like cells. Biomaterials. Feb; 21(4):369-76; 2000.

Nogami H, Urist MR. Explants, transplants and implants of a cartilage and bone morphogenetic matrix. Clin Orthop. (103): 235-51; 1974.

Oliveira RC, Sicca CM, Silva TL, Cestari TM, Oliveira OT, Buzalaf MAR, et al. Temperature effect on the denaturation of microgranular cortical bone of bovine origin. Microscopic and biochemistry assessment of cell response in rats. Revista FOB. Jul/Dez; 7(3/4): 85-93; 1999 (in Portuguese).

Palmer SH, Gibbons CL, Athanasou NA. The pathology of bone allograft [abstract]. J Bone Joint Surg Br. Mar; 81(2):333-5; 1999.

Poumarat G, Squire P. Comparison of mechanical properties of human, bovine bone and a new processed bone xenograft. Biomaterials. Apr; 14(5):337-40; 1993.

Reddi AH, Cunningham NS. Initiation and promotion of bone differentiation by bone morphogenetic proteins [abstract]. J Bone Miner Res. Dec; 8 Suppl 2:S499-502; 1993.

Seiler 3rd JG, Johnson J, Hand G, Microsurgery Clinic. Iliac crest autogenous bone grafting: donor site complications. J Southern Orthopedic Association [online]. Internet:http://www.medscape.com/viewarticle/410431 [Accessed Sept. 7th, 2011].

Slooff TJ, Buma P, Schreurs BW, Schimmel JW, Huiskes R, Gardeniers J. Acetabular and femoral reconstruction with impacted graft and cement. Clin Orthop. Mar; (324):108-15; 1996.

Slooff TJ, Huiskes R, van Horn J, Lemmens AJ. Bone grafting in total hip replacement for acetabular protrusion [abstract]. Acta Orthop Scand. Dec; 55(6):593-96; 1984.

Sommerville SM, Johnson N, Bryce SL, Journeaux SF, Morgan DA. Contamination of banked femoral head allograft: incidence, bacteriology and donor follow up [abstract]. Aust N Z J Surg. Jul; 70(7):480-4; 2000.

Springfield DS. Massive autogenous bone grafts. Orthop Clin North Am. Apr; 18(2):249-56; 1987.

Sugihara S, van Ginkel AD, Jiya TU, van Royen BJ, van Diest PJ, Wuisman PI. Histopathology of retrieved allografts of the femoral head. J Bone Joint Surg Br. Mar; 81(2):336-41; 1999.

Tägil M. The morselized and impacted bone graft. Animal experiments on proteins, impaction and load [Thesis]. Lund (Sweden): Lund University Hospital; 2000.

Taylor D. Inactivation of the BSE agent. C R Acad Sci III. Jan; 325(1):75-6; 2002.

Thien TM, Welten ML, Verdonschot N, Buma P, Yong P, Schreurs BW. Acetabular revision with impacted freeze-dried cancellous bone chips and a cemented cup: a report of 7 cases at 5 to 9 years' follow-up. J Arthroplasty. Aug; 16(5):666-70; 2001.

Turek SL. Orthopaedics: Principles and applications. 4th ed. Editora Manole Ltda, Rio de Janeiro, RJ, Brazil. p.756; 1991 (in Portuguese).

Ullmark G, Obrant KJ. Histology of impacted bone-graft incorporation. J Arthroplasty. Feb; 17(2):150-7; 2002.

Update: Allograft-associated bacterial infections - United States, 2002. Nov., 4th, 2002. http://www.medscape.com/viewarticle/430131 [accessed Jun, 9th, 2011].

Urist MR, Hernandez A. Excitation transfer in bone. Deleterious effects of cobalt 60 radiation-sterilization of bank bone. Arch Surg. Oct; 109(4):486-93; 1974.

Vajaradul Y. Bone banking in Thailand. A 10-year experience (1984-1994).Clin Orthop. Feb; (323):173-80; 1996.

Viceconti M, Toni A, Brizio L, Rubbini L, Borrelli A. The effect of autoclaving on the mechanical properties of bank bovine bone [abstract]. Chir Organi Mov. Jan-Mar; 81(1):63-8; 1996.

Zhang Q, Cornu O, Delloye C. Ethylene oxide does not extinguish the osteoinductive capacity of demineralized bone. A reappraisal in rats. Acta Orthop Scand. Apr; 68(2):104-8; 1997.

13

Cross-Linked Gelatin Microcapsules for Drug Delivery in a Arthritic TMJ

P. R. Kramer[1], Brian Windsor[2], Kenneth Carson[3] and Larry Bellinger[1]
[1]*Department of Biomedical Sciences, Baylor College of Dentistry, Texas A&M Health Science Center, Dallas, TX*
[2]*Appian Labs Bee Caves Road l Austin, Texas*
[3]*Southwest Research Institute Culebra RdSan Antonio, TX*
USA

1. Introduction

A majority of individuals reporting temporomandibular joint (TMJ) disorders have joint damage, inflammation or arthritis (Manfredini, Chiappe & Bosco, 2006; Plesh, Sinisi, Crawford & Gansky, 2005). The joint will show loss of extra-cellular matrix components in the articular cartilage and subchondral bone resulting in destruction of cartilage and bone, such processes lead to inflammation and exacerbation of joint tissue catabolism (Tanaka, Detamore & Mercuri, 2008). Matrix metalloproteinases 1 and 9 (MMP-1 and MMP-9) are two major enzymes that contribute to tissue catabolism and have been observed in patients with TMJ disorders (Kanyama, Kuboki, Kojima, Fujisawa, Hattori, Takigawa & Yamashita, 2000; Srinivas, Sorsa, Tjaderhane, Niemi, Raustia, Pernu, Teronen & Salo, 2001; Yoshida, Takatsuka, Hatada, Nakamura, Tanaka, Ueki, Nakagawa, Okada, Yamamoto & Fukuda, 2006). Reversal of these disease processes and treatment of the joint to reduce pain are effective in the early stages of the disease, but treatment often fails to alleviate the severe, chronic pain caused by advanced joint degeneration (Gerwin, Hops & Lucke, 2006; Tanaka, Detamore & Mercuri, 2008).

Treatment of TMJ osteoarthritis with intra-articular injections of non-steroidal anti-inflammatory drugs (NSAIDs) and opiates into the superior joint space have shown efficacy (Bryant, Harrison, Hopper & Harris, 1999; Swift, Roszkowski, Alton & Hargreaves, 1998; Zuniga, Ibanez & Kozacko, 2007). Intra-articular administration versus systemic administration of NSAID or opiates would be advantageous for treatment of TMJ inflammation and pain because local administration avoids the ectopic effects seen with NSAIDs like rofecoxib (i.e., Vioxx) (Lin, Weisdorf, Solovey & Hebbel, 2000) or opiates. For example, nonselective NSAIDS can cause intestinal bleeding, whereas some selective cyclooxygenase-2 inhibitors have significant cardiovascular and renal safety risks (Davies & Jamali, 2004; Mukherjee, Nissen & Topol, 2001). Moreover, opioids frequently cause constipation, sedation, nausea, vomiting, and respiratory depression (Mercadante, 1999).

Intra-articular injection remains controversial in light of decades of mixed reports demonstrating intra-articular injections either accelerate or trigger destruction of tissues within the TMJ and the surrounding area (Bjornland, Rorvik, Haanaes & Teige, 1994; Sugisaki, Ikai & Tanabe, 1995; Westesson, Eriksson & Liedberg, 1986). Recent reports demonstrate that the risks of intra-articular TMJ injection can be minimized by utilizing magnetic resonance imaging (MRI) for visualizing the needle during the injection procedure (Fritz, Thomas, Tzaribachev, Horger, Claussen, Lewin & Pereira, 2009; Hayakawa, Kober, Otonari-Yamamoto, Otonari, Wakoh & Sano, 2007). Current treatment protocols that utilize intra-articular drug delivery can require frequent injections, increasing the risk of infection and damage to the joint and, in the event MRI or some other form of imaging is utilized, dramatically increase the expense of the procedure. Alternatively, if drug delivery could be sustained after a single injection these risks from a multi-injection protocol could be minimized.

A variety of methods have been tested for sustained drug delivery in a joint space, including encapsulating or incorporating drugs into nano- or microparticles consisting of organic polymers (Deasy, 1994; Mountziaris, Kramer & Mikos, 2009). In this report we test a crosslinked fluid filled gelatin capsule for intra-articular injection. This capsule has a gelatin shell with a core of oil containing the drug ibuprofen or morphine. Other studies used uncrosslinked gelatin microcapsules, in contrast to our crosslinked capsules. The capsules were given orally but only released drug for 24-48 hours (Jizomoto, Kanaoka, Sugita & Hirano, 1993). Most intra-articular studies testing sustained release of NSAIDs utilized poly(lactide-co-glycolide) (PLGA) (Bozdag, Calis, Kas, Ercan, Peksoy & Hincal, 2001; Fernandez-Carballido, Herrero-Vanrell, Molina-Martinez & Pastoriza, 2004a; Fernandez-Carballido, Herrero-Vanrell, Molina-Martinez & Pastoriza, 2004b; Liggins, Cruz, Min, Liang, Hunter & Burt, 2004; Puebla, Pastoriza, Barcia & Fernandez-Carballido, 2005; Tuncay, Calis, Kas, Ercan, Peksoy & Hincal, 2000). PLGA has a rigid structure and may be irritating to the joint when injected intra-articularly, particularly when smaller than 20 microns (Liggins, Cruz, Min, Liang, Hunter & Burt, 2004). Importantly, in vivo studies injecting solid gelatin spheres have shown that they do not induce an inflammatory response in vivo suggesting gelatin in these studies should not induce an immune response (Brown, Leong, Huang, Dalal, Green, Haimes, Jimenez & Bathon, 1998).

Testing the rate of gelatin microcapsule degradation, as a result of MMP degradation, and the level of inflammation induced by the microcapsules in the TMJ are necessary. Also an important question to address was does sustained release improve pain reduction when administering NSAIDs or opiates to treat a TMJ disorder? To address these questions we used a rat model for TMJ arthritis.

In this model we inject the TMJ with the adjuvant complete Freund's adjuvant (CFA) and the rat's meal duration will lengthen in male and female rats as a result of this injection (Kerins, Carlson, Hinton, Grogan, Marr, Kramer, Spears & Bellinger, 2005; Kerins, Carlson, McIntosh & Bellinger, 2003; Kerins, Carlson, McIntosh & Bellinger, 2004; Kramer & Bellinger, 2009; Thut, Hermanstyne, Flake & Gold, 2007). Microcapsules containing vehicle or the NSAID ibuprofen or morphine were injected into the TMJ of rats that had no joint arthritis or had adjuvant (i.e., CFA) induce arthritis. Degradation of the microcapsules was monitored and the level of inflammatory cytokine IL-1β in the joint tissues was quantitated. In addition, the nociceptive response to the microcapsules loaded with vehicle or NSAID or morphine were measured in a non-arthritic and arthritic TMJ after intra-articular injection.

2. Materials and methods

2.1 Microcapsule production

To produce the loaded microcapsules canola oil was sonicated in water to induce formation of droplets 20-50 micrometers in size. Before sonication the canola oil was mixed with

2.5µl/ml of 1mM Alexa 488 dye (Invitrogen, Carlsbad CA) dissolved in toluene. Or a saturated solution of ibuprofen in canola oil was used containing ~15% (w/v) ibuprofen. A solution of Type A gelatin with a Bloom strength of 300 was added after sonication. The collagen gelatin was allowed to coat the oil droplets such that 80% of the microcapsule mass was canola oil and 20% was a gelatin shell by weight. Amino acids in the gelatin coated oil droplets were then cross-linked by addition of 15% 1-ethyl-3-(3-dimethylaminopropyl) carbodiimide) [EDC] (dry wt. of gelatin) to induce stable microcapsules. EDC is a water soluble carbodiimide usually obtained as the hydrochloride that can generally be used as a carboxyl activating agent for the coupling of primary amines to yield amide bonds between a free amine group (e.g., protein- or peptide-bound lysine) and the gamma-carboxamid group of protein- or peptide-bound glutamine. The cross-linking reaction was performed at room temperature for 12 hr. After crosslinking the microcapsules were washed 4 times with Tris Buffer pH 7.0, dried, sterilized with ethylene oxide and then hydrated with 0.9% saline.
The morphine capsules were produced in a similar manner with some modifications. Morphine alkaloid crystals were ground to a small size (less than 50 microns) and suspended in canola oil. This suspension was emulsified in a solution of the gelatin at 60°C. A complexing agent (hexametaphosphate) was added to the aqueous phase and the pH was adjusted to approximately 4.75 with acetic acid to allow coacervation to occur. The microcapsules were crosslinked, lyophilized until dry and sterilized.

2.2 Detection of Ibuprofen and morphine by HPLC

Known weights of beads were dissolved in acetonitrile and analyzed via high performance liquid chromatography (HPLC) as follows. A six point calibration curve was prepared by serial dilution and HPLC analysis. The stock solution of 1mg/mL was prepared in 1:1 deionized water (pH 2.5) and acetonitrile. Concentrations of 1, 5, 10, 25, 50 and 100 µg/mL were made in methanol. Samples of 20 µL were injected onto a C-18 column (Supelco Discovery C-18, 4.6 x 15 cm). The isocratic separation was carried out at 30°C using a mobile phase of 1:1 deionized water (pH 2.5) and acetonitrile. The flow rate was 2.0 ml/min with a run time of 10 minutes. Absorbance at 214 nm was taken using a Waters 486 UV detector. The absorbance of the sample was compared to a six-point standard curve from which concentration and percent loading in capsules was determined.

2.3 In vitro assay for microcapsule degradation

In 24 well tissue culture plates approximately 80,000 microcapsules were placed in each well with either 0.9% saline, 15 µg/ml CFA (paraffin oil/15µg *Mycobacterium tuberculosis*) mixed in water, or a 50:50 mixture of 0.9% saline and 15 µg/ml CFA. A homogenate of the water and oil was created by passing the solution through a 20 gauge needle 5 times. The plates were placed in a 5% CO_2 chamber at 37°C. The microcapsules were counted in triplicate in a hemacytometer chamber 0, 5 and 10 days following addition to the different solutions.

2.4 TMJ Injections

The Baylor College of Dentistry Institutional Animal Care and Use Committee approved the experimental protocol. Male (250 grams) Sprague-Dawley rats from Harlan Industries, Houston, TX were kept on a 12:12 light/dark cycle with lights on at 08:00 hours. The animals were housed individually in our computerized feeding modules and given food and water ad libitum. They were acclimated to the surroundings for two days before receiving injections. Prior to the TMJ injections, the rats were removed from their cages and anesthetized with a 5% gas flow of isoflurane. Following the TMJ injections and removal from anesthesia, the rats began freely moving within two minutes.

2.4.1 Bead degradation study

Saline or 15 µg of CFA in 15 µl was injected into the upper joint space of the TMJ followed by a second injection 24 hours later of 30 µl of dye loaded microcapsules (90 mg microcapsules [dry weight]/1 mlTris buffer or 0.9% saline) into the same location. The animals were sacrificed 5 hours (day 0), 5 and 10 days after injection of microcapsules and TMJ was removed en bloc, fixed in paraformaldehyde, sectioned and stained as described below.

2.4.2 Microcapsules affect nociceptive response study

Rats were injected with 30 µl 0.9% saline or 15 µg CFA and then 24 hours later the rats were injected with either saline or 30 µl of the microcapsule slurry (20% w/v) in 0.9% saline. Before and after injection of the microcapsules the meal duration was recorded.

2.4.3 MMP effect on degradation study

Rats were injected with 30 µl saline or 15 µg CFA or saline with an MMP inhibitor or CFA with an MMP inhibitor added and then 24 hours later these groups of rats were injected with 30 µl microcapsules or microcapsules plus the MMP inhibitor. The MMP inhibitor was a 1 µM solution of the MMP-2,9 inhibitor IV (EMD Biosciences, cataloge # 444274). In the first experiment the rats were sacrificed 0, 5 and 10 days following microcapsule injection, the TMJ was removed, sectioned and the microcapsules counted. In the second experiment the rats nociceptive response was assayed in the pellet feeders, as described below.

2.4.4 Drug loaded microcapsules study

Rats were injected into the upper joint space of the TMJ with a 30 µl slurry of microcapsules containing 15% ibuprofen or 1% morphine in oil or aslurry of microcapsules containing just oil. After twenty-four hours a portion of these animals were subdivided further; one group received bilateral injections of 0.9% saline (30 µl) and the other group received an injection of CFA into the upper joint space. Before and after injection the nociceptive response (i.e., meal duration) was assayed by placing the rats in pellet feeders. Also, on day 7 post-injection the TMJ tissue of a portion of these rats was harvested for quantitation of the cytokine IL-1β.

2.5 Nociceptive assay

The rats were housed individually in sound-attenuated chambers equipped with photobeam computer-activated pellet feeders (Med Assoc. Inc., East Fairfield, VT). The rats were given 45 mg rodent chow pellets (Product No. FO 165, Bioserv, Frenchtown, NJ). When a rat removes a pellet from the feeder trough, a photobeam placed at the bottom of the trough is no longer blocked, signaling the computer to drop another pellet, record the date and time, and keep a running tally of the total daily food consumption. The computer record of pellets dropped over time establishes the meal duration, which is a continuous non-invasive biological marker of TMJ nociception (surface and deep) in undisturbed male and female rats (Kerins, Carlson, Hinton, Grogan, Marr, Kramer, Spears & Bellinger, 2005; Kerins, Carlson, McIntosh & Bellinger, 2003).

2.6 Animals and tissue preparation

Rats were sacrificed within 20 sec to minimize stress. For the cytokine study the TMJ anterior, disc, retrodiscal and synovium were dissected from one side by performing a superficial, horizontal skin incision parallel and just inferior to the zygomatic arch. The masseter and temporalis muscles were cut away from the arch and the ramus of the mandible so that the arch could be removed with ronjeurs. The neck of the condyle was grasped with hemostats and the condylar neck fractured to allow removal of any remaining musculature and access to the anterior, disc, retrodiscal and synovial tissues. Dissected TMJ tissue was excised from the posterior neck of the condyle, and all anterior tissue, articular disc, retrodiscal tissue and synovium were removed, placed in liquid nitrogen and stored at -80°C. To count the number of microcapsules in the TMJ a 0.5 cm cube of TMJ tissue centered on the condyle from the other side was removed and placed in 4% paraformaldehyde at 4°C overnight. The tissue was then decalcified in 0.5 M EDTA in a Pelco microwave (Ted Pella Inc., Redding CA) for 2 weeks, frozen and 20 µm sections were cut and mounted on Superfrost glass slides (Fisher Scientific, Pittsburgh, PA). Every 5th section was stained with hematoxylin and eosin for counting and a small number of the slides were mounted with fluormount and DAPI. Microcapsules were counted on every 5th section to obtain a representative sample through the entire TMJ region (West & Slomanka, 2001). The fluorescent signal was imaged using MetaMorph Imaging System software (Molecular Devices Corporation, Sunnyvale, CA), a Photometrics CoolSnap K4 CCD camera (Roper Scientific, Inc, Duluth, GA) and a fluorescent microscope using a DAPI filter with excitation between 395-410 nm and an emission between 450-470 nm, as well as, a FITC filter with excitation between 490-505 nm and an emission between 515-545 nm.

2.7 Cytokine assay

The TMJ tissue was homogenized in buffer (75 mM potassium acetate pH 7.4, 300 mM NaCL, 10 mM EDTA, 0.25% Triton X-100, protease inhibitors). It has previously been shown that TMJ-injected CFA can increase IL-1β (Kerins, Carlson, McIntosh & Bellinger, 2003) . Therefore, the cytokines IL-1β were quantitated from this homogenate using ELISA kits according to the manufacturer's directions (R&D Systems, Minneapolis, MN).

3. Statistics

The data were analyzed using a two-way analysis of variance with repeated measurement. Independent variables were treatment and time. The dependent variable was either the bead count or meal duration. The data found to be significant were further analyzed by Bonferonni pos-hoc test.

4. Results

Images of the microcapsules in solution show that the capsules average size was 30 µm (Fig. 1A) and that the inside of the microcapsule is loaded with the dye/mineral oil mixture (Fig. 1B). About 80% of the mass of these microcapsules is the fluid mineral oil and about 20% of the mass consists of the gelatin shell.

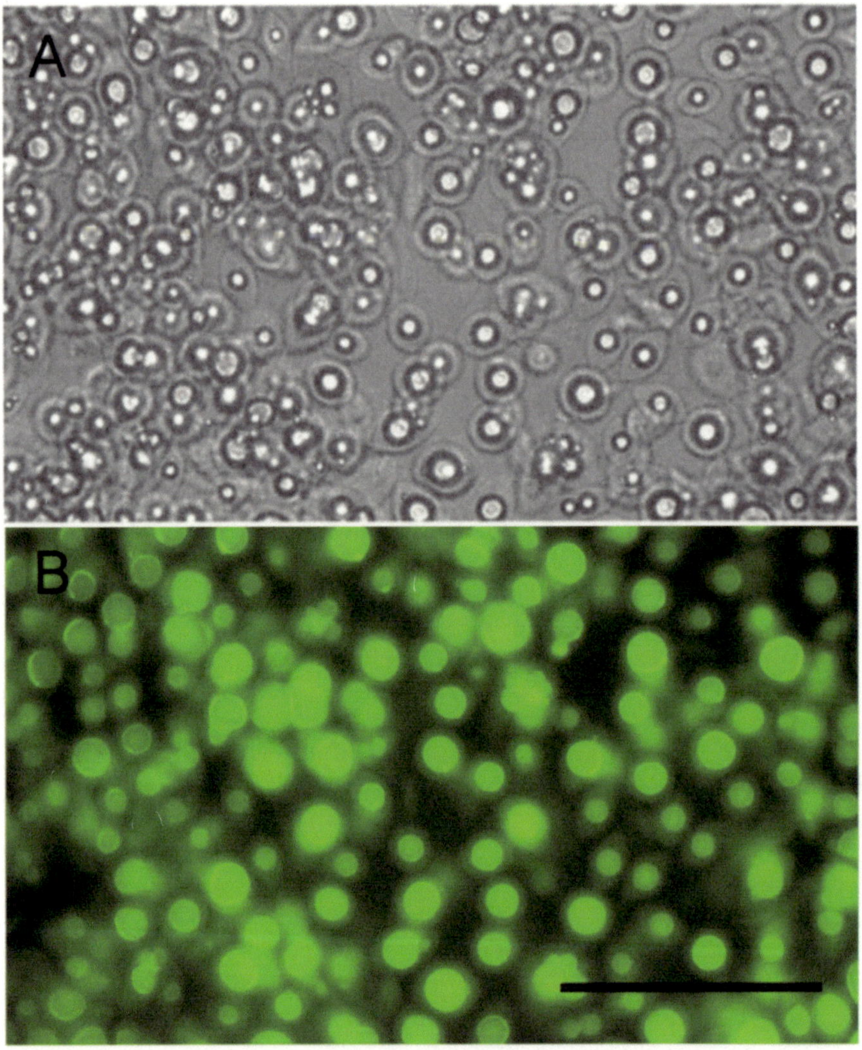

Fig. 1. Gelatin microcapsules containing canola oil mixed with Alexa 488 dye range in size between 15-30 micrometers. Microcapsules are loaded with canola oil (80% by weight) mixed with 1mM Alexa 488 dye. A) Bright field image of the microcapsules in solution. B) Fluorescent image of the same microcapsules before injection into the TMJ. Bar equals 100 μM.

To initially assess the degradation characteristics of the gelatin shell the microcapsules were placed in 24 well tissue culture plates containing saline and CFA solutions. Over a period of 10 days the beads did significantly degrade in a mixture of isotonic saline and 15 μg of CFA (Fig. 2).

Injection of dye loaded microcapsules (30 μl) into the upper joint space, a region between the articular fossa and condyle (Fig. 3A) produced an area of beads 2-3 mm in diameter (dotted line, Fig. 3B) in the upper joint space of the rat TMJ. Cells (e.g. neutrophils) were adjacent to the microcapsules 5 hours after injection (blue nuclei, Fig. 3C-E). In the TMJ the microcapsules appeared to degrade as a result of inducing an arthritic response (i.e., CFA injection), compare Fig. 4A to Fig. 4B and compare Fig. 4C to Fig. 4D. Time also reduced the number of microcapsules in the joint, compare 5 day and 10 day saline injected rats (compare Fig. 4A to Fig. 4C) and 5 day and 10 day CFA injected rats (compare Fig. 4B to Fig. 4D). A significant decrease in the number of intact beads was observed in the inflamed TMJ when comparing the 5 day time point to the 10 day time point (Fig. 4E).

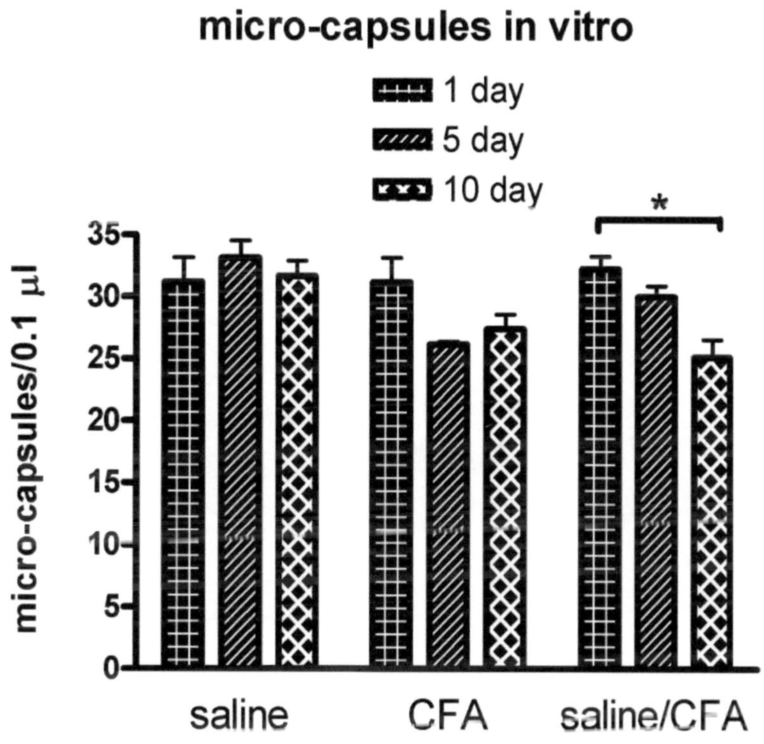

Fig. 2. Microcapsule breakdown in vitro. Microcapsules (approximately 80,000) were placed in 200 µl of three different solutions at a temperature of 37°C and the degradation of the microcapsules was monitored by counting the number of intact microcapsules remaining after 1, 5 and 10 days. The solutions the microcapsules were placed in consisted of either 1) 0.9% saline or 2) 15 µg/ml of CFA/water homogenate or 3) a 50%/50% homogenate of 0.9% saline and 15 µg/ml CFA. At each time point a 10 µl aliquote was removed and the number of microcapsules was counted in triplicate in a hemacytometer chamber. Values are the mean ± SEM.

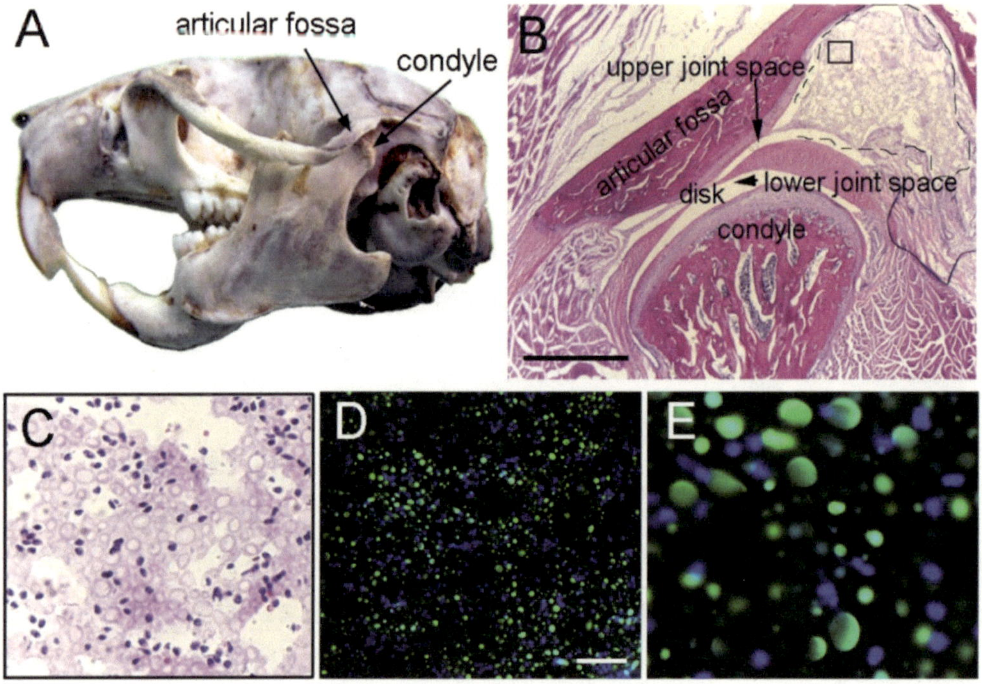

Fig. 3. Injection of gelatin microcapsules containing canola oil with Alexa 488 dye were injected into the upper joint space of a rat temporomandibular joint (TMJ). A) Sagittal view of a rat skull, arrows point to the TMJ condyle and articular fossa. In this experiment the TMJ upper joint space was injected with 30 μl of dye loaded microcapsules (90 mg microcapsules [dry weight] in 1 ml of Tris buffer or 0.9% saline and then the rats were sacrificed 5 hours later. B) Saggittal section of a rat TMJ 5 hours after injection of microcapsules into the upper joint space (arrow) stained with hemotoxylin and eosin. Dotted line in the upper joint space outlines the region containing the injected microcapsules. C) High magnification image of boxed region in panel B. D) Fluorescent image of Alexa 488 loaded microcapsules 5 hours after injection into the TMJ. Green is the Alexa 488 loaded microcapsules and blue is the DAPI stained cell nuclei. E) High magnification of image from panel D. Bar in panel B equals 1 mm and bar in panel D equals 100 μm.

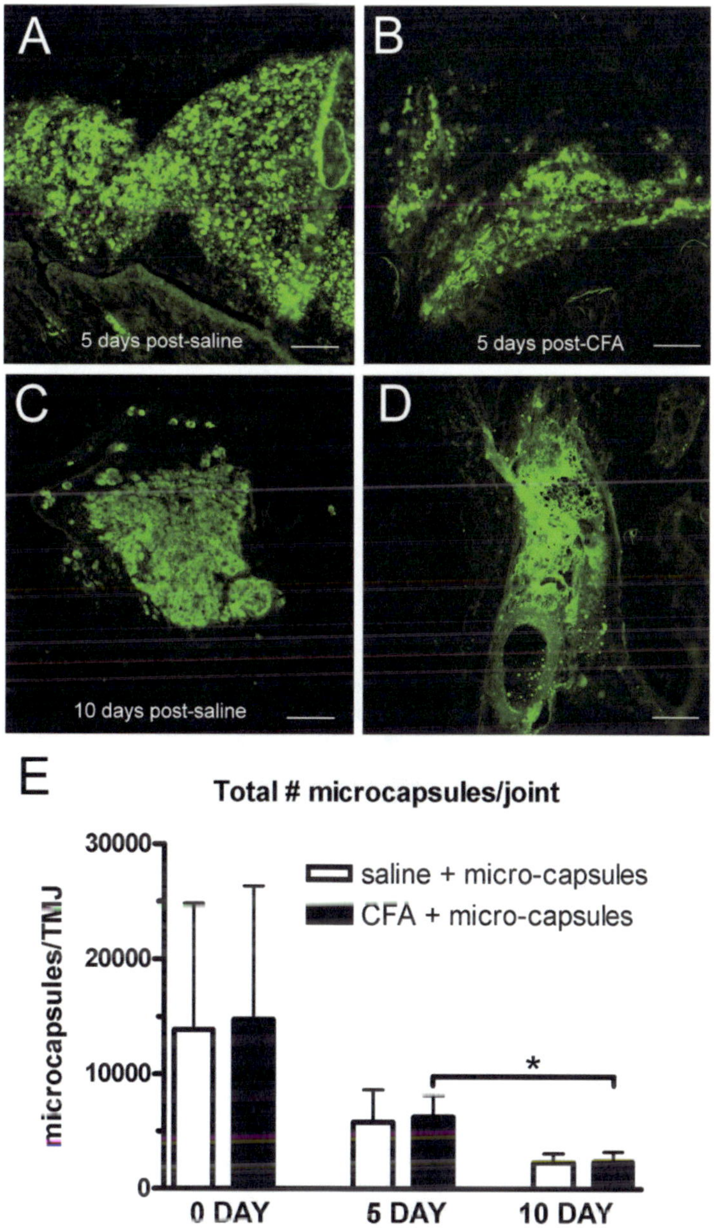

Fig. 4. Microcapsule breakdown in a non-arthritic and arthritic TMJ. Saline or 15 µg of CFA in 15 µl was injected into the TMJ followed by a second injection 24 hours later of 30 µl of dye loaded microcapsules. Microcapsules in the upper joint space/synovial tissue were imaged in sagittal sections of the TMJ tissue 5 and 10 days after injection of microcapsules. Images were captured 5 days after injecting the TMJ with microcapsules and saline (A) or CFA (B). Microcapsules in the upper joint space/synovial tissue was imaged 10 days after injection of microcapsules in a joint previously injected with saline (C) or CFA (D). The histogram below indicates the number of microcapsules counted per joint in rats sacrificed 0, 5 and 10 days after injection. There were 5 animals per group. Asterisk indicates $P<0.05$.

We next asked the question, would injection of microcapsules into the TMJ induce a pain response in the rat with a non-arthritic or an arthritic joint. To test the response to microcapsule injection we measured a behavioral correlate of nociception (meal duration) before and after injecting microcapsules into the TMJ of a rat previously injected with saline (non-arthritis) or CFA (arthritic). Microcapsule injection did not significantly increase the pain response in either the non-arthritic or arthritic joint (Fig. 5).

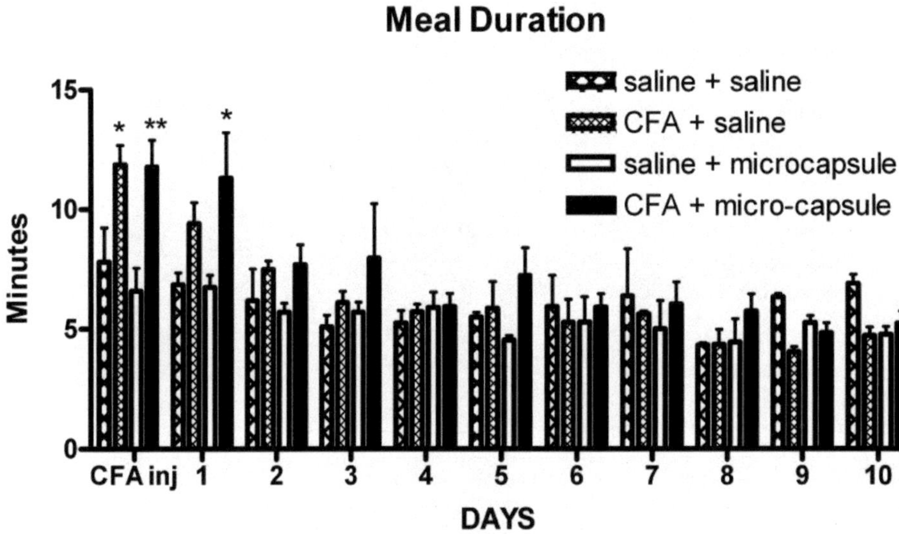

Fig. 5. Nociceptive response after injecting microcapsules into a non-arthritic and arthritic TMJ. Rats were injected with 30 μl 0.9% saline or 15 μg CFA (CFA inj) and then 24 hours later the rats were injected with either saline or 30 μl microcapsules in 0.9% saline. After injection of the microcapsules the meal duration was recorded for 10 days (1 through 10). There were 8 animals per group. *=P<0.05, **=P<0.01 when comparing the CFA + saline group to the saline + saline group and when comparing the CFA + microcapsule group to the saline + microcapsule group.

To test that the breakdown of beads in vivo may be due the presence of MMP-2 and MMP-9 we injected the microcapsules with an MMP-2/9 inhibitor. The number of microcapsules decreased over time in vivo but addition of a MMP-2/9 inhibitor had no significant effect on microcapsules degradation after injection into a rat TMJ (Fig. 6). The inhibition of the MMP-2/9 also did not affect the nociceptive response after injecting the TMJ with microcapsules (Fig. 7).

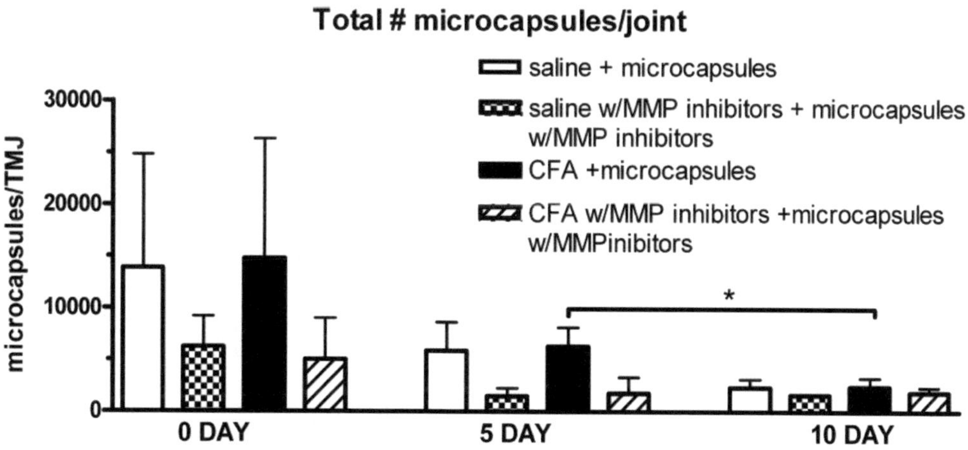

Fig. 6. Effect of metalloprotease inhibitor 2 and 9 on microcapsule breakdown in vivo Rats were injected with saline or CFA or saline with an MMP inhibitor or CFA with an MMP inhibitor added and then 24 hours later these groups of rats were injected with 30 μl microcapsules or microcapsules plus MMP inhibitor. All injections were into the superior joint space of the TMJ. The inhibitor was a 1 μM solution of the MMP-2/9 inhibitor IV. The histogram shows the total number of beads per joint after 0, 5 and 10 days after bead injection. There were 3-5 animals per group. *=P<0.05.

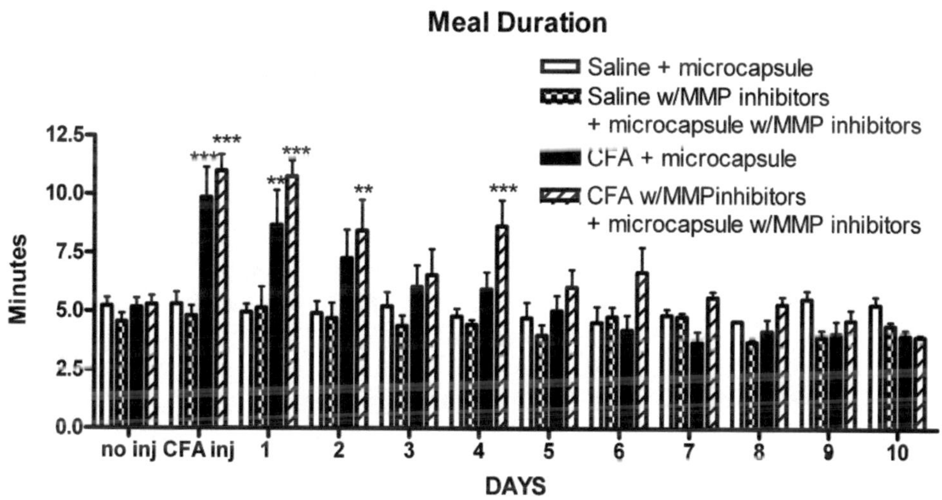

Fig. 7. Nociceptive response after injecting microcapsules along with metalloprotease inhibitors Rats were injected into the upper joint space of the TMJ with 30 μl saline or 15 μg CFA (CFA inj), some in combination with a MMP-2/9 inhibitor. One day after this injection a second 30 μl injection of microcapsules or microcapsules containing MMP-2/9 inhibitor was performed. Before and after injection the meal duration was recorded. No inj= before animal were injected. There were 8 animals per group. *=P<0.05, **=P<0.01, ***=P<0.001 when comparing CFA injected rats to the saline injected rats.

Ibuprofen drug loaded microcapsules did not significantly affect the nociceptive response (Fig. 8A) or the immune response (Fig. 8B) of CFA injected rats. Morphine loaded microcapsules did significantly decrease the nociceptive response ($p<0.05$, days 4 and 5) and post-hoc testing showed a significant decrease on the fourth day post-CFA injection (Fig. 8A).

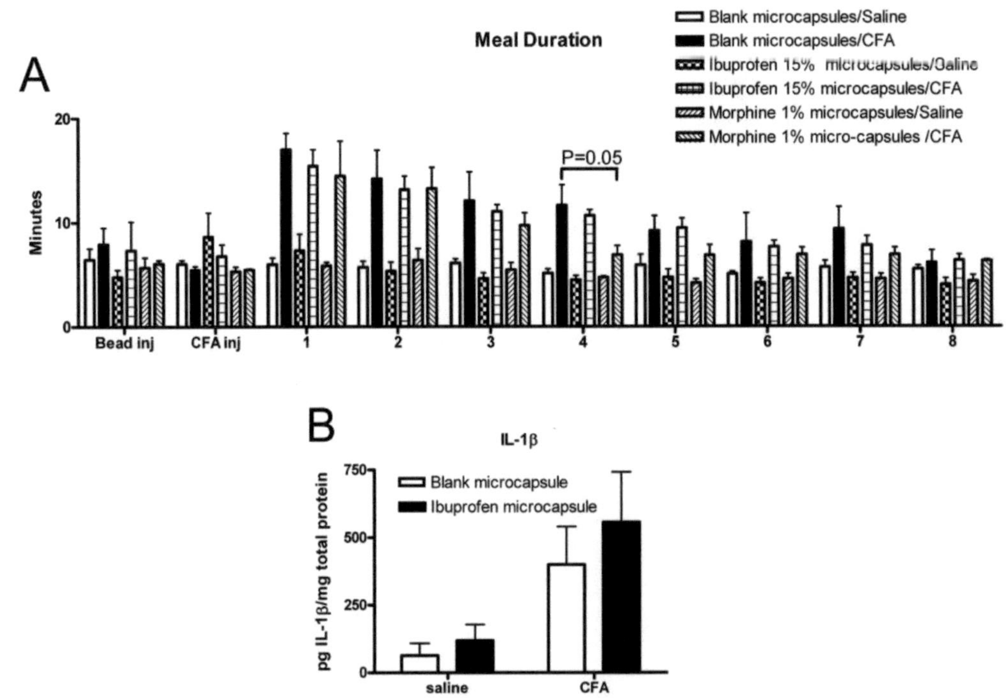

Fig. 8. Nociceptive and inflammatory response after injecting microcapsules containing ibuprofen or morphine. Rats TMJs were injected with a 30 μl solution of microcapsules (bead inj). The microcapsules contained oil (Blank microcapsules) or oil with 15% ibuprofen (Ibuprofen microcapsules) or oil containing 1% morphine (Morphine microcapsules). 24 hours after microcapsule injection the rats were subdivided further for TMJ injection of either saline or 15 μg CFA (CFA inj). A) Before and 8 days after injection of the saline/CFA the daily meal duration was recorded. There were 8 animals in each of the four treatment groups. B) The amount of IL-1β in the TMJ retrodiscal, synovial and disc tissue 7 days after injection with microcapsules. There were 3-4 animals in each of the four treatment groups for the cytokine analysis.

5. Discussion

Gelatin microcapsules have the capability for sustained drug release after intra-articular injection (Inoue, Takahashi, Arai, Tonomura, Sakao, Saito, Fujioka, Fujiwara, Tabata & Kubo, 2006; Lu, Zhang, Sun & Zhong, 2007; Saito, Takahashi, Arai, Inoue, Sakao, Tonomura, Honjo, Nakagawa, Inoue, Tabata & Kubo, 2009). Sustained drug delivery into a diseased TMJ has the potential to improve the treatment of TMJ pain and inflammation. In this report a rat model of TMJ inflammatory arthritis was used and we tested the effect of intra-articularly injected gelatin microcapsules on the nociceptive response as well as on the inflammatory response. Loading the gelatin microcapsules with the ibuprofen or morphine was accomplished because we hypothesized that intra-articular injection of drug loaded beads would reduce the nociceptive response. We determined that gelatin microcapsules do not increase IL-1β levels in the disc and synovial tissues after injection into the TMJ. Nor do the capsules increase the nociceptive response in an arthritic joint. Importantly, injection of morphine but not ibuprofen loaded microcapsules decreased the nociceptive response of a rat with an arthritic TMJ. Because injection of microcapsules loaded with morphine decreased the nociceptive response of a rat with inflammatory arthritis we expect that the microcapsules will amealorate the pain response in patients with TMJ disease.

5.1 TMJ intra-articular model for testing microcapsules

The premise of our animal (i.e., meal duration) model is that the CFA induced TMJ pain would affect the rat, such that, when a hungry animal initiated a meal the animal would eat slowly due to the TMJ pain associated with the movement of the mandible during the chewing process. This is exactly what we observed following bilateral TMJ CFA injections in males and females, i.e., the rats had longer meal durations (Harper, Kerins, Talwar, Spears, Hutchins, Carlson, McIntosh & Bellinger, 2000; Kerins, Carlson, Hinton, Grogan, Marr, Kramer, Spears & Bellinger, 2005; Kerins, Carlson, McIntosh & Bellinger, 2003). Support that meal duration is a measure for orofacial pain it that when ibuprofen is administered directly into a inflamed, CFA-injected TMJ meal duration was normal in both male and female rats (Kerins, Carlson, McIntosh & Bellinger, 2003). Our selection of CFA was made because it produces a persistent arthritic pain response that last for over two weeks (Hill, Bellinger, Spears, Hutchins, Kerins & Kramer, 2007; Ren, 1999). Thus, of all the agents, CFA was best when trying to establish long duration pain. Injection of CFA into the TMJ significantly lengthened meal duration in rats, while the same amount of CFA in the knee did not affect meal duration (Kerins, Carlson, Hinton, Grogan, Marr, Kramer, Spears & Bellinger, 2005) indicating meal duration is a specific measure of orofacial pain. Interestingly IL-1β remained significantly elevated in the TMJ of the ibuprofen treated animals injected with CFA (Kerins, Carlson, McIntosh & Bellinger, 2003), suggesting that some inflammation from the CFA injection remained. In another study, cyclooxgenase-II (COX-2) inhibitors normalized meal duration in rats after CFA injection (Kerins, Carlson, McIntosh & Bellinger, 2004). In this study the COX-2 inhibitor also attenuated the inflammation, i.e., TMJ tissue IL-1β normalized (Kerins, Carlson, McIntosh & Bellinger, 2004). In still another study, rats were given capsaicin or vehicle at 2 and 10 days of age; capsaicin permanently destroyed afferent nociceptive fibers in these animals (Bellinger, Spears, King, Dahm, Hutchins, Kerins & Kramer, 2007). When these male rats reached adulthood saline or CFA was injected into the TMJ and their meal duration was measured. Capsaicin treatment alone had no effect on meal duration, because saline injected, non-capsaicin treated rats had the same meal duration as saline injected, capsaicin treated rats. Non-capsaicin treated rats injected with CFA had longer meal durations than rats that were pre-treated with capsaicin, which demonstrated meal duration after CFA injection was normalized due to a capsaicin-induced loss of afferent nociceptive neuronal fibers (Bellinger, Spears, King, Dahm, Hutchins, Kerins & Kramer, 2007). The lack of change in meal duration in these capsaicin treated male rats occurred despite CFA inducing greater TMJ swelling, which demonstrated that the physical and mechanical changes in the inflamed TMJ synovial joint did not affect meal duration measurements. Another rationale for suggesting that meal duration is a measure of nociception stems from the finding that eating is impaired in patients with TMD (Haketa, Kino, Sugisaki, Amemori, Ishikawa, Shibuya, Sato & Yoshida, 2006) and from a clinical study of juvenile rheumatoid arthritic children (Harper, Brown, Triplett, Villasenor & Gatchel, 2000) that examined chewing performance as an objective measure of masticatory function. It showed that the juvenile rheumatoid arthritic children with TMD symptoms changed their chewing habits presumably to "guard" against pain. Most recently, meal duration in the rat was shown to be increased over the course of a week following pulp exposures demonstrating meal duration can also be used as a measure of tooth nociception (Bellinger, He & Kramer, 2010).

5.2 Sustained drug release by gelatin is safe and effective

Gelatin microcapsules are one type of sustained drug release mechanism that incorporates a shell of gelatin around a core of oil containing drug. One advantage of gelatin is it has been shown to be a safe means for sustained drug delivery because in vivo there is no inflammatory response (Brown, Leong, Huang, Dalal, Green, Haimes, Jimenez & Bathon, 1998; Tuncay, Calis, Kas, Ercan, Peksoy & Hincal, 2000) consistent with our result in the TMJ of a rat that showed injection of microcapsules did not increase the nociceptive response nor increased IL-1β levels in the TMJ. Studies using a shell of gelatin encapsulating oil containing drug demonstrated that uncrosslinked gelatin was effective when given orally (Jizomoto, Kanaoka, Sugita & Hirano, 1993). A previous pharmacokinetic study injecting gelatin microspheres containing NSAID show that the intra-articular concentration of NSAID was 8-fold higher 8 hours after injection versus the concentration of NSAID in a joint injected with a non-encapsulated solution of NSAID (Lu, Zhang, Sun & Zhong, 2007). Another recent study in a rabbit model indicated that intra-articular delivery of basic fibroblast growth factor or platelets via gelatin microspheres improved knee joint swelling, proteoglycan expression, and histological appearance of arthritic knee tissue (Inoue, Takahashi, Arai, Tonomura, Sakao, Saito, Fujioka, Fujiwara, Tabata & Kubo, 2006; Saito, Takahashi, Arai, Inoue, Sakao, Tonomura, Honjo, Nakagawa, Inoue, Tabata & Kubo, 2009). Our work is consistent with these results demonstrating microcapsule drug release can ameliorate arthritic TMJ pain. Future work would focus on encapsulating alternative drugs shown to be effective in relieving TMJ pain, such as mepivacaine (Zuniga, Ibanez & Kozacko, 2007).

5.3 Microcapsule size and thickness for in vivo injection

Thickness of the microcapsule wall can be varied and the timing of drug release would be based on the capsule cell wall thickness. What is important to keep in mind is that the microcapsules for this application need to be injectable and thus the diameter should not exceed the inner bore of the needle (e.g. 165 μM for a 29 gauge needle). As the wall of the bead becomes thicker the amount of loaded drug decreases thus, you inject less drug when using beads with a thicker wall diameter. Thus, a balance between the amount of time you want before drug release and the total amount of drug administered must be obtained. The diameter of the sphere is also important, with spheres greater than 26 μM remaining in the interstitial fluid of the tissue because they are not phagocytosed by cells (e.g., macrophages) (Horisawa, Kubota, Tuboi, Sato, Yamamoto, Takeuchi & Kawashima, 2002). The optimal size range for intra-articular drug delivery systems is application specific (Horisawa, Hirota, Kawazoe, Yamada, Yamamoto, Takeuchi & Kawashima, 2002; Horisawa, Kubota, Tuboi, Sato, Yamamoto, Takeuchi & Kawashima, 2002; Liggins, Cruz, Min, Liang, Hunter & Burt,

2004) but in this intra-articular paradigm we did not want intracellular drug release thus the bead diameter was approximately 30 μM.
In conclusion drug loaded gelatin microcapsules reduce the nociceptive response of an arthritic TMJ. These microcapsules are expected to be useful not only for the treatment of pain but also to modify the joint environment prior to implantation by delivering pro-regenerative signals in a spatially and temporally controlled fashion. The limitations of current therapeutic strategies for TMJ disorders have led to increased interest in tissue engineering strategies, which combine cells, bioactive factors, and implantable scaffolds to trigger joint regeneration (Detamore & Athanasiou, 2003). In addition to the added benefit of sustained drug release local administration of drug has the added benefit of avoiding systemic drug release which can result in ectopic effects.

6. References

[1] Bellinger, L. L., He, L., and Kramer, P. R., 2010, Meal duration; a measure of tooth and temporomadibular joint nociception.: American Association of Dental Research CD-ROM, p. 1267.5/AA31, Washington, DC.
[2] Bellinger, L. L. Spears, R. King, C. M. Dahm, F. Hutchins, B. Kerins, C. A. & Kramer, P. R. (2007), Capsaicin sensitive neurons role in the inflamed TMJ acute nociceptive response of female and male rats: *Physiology and Behavior*, Vol. 90, pp. 782-789.
[3] Bjornland, T. Rorvik, M. Haanaes, H. R. & Teige, J. (1994), Degenerative changes in the temporomandibular joint after diagnostic arthroscopy. An experimental study in goats.
[4] Bozdag, S. Calis, S. Kas, H. S. Ercan, M. T. Peksoy, I. & Hincal, A. A. (2001), In vitro evaluation and intra-articular administration of biodegradable microspheres containing naproxen sodium: *J Microencapsul.*, Vol. 18, pp. 443-456.
[5] Brown, K. E. Leong, K. Huang, C. H. Dalal, R. Green, G. D. Haimes, H. B. Jimenez, P. A. & Bathon, J. (1998), Gelatin/chondroitin 6-sulfate microspheres for the delivery of therapeutic proteins to the joint: *Arthritis Rheum*, Vol. 41, pp. 2185-2195.
[6] Bryant, C. J. Harrison, S. D. Hopper, C. & Harris, M. (1999), Use of intra-articular morphine for postoperative analgesia following TMJ arthroscopy: *British Journal of Oral and Maxillofacial Surgery*, Vol. 37, pp. 391-396.
[7] Davies, N. M. & Jamali, F. (2004), COX-2 selective inhibitors cardiac toxicity: getting to the heart of the matter: *J Pharm.Pharm.Sci*, Vol. 7, pp. 332-336.
[8] Deasy, P. B. (1994), Evaluation of drug-containing microcapsules: *J Microencapsul.*, Vol. 11, pp. 487-505.
[9] Detamore, M. S. & Athanasiou, K. A. (2003), Motivation, characterization, and strategy for tissue engineering the temporomandibular joint disc: *Tissue Eng*, Vol. 9, pp. 1065-1087.
[10] Fernandez-Carballido, A. Herrero-Vanrell, R. Molina-Martinez, I. T. & Pastoriza, P. (2004a), Biodegradable ibuprofen-loaded PLGA microspheres for intraarticular administration. Effect of Labrafil addition on release in vitro: *Int.J Pharm.*, Vol. 279, pp. 33-41.
[11] Fernandez-Carballido, A. Herrero-Vanrell, R. Molina-Martinez, I. T. & Pastoriza, P. (2004b), Sterilized ibuprofen-loaded poly(D,L-lactide-co-glycolide) microspheres for intra-articular administration: effect of gamma-irradiation and storage: *J Microencapsul.*, Vol. 21, pp. 653-665.

[12] Fritz, J. Thomas, C. Tzaribachev, N. Horger, M. S. Claussen, C. D. Lewin, J. S. & Pereira, P. L. (2009), MRI-guided injection procedures of the temporomandibular joints in children and adults: technique, accuracy, and safety.

[13] Gerwin, N. Hops, C. & Lucke, A. (2006), Intraarticular drug delivery in osteoarthritis: *Adv.Drug Deliv.Rev.*, Vol. 58, pp. 226-242.

[14] Haketa, T. Kino, K. Sugisaki, M. Amemori, Y. Ishikawa, T. Shibuya, T. Sato, F. & Yoshida, N. (2006), Difficulty of food intake in patients with temporomandibular disorders: *Int J Prosthodont.*, Vol. 19, pp. 266-270

[15] Harper, R. P. Brown, C. M. Triplett, M. M. Villasenor, A. & Gatchel, R. J. (2000), Masticatory function in patients with juvenile rheumatoid arthritis: *Pediatr.Dent.*, Vol. 22, pp. 200-206.

[16] Harper, R. P. Kerins, C. A. Talwar, R. Spears, R. Hutchins, B. Carlson, D. S. McIntosh, J. E. & Bellinger, L. L. (2000), Meal pattern analysis in response to temporomandibular joint inflammation in the rat: *J.Dent.Res.*, Vol. 79, pp. 1704-1711.

[17] Hayakawa, Y. Kober, C. Otonari-Yamamoto, M. Otonari, T. Wakoh, M. & Sano, T. (2007), An approach for three-dimensional visualization using high-resolution MRI of the temporomandibular joint: *Dentomaxillofac.Radiol.*, Vol. 36, pp. 341-347.

[18] Hill, G., Bellinger, L. L., Spears, R., Hutchins, B., Kerins, C., and Kramer, P. R., 2007, Operant behavioral model for studying persistent orofacial nociception: The Winter Conference on Animal Learning and Behavior, Winter Park, CO.

[19] Horisawa, E. Hirota, T. Kawazoe, S. Yamada, J. Yamamoto, H. Takeuchi, H. & Kawashima, Y. (2002), Prolonged anti-inflammatory action of DL-lactide/glycolide copolymer nanospheres containing betamethasone sodium phosphate for an intra-articular delivery system in antigen-induced arthritic rabbit: *Pharm.Res*, Vol. 19, pp. 403-410.

[20] Horisawa, E. Kubota, K. Tuboi, I. Sato, K. Yamamoto, H. Takeuchi, H. & Kawashima, Y. (2002), Size-dependency of DL-lactide/glycolide copolymer particulates for intra-articular delivery system on phagocytosis in rat synovium: *Pharm.Res.*, Vol. 19, pp. 132-139.

[21] Inoue, A. Takahashi, K. A. Arai, Y. Tonomura, H. Sakao, K. Saito, M. Fujioka, M. Fujiwara, H. Tabata, Y. & Kubo, T. (2006), The therapeutic effects of basic fibroblast growth factor contained in gelatin hydrogel microspheres on experimental osteoarthritis in the rabbit knee: *Arthritis Rheum*, Vol. 54, pp. 264-270.

[22] Jizomoto, H. Kanaoka, E. Sugita, K. & Hirano, K. (1993), Gelatin-acacia microcapsules for trapping micro oil droplets containing lipophilic drugs and ready disintegration in the gastrointestinal tract: *Pharm.Res*, Vol. 10, pp. 1115-1122.

[23] Kanyama, M. Kuboki, T. Kojima, S. Fujisawa, T. Hattori, T. Takigawa, M. & Yamashita, A. (2000), Matrix metalloproteinases and tissue inhibitors of metalloproteinases in synovial fluids of patients with temporomandibular joint osteoarthritis: *J Orofac.Pain.*, Vol. 14, pp. 20-30.

[24] Kerins, C. A. Carlson, D. S. Hinton, R. J. Grogan, D. M. Marr, K. Kramer, P. R. Spears, R. D. & Bellinger, L. L. (2005), Specificity of meal pattern analysis as an animal model of dermining temporomandibular joint inflammation/pain: *International Journal of Oral Maxiollofacial Surgery*, Vol. 34, pp. 425-431.

[25] Kerins, C. A. Carlson, D. S. McIntosh, J. E. & Bellinger, L. L. (2003), Meal pattern changes associated with temporomandibular joint inflammation/pain in rats; analgesic effects: *Pharmacology Biochemistry and Behavior*, Vol. 75, pp. 181-189.

[26] Kerins, C. Carlson, D. McIntosh, J. & Bellinger, L. (2004), A role for cyclooxygenase II inhibitors in modulating temporomandibular joint inflammation from a meal pattern analysis perspective: *J Oral Maxillofac Surg*, Vol. 62, pp. 989-995.

[27] Kramer, P. R. & Bellinger, L. L. (2009), The effects of cycling levels of 17beta-estradiol and progesterone on the magnitude of temporomandibular joint-induced nociception: *Endocrinology*, Vol. 150, pp. 3680-3689.

[28] Liggins, R. T. Cruz, T. Min, W. Liang, L. Hunter, W. L. & Burt, H. M. (2004), Intra-articular treatment of arthritis with microsphere formulations of paclitaxel: biocompatibility and efficacy determinations in rabbits: *Inflamm.Res*, Vol. 53, pp. 363-372.

[29] Lin, Y. Weisdorf, D. J. Solovey, A. & Hebbel, R. P. (2000), Origins of circulating endothelial cells and endothelial outgrowth from blood: *J.Clin.Invest*, Vol. 105, pp. 71-77.

[30] Lu, Y. Zhang, G. Sun, D. & Zhong, Y. (2007), Preparation and evaluation of biodegradable flubiprofen gelatin micro-spheres for intra-articular administration: *J Microencapsul.*, Vol. 24, pp. 515-524.

[31] Manfredini, D. Chiappe, G. & Bosco, M. (2006), Research diagnostic criteria for temporomandibular disorders (RDC/TMD) axis I diagnoses in an Italian patient population: *J Oral Rehabil.*, Vol. 33, pp. 551-558.

[32] Mercadante, S. (1999), Problems of long-term spinal opioid treatment in advanced cancer patients: *Pain*, Vol. 79, pp. 1-13.

[33] Mountziaris, P. M. Kramer, P. R. & Mikos, A. G. (2009), Emerging intra-articular drug delivery systems for the temporomandibular joint: *Methods*, Vol. 47, pp. 134-140.

[34] Mukherjee, D. Nissen, S. E. & Topol, E. J. (2001), Risk of cardiovascular events associated with selective COX-2 inhibitors: *JAMA: The Journal of the American Medical Association*, Vol. 286, pp. 954-959.

[35] Plesh, O. Sinisi, S. E. Crawford, P. B. & Gansky, S. A. (2005), Diagnoses based on the Research Diagnostic Criteria for Temporomandibular Disorders in a biracial population of young women: *J Orofac.Pain.*, Vol. 19, pp. 65-75.

[36] Puebla, P. Pastoriza, P. Barcia, E. & Fernandez-Carballido, A. (2005), PEG-derivative effectively modifies the characteristics of indomethacin PLGA microspheres destined to intra-articular administration: *J Microencapsul.*, Vol. 22, pp. 793-808.

[37] Ren, K. (1999), An improved method for assessing mechanical allodynia in the rat: *Physiology and Behavior*, Vol. 67, pp. 711-716.

[38] Saito, M. Takahashi, K. A. Arai, Y. Inoue, A. Sakao, K. Tonomura, H. Honjo, K. Nakagawa, S. Inoue, H. Tabata, Y. & Kubo, T. (2009), Intraarticular administration of platelet-rich plasma with biodegradable gelatin hydrogel microspheres prevents osteoarthritis progression in the rabbit knee: *Clin Exp Rheumatol.*, Vol. 27, pp. 201-207.

[39] Srinivas, R. Sorsa, T. Tjaderhane, L. Niemi, E. Raustia, A. Pernu, H. Teronen, O. & Salo, T. (2001), Matrix metalloproteinases in mild and severe temporomandibular joint internal derangement synovial fluid: *Oral Surg.Oral Med Oral Pathol.Oral Radiol.Endod.*, Vol. 91, pp. 517-525.

[40] Sugisaki, M. Ikai, A. & Tanabe, H. (1995), Dangerous angles and depths for middle ear and middle cranial fossa injury during arthroscopy of the temporomandibular joint.
[41] Swift, J. Q. Roszkowski, M. T. Alton, T. & Hargreaves, K. M. (1998), Effect of intra-articular versus systemic anti-inflammatory drugs in a rabbit model of temporomandibular joint inflammation: *J Oral Maxillofac Surg*, Vol. 56, pp. 1288-1295.
[42] Tanaka, E. Detamore, M. S. & Mercuri, L. G. (2008), Degenerative disorders of the temporomandibular joint: etiology, diagnosis, and treatment: *J Dent Res*, Vol. 87, pp. 296-307.
[43] Thut, P. D. Hermanstyne, T. O. Flake, N. M. & Gold, M. S. (2007), An operant conditioning model to assess changes in feeding behavior associated with temporomandibular joint inflammation in the rat: *J Orofac.Pain*, Vol. 21, pp. 7-18.
[44] Tuncay, M. Calis, S. Kas, H. S. Ercan, M. T. Peksoy, I. & Hincal, A. A. (2000), Diclofenac sodium incorporated PLGA (50:50) microspheres: formulation considerations and in vitro/in vivo evaluation: *Int.J Pharm.*, Vol. 195, pp. 179-188.
[45] West, M. J. & Slomanka, L. (2001), 2-D versus 3-D cell counting--a debate. What is an optical disector?: *Trends Neurosci.*, Vol. 24, pp. 374-380.
[46] Westesson, P. L. Eriksson, L. & Liedberg, J. (1986), The risk of damage to facial nerve, superficial temporal vessels, disk, and articular surfaces during arthroscopic examination of the temporomandibular joint.
[47] Yoshida, K. Takatsuka, S. Hatada, E. Nakamura, H. Tanaka, A. Ueki, K. Nakagawa, K. Okada, Y. Yamamoto, E. & Fukuda, R. (2006), Expression of matrix metalloproteinases and aggrecanase in the synovial fluids of patients with symptomatic temporomandibular disorders: *Oral Surg.Oral Med Oral Pathol.Oral Radiol.Endod.*, Vol. 102, pp. 22-27.
[48] Zuniga, J. R. Ibanez, C. & Kozacko, M. (2007), The analgesic efficacy and safety of intra-articular morphine and mepivicaine following temporomandibular joint arthroplasty: *J Oral Maxillofac Surg*, Vol. 65, pp. 1477-1485.

Part 3

Loosening

14

Risk Factors for Aseptic Loosening Following Total Hip Arthroplasty

Scott J. MacInnes, Andrew Gordon and J. Mark Wilkinson
Academic Unit of Bone Metabolism and Department of Orthopaedics, University of Sheffield, Sheffield, United Kingdom

1. Introduction

Total hip arthroplasty (THA) is one of the most successful orthopaedic procedures and has relieved pain and improved hip function in millions of patients worldwide. Despite the success of modern prosthetic designs and bearing surfaces, around 10% of THA prostheses still fail within 10 years[1]. Improvements in surgical technique and prosthesis design have decreased the incidence of deep sepsis, dislocation and fracture, however aseptic loosening, the clinical end point of osteolysis, remains the most frequent complication and in the UK accounts for 63% of all revision surgery (Table 1)[2]. Prosthesis loosening results in pain and disability, requiring revision surgery. Revision THA is associated with a 3 to 8-fold greater in-hospital mortality, poorer functional outcome, longer hospital stay, and higher cost than primary surgery[1,3-5].

The problem of osteolysis has been recognized in Judet's acrylic hemiarthroplasty introduced in the 1940s. Prosthesis loosening complicating THA in the 1950's and 1960's was poorly understood and attributed to unconfirmed sepsis[6] and prosthesis motion[7]. In the 1980's loosening was thought to be the result of "cement disease"[8], arising due to a foreign body reaction to methyl methacrylate. When the development of cementless prostheses

National Joint Registry hip Annual Report Data 2009		
	Number	%
Total procedures	72,432	
Primary procedures	65,229	90%
Revision procedures	7,203	10%
Indication for revision		
Aseptic Loosening	3,524	49%
Osteolysis	999	14%
Pain	2,035	29%
Infection	1,020	14%
Dislocation/ subluxation	1,141	16%
Periprosthetic fracture	618	9%

Table 1. Summary of hip surgery data from 7th Annual Report National Joint Registry for England and Wales[2]

failed to eliminate this problem, wear at the bearing couple was subsequently identified as the main source of particulate debris giving rise to osteolysis.

Advances in prosthesis materials, design and surgical technique have improved the wear performance of prostheses, which will decrease the future incidence of osteolysis. However, an ageing population combined with younger more active patients now undergoing joint arthroplasty suggests that osteolysis and resulting prosthesis loosening will continue to be the major complication of THA.

2. Pathophysiology of osteolysis

The term aseptic loosening describes mechanical failure of the prosthesis-host interface, and arises primarily as the end result of focal periprosthetic inflammatory bone loss occurring at this interface. This pro-inflammatory microenvironment is driven by particulate wear debris, which is generated primarily at the articular bearing surface and at other non-articular prosthesis or cement surfaces[9]. Willert first proposed the involvement of prosthetic debris in the development of oesteolysis. He identified a resultant foreign body reaction and granuloma formation which included macrophages and multinucleated giant cells[10]. This foreign body reaction has subsequently been reproduced in animal models[11]. Once particulate wear debris has been dispersed into the joint fluid it may initiate a foreign body reaction at contact surfaces with the host tissues. Schmalzried coined the term "effective joint space" to describe all areas where open communication with the joint pseudo-capsule may allow circulation of the joint fluid and particulate debris[12]. The effective joint space is thus dynamic and may advance along a tissue plane as osteolysis progresses. Variations in hydrostatic pressure within the joint space during activity may contribute to this circulation[12].

As well as its role in the migration of wear particles, hydrostatic fluid pressure changes within the joint have been implicated as an osteolytic stimulus. Aspenberg showed in an animal model that fluid pressure alone can lead to osteolysis[13]. Skoglund also showed that the osteolytic effect of fluid pressure on the bone was greater than that of particles[14]. However, it remains unclear what contribution this potential mechanism makes to the development of osteolysis clinically. Early migration of the femoral component may predict early and mid-term prosthesis failure. It has been suggested that this migration may lead to instability resulting in locally high fluid pressures which may, in turn, lead to osteolysis[15]. However, it is also likely that the predictive value of early migration measurements is due to the identification of failures of initial prosthesis fixation, resulting in loosening due to technical failure.

3. The biology of osteolysis

The process of aseptic loosening is characteristically accompanied with the development of a fibrous membrane at the bone-cement interface. Histological analysis of this membrane has shown a synovial-like fibrovascular tissue containing cells including macrophages, fibroblasts and foreign body giant cells[9,16]. The predominant cell types driving osteolysis, the macrophage and fibroblast, signal through various pro-inflammatory cytokines (including the interleukins, TNF alpha, and vascular endothelial growth factor VEGF) following either phagocytosis of the particles or through surface contact[17].

The biological process through which wear particles induce this inflammatory response is still not fully understood. It has become clear that the innate immune system is involved in the initiation of the biological response. The innate immune system is the body's first defense against foreign pathogens. Its ability to recognize and eliminate pathogens relies on pattern recognition receptors (PRR). PRRs are expressed by several cells in the monocyte cell lineage and include toll-like receptors (TLR) and the NOD-like receptors (NLR). These subfamilies evoke an inflammatory response either through the activation of transcription factors or through the formation of inflammasomes (Figure 1). Inflammasomes are large cytoplasmic complexes that activate inflammatory caspases required for the catalysis of pro-IL-1β and pro-IL-18 into their active forms[18]. Disorders of inflammasome signaling are associated with a number of auto-inflammatory conditions.

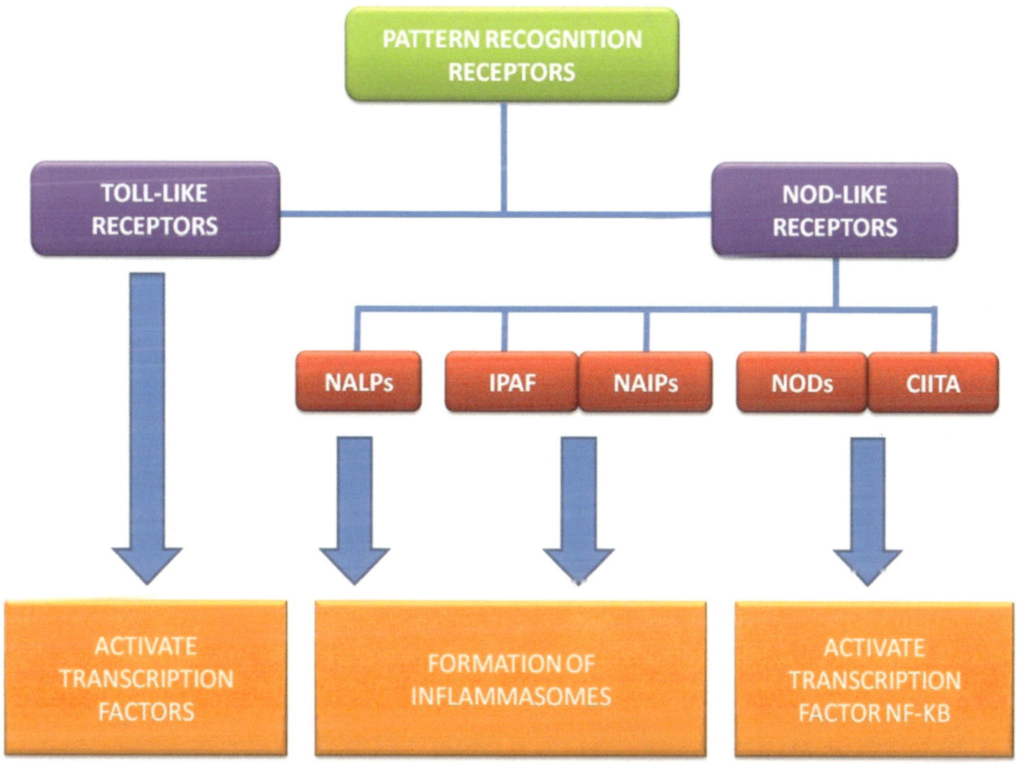

Fig. 1. Summary of pattern recognition receptors and their effector pathways. NALP = NACHT, LRR and PYD domain-containing proteins, IPAF = Ice protease activating factor, NAIP = neuronal apoptosis inhibitory protein, NOD = nucleotide-binding oligomerization domain proteins, CIITA = Major histocompatibility complex class-2 transactivator

Caicedo et al found that metal implant debris stimulated an inflammatory response in macrophages through inflammasome signaling (Figure 2)[19]. Maitra found that UHMWPE wear particles are phagocytosed causing intracellular activation of NACHT, LRR and PYD domains-containing protein 3 (NLRP3) leading to inflammasome formation. In addition alkane polymers generated by UHMWPE activate TLRs through cell surface contact. This leads to the activation of transcription factors including NF-KB resulting in cytokine release[20]. St Pierre *et al* showed in a mouse model that titanium particles also induce an inflammatory response through the activation of the NLRP3 inflammasome[21].

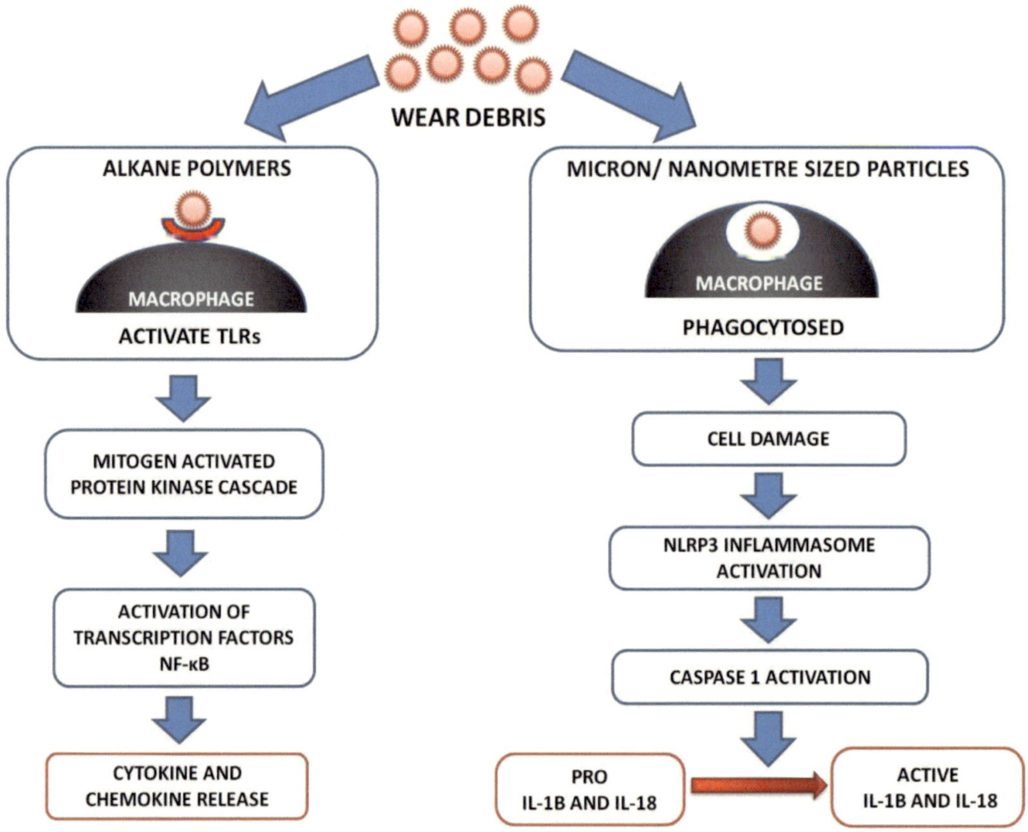

Fig. 2. Toll-like receptor and inflammasome signaling in response to wear debris

The released pro-inflammatory cytokines, in turn, modulate the activation of other cell types in the periprosthetic environment, including osteoblasts. Osteoblasts closely interact with osteoclasts in coupled bone remodeling, regulating bone resorption through the activation of osteoclasts[22]. Activated osteoblasts stimulate the monocyte / macrophage cell lineage through activation of receptor activator of nuclear factor κ B (RANK) by its ligand (RANKL) and macrophage colony stimulating factor (M-CSF). Together these induce expression of genes required for the development and maturation of polykaryon osteoclasts and activation of their function of bone resorption[23]. This upregulation of periprosthetic bone resorption results in failure of the integrity of the prosthesis-host construct and loosening of the prosthesis. Activated macrophages also produce matrix metalloproteinases (MMPs) that directly degrade demineralized collagen matrix.

Fibroblasts are the most frequent cell type found in the loosening membrane, and also play a role in the pathogenesis of osteolysis. They produce the fibrous collagenous matrix which surrounds the prosthesis and in addition, secrete RANKL and IL-6 which are both osteoclastogenic and stimulate the formation of multinucleated giant cells[24,25]. In addition to upregulation of the osteoclastic response, particulate debris suppresses differentiation of mesenchymal stem cells (MSC) into mature functioning osteoblasts and reduces synthetic activity of mature osteoblasts further shifting turnover balance in favor of net bone loss[26].

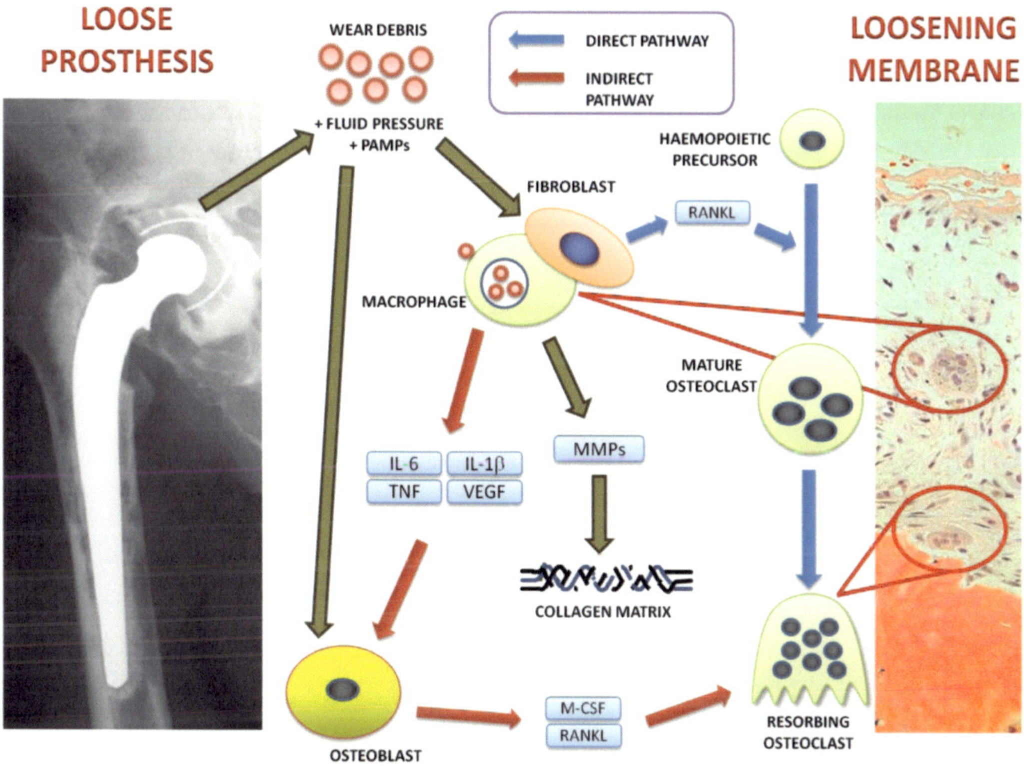

Fig. 3. Summary of biological response to wear debris. Recruitment and activation of osteoclasts may occur directly through the production of RANKL by fibroblasts, or indirectly through the production of pro-inflammatory cytokines that stimulate the production of RANKL by the osteoblast. TNF may stimulate osteoclast differentiation and activation through both routes.

other cell types may also be involved in the inflammatory response to wear particulate debris. These include lymphocytes and mast cells. The presence of lymphocytes suggests involvement of the adaptive immune system. It is suggested that particulate debris may undergo opsonisation which allows them to be targeted by B and T lymphocytes. Degranulated mast cells have been found in the periprosthetic tissue surrounding loose prostheses confirming their activation in the process of osteolysis[27]

Although aseptic loosening, by definition, occurs in the absence of bacterial infection, recent evidence suggests that bacterial endotoxin may contribute. Gram-positive and gram-negative bacteria produce (as constituent components of their cell walls or as toxins) a number of molecules including endotoxins and peptidoglycans, collectively termed pathogen associated molecular patterns (PAMPs) that act as ligands for PRRs. The presence of PAMPs has been confirmed in the periprosthetic tissue of patients undergoing revision surgery for aseptic loosening[28]. Using RNA gene sequencing, the presence of bacteria in the periprosthetic biofilm surrounding loose prostheses has also now been confirmed[29]. It has been shown both in vitro and in animal models that PAMPs adherent to particulate debris activate PRRs on macrophages, increasing the biological activity of wear particles[30].

4. Risk factors for osteolysis

Although the final pathway to the development of aseptic loosening is process of mechanical failure of the construct driven by inflammatory-mediated bone loss, multiple factors mediate an individual's susceptibility to this process. These may broadly be divided into patient, surgical, and prosthesis-related factors (Figure 4). Although not an exhaustive list, some of these proposed factors that have been identified and validated will be discussed.

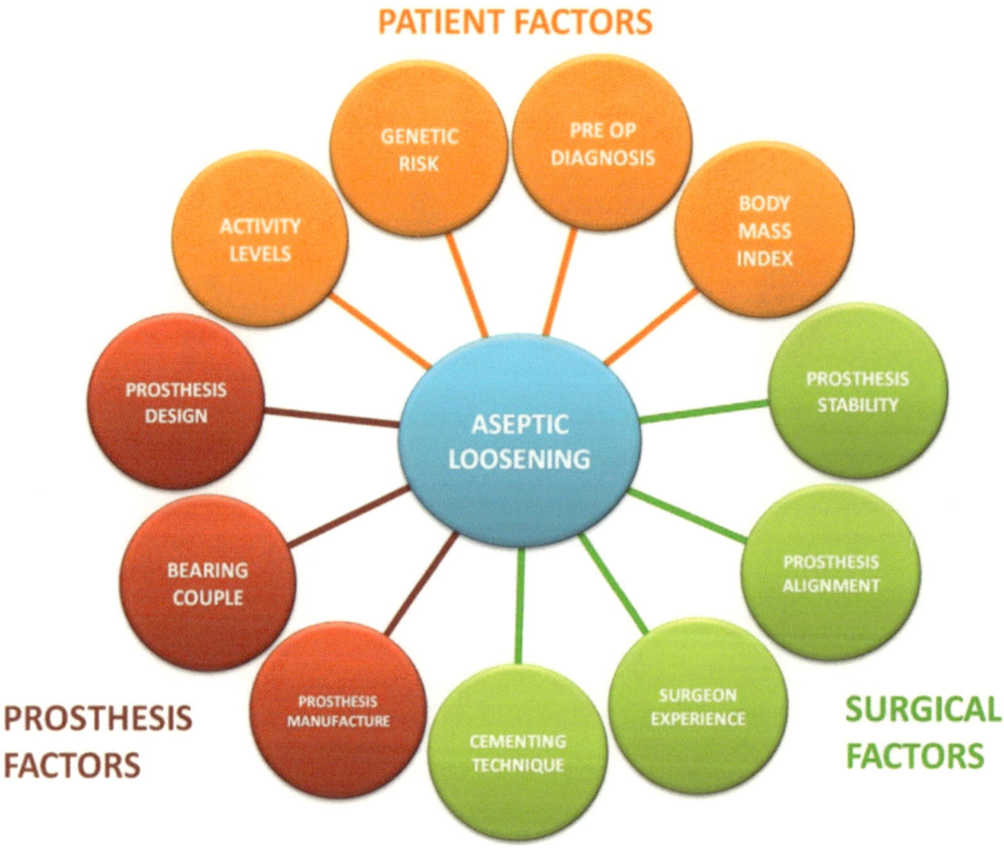

Fig. 4. Summary of risk factors that influence the development of aseptic loosening

5. Patient risk factors

5.1 Preoperative diagnosis

The most common indication for THA is idiopathic osteoarthritis. Within this diagnosis group, those with an atrophic pattern of bone response to osteoarthritis are at increased risk of acetabular prosthesis loosening[31]. Proximal femoral bone geometry may also affect prosthesis survival, with large non-tapering femoral canal shape (stove-pipe) being associated with an increased risk of aseptic loosening[31].

Higher rates of prosthesis loosening also occur in patients who have undergone arthroplasty for post-traumatic arthritis and osteonecrosis when compared with primary osteoarthritis. However, it is thought that this finding may relate to higher activity levels and increased bearing surface wear, rather than being a function of the pre-operative diagnosis[32,33].

A number of preoperative diagnoses carry a possible increased risk of prosthesis failure through associated medication. Patients taking systemic steroids have been found to have a higher risk of reoperation[34]. Non-steroidal anti-inflammatory drugs (NSAIDs) have been implicated in impaired bone healing, and patients taking NSAIDs have higher reoperation rates, although NSAID use may be acting as a marker of a painful prosthesis rather than contributing directly to prosthesis failure[34].

Poorer prosthesis survival might be expected in patients with inflammatory arthropathy due to its inflammatory pathogenesis and the historic frequent use of corticosteroids in its treatment (that are associated with loss of bone mass through osteoblast suppression). However, Furnes *et al*, in a large arthroplasty registry-based study, found no difference in THA survival between patients with rheumatoid arthritis versus those with osteoarthritis[35]. Rud-Sorensen *et al* found that the risk of stem revision due to aseptic loosening was lower in rheumatoid patients versus primary osteoarthritis, whilst acetabular prosthesis survival was similar[36].

Furnes *et al* and Bordini *et al* have reported higher acetabular revision rates due to aseptic loosening in patients with a primary diagnosis of developmental dyplasia of the hip compared to primary osteoarthritis[37,38]. Rates of acetabular prosthesis failure are higher in younger patients and those with greater graft coverage of the cup[39]. The role of these factors is unclear, but may relate to activity levels, or mechanical factors influencing prosthesis support.

5.2 Body mass index and obesity

The Health Survey for England 2009 showed that over the last 16 years there has been marked increase in the proportion of the population that are obese. This proportion increased from 13% of men in 1993 to 22% in 2009 and from 16% of women in 1993 to 24% in 2009[40]. The mean BMI of a patient undergoing THA in England and Wales has increased over the last 5 years from 27.4 to 28.4. Likewise the percentage of patients classed as either obese or morbidly obese has risen from 29% in 2004 to 37%

Historically, obesity has been deemed a relative contraindication for THA[41], as the joint reaction force experienced at the hip is directly proportional to body weight, and thus obesity was considered a risk factor for prosthesis failure. Obesity is associated with a higher incidence of perioperative complications including cardiovascular and respiratory events[42], venous thrombosis[43], wound infection[44], and dislocation[45]. However, despite the increase in joint load in these patients, no consistent increase in bearing wear or osteolysis has been shown across study populations[46,47] and thus obesity is not a clear risk factor for osteolysis.

5.3 Bearing-surface wear and activity level

Patient activity level associates with osteolysis. It is thought this association operates primarily though the production of wear of the bearing surface. Flugsrud showed that patients who undertake intermediate to intense activity are four times more likely than the less-active to develop acetabular prosthesis loosening[48]. A recent study with five to ten year

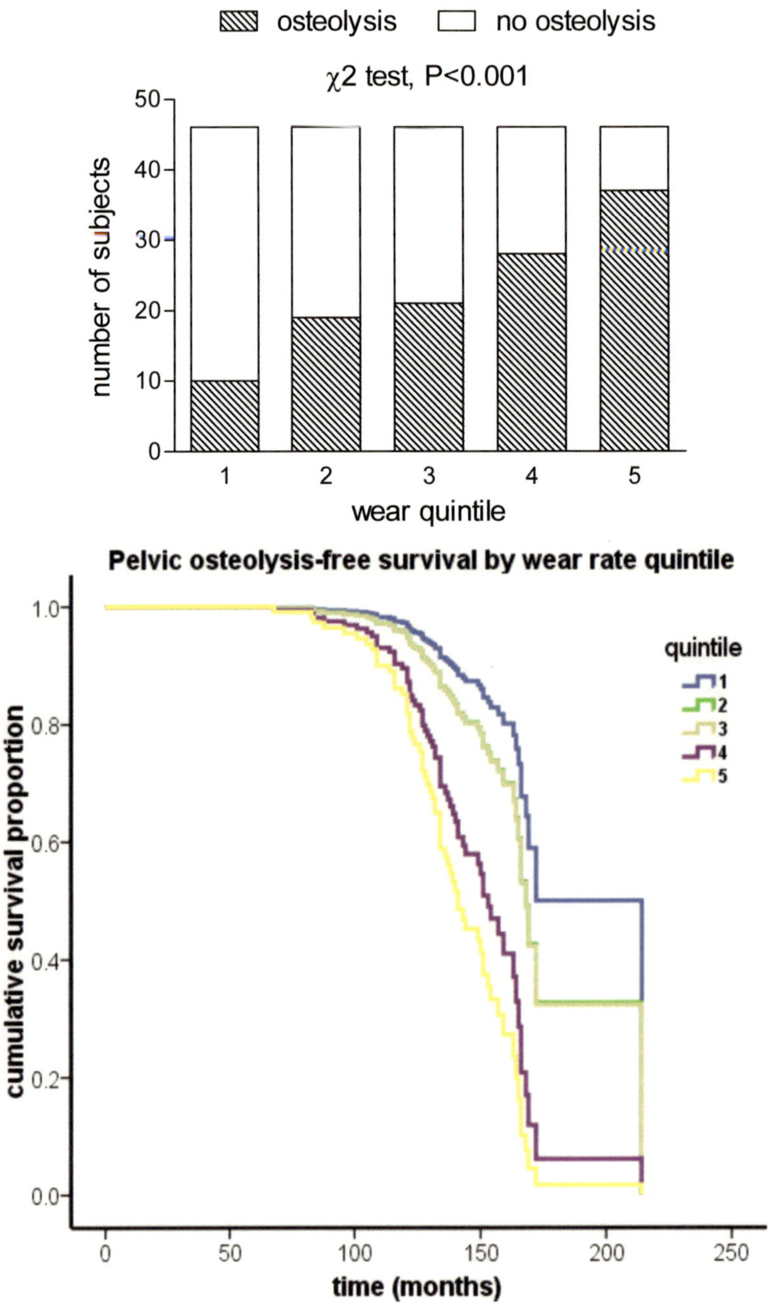

Fig. 5. Continuous dose-response relationship between prosthesis bearing wear and risk of osteolysis. Top panel shows data from a study of 115 cases and 115 controls after Charnley THA with consistent increase in proportion of subjects with osteolysis with increasing wear rate (by quintile)[57]. Bottom panel shows survivorship analysis in a cohort study of 319 hybrid THAs followed for a minimum of 10 years, and showing a similar dose-response relationship between osteolysis and polyethylene wear[58].

follow up has shown that 24% of patients who have engaged in high levels of activity developed femoral osteolysis, and had higher revision rates[49].

Traditionally the rate of polyethylene wear has been reported as a function of time. The results from ex-vivo hip simulator experiments have shown that the number of hip cycles is proportional to the rate of wear of prosthesis surface[50]. In vivo, there is a great range of wear rates between individual as a consequence of differing activity levels[51]. Several validated assessment tools have been developed to measure activity levels in arthroplasty populations[52], and Schmalzried *et al* showed that wear in patients is a function of activity[53]. There are no clear guidelines outlining what levels of activity can be undertaken following THA although the proportion of patients participating in athletic activity following THA ranges between 52 - 83%[54-56]. Whilst low-impact activities such as walking, swimming and cycling have always been recommended following THA, some patients participate in more high-impact and competitive sports. The increasing participation in athletic activity and higher post-operative expectations can partly be explained by the increasing numbers of younger patients undergoing THA. 42% of men and 31% of women who underwent THA in England and Wales in 2009 were under the age of 65 years[2]. A large number of patients over the age of 65 are also participating in high levels of activity[49].

Several investigators have shown a relationship between high levels of polyethylene wear and osteolysis/aseptic loosening, and the concept of a wear-rate 'threshold' (commonly defined as 0.1mm/year) below which osteolysis occurs very rarely, has been suggested. Wilkinson et al quantitated the association between wear and osteolysis and found no evidence to support this concept. In a case-control study of 230 hips after cemented Charnley THA with a metal on polyethylene bearing they showed that the risk of osteolysis increased with each quintile increase in wear, from very low levels of wear, below the suggested threshold, through to high levels[57]. They subsequently showed that the risk of osteolysis showed a similar pattern of consistently increasing risk ratio with each wear rate quintile in a separate cohort study of patients with 319 hybrid THAs using a metal on conventional polyethylene bearing (Figure 5).

5.4 Genetic factors

Within a given ethnic population the sequence of DNA between individuals is 99.5% identical. However, variability within the code does occur and gives rises to the phenotypic variability within the population. These variants occur at approximately every 1000 nucleotide base pairs of the code. This variation, where it occurs in >1% of the population is termed a polymorphism. The most common type of variant is a single letter change in the DNA sequence, termed a single nucleotide polymorphism (SNP). There are thought to be around 10 million common SNPs in the human genome. The individual specific risk of common diseases is thought to be influenced by the sum of many genetic variations, each potentially causing small changes in biological function and consequently subtle changes in phenotype[59].

Patients vary in their osteolytic response to particulate wear debris. Some show little bone resorption in the presence of marked prosthesis wear whereas others undergo marked osteolysis following a small amount of prosthesis wear (Figure 6)[57]. Macrophage responsiveness to in-vitro particulate debris stimulation also varies between individual[60], and monocytes (PBMCs) taken from patients with a susceptibility to osteolysis exhibit quantitatively greater inducible cytokine responses to particulate debris in-vitro versus patients without this susceptibility[61] . It is suggested that this inter-patient variability may have a genctic basis.

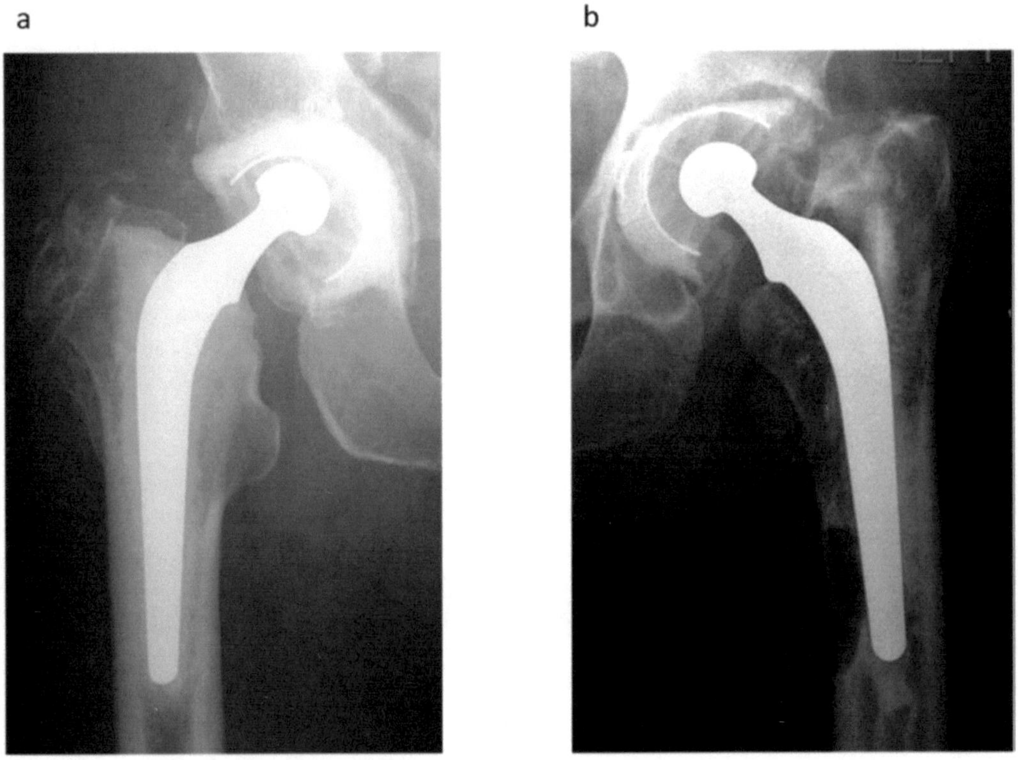

Fig. 6. Patients exhibit variable osteolytic responses to wear debris. a) radiograph showing marked polyethylene wear, but no osteolytic response, b) radiograph showing mild wear but pronounced femoral and acetabular osteolysis with prosthesis loosening.

Variation within the genes encoding inflammatory cytokines have been associated with osteolysis. Wilkinson *et al* showed an association between variability within the DNA encoding the tumor necrosis factor (TNF) promoter region (dbSNP rs361525) and risk of osteolysis following THA[62]. Subjects with osteolysis were approximately twice as likely to carry the variant DNA code as those subjects with no osteolysis. This association has been replicated in an independent population by Ambruzova *et al*[63]. Gordon *et al* have reported genetic variation within the genes encoding Interleukin-1 receptor antagonist (IL-1RN) and IL-6 is also associated with osteolysis[64]. Similar associations have also been identified in other populations[65-67].

Variation within genes that regulate bone turnover also associate with osteolysis. Gordon *et al* showed that carriage of the dbSNP rs288326 variant in the FRZB gene encoding secreted frizzled-related protein-3 (Frp3), a regulatory glycoprotein within the osteogenic Wnt signaling pathway that modulates mesenchymal stem cell differentiation of osteoblasts[68], associated with susceptibility to osteolysis following THA[69]. Its carriage also associated with the development of heterotopic ossification following THA. Malik *et al* have also shown associations between aseptic loosening and other candidate loci within the genes encoding matrix metalloproteinase 1 and the vitamin D receptor[67], mannose-binding lectin[70], and the RANK/OPG pathway[71].

Recent studies using beadchip assays have shown that many genes are differentially expressed in wear debris-induced cells and tissues[72-74], and have highlighted our limited understanding of the spectrum of biological mediators involved in the pathogenesis of osteolysis. The identification of further risk loci is required to further understanding of the pathogenesis of aseptic loosening. This would potentially allow for the development of screening tools, and provide investigational targets for prophylaxis or treatment with the aim of reducing the need for revision surgery, and its associated morbidity and mortality.

6. Prosthesis risk factors

6.1 Prosthesis design

Prosthesis design factors, aside from those that modulate wear, contribute to risk of osteolysis. Modularity allows intra-operative adjustment of bearing surfaces, prosthesis length and offset. However, it also creates additional interfaces within the construct at which generation of debris through wear may occur. Such interfaces include the trunion between the femoral head and stem at which corrosive wear may occur, and backside wear between an acetabular liner and its shell at which abrasive wear may occur, and potentially several other prosthetic component junctions in highly modular systems. Hydroxyapatite coating of the prosthesis may prevent osteolysis following injection of intra-articular particles by sealing the implant-bone interface from their ingression though the promotion of osseointegration at this interface[75,76], but may also be a source of third-body wear. Selection of bearing diameter is also a factor. The use of larger head sizes reduces the risk of dislocation, but increase volumetric wear[77]. The need for a thinner liner to accommodate the larger head may also cause increased contact stresses and an increase in wear

6.2 Polyethylene wear

The metal on polyethylene bearing couple remains the gold standard for THA. However, the manufacturing and sterilization process of polyethylene has changed over time with the aim of improving its wear rate characteristics. The earliest prostheses were made with non-cross-linked ultra-high molecular weight polyethylene (UHWPE) that was irradiated to render it sterile for patient use. The process of sterilization with ionizing radiation leads to cross-linking within the polymer. Cross-linking improves wear resistance of the material, but also causes the formation of free radicals. Free radical species cause the oxidation of UHMWPE over time. Polyethylene oxidation degrades UHMWPE, and decreases its wear resistance.

Several production techniques have been developed to reduce the generation of free radicals, including annealing and melting. Melting reduces free radical concentration more than annealing but adversely affects the yield stress and fatigue resistance of the polymer. Annealing below melting point has a less adverse effect on the mechanical properties, but is less effective than melting at free radical removal. Sterilization in an oxygen-free environment also produces more cross-linking and reduces free radical production[78]. Irradiation in an inert gas and vacuum packing is also now routinely carried out to reduce pre-implantation oxidation, however this does not prevent oxidation occurring in vivo. Faris *et al* compared the wear rates of UHMWPE produced using three combinations of polyethylene production and sterilization techniques[79] and found the best wear rates were achieved in sterilization by radiation in an inert gas with molded polyethylene. Irradiation sterilization of ram extruded components in an inert gas and in air had 11% and 16% more wear respectively.

Highly cross-linked polyethylene has exhibited reduced wear rates clinically in short-term studies[80,81], and thus their potential role in reducing the incidence of osteolysis is promising. Further developments in polyethylene modification techniques are currently being explored to further reduce oxidization in-vivo and optimize the wear performance of UHMWPE without compromising its other mechanical properties, and include doping with anti-oxidants such as vitamin E and cycling of annealing and irradiating. However, the macrophage response in osteolysis is influenced by the size, composition and number of wear particles[82,83]. Particle size and number vary with the extent of cross-linking within the material. Although cross-linking reduces the total amount of wear debris generated versus conventional UHMWPE, the particle size produced is smaller, and the number of particles is increased, which may enhance their osteolytic potential *in-vivo*. Also, whilst increased cross-linking results in enhanced wear resistance there is a reduction in fatigue strength potentially leading to mechanical failure[84].

6.3 Alternate bearing couples

Although metal on polyethylene bearings have most commonly been used in THA, there is a long history of use of other bearing couples, including metal on metal, ceramic on ceramic, and ceramic on polyethylene.

Metal on metal bearings have reduced wear rates compared with metal on polyethylene. Jacobbson reported a 77% 20-year survivorship of the metal on metal McKee Farrar THA compared to 73% for the Charnley THA[85]. Metal on metal prostheses also have the advantages of allowing a larger bearing diameter, improving stability characteristics, and are self-polishing. Although the volumetric wear rate of metal on metal bearings is low, the particles generated are in the nanometer range and the number of particles is far greater[86]. These particles circulate widely within the body and their systemic effects remain unclear. At a local level metal release can cause an adverse surrounding tissue reaction, termed aseptic lymphocytic vasculitis associated lesions (ALVAL), and inflammatory masses[87,88]. Metal hypersensitivity may also occur[87].

Ceramic on polyethylene and ceramic on ceramic bearing couples have lower wear and osteolysis rates versus metal on polyethylene bearings in some long-term studies[89,90]. Most ceramic wear particles are also in the nanometer range and wear volume is lower than that of metal on metal bearing couples. A prospective randomized multicenter study of 930 hips comparing alumina-on-alumina with cobalt chromium-on-polyethylene bearing couples reported an alumina-alumina survival rate of 96.8% at 10 years[91]. However, cases of osteolysis have also been reported in poorly functioning ceramic on ceramic prostheses. Yoon reported osteolysis rates of 22% in a series of patients with ceramic on ceramic prostheses[92]. Nam reported a case of alumina debris induced pelvic and femoral osteolysis in a well-functioning prosthesis[93]. Ceramics are also expensive, have a small fracture risk due to their brittleness, and are sensitive to component mal-positioning that may result in impingement damage and stripe wear. There are also some reports of squeaking associated with ceramic on ceramic bearing couples[94].

7. Surgical risk factors

Regardless of prosthesis design and bearing surface, surgical technique is an important factor that affects prosthesis survival. Data from large national joint registries has recently facilitated examination of these factors in relation to prosthesis survival.

7.1 Hospital type and surgeon operating volume

Type of hospital and the surgeon undertaking the procedure can influence THA survival. Fowles *et al* showed that low operating volume is associated with increased risk of THA revision[95]. Similarly, Espehaug *et al,* using data from the Norwegian arthroplasty register, found the lowest revision rates amongst surgeons with the highest THA volume[96]. In the same study, university hospitals had higher revision rates than local and central hospitals. This may be attributed to the lower number of operations per surgeon at these hospitals or possible centralization of high-risk patients and more complex cases. Bordini *et al* found that prosthesis survival was negatively associated with lower surgeon skill[38].

7.2 Prosthesis alignment and soft tissue balancing

Malalignment of prostheses may alter the articulation of prosthesis components with the potential to increase contact stresses and increase wear, this increases the incidence of edge loading and results in stripe wear in hard on hard bearing couples. Despite the advantage of larger femoral head size, soft tissue balancing remains important in the reduction of dislocation of the femoral head. Subluxation of the femoral head during the swing phase of gait, especially in metal on polyethylene couples, causes socket edge contact resulting in wear[97]. Complete dislocation of the femoral head may damage the head during dislocation-relocation, and can increase wear rates.

7.3 Prosthesis dislocation and interface micromotion

Prosthesis stability influences the development of aseptic loosening. Motion between the prosthesis and bone contributes to the formation of a fibrous membrane rather than bone[98]. Bechtold et al found that particulate wear debris prevents bone formation in the presence of prosthesis instability [99]. In addition, prosthesis motion alters local joint fluid pressures and can transport particles along the periprosthetic space.

7.4 Cementing techniques

Improvements in prosthesis survival have accompanied advances in cementation technique[100]. First generation cementing techniques involved finger packing of the cement without bone preparation, pressurization or use of a medullary plug. In the mid-seventies second generation techniques were adopted which involved improved canal preparation by pulsatile lavage that increased cement penetration and interdigitation, retrograde insertion of cement using a gun to reduce blood lamination, and the use of an intramedullary plug to limit the size of the cement column. Studies with 10 year follow up have shown that 2nd generation techniques were associated with a reduced the incidence in femoral loosening with rates of 3 to 7%[101,102] compared with rates of approximately 30% at 10 years in first generation reports[103,104]. Third generation techniques included vacuum mixing of cement to reduce cement porosity and increase fatigue strength[105], and cement pressurization to further improve cement interdigitation. Subsequently 4th generation cementation techniques have added distal and proximal prosthesis centralizers to improve the stem position allowing for an optimal and even cement mantle. Herbert, in a review of the Swedish THA Register examining 160,000 cases, reported that the evolution from 1st to 3rd generation cementing techniques over a 20 year period was associated with a reduced incidence of revision for aseptic loosening[100].

8. Summary and future directions

Aseptic loosening is the end result of a complex interaction of variables leading to development of osteolysis. Although the last 30 years has seen many advances in the understanding of these factors, osteolysis will remain a problem for the foreseeable future. Newer bearing surfaces have shown potential in wear rate reduction. However, wear particles from all materials have the potential to trigger an inflammatory response. The local and systemic consequences of metal release also need to be more clearly defined and quantitated. Further studies looking at prosthesis bone anchorage in conjuction with particle and pressure effects need to be explored, and the factors that influence loosening membrane formation.

Currently the only effective treatment for aseptic loosening is revision surgery. Future advances in our understanding of the biological response to wear particles may lead to the development of biological markers for better prediction and early detection of osteolysis, and the development of non-surgical solutions for prophylaxis and therapy. Advances in genomic and bioinformatics technology have provided us with the opportunity to identify investigational targets for prophylaxis or treatment. Pharmocological and biological agents used in the treatment of osteolysis in metastatic disease and metabolic bone disease may have potential in osteolysis following THA.

9. References

[1] Kurtz SM, Ong KL, Schmier J, Mowat F, Saleh K, Dybvik E, et al. Future clinical and economic impact of revision total hip and knee arthroplasty. J Bone Joint Surg 2007 Oct;89-A Suppl 3:144-51.

[2] The NJR centre HH. National joint registry for England and Wales. 7th annual report, 2010. Available from URL: www.njrcentre.co.uk.

[3] Mahomed NN, Barrett JA, Katz JN, Phillips CB, Losina E, Lew RA, et al. Rates and outcomes of primary and revision total hip replacement in the United States medicare population. J Bone Joint Surg 2003 Jan;85-A(1):27-32.

[4] Doro C, Dimick J, Wainess R, Upchurch G, Urquhart A. Hospital volume and inpatient mortality outcomes of total hip arthroplasty in the United States. J Arthroplasty 2006 Sep;21(6 Suppl 2):10-6.

[5] Zhan C, Kaczmarek R, Loyo-Berrios N, Sangl J, Bright RA. Incidence and short-term outcomes of primary and revision hip replacement in the United States. J Bone Joint Surg 2007 Mar;89-A(3):526-33.

[6] Charnley J, Follacci FM, Hammond BT. The long-term reaction of bone to self-curing acrylic cement. J Bone Joint Surg. Br. 1968: 50; 822-29.

[7] McKee GK, Watson-Farrar J. Replacement of arthritic hips by the McKee Farrar prosthesis. J Bone Joint Surg. Br. 1966; 48 (2): 245-59.

[8] Jones LC, Hungerford DS. "Cement disease." Clin Orthop 1987; 225: 192-206.

[9] Goldring SR, Schiller AL, Roelke M, Rourke CM, O'Neill DA, Harris WH. The synovial-like membrane at the bone-cement interface in loose total hip replacements and its proposed role in bone lysis. J Bone Joint Surg 1983 Jun;65-A(5):575-84.
[10] Willert HG, Semlich M. Reactions of the articular capsule to wear products of artificial joint prostheses. J Biomed Mater Res. 1977; 11:157-164.
[11] Goodman SB, Fornasier VL, Lee J, Kei J. The histological effects of the implantation of different sizes of polyethylene particles in the rabbit tibia. J Biomed Mater Res. 1990; 24: 517 – 524.
[12] Schmalzried TP, Jasty M, Harris WH. Periprosthetic bone loss in total hip arthroplasty. Polyethylene wear debris and the concept of the effective joint space. J Bone Joint Surg Am 1992a; 74: 849 – 63.
[13] Aspenberg P, Van der Vis H. Fluid pressure may cause periprosthetic osteolysis. Particles are not the only thing. Acta Orthop Scand 1998; 69: 1-4.
[14] Skoglund B, Aspenberg P. PMMA particles and pressure – a study of the osteolytic properties of two agents proposed to cause prosthetic loosening. J Orthop Res 2003; 21: 196-201.
[15] Aspenberg P, Van der Vis H. Migration, particles, and fluid pressure. A discussion of causes of prosthetic loosening. Clin Orthop Rel Res 1998; 352: 75-80.
[16] Harris WH, Schiller AL, Scholler J, Freiberg RA, Scott R. Extensive localized bone resorption in the femur following total hip replacement. J Bone Joint Surg Am 1976; 58: 612-618. .
[17] Tuan RS, Lee FY, Konttinen YT, Wilkinson JM, Smith RL. What are the local and systemic biologic reactions and mediators to wear debris, and what host factors determine or modulate the biologic response to wear particles? J Am Acad Orthop Surg 2008; 16(supl 1): S42-S48.
[18] Martinon F, Mayor A, Tschopp J. The inflammasomes: guardians of the body. Annu Rev Immunol. 2009; 27: 229-65.
[19] Caicedo, M. S. *et al.* Soluble and particulate Co-Cr-Mo alloy implant metals activate the inflammasome danger signaling pathway in human macrophages: a novel mechanism for implant debris reactivity. *J Orthop Res* 27, 847-854, doi:10.1002/jor.20826 (2009).
[20] Maitra R, Clement CC, Scharf B, Crisi GM, Chitta S, Paget D, Purdue PE, Cobelli N, Santambrogio L. Endosomal damage and TLR2 mediated inflammasome activation by alkane particles in the generation of aseptic osteolysis. Mol Immunol 2009 Dec;47(2-3):175-84.
[21] St Pierre CA, Chan M, Iwakura Y, Ayers DC, Kurt-Jones EA, Finberg RW. Periprosthetic osteolysis: characterizing the innate immune response to titanium wear-particles. J Orthop Res. 2010 Nov; 28(11): 1418-1424.
[22] Rodan GA, Martin TJ. Role of osteoblasts in hormonal control of bone resorption- A hypothesis. Calcif Tissue Int 1981;33: 349-351.
[23] Boyle WJ, Simone WS, Lacey DL. Osteoclast differentation and activation. Nature 2003, 423. 337-342.
[24] Wei X, Zhang X, Zuscik MJ, Drissi MH, Schwarz EM, O'Keefe RJ Fibroblasts express RANKL and support osteoclastogenesis in a COX-2-dependent manner after stimulation with titanium particles. J Bone Miner Res 2005;20:1136-48.
[25] Sakai H, Jingushi S, Shuto T, Urabe K, Ikenoue T, Okazaki K, Kukita T Fibroblasts from the inner granulation tissue of the pseudocapsule in hips at revision

arthroplasty induce osteoclast differentiation, as do stromal cells. Ann Rheum Dis 2002;61:103-9).
[26] Wang ML, Tuli R, Manner PA, Sharkey PF, Hall DJ, Tuan RS. Direct and indirect induction of apoptosis in human mesenchymal stem cells in response to titanium particles. J Orthop Res 2003; 21: 697-707.
[27] Solovieva SA, Ceponis A, Konttinen YT, Takagi M, Suda A, Eklund KK, Sorsa T, Santavirta S. Mast cells in loosening of totally replaced hips. Clin Orthop Rel Res. 1996 Jan;(322): 158-165.
[28] Nalepka JL, Lee MJ, Kraay MJ, Marcus RE, Goldberg VM, Chen X, Greenfield E. Lipopolysaccharide found in aseptic loosening of patients with inflammatory arthritis. Clin Orthop Rel Res 2006; 451: 229-235.
[29] Dempsey KE, Riggio MP, Lennon A, Hannah VE, Ramage G, Allan D, Bagg J. Identification of bacteria on the surface of clinically infected and non-infected prosthetic hip joints removed during revision arthroplasties by 16S rRNA gene sequencing and by microbiological culture. Arthritis Res Ther 2007; 9:R46.
[30] Greenfield EM, Bechtold J. What other biologic and mechanical factors might contribute to osteolysis? J Am Acad Orthop Surg 2008; 16 (suppl 1): S56-S62.
[31] Kobayashi S, Saito N, Horiuchi H, Iorio R, Takaoka K Poor bone quality or hip structure as risk factors affecting survival of total-hip arthroplasty. Lancet 2000;355:1499-504.
[32] Tsao AK. What patient and surgical factors contribute to implant wear and osteolysis in total joint arthroplasty. J Am Acad Orthop Surg 2008; 16 (suppl 1):S7–S13.
[33] Letson GD. Activity relationships of THA in patients with osteonecrosis and osteonecrosis. Orthopedics. 1996 Aug; 19 (8):665-8.
[34] Espehaug B, Havelin LI, Engesaeter LB, Langeland N, Vollset SE Patient-related risk factors for early revision of total hip replacements. A population register-based case-control study of 674 revised hips. Acta Orthop Scand 1997;68:207-15.
[35] Furnes, O. *et al.* Hip disease and the prognosis of total hip replacements. A review of 53,698 primary total hip replacements reported to the Norwegian Arthroplasty Register 1987-99. *J Bone Joint Surg Br* 83, 579-586 (2001).
[36] Rud-Sorensen, C., Pedersen, A. B., Johnsen, S. P., Riis, A. H. & Overgaard, S. Survival of primary total hip arthroplasty in rheumatoid arthritis patients. *Acta Orthop* 81, 60-65, doi:10.3109/17453671003685418 (2010).
[37] Furnes O, Lie SA, Vollset, Engesater LB, Havelin LI. Hip disease and the survival of hip prostheses in the Norwegian Arthroplasty Register. Acta Orthop Scand (Suppl 280) 1998;69.
[38] Bordini, B. *et al.* Factors affecting aseptic loosening of 4750 total hip arthroplasties: multivariate survival analysis. *BMC Musculoskelet Disord* 8, 69 (2007).
[39] Papachristou G, Hatzigigoris P, Panousis K, Plessas S, Sourlas J, Levidiotis C, Chronopoulos E. Total hip arthroplasty for developmental hip dysplasia. International Orthopaedics. 2006; 30: 21-25.
[40] Health Survey for Enlgland 2009: Trend Tables. The Health and Social Care Information Centre, 2010.
[41] Charnley J. Long term results of low friction arthroplasty. Hip 1982: 42-9.
[42] Adams JP, Murphy PG. Obesity in anaesthesia and intensive care. Br J Anaesth 2000; 85: 91-108.

[43] LoweGD, HaverkateF, Thompson SG. Prediction of deep venous thrombosis after hip replacement surgery by preoperative clinical and haemostatic variables: the ECAT DVT study: European concerted action on thrombosis. Thromb Haemostat 2003; 89: 493-498.
[44] Namba RS, Paxton L, Fithian DC, Stone ML. Obesity and perioperative morbidity in total hip and knee arthroplasty patients. J Arthroplasty 2005; 20 (suppl 3): 46-50.
[45] Chee YH. Total hip replacement in the morbidly obese patient with OA. JBJS 2010; 92-B(8): 1066-1071.
[46] Lubbeke A, Garavaglia G, Barea C, Roussos C, Stern R, Hoffmeyet P. Influence of obesity on femoral osteolysis five and ten years following total hip arthroplasty. J Bone Joint Surg Am 2010; 92: 1964 - 1972.
[47] Andrew JG, Palan J, Kurup HV, Gibson P, Murray DW, Beard DJ. Obesity in toal hip replacement. J Bone Joint Surg Br 2008; 90: 424-429.
[48] Flugsrud GB, Nrdsletten L, Espenhaug B, Havelin LI, Meyer HE. The effect of middle-age body weight and physical activity on the risk of early revision hip arthroplasty: a cohort study of 1,535 individuals. Acta Orthop 2007; 86: 963-974.
[49] Lubbeke A, Garavaglia G, Barea, Stern R, Peter R, Hoffmeyer P. Influence of patient activity on femoral osteolysis at five and ten years following hybrid total hip replacement. J Bone Joint Surg Br 2011; 93: 456-463. .
[50] Clark, I C Wear of artificial joint materials. Friction and wear studies. Eng Med 10: 115 - 122, 1981.
[51] Schmalzried TP, Szuszczewicz ES, Northfield MR, Akizuki KH, Frankel RE, Belcher G, Amstutz HC. Quantitative assessment of walking activity after total hip or knee replacement. J Bone Joint Surg Am 1998; 80: 54-59.
[52] Naal FD, Impellizzeri FM, Leunig M. Which is the best activity rayting scale for patient undergoing total joint arthoplasty? Clin Orthop Rel Res 2009; 467: 958-965.
[53] Schmalzried TP, Shepherd EF, Dorey FJ, Jackson WO, dela Rosa M, Fa'vae F, McKellop HA, McClung CD, Martell J, Moreland JR, Amstutz HC. Wear is a function of use, not time. Clin Orthop Rel Res 2000; 381: 36-46.
[54] Huch K, Muller KAC, Sturmer T, Brenner H, Puhl W, Gunther K-P. Sports activities 5 years after total hip or knee arthroplasty: the Ulm osteoarthritis study. Ann Rheum Dis 2005; 64: 1715–1720.
[55] Wylde V, Blom A, Dieppe P, Hewlett S, Learmonth I. Return to sport after joint replacement. J bone Joint Surg Br 2008; 90: 920-923.
[56] Chatterji U, Asworth MJ, Lewis PL, Dobson PJ. Effect of total hip arthroplasty on recreational and sporting activity. ANZ J Surg 2004; 74: 446-449.
[57] Wilkinson JM, Hamer AJ, Stockley I, Eastell R. Polyethylene wear rate and osteolysis: critical threshold versus continuous dose-response relationship. J Orthop Res 2005 May;23(3):520-5.
[58] Emms, N. W., Stockley, I., Hamer, A. J. & Wilkinson, J. M. Long-term outcome of a cementless, hemispherical, press-fit acetabular component: survivorship analysis and dose-response relationship to linear polyethylene wear. *J Bone Joint Surg Br* 92, 856-861, doi:92-B/6/856 [pii] 10.1302/0301-620X.92B6.23666 (2010).
[59] Misch EA, Hawn TR. Toll -like receptor polymorphisms and susceptibility to human disease. Clin Sci. 2008; 114: 347-360.
[60] Matthews JB, Green TR, Stone MH, Wroblewski BM, Fisher, J, et al. Comparison of the response of primary human peripheral blood mononuclear phagocytes from

different donors to challenge with model polyethylene particles of known size and dose. Biomaterials 2000 Oct;21(20):2033-44.

[61] Gordon A, Kiss-Toth E, Greenfield E, Eastell R, Wilkinson J. Differences in cytokine mRNA expression in stimulated mononuclear cells from subjects with previous osteolysis versus non-osteolysis subjects after total hip arthroplasty. Trans ORS 33, 424. 2008.

[62] Wilkinson JM, Wilson AG, Stockley I, Scott IR, Macdonald DA, Hamer AJ, et al. Variation in the TNF gene promoter and risk of osteolysis after total hip arthroplasty. J Bone Miner Res 2003;18(11):1995-2001.

[63] Ambruzova Z, Gallo J, Mrazek F, Kubistova Z, Onderkova J, Petrek M. Association of cytokine gene polymorphisms with expansile periprosthetic osteolysis in total hip arthroplasty. Tissue Antigens 2006;67(6):528.

[64] Gordon A, Kiss-Toth E, Stockley I, Eastell R, Wilkinson JM. Polymorphisms in the Interleukin-1 Receptor Antagonist and Interleukin-6 Genes Affect Risk of Osteolysis in Patients with Total Hip Arthroplasty. Arthritis Rheum 2008;58:3157-65.

[65] Kolundiz R, Orlic D, Truklja V, Pavelic K, Troselj KG. Single nucleotide polymorphisms in the interleukin-6 gene promoter, tumour necrosis factor-α gene promoter, and transforming growth factor-β1 gene signal sequence as predictors of time to onset of aseptic loosening after total hip arthrolasty: preliminary study. J Orthop Sci 2006; 11: 592-600.

[66] Gallo J, Mrazek F, Petrek M. Variation in cytokine genes can contribute to severity of acetabular osteolysis and risk for revision in patients with ABG 1 total hip arthroplasty: a genetic association study. BMC Med Genet 2009; 10:109.

[67] Malik MH, Jury F, Bayat A, Ollier WE, Kay PR. Genetic susceptibility to total hip arthroplasty failure: a preliminary study on the influence of matrix metalloproteinase 1, interleukin 6 polymorphisms and vitamin D receptor. Ann Rheum Dis 2007 Aug;66(8):1116-20.

[68] Martin TJ, Sims NA, Ng KW. Regulatory pathways revealing new approaches to the devlopment of anabolic drugs for osteoporosis. Osteoporos Int 2008; 19: 1125-1138.

[69] Gordon A, Southam L, Loughlin J, Wilson AG, Stockley I, Hamer AJ, et al. Variation in the secreted frizzled-related protein-3 gene and risk of osteolysis and heterotopic ossification after total hip arthroplasty. J Orthop Res 2007 Dec 12;25(12):1665-70.

[70] Malik MH, Bayat A, Jury F, Kay PR, Ollier WE. Genetic susceptibility to total hip arthroplasty failure--positive association with mannose-binding lectin. J Arthroplasty 2007 Feb;22(2):265-70.

[71] Malik MH, Bayat A, Jury F, Ollier WE, Kay PR. Genetic susceptibility to hip arthroplasty failure--association with the RANK/OPG pathway. Int Orthop 2006 Jun;30(3):177-81.

[72] Garrigues GE, Cho DR, Rubash HE, Goldring SR, Herndon JH, Shanbhag AS. Gene expression clustering using self-organizing maps: analysis of the macrophage response to particulate biomaterials. Biomaterials 2005 Jun;26(16):2933-45.

[73] Shanbhag AS, Kaufman AM, Hayata K, Rubash HE. Assessing osteolysis with use of high-throughput protein chips. J Bone Joint Surg 2007 May;89-A(5):1081-9.

[74] Koulouvaris P, Ly K, Ivashkiv LB, Bostrom MP, Nestor BJ, Sculco TP, et al. Expression profiling reveals alternative macrophage activation and impaired osteogenesis in periprosthetic osteolysis. J Orthop Res 2008 Jan;26(1):106-16.

[75] Rahbek O, Kold S, Bendix K, Overgaard S, Soballe K. Superior sealing effect of hydroxyapatite in porous-coated implants: Experimental studies on the migration of polyethylene particles around stable and unstable implants in dogs. Acta Orthop 2005; 76: 375 - 385.
[76] Soballe K, Hansen ES, Brockstedt-Rasmussen H, Bunger C. Hydroxyapatite coating converts fibrous tissue to bone around loaded implants. J Bone Joint Surg Br 1993; 75: 270-278.
[77] Charnley J, Kamangar A, Longfield MD: The optimum size of prosthetic heads in relation to the wear of plastic sockets in total replacement of the hip. Med Biol Eng 1969; 7: 31-39.
[78] Mckellop HA, Shen FW,Campbell P, Ota T. Effect of molecular weight, calcium stearate, and sterilization methods on the wear of ultra high molecular weight polyethylene acetabular cups in a joint simulator. J Orthop Res 1999; 17:329-339.
[79] Faris PM, Ritter MA, Pierce AL, Davis KE, Faris GW. Polyethylene sterilization and production effects wear in total hip arthroplasties. Clin Orthop Rel Res 2006; 453: 305-308.
[80] Dorr LD, Wan Z, Shahrdar C, Sirianni L, Boutary M, Yun A. Clinical performance of a Durasul highly cross linked polyethylene acetabular liner for total hip arthroplasty at five years. J Bone Joint Surg Am 2005; 87: 1816-1821.
[81] Digas G, Karrholm J, Thanner J, Malchau H, Herberts P. The Otto Aufranc Award: Highly cross-linked polyethylene in total hip arthroplasty. Randomized evaluation of penetration rate in cemented and uncemented sockets using radiostereometric analysis. Clin Orthop Rel Res 2004; 429: 6-16.
[82] Shanbhag AS, Jacobs JJ, Black J, Galante JO, Glant TT: Human monocyte response to particlute biomaterials generated in vivo and in vitro. J Orthop Res 1995;13:792-801.
[83] Shanbhag AS, Jacobs JJ, Glant TT, Gilbert JL, Black J, Galante JO. Composition and morphology of wear debris in failed uncemented total hip replacement. J Bone Joint Surg Br; 76: 60-67.
[84] Bradford, L., Baker, D., Ries, M. D. & Pruitt, L. A. Fatigue crack propagation resistance of highly crosslinked polyethylene. *Clin Orthop Relat Res*, 68-72, doi:00003086-200412000-00011 [pii] (2004).
[85] Jacobsson SA, Djerf K, Wahlstrom O. Tewenty-year results of McKee Farrar versus Charnley prosthesis. Clin Orthop Rel Res 1996; 329: S60-S68.
[86] Doorn PF, Campbell PA, Worrall J, Benya PD, McKellop HA, Amstutz HC. Metal wear particle characterization from metal on metal total hip replacements: Transmission electron microscopy study of periprosthetic tissues and isolated particles. J Biomed Mater Res 1998; 42: 103-111.
[87] Willert, H. G. *et al.* Metal-on-metal bearings and hypersensitivity in patients with artificial hip joints. A clinical and histomorphological study. *J Bone Joint Surg Am* 87, 28-36, doi:87/1/28 [pii] 10.2106/JBJS.A.02039pp (2005).
[88] Pandit, H. *et al.* Pseudotumours associated with metal-on-metal hip resurfacings. *J Bone Joint Surg Br* 90, 847-851, doi:10.1302/0301-620X.90B7.20213 90-B/7/847 [pii] (2008).
[89] Urban JA, Garvin KL, Boese CK, Bryson L, Pederson DR, Callaghan JJ, Miller RK. Ceramic-on-polyethylene bearing surfaces in total hip arthroplasty. Seventeen to twenty-one-year results. J Bone Joint Surg Am 2001; 83: 1688-1694.
[90] Hannouche D, Hamadouche M, Nizard R, Bozot P, Sedel L. Ceramics in total hip replacement. Clin Orthop Rel Res. 2005; 430: 62-71.

[91] Mesko, J. W., D'Antonio, J. A., Capello, W. N., Bierbaum, B. E. & Naughton, M. Ceramic-on-ceramic hip outcome at a 5- to 10-year interval: has it lived up to its expectations? *J Arthroplasty* 26, 172-177, doi:S0883-5403(10)00261-5 [pii]10.1016/ j.arth.2010.04.029 (2011).

[92] Yoon, TR, Rowe SM, Jung ST, Seon KJ, Maloney WJ. Osteolysis in association with a total hip arthroplasty with ceramic bearing surfaces. J Bone Joint Surg Am 1998; 80: 1459-1468.

[93] Nam KW, Yoo JJ, Lae Kim Y, Kim YM, Lee MH, Kim HJ. Alumina-debris-induced osteolysis in contemporary alumina-on-alumina total hip arthroplasty. A case report. J Bone Joint Surg Am 2007; 89: 2499-2503.

[94] Jarrett, C. A. *et al.* The squeaking hip: a phenomenon of ceramic-on-ceramic total hip arthroplasty. *J Bone Joint Surg Am* 91, 1344-1349, doi:91/6/1344 [pii] 10.2106/ JBJS.F.00970 (2009).

[95] Fowles, J., Bunker, J. P. & Schurman, D. J. Hip surgery data yield quality indicators. *Bus Health* 4, 44-46 (1987).

[96] Espehaug, B., Havelin, L. I., Engesaeter, L. B. & Vollset, S. E. The effect of hospital-type and operating volume on the survival of hip replacements. A review of 39,505 primary total hip replacements reported to the Norwegian Arthroplasty Register, 1988-1996. *Acta Orthop Scand* 70, 12-18 (1999).

[97] McKellop HA, D'Lima Darryl. How have wear testing and joint simulator studies helped to discriminate among materials and designs? J AM Acad Orthop Surg 2008; 16 (suppl 1): S111-S119.

[98] Bragdon CR, Jasty M, Greene M, Rubash HE, Harris WH. Biologic fixation of total hip implants: Insights gained from a series of canine studies. J Bone Joint Surg Am 2004; 86 (suppl 2): 105-117.

[99] Bechtold JE, Kubic V, Soballe K. Bone ingrowth in the presence of particulate polyethylene: Synergy between interface motion and particulate polyethylene in periprosthetic tissue response. J Bone Joint Surg Br 2002; 84: 915-919.

[100] Herberts P, Malchau H. Long-term registration has improved the quality of hip replacement. A review of the Swedish THR Register comparing 160,000 case. Acta Orthop Scand 2009; 71: 111-121.

[101] Mulroy RD, Harris WH. The effect of inproved cementing techniques on component loosening in total hip replacement: An 11-year radiographic rebiew. J Bone Joint Surg Br 1990; 72: 757-760.

[102] Stauffer RN. Ten year results of second generation femoral cementing in total hip replacement surgery. Read at the Harvard Medical School Postgraduate Course on Total Hip Surgery. Cambridge, MA, Oct, 1991.

[103] Stauffer RN. Ten year follow up study of total hip replacement. J Bone Joint Surg Am 1982; 7: 983-990.

[104] Barrack RL, Mulroy RD, Harris WH. Improved cementing techniques and femoral component loosening in young patients with hip arthroplasty. J Bone Joint Surg 1992; 74: 385-389.

[105] Davies JP, Jasty M, O'Connor DO, Burke DW, Harrigan TP, Harris WH. The effect of centrifuging bone cement. J Bone Joint Surg Br 1989; 71: 39-42.

15

Evidence Linking Elevated Oxidative Stress and Aseptic Loosening of Hip Arthroplasty

Plamen Kinov and Peter Tivchev
Queen Giovanna – ISUL University Hospital, Department of Orthopedics and Traumatology, Medical University of Sofia
Bulgaria

1. Introduction

Aseptic loosening is still the most common late complication after total hip arthroplasty (THA) and one of the main reasons for its failure. Artificial joints are made of metallic, polymeric and ceramic components. In the process of prosthesis functioning in the recipient's body implant materials are subject to wear and fretting as well as of influence of aggressive biological fluids. Wear debris particles, corrosion products and metal ions from the bearing and contact surfaces of the implant are released in the periprosthetic tissues. As a result of the processes taking part at the implant-bone interface osteolysis develops with subsequent loosening of the implant.

Today, the most widely used bearing surface is a metal femoral head made of cobalt chromium molybdenum alloy coupled with a polymeric inlay fabricated from ultra-high molecular weight polyethylene (UHMWPE). For decades in clinical use, metal on polyethylene (MoPE) bearings in total hip arthroplasty provided consistent results. Despite the widespread use of UHMWPE as a bearing surface its wear is the main obstacle restricting the longevity of the artificial joint. With an average rate of polyethylene (PE) wear of 0.1mm per year, 100 million UHMWPE particles (assumed diameter of 1 μm) are liberated into the joint space on a daily basis (Muratoglu & Kurtz, 2002). It is now well established that cyclic mechanical loading, production of wear particles, and the ensuing cascade of adverse tissue response are all significant contributors to local osteolysis at the prosthesis–bone interface and in certain cases loosening of the prosthesis (Aspenberg & Herbertsson, 1996, Goldring et al., 1986, Schmalzried et al., 1992, Willert & Semtlitsch, 1977). Deterioration of clinical results with time and eventually revision of the arthroplasty were a very strong impetus for the search for the "ideal bearing" (Muratoglu & Kurtz, 2002). Improving longevity of the total hip arthroplasty by engineering of new bearing couples with improved biomechanical characteristics and lower rate of wear has been the main line of ongoing research in the orthopedic community. Today, orthopedic surgeons have a wide choice of implants and bearing couples for a particular patient. The new generation of joint bearings provides significantly lower wear rates and is anticipated to diminish the incidence of osteolysis and subsequent revisions.

Next to development of new bearing surfaces, the second line of research focuses on understanding of the underlying mechanisms of the process aseptic loosening of THA. Aseptic loosening is characterized with osteolysis and formation of thick membrane around the prostheses that eventually leads to its loosening. Currently, it is well established fact that loosening is a result of host response to wear debris and corrosion products of implant materials. Particles can readily be detected in the periprosthetic tissues as well as at remote locations such as lymph nodes, liver, spleen or bone marrow. Wear debris induce inflammation in the periprosthetic tissues that is sustained through the functioning of the implant as long as wear particles are produced.

Metal wear debris, degradation and corrosion products, such as ions and reactive oxygen species (ROS), has been considered to be crucial factors in the process of loosening leading to the failure of metal implants (Tsaryk, 2009). Metal debris could induce inflammatory responses mediated by neutrophils, macrophages, fibroblasts and other cells. Metal ions and corrosion products are potentially toxic, can cause allergic reactions of hypersensitivity, chromosomal aberrations, and eventually malignancy (Keegan et al., 2007).

Elevated oxidative stress has been proposed to be a causative factor in many inflammatory and degenerative disorders with tissue damage and fibrosis in different organs and systems (Hogg, 1998, Park et al., 2001). In addition, recent in vitro studies showed the combined effect of particles and macrophage and osteoclast activation on the increase of oxidative stress (Fleury et al., 2006, Petit et al., 2005, Wei et al., 2009). This suggests involvement of reactive oxygen species (ROS) in the mechanism of aseptic loosening of hip arthroplasty. The chronic inflammation state with the elevated oxidative stress results in extensive formation of granulation tissue and fibrous capsule, periprosthetic bone resorption due to osteoclast activation by inflammatory stimuli and finally aseptic loosening of the implant (Tsaryk, 2009). In support of this hypothesis we proved the involvement of ROS in excessive fibrosis around loose hip prostheses (Kinov et al., 2006). This suggests involvement of reactive oxygen species in the mechanism of aseptic loosening of hip arthroplasty leading to formation of the fibrous pseudocapsule that typically consists of a combination of fibrous tissue and macrophages. However, the mechanisms of involvement of ROS in aseptic loosening of THA are still to be elucidated.

Some researchers further implicated that free radicals may be involved in the induction and maintenance of chronic inflammation with resulting periprosthetic bone resorption. In support of this hypothesis, recent studies on osteoporosis (Hamel et al., 2008, Li et al., 2009) show that elevated oxidative stress is involved in inhibiting osteoblastic differentiation and stimulating osteoclastogenesis. In addition, in vitro study showed the combined effect of particles and macrophage and osteoclast activation on release of reactive oxygen and nitrogen species (Wang et al., 2002). Different studies investigate the mechanisms of action of oxidative stress on bone formation (Bai et al., 2004, 2005, Chen et al., 2010, Kim et al., 2010, Mazière et al., 2010, Rached et al., 2010). However, the exact mechanism and actions of ROS on inhibition of osteoblasts are still largely unknown. Considering the fact that elevated oxidative stress induces bone loss in postmenopausal osteoporosis (Lean et al., 2005) whereas antioxidants suppress osteoclast activity and enhance differentiation of osteoblasts (Aitken et al., 2004, Mody et al., 2001) it is possible that ROS are involved in aseptic loosening of total hip arthroplasty. In support of this, in two previous studies, we have shown direct evidence for involvement of elevated oxidative stress in aseptic loosening of THA (Kinov et al., 2006, 2010).

2. Materials for bearings of hip prostheses

Materials are very important for the long-term success of THA. Since the introduction of low friction arthroplasty (LFA) by Sir John Charnley in the 1960's, much has been learned about the durability and biocompatibility of materials used in joint replacement. Concerns about higher rates of aseptic loosening and subsequent prosthesis revision among young and active patients have lead to the development of new implant designs and alternative bearings (Muratoglu & Kurtz, 2002). Strength and endurance, friction and wear properties, inertness and biocompatibility of the materials should be optimized in order to eliminate or diminish to a negligible extent the reaction of the organism to wear debris.

2.1 Brief historical remarks

Aseptic loosening has been observed since the beginning of hip replacement. Metal bearings were first introduced by Wiles in the 1930s (Wiles, 1957), but they received wider application in the 1950s and 1960s with the pioneer works of McKee-Farrar and Ring (McKee & Watson-Farrar, 1966, Ring, 1967). The earlier prototypes were manufactured of stainless steel and fracture of the prostheses was a frequent complication (McKee & Watson-Farrar, 1966, Ring, 1967). To solve this problem the cobalt chromium molybdenum (CoCrMo/CoCrMo) articulation was developed. However, the metal-on-metal (MoM) bearing was eventually abandoned in the 1970's in favor of the Charnley's low friction arthroplasty. Next to biomechanical factors associated with the joint center and surgical implementation technique, two main reasons for shift from MoM bearing were manufacturing problems and long-term concerns associated with metal toxicity (Muratoglu & Kurtz, 2002).

In 1958, Charnley introduced the "low friction arthroplasty" in which the initial bearing material was polytetrafluoroethylene (Charnley, 1979). Because of high rate of wear and "intense foreign-body reaction", in 1962, polytetrafluoroethylene was replaced with ultra-high molecular weight polyethylene. After use of UHMWPE the rate of wear and the need for revision decreased tremendously. In the cases that required revision the implant-bone interface was surrounded by granulomatous tissue rich of inflammatory cells. Charnley believed that those findings were a result of infection (Charnley et al., 1968). A benign, noninflammatory adverse tissue response was suggested (Harris et al., 1976). Willert and Semlitsch proposed that aseptic loosening resulted from reaction to wear debris ingested by the macrophages in the periprosthetic tissue (Willert & Semlitsch, 1977). Their findings were supported by Mirra et al. (Mirra et al., 1976), and Goldring et al. demonstrated that the periprosthetic membranes were capable of producing collagenase and prostaglandin E2, a powerful stimulator of bone resorption in vivo (Goldring et al., 1986). Polymethylmethacylate (PMMA) was proposed as a cause for osteolysis and loosening and the term "cement disease" was introduced (Jones & Hungerford, 1987). However, the problems of osteolysis and aseptic loosening persisted after the implementation of improved cementing techniques and cementless implants. This led researchers and clinicians to propose other causes for osteolysis and subsequent loosening such as polyethylene and metal debris.

The first ceramic-on-ceramic (CoC) total hip arthroplasty was developed by Boutin in 1970 (Boutin, 1971, Boutin & Blanquaert, 1981). The main advantages of ceramics are its superior wear characteristics and biocompatibility, along with better corrosion resistance compared to metallic alloys. Initially, application of ceramics in total hip arthroplasty exclusively included use of alumina (Al_2O_3) (Boutin & Blanquaert, 1981). In the late 1980s, alumina was replaced with zirconia (ZrO_2) due to its superior strength and toughness as compared with alumina (Willmann, 1998). Drawback of ceramic materials used for bearing couples is their inherently lower strength and toughness under tension and bending. Fracture of the ceramic bearing component is the main mode of failure that occurs even with modern ceramic composites.

2.2 Ultra-high molecular weight polyethylene

Since 1962, ultra-high molecular weight polyethylene has been successfully used in hip replacement for four decades. UHMWPE is a polymer with outstanding chemical and mechanical characteristics. The chemical composition of polyethylene is simple, consisting only of carbon and hydrogen. However, at molecular level the polymer is a complex crystalline structure and at super-molecular level it is in the form of powder (also known as resin) than must be consolidated by melting or pressure to form a solid body. By further processing complexity could be added to the chemical structure of the polymer. In joint replacement, of special importance are its chemical inertness, low friction, lubricity, impact resistance, and abrasion resistance (Muratoglu & Kurtz, 2002, Kurtz, 2004).

After recognition of the problem of wear of the artificial bearing and the ensuing adverse tissue reaction to wear debris the issue is a focus of ongoing research. Alternative bearings were proposed with the goal of elongating longevity of the hip arthroplasty. Polyethylene is a crystalline polymer and its mechanical properties are dependent on its molecular weight and crystalinity. In its solid state, UHMWPE is a two-phase material with crystalline domains embedded within an amorphous phase. The complexities in the microstructure of UHMWPE give rise to a range in mechanical behavior depending upon the processing, thermal and radiation exposure, storage, and prior mechanical history of the polymer (Muratoglu & Kurtz, 2002).

In the 1990s, radiation crosslinking combined with thermal treatment has emerged as a technology to improve the wear and oxidation resistance of UHMWPE acetabular components (McKellop et al., 1999, Muratoglu et al., 2001). The new bearing showed reduced wear rate in numerous in vitro and clinical studies (McKellop et al., 1999, Muratoglu et al., 2001, Campbell et al., 2010, Kurtz et al., 2010). The wear rate of the alternative bearing of highly cross-linked polyethylene and CoCr was significantly lower compared to conventional articulation (UHMWPE/CoCr) (McKellop et al., 1999). The reduced wear rates and enhanced strength allow wider clinical application of the highly cross-linked polyethylene. There is an opportunity to enlarge the diameter of the femoral head used in total hip arthroplasty. This will allow increased range of motion of the joint, increased activities in daily living, greater stability of the joint and reduced incidence of subluxation and dislocation, and less frequent impingement.

2.3 Metal-on-metal bearings in hip arthroplasty

Metal-on-metal hip prostheses made of cobalt-chromium-molybdenum alloys represent an alternative to metal-on-polyethylene bearings because of their substantially lower wear rates (Kurtz, 2004). MoM bearings were proposed in an effort to eliminate wear-induced osteolysis. However, the size, the shape, the number and the chemical characteristics of ion particles are different from the polyethylene particles (Sieber et al., 1999). Because of the difference in particle size, metal-on-metal bearings have been estimated to produce about

100 times more wear debris particles than CoCr/UHMWPE bearings (Doorn et al., 1999, Firkins et al., 2001). As a result of increased biological activity of the smaller metal particles different problems from those of MoPE bearings emerged. Adverse reactions to metal debris have been reported to be a cause of pain in metal-on-metal hip arthroplasty (Wynn-Jones et al., 2011) and potential carcinogenesis raised concerns (Keegan et al., 2007). Two important features determine the survivorship of each type of metal implant: metallurgy and implant design. They are interrelated and determine the biological response to an implant and the survivorship of THA. The properties of the bearing surface are dependent on the manufacturing process. This will result in different wear pattern and metal ion release (Catelas et al., 2003).

Large femoral heads used with MoM bearing have certain advantages: allow accelerated rehabilitation, good range of motion, lesser possibility for impingement, greater intrinsic stability. However, MoM bearing is very sensitive to improper surgical technique. Suboptimal or improper positioning of the components of the arthroplasty leads to impingement, edge loading, reduced clearance that subsequently results in elevated production of metal wear debris.

2.4 Ceramics in hip arthroplasty

After the drawback of implant fracture in the 1970's and early 1980's, the very low wear rate of ceramic materials renewed interest in developing new designs of CoC bearings for clinical use in the 1990's. Ceramics are brittle, polycrystalline hard bodies, characterized with high hardness and friction endurance. Particles produced by CoC articulations are considered biologically inert and could reduce the rate of osteolysis observed with conventional PE bearings. Despite their brittleness, ceramic materials have several tribological properties, including hardness, which contribute to wear and scratch resistance (Kurtz, 2004). There are three types of ceramics that are of interest in THA, including alumina, zirconia, and alumina matrix composites (Kurtz, 2004). The strength of the ceramics depends on the size of the alumina or zirconia powder grains and the distribution of internal defects, as well as on its composition (i.e., percentage of alumina versus zirconia). Advances in technology with diminishing of grain size have resulted in improved strength. However, the survival of the CoC hip arthroplasty is highly dependent on surgical implantation technique. This articulation is less forgiving than conventional UHMWPE bearing to improper positioning of the components with a subsequent risk of fracture. Although fracture risk is low, it continues to be an issue of debate among orthopedic surgeons. Another potential problem is chipping of the liner that occurs with impingement or during insertion with improper placement.

Biomechanical studies show excellent wear resistance of ceramic bearings. However, clinical studies do not show significant advantage of ceramics compared to polyethylene. In two randomized studies, an alumina-on-alumina bearing was compared with cobalt-chrome-on-polyethylene bearing (Bierbaum et al., 2002, Capello et al., 2005). There was no significant difference in clinical outcome between CoC and MoPE bearings.

3. Wear debris and aseptic loosening of total hip arthroplasty

Osteolysis and subsequent loosening remain the most frequent complication after THA and the main cause for its failure. Wear-induced particle debris and the associated host response is principle factor in this process. Abundant evidence show that the macrophages play a key role in wear debris induced periprosthetic osteolysis (Brooks et al., 2002, Park et al., 2005, Purdue et al., 2006, Sabokbar et al., 1997, Wang et al., 2002). Phagocytosis of wear particles induces secretion of various proinflammatory cytokines such as tumor necrosis factor alpha (TNF-α), IL-1 and PGE_2 (Goldring, Lam et al., 2000, Yao et al., 2008). This inflammatory response is modulated by various factors including chemical composition, size, shape, and volume of the particles (Sieber et al., 1999, Yang et al., 2002). The prostheses-bone interface could be also influenced by other factors such as endotoxins (Kido et al., 2001), matrix metaloproreinases secreted from activated macrophages that directly resorb bone (Brooks et al., 2002), and mechanical factors such as high fluid pressure (Aspenberg & Van der Vis, 1998, Van der Vis et al., 1998). Although the inflammatory response to wear debris is central to the process of aseptic loosening, the detailed nature of the local response may vary based upon several parameters, including prosthetic type and material, patterns of wear, and patient-related factors (Purdue et al., 2006).

Similar to polyethylene debris, metallic debris migrate in the periprosthetic tissues, and because of its smaller size is easily phagocytosed by histiocytes (Doorn et al., 1999). Metal ions can be involved in various cellular, local and systemic biological reactions. However, the mechanism of metal toxicity is not fully understood today. It is well known fact that metals are involved in production of reactive oxygen species (ROS), such as superoxide ions ($O_2^{\cdot-}$), hydrogen peroxide (H_2O_2), hydroxyl radical ($OH^{\cdot}$), and nitrogen oxide ($NO^{\cdot}$) via Fenton/Haber-Weiss chemistry (Sawyer, 1990). Free radicals may damage purine and pyrimidine bases of DNA (Valko et al., 2006). Moreover, direct binding of Cr to DNA is reported (Wolf et al., 1989) that may inhibit the process of DNA repair (Witkiewicz-Kucharczyk & Bal, 2006). These gene modifications and eventual mutations can lead to carcinogenesis. Metal ions have been also associated with a delayed immune reaction (hypersensitivity) (Hallab et al., 2001). It was suggested that a vicious circle of particle phagocytosis, cellular lysis and subsequent release of particles by the involved cells may play role in delayed hypersensitivity reaction mediated by T-lymphocytes (Hallab et al., 2005). In addition to systemic and cellular reactions various local adverse reactions such as extensive necrosis (Ollivere et al., 2009), periprosthetic osteolysis (Amstutz et al., 2011) and pseudotumour reactions (either cystic or solid) (De Haan et al., 2008, Wynn-Jones et al., 2011) have been reported with MoM bearings. Perivascular accumulation of activated macrophages and T-lymphocytes has also been associated with periprosthetic osteolysis (Park et al., 2005). In addition, direct toxicity may also be involved in bone loss (Fleury et al., 2006, McKay et al., 1996).

Cells in synovial membrane of the artificial hip joint generate synovial fluid that is called pseudosynovial fluid and secrete the mediators of inflammation into it. Schmalzried et al. hypothesized that wear debris is dispersed into the joint fluid (Schmalzried et al., 1992). Access to the joint fluid for the wear particles is dependent on the contact between implant and bone. Wear debris activates macrophages, which activate osteoclasts or become osteoclasts themselves and initiate bone resorption (Sabokbar et al., 1997). The resulting bone loss will enlarge the interface and ease the flow of joint fluid, resulting in higher transportation capacity of the debris and gradual loosening of the implant. This concept is in concordance with the high pressure theory that was suggested by Aspenberg and Van der Vis (Aspenberg & Van der Vis, 1998).

4. Oxidative stress

Oxidative stress is a condition when the balance of formation of oxidants exceeds the rate of metabolism and the ability of antioxidant systems to remove ROS. High levels of ROS can damage proteins, lipids, and DNA, and eventually cause cell death.

Alternatively, oxidative stress can trigger activation of specific physiologic signaling pathways (Rached et al., 2010). In several studies, reactive oxygen species have been demonstrated as one of the key factors in inflammation (Kamikawa et al., 2001, Wang et al., 2002, Tsaryk, 2009). Because of the inflammatory nature of aseptic loosening of total hip replacement, arthroplasty, it is likely that free radicals play a major role in this condition as well. In the periprosthetic tissues, detection of reactive oxygen species provides evidence for the formation and activity of free radicals (Windhager et al., 1998, Kinov et al., 2006). Under physiological conditions, ROS are part of normal regulatory circuits, and the cellular redox state is tightly controlled by antioxidants. However, increased concentrations of ROS and loss of cellular redox homeostasis following extensive particulate challenge can lead to up-regulation of inflammatory processes in the interface membrane.

The interface between implant and bone is rich of transitional metals from the alloy of the implant. Transition elements like vanadium (V), chromium (Cr), manganese (Mn), iron (Fe), cobalt (Co), nickel (Ni), molybdenum (Mo), so-called d-block elements, show variable valence, which allow them to undergo changes in oxidation state involving one electron. If free radicals have a causative role in aseptic loosening than transition metals would have a strong promotional effect (Windhager et al., 1998). Via the Fenton reaction they would greatly stimulate inflammation and loosening. Iron i.e., exerts its toxicity through a series of reactions with reactive oxygen species called modified Haber-Weiss or Fenton reaction (Fe2+ + H2O2 → Fe3+ [H2O2-] → .OH + -OH), generating the highly toxic hydroxyl radical (.OH) (Lubec, 1996).

The generation of hydroxyl radicals via Fenton chemistry represents one of the most important mechanisms in various pathologic conditions. Hydroxyl radicals can lead to DNA and protein damage and impairment of normal DNA and protein synthesis and cell proliferation and thus has been thought to be casually involved in the multistep process of loosening (Wang et al., 2002). Furthermore, ferrous/ferric ion has a decisive function in lipid peroxidation process by direct reaction with unsaturated fatty acids or reaction with preformed lipid hydroperoxides to form chain-carrying alkoxyl and peroxyl radicals, leading to severe damage of cellular integrity (Lin & Girotti, 1993, Minotti & Aust, 1992, Schaich, 1992).

The effects of the metal wear particles on oxidative stress are not augmented by polyethylene and cement wear debris, originating from materials used for implant fixation. In an in vitro study, Petit et al. compared the effects of different wear products from hip prostheses on the nitration of proteins (an evidence for oxidative damage) in macrophages (Petit et al., 2005). The effect of both Co(2+) and Cr(3+) ions was inhibited by glutathione monoethyl-ester that provides protection against oxidative stress. However, ultra-high molecular weight-polyethylene and alumina ceramic particles had no significant effect on the nitration of proteins.

Because of their excellent mechanical properties, titanium and titanium alloys are widely used in orthopedic implants. Moreover, superb corrosion resistance and biocompatibility are characteristic for titanium and are the main reasons for its wide use in various biomaterials. However, as a result of wear and corrosion, titanium ions are released in the periprosthetic tissues and can be found in systemic circulation. Titanium may be directly involved in ROS production interacting with H_2O_2 leading to formation of hydroxyl radicals

(Lee et al., 2005). ROS production may exceed physiological protection mechanisms and can thus be referred to as oxidative stress (Tsaryk, 2009).
CoCr alloys have higher corrosion rate compared to titanium and titanium alloys and release toxic Co and Cr ions. Furthermore, Co ions mediate oxidative stress and could increase up to eight times oxidative stress in the cell (Limbach et al., 2007).
It proves that elevated oxidative stress in the setting of aseptic loosening is a local phenomenon. Recent studies showed that increased levels of Co and Cr ions are not connected with elevation of the level of oxidative stress in the blood of patients (Antoniou et al., 2008, Tkaczyk et al., 2010).

4.1 Response to oxidative stress - oxidative stress and bone

Excessive amounts of ROS are toxic to the organism and cells have specific protection mechanisms against oxidative stress. In ROS deactivation, superoxide dismutase (SOD), catalase and gluthatione (GSH-GSSG) system play central role. In one of the most important systems, glutathione peroxidases detoxifies peroxides with GSH acting as an electron donor in the reduction reaction, producing GSSG as an end product (Townsend et al., 2003). Hence, the balance between reduced (GSH) and oxidized gluthatione (GSSG) is very important for protection against oxidative stress. A deficiency of GSH puts the cell at risk for oxidative damage. It is not surprising that an imbalance of protection mechanisms against oxidative stress is observed in wide range of pathologies including inflammatory and degenerative disorders with tissue fibrosis.
Elevated oxidative stress was associated with low bone mineral density (Ozgocmen et al., 2007, Basu et al., 2001) and gene polymorphisms in antioxidant enzymes were also associated with low bone mineral density (Mlakar et al., 2010). Further research elucidated oxidative stress as a potential modulator of osteogenesis in different skeletal diseases (Liu et al., 2010). ROS have been involved in osteoporosis by causing cellular death and by inhibiting osteoblast proliferation and stimulating osteoclast differentiation (Hamel et al., 2008, Weitzmann & Pacifici, 2006). It was proven that H_2O_2 inhibits osteoblast proliferation time- and dose-dependently (Li et al., 2009) and that decreasing oxidative stress normalizes bone formation and bone mass in mice (Rached et al., 2010). Although extensively studied (Bai et al., 2005, Basu et al., 2001, Mody et al., 2001, Rached et al., 2010)., the mechanisms of action of ROS on bone formation are not completely understood. (Bai et al., 2005, Basu et al., 2001, Mody et al., 2001, Rached et al., 2010).

5. Material and methods

5.1 Patients

In two studies, we investigated 58 total hip arthroplasties revised for aseptic loosening or high rate of wear of the polyethylene (40 hips) and osteolysis (12 hips) in order to clarify the involvement of ROS in the process of aseptic loosening.
Between August 1999 and October 2002, periprosthetic tissues were consecutively obtained at revision of 40 primary THAs at the Department of Orthopedic Surgery, Medical University of Graz. Group I consisted of 8 men and 20 women, with mean age 66 years (range, 32–88 years) at the time of revision. The mean interval between primary THA and revision was 126 months (range, 11–320 months). In Group II, there were three men and nine women with mean age 69 years (range, 54–84 years). In this group, the

mean interval between primary THA and revision was 97 months (range, 14–157 months) (p=0.405). As a control group, 16 samples of fascia lata were obtained from 16 patients during primary THA.

In a second study, periprosthetic tissues and pseudosynovial fluid were obtained at revision of 18 consecutive primary THA performed at the Department of Orthopedics and Traumatology, Medical University of Sofia. The eight men and 10 women in the series had mean age 63.2 years (range, 52 to 78 years) at the time of revision. The mean interval between primary THA and revision was 10.8 years (range, 2.1 to 22.3 years). The pseudosynovial fluid was immediately deep frozen at -80°C until analysis. The periprosthetic samples were fixed in 10% formalin until being processed. Patients with multiple revisions and infections were excluded from the studies. As a control group, 18 samples of joint fluid were obtained from 18 patients during primary TKA.

5.2 Radiographic analysis

Prostheses fixation was graded according to the criteria of Engh et al. (Engh et al., 1989) for the cementless and Harris & Penenberg (Harris & Penenberg, 1987) for the cemented components. Osteolysis was graded according to Paprosky (Paprosky & Burnett, 2002). Annual polyethylene wear was measured as described by Livermore et al. (Livermore et al., 1990) and corrected for magnification.

5.3 Histological examination

A portion of each specimen was embedded in paraffin, processed with xylene, cut into 5-mm thick sections, and stained with hematoxylin and eosin. All sections were studied blindly at a maximum magnification of 600x and were graded in a semiquantitative fashion for cellular constituents and particulate debris according to Mirra et al. (Mirra et al., 1976). Tissue necrosis was recorded as present or absent.

5.4 Electron microscopic examination

Evaluation of the ultrastructure of collagen was obtained by examination of ten representative cases with electron microscopy. These samples were fixed in glutharaldehyde and were processed with standard techniques.

5.5 GSH and GSSG determination

Reduced glutathione and oxidized glutathione was measured by spectrophotometry (Beckman Instruments, Fullerton, CA) according to the method of Tietze (Tietze, 1969). Measurements with GSH concentrations bellow 200 μmol/g wet weight were excluded from calculation because of high possibility for error. Results were then weighted for hydroxyproline content and expressed as μmol/mg. Samples were run in duplicates and run according to supplier's instructions (OxisResearch, Portland, OR).

5.6 Malondialdehyde determination

5.6.1 Malondialdehyde determination in periprosthetic tissue

Tissue malondialdehyde levels were determined by Khoschsorur's method (Khoschsorur et al., 2000). The samples were chromatographed on a high performance liquid chromatographer (HPLC) (Spectrochrom, Brackley, UK) interfaced to a LiChrosorb RP18 column. Fluorometric detection was performed with excitation at 527 nm and emission at 551 nm.

Arbitrary values obtained were compared with a series of standard solutions (Sigma-Aldrich, St. Louis, MO). Results were expressed as nmol/mg hydroxyproline.

5.6.2 Malondialdehyde determination in pseudojoint fluid

Joint fluid malondialdehyde levels were determined by the modified method of Yagi (Yagi, 1982). The samples were read with fluorometric detection at 515/553 nm. As a standard solution Tetraetoxypropane in concentration of 0.1 µmol/L was used. Results were expressed as nmol/L.

5.7 Collagen determination

Hydroxyproline content was evaluated according to the method of Reddy & Enwemeka (Reddy & Enwemeka, 1996). Absorbance of each sample was read at 550 nm using HPLC (Spectrochrom). Serial dilutions of commercial pure hydroxyproline (Sigma-Aldrich) were used as standard. All samples were assayed in duplicates. Results were expressed as mg/g wet tissue.

5.8 Metal particle analysis

Elemental concentrations were determined by Inductively Coupled Plasma-Mass Spectrometry (HP-4500; Agilent Technologies, Waldbronn, Germany). Standard reference material was obtained from NIST (RF 1577b, NIST, Gaithersburg, MD). Values were measured in µg/g wet weight.

6. Results

6.1 Histological examination

Histological examination of the periprosthetic tissues showed large amounts of metal and polyethylene debris and a nonspecific chronic inflammatory reaction. Wear debris, macrophages that had phagocytosed small metal and polyethylene particles, fibroid necrosis, and proliferation of capillaries were seen more commonly in granulomas (Fig. 1).

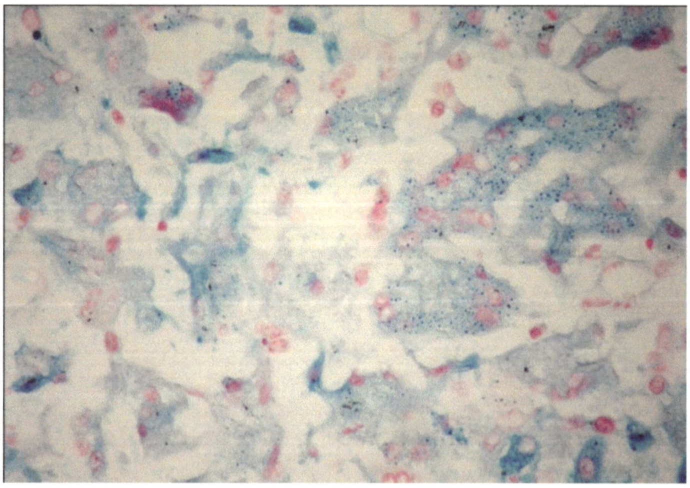

Fig. 1. Polyethylene and metal particles in the interstitium, giant cells and macrophages (Perle's iron stain, x500)

In contrast, stroma rich of connective tissue, abundance of fibroblasts with less frequent macrophages were more prevalent in the fibrous pseudocapsule (Fig. 2).

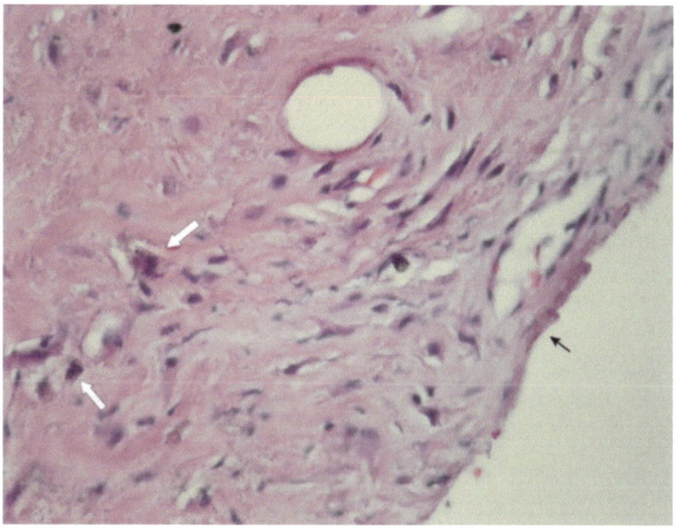

Fig. 2. Periprosthetic tissue from 72-year-old male, 9 years after implantation of cementless prosthesis. Adjacent to the implant synovia-like membrane with 1-2 cell layers (arrow), interstitial matrix rich of fibrous tissue with abundance of fibroblasts and macrophages digested wear debris (open arrow) (haematoxylene staining, x500).

6.2 Electron microscopic examination

Analysis of selected sections from ten representative cases by electron microscopy established damaged collagen fibers and presence of collagen cross-links. Their relative

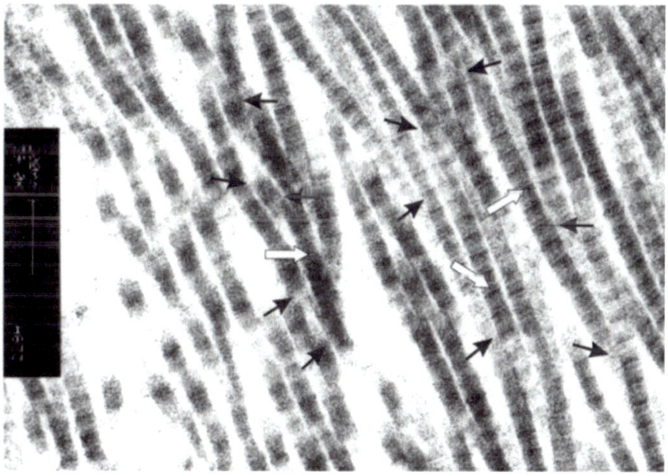

Fig. 3. Electron micrograph (x39 000) showing periprosthetic tissue taken from stable cementless hip replacement 86 months after implantation. The picture shows damaged collagen fibers (open arrows) with numerous cross-links (black arrows).

abundance compared to control samples taken from fascia lata supported the proposal that these findings were a result of ROS damage (Fig. 3). Wear debris inclusions were demonstrated in the various cells (Fig. 4).

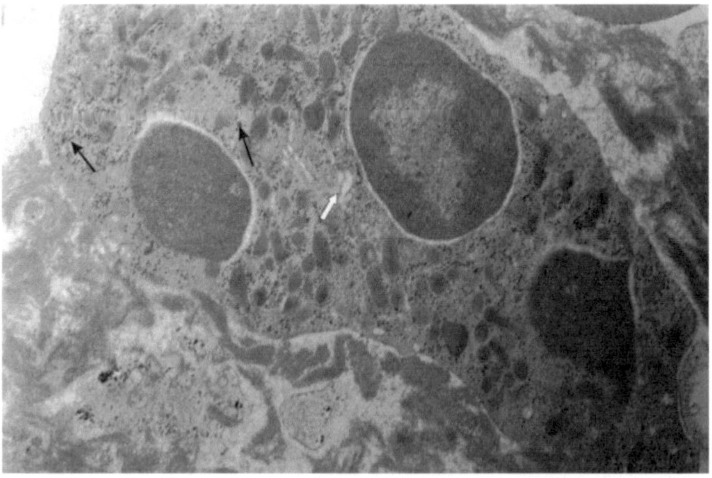

Fig. 4. Electron micrograph (x12 000) showing giant cell with ingested polyethylene (open arrow) and metal (black arrow) particles.

6.3 Glutathione determination

Level of reduced and oxidized glutathione was elevated in both groups compared to controls. However, a lower statistically significant GSH/GSSG ratio was detected only in Group II compared to Group I and controls ($p=0.005$ and $p=0.024$, respectively). GSH and GSSG concentrations and GSH/GSSG ratio in the two groups and controls are given in Table 1.

Analyzed parameter	***Group I*** (N 28)	***Group II*** (N 12)	***Controls*** (N 16)
GSH	74.1 ±67.3 *	58.7 ±35 *	18.9 ±20.9
GSSG	19.3 ±26.4 *	21.8 ±12.6 */***	4.3 ±4.4
GSH/GSSG	5.4 ±3.6	3.1 ±1.4 **/****	4.4 ±1.5

* $p<0.0001$, ** $p<0.024$ versus the control group; *** $p<0.045$, **** $p<0.005$ versus Group I

Table 1. The levels of GSH, GSSG, as well as GSH/GSSG ratio in periprosthetic tissues and controls. Values measured in µmol/mg hydroxyproline. Data represented as mean ±SD.

6.4 Malondialdehyde determination

6.4.1 Malondialdehyde determination in periprosthetic tissues

Determination of oxidative stress assessed by level of lipid peroxidation product MDA in periprosthetic tissues obtained from 40 primary THA, revised for loosening or high rate of wear, showed higher oxidative stress in the two groups. The mean MDA value of the 28 patients in Group I was 0.052 nmol/mg (±0.09 SD), and of the 12 patients with high rate of wear and osteolysis in Group II, 0.031 nmol/mg (±0.014 SD) (p=0.74). MDA levels in the control tissues (0.009 nmol/mg, ±0.0093 SD) were significantly lower than those in Group I (p<0.0001) and Group II (p<0.0001). Figure 5 shows the comparisons between the two groups and controls in graphical form.

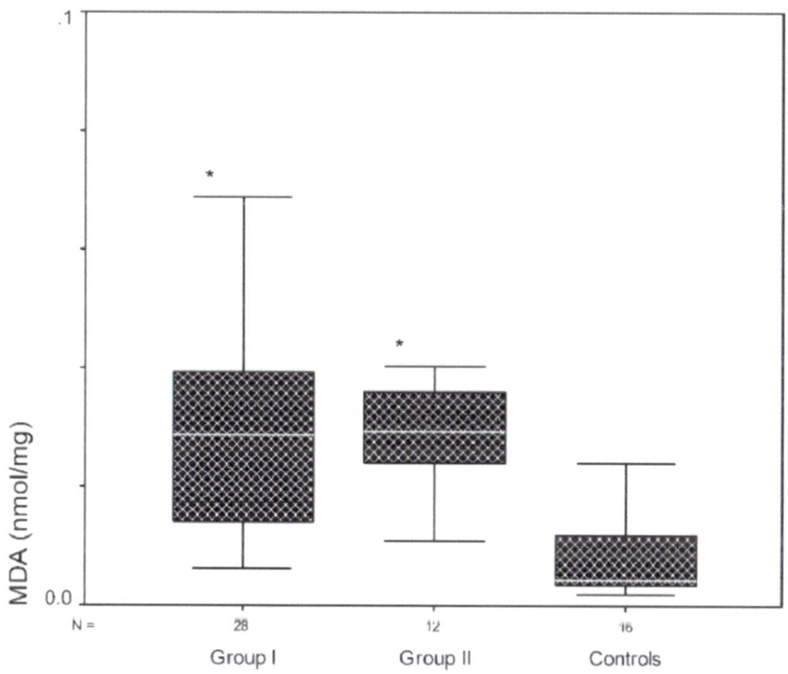

*p<0.0001 in comparison with controls.

Fig. 5. The concentration of lipid peroxidation product, malondialdehyde (MDA), in periprosthetic tissues and controls. Values were measured in nmol/mg hydroxyproline. The lower and upper lines in the boxes represent the 25th and 75th percentiles, respectively, with the median marked in the box.

6.4.2 Malondialdehyde determination in pseudosynovial fluid

Determination of oxidative stress assessed by level of lipid peroxidation product MDA in pseudojoint fluid showed higher oxidative stress in revision cases. The mean MDA value of the 18 patients with loose hip prostheses was 27.5 nmol/L (±17.6 SD, range 13.5 to 82.9). MDA level in the pseudojoint fluid from controls was significantly lower - 14.9 nmol/L (±4.5 SD, range 10.7 to 28.9) (p=0.001). Figure 6 shows the comparison between patients and controls in graphical form. Although not significantly, MDA level correlated moderately with linear polyethylene wear and grade of femoral osteolysis (Spearman's rho=0.321 and rho=0.315, respectively). Oxidative stress measured by MDA level in pseudosynovial fluid did not correlate with pelvic osteolysis or time elapsed from previous surgery.

6.5 Hydroxyproline determination

Mean value of hydroxyproline in both groups was 13.9 mg/g (±10.2 SD), and in controls, 55.6 mg/g (±38.6 SD) ($p<0.013$).

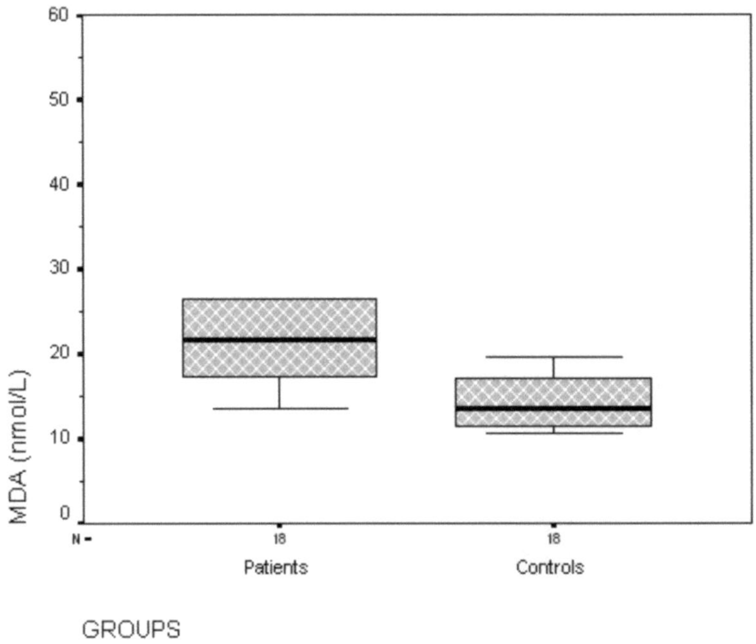

$p<0.001$

Fig. 6. The concentration of lipid peroxidation product - malondialdehyde in joint fluid. Values were measured in nmol/L. The lower and upper lines in the boxes represent the 25th and 75th percentiles, respectively, with the median marked in the box.

6.6 Metal particle analysis

The tissue concentrations of the different metals for the Co-Cr and Ti-alloy prostheses are shown in Table 2. The mean level of MDA in the 23 implants made of titanium alloy was 0.059 µg/mg, and of the 9 implants made of Co-Cr alloy, 0.023 µg/mg. However, this difference was not significant (p=0.145).

Composition Stem/Cup	Ti	V	Fe	Cr	Co
Co-Cr/Co-Cr alloy (N 9)	na	na	13.5 ±11.2	75.3 ±160 *	33.2 ±34.5
Ti/Ti alloy (N 23)	70.1 ±189.5	4.4 ±8.7	na	na	na
Co-Cr/Ti alloy (N 8)	381.8 ±911.9	20.6 ±46.5	11.2 ±12.2	2.7 ±4 *	4.1 ±5.6

* $p<0.013$ in comparison between groups

Table 2. Concentrations of various metals in periprosthetic tissues from Co-Cr alloy and titanium alloy prostheses. Values measured in µg/g wet tissue. Data represented as mean ±SD.

6.7 Correlations

In the 40 hips, levels of MDA correlated with levels of GSH and GSSG (rho=0.509, p<0.0001, and rho=0.421, p<0.001, respectively). Because oxidative stress is a significant contributor to tissue fibrosis, a second set of correlations was calculated that measured the correlation between oxidative stress and hydroxyproline content. There was a correlation between GSH, GSSG, as well as MDA levels and periprosthetic collagen content. GSH/GSSG ratio and MDA level correlated with degree of osteolysis (rho=0.337, p=0.007, and rho=0.374, p=0.017, respectively). GSSG and MDA levels were higher in hips with greater annual wear of the polyethylene.

7. Rationale of oxidative stress and aseptic loosening

Three different mechanisms are mainly responsible for osteolysis and loosening: exacerbated inflammation caused by ROS production in the periprosthetic tissue; cascade of cellular and molecular interactions ultimately resulting in osteoclasts activation; and, compromised bone formation resulting from increased cytotoxicity on mesenchymal osteoprogenitors.

Wear debris such as polyethylene, PMMA and metal particles, metal degradation products and ions may be exposed to the ROS produced by the inflammatory cells in the periprosthetic tissues. Mediators such as H_2O_2, NO and ONOO− are released by the macrophages and the inflammatory cells. Metal debris and metal degradation products could react with the free radicals resulting in elevation of oxidative stress. H_2O_2 in the cells can also undergo the Fenton reaction in the presence of metal ions with subsequent formation of highly toxic hydroxyl radical (Lubec, 1996, Sawyer, 1990). Various studies have reported that ROS are connected with tissue damage and fibrosis (Park et al., 2001, Riedle & Kerjaschki, 1997, Wang et al., 2002, Windhager et al., 1998). On the other hand, the effect of submicron wear debris on macrophage production of reactive oxygen species is largely unexplored. Thus, these facts led to the hypothesis that ROS play a role in aseptic loosening and formation of fibrous pseudocapsule around hip implants. Our results demonstrated in vivo elevated oxidative stress in periprosthetic tissues and pseudosynovial fluid from loose hip prostheses and hip implants with high rate of wear. This added further insight into the mechanism of aseptic loosening of hip arthroplasty.

When the cells are exposed to a large amount of oxidants, the capacity of the regulatory mechanisms of cellular response to oxidative stress may be exceeded by the rate of ROS production, resulting in a condition of "oxidative stress". In the present study, we found increased levels of markers of oxidative stress in periprosthetic tissues and pseudosynovial fluid from loose THAs. Our results are difficult to compare as the available studies on the possible role of oxidative stress in aseptic loosening of THA are in vitro experiments. We believe that, in the early stage of aseptic loosening, the exposure to wear debris could be responsible for the increase in the values of markers of oxidative stress in total hip arthroplasties with high rate of wear and osteolysis. Moreover, free radicals may be involved in sustaining the foreign-body reaction to wear debris. Later on, chronic exposure would result in a triggering of compensatory mechanisms leading to progressive increase in antioxidants and low oxidative stress as observed in the beginning of loosening (Table 1). This is consistent with the conception of oxidative stress regulation. However, other mechanisms may play role, too.

Lipids of cell membranes are a prominent target for free radicals generated in a complex series of oxygen-dependant reactions via Fenton's chemistry (Sawyer, 1990). Iron-induced lipid peroxidation has been demonstrated in various studies (Marmunti et al., 2004, Lim & Vaziri, 2004). However, we could not establish correlation between levels of MDA and iron. As metal-catalyzed lipid peroxidation is dependent on metal as a catalyst, there might be little influence of metal concentrations, and many other factors might also contribute to MDA formation. On the opposite, we found elevated MDA level in hips with prostheses made of titanium alloy. This finding might be explained by higher rate of wear of titanium implants compared to Co-Cr implants (Table 2) (Wang et al., 2002). We hypothesized that the process of wear debris-mediated loosening leads to elevation of oxidative stress. In support of this, Wang et al. found that exposure to particles stimulates superoxide production by macrophages and osteoclasts (Wang et al., 2002). Furthermore, it was observed that the increase of free radicals on polyethylene correlated with the degree of inflammation of synovial cells in culture (Fiorito et al., 2001). The correlation between markers of oxidative stress and hydroxyproline levels suggest, first of all, that the increase of collagen in periprosthetic tissues in the presence of wear debris is due to elevated oxidative stress. Connective tissue metabolism is normally characterized by equilibrium between degradation and synthesis of extracellular matrix. Deviation from the equilibrium may lead to the replacement of extracellular matrix by fibrous tissue (Park et al., 2001, Riedle & Kerjaschki, 1997, Wang et al., 2002, Windhager et al., 1998). The fibrous pseudocapsule formed is probably related to high intraarticular pressure and expansion of the effective joint space as well as production of inflammatory substances and subsequent loosening of the implant (El-Warrak et al., 2004, Van der Vis et al., 1998).
Most of the studies elucidating the mechanism of loosening of hip arthroplasty are performed on animal models or are in vitro studies. However, the results from in vitro or animal studies could not be easily translated to humans. The findings of our in vivo studies provide further insight into the possible mechanisms of aseptic loosening. The number of cases in the studies was relatively small but the differences in measurements of markers of oxidative stress between patients and controls were high which compensated for small sample size.

8. Future perspectives

Clinical results of total hip arthroplasty deteriorate with time with aseptic loosening being the main reason for its failure. Clinical and experimental studies show that aseptic loosening is a failure of fixation of the implant secondary to wear of the components of the prostheses (Bechtold et al., 2002, El-Warrak et al., 2004, Willert & Semlitsch, 1977).
Improvements in bearing surfaces may diminish implant wear and associated osteolysis. For forty years, MoPE is the bearing of choice in THA. After recognition of the problem of wear alternative bearings were proposed. Metal-on-high cross-linked polyethylene, ceramic-on-polyethylene, ceramic-on-ceramic, and metal-on-metal are becoming increasingly popular.
However, reducing particle size may increase its biological activity (Sieber et al., 1999, Yang et al., 2002). Moreover, some of the new alternative bearings are very sensitive to improper surgical technique.
The initial bone-implant interface is of paramount importance for the longevity of the joint reconstruction. After implantation the prosthesis is in contact with the bone, but as the

contact is not uniform along the entire surface there are gaps between the surfaces. During the healing phase, these gaps are filled with callus tissue which may mature in different directions, i.e. by bony healing or osseointegration, where there is no fibrous lining between the implant and the bone, or by soft tissue encapsulation with formation of synovial-like membrane (Albrektsson, 1990). In osseointegration of the prosthesis the interface can resist shearing as well as tensile loads whereas the fibrous tissue interface can withstand compressive and, to lesser extent, shear loads, but fails with tensile loads. In the case of soft tissue anchorage when the prosthesis is loaded there will be movements. As far as they are micro-movements the implant will be stable. Some bone resorption will occur, but it is usually compensated for by new bone formation to maintain equilibrium between applied load and strength of tissue. But even in the physiological range of movement there is a constant risk of overloading the device which will result in macro-movements and implant failure. Improving initial implant fixation with bisphosphonates may represent a promising strategy for improving initial fixation and clinical outcome after THA (Friedl et al., 2009, Kinov et al., 2006).

Successful inhibition of osteoclast activity in postmenopausal osteoporosis and increase of bone mineral density with use of bisphosphonates turn research efforts in this direction. Osteoclast is the ultimate cell in the cascade of events that lead to periprosthetic osteolysis. Various in vitro and animal studies have shown encouraging results (Horowitz et al., 1996, Millett et al., 2002, Shanbhag et al., 1997, von Knoch et al., 2005). However currently, convincing results from clinical studies supporting the use of bisphosphonates are still lacking.

The local inflammatory response to wear debris particles with cascade of cellular and molecular interactions ultimately results in periprosthetic osteolysis and aseptic loosening. Biological approach to prevention of this deleterious complication of THA seems promising. In-depth research into bone biology and molecular mechanisms of bone metabolism has led to the identification of novel possible strategies. Receptor activator of nuclear factor kappa-B ligand (RANKL) plays a key role in osteoclastogenesis which makes this cytokine an attractive target in efforts for prevention of osteolysis. Clinical studies have demonstrated its effectiveness in decreasing bone turnover and fracture prevention (Bekker et al., 2004, Cummings et al., 2009). However, its potent effect on osteoclast function has not been evaluated in periprosthetic osteolysis.

Other promising novel therapeutical targets include: osteoclast protease cathepsin K; sclerostin and dickkopf-1, two endogenous inhibitors of bone formation; the osteoclast ATPase proton pump, vitronectin receptor, and src tyrosine kinase, all of which are required for resorption (Purdue et al., 2006).

Such approaches would be expected to decrease bone loss, but not influence inflammation. It was proven that tumor necrosis factor alpha (TNF α) is capable of inducing osteoclastogenesis in presence of small amounts of RANKL (Lam et al., 2000) whereas interleukin-1 (IL-1) is directly involved into osteoclast differentiation (Yao et al., 2008). This suggests that effective inhibition of osteolysis includes blockade of proinflammatory mediators. In support of this direct evidence that cyclo-oxygenase 2 (COX-2) inhibits wear induced osteolysis in an animal model were provided (Zhang et al., 2001). However, these treatment possibilities should be approached with caution as signaling molecules are involved in variety of processes and their inconsiderate manipulation may have deleterious effects.

The local inflammatory response of the organism to wear debris is the main cause for osteolysis and prostheses loosening. However, current knowledge of wear-induced mechanism of aseptic loosening is not complete. Understanding of the mechanisms of wear-induced osteolysis will help control undesirable processes at the implant-bone interface and extend longevity of hip arthroplasty.

9. Conclusion

Our study provided further insight into the mechanism of aseptic loosening of hip arthroplasty. The most interesting aspect of this study is the evidence of elevated production of ROS, which are known to cause tissue fibrosis and may help explain the initiation of aseptic loosening. We feel that the thick pseudocapsule around loose prostheses is not an adaptive but a reactive tissue as a result of decreased degradation and increased formation of collagen matrix and proliferation of fibroblasts due to high oxidative stress. Furthermore, we demonstrated that elevated oxidative stress is associated with aseptic loosening of hip arthroplasty, suggesting that oxidative stress might induce periprosthetic osteolysis and subsequent loosening. Research in this line may help introducing new strategies for therapeutic prevention and/or treatment of osteolysis and subsequent aseptic loosening of total hip arthroplasty.

10. References

Aitken, C., Hodge, J., Nishinaka, Y., Vaughan, T., Yodoi, J., Day, C., Morrison, N. & Nicholson, G. (2004). Regulation of human osteoclast differentiation by thioredoxin binding protein-2 and redoxsensitive signaling, *J Bone Miner Res* Vol.19:2057–2064.

Albrektsson, T. (1990). Biological factors of importance for bone integration of implanted devices, *in* Older MWJ (ed.), *Implant bone interface*, Springer-Velag, London.

Amstutz, H., Wisk, L. & Le Duff, M. (2011). Sex as a patient selection criterion for metal-on-metal hip resurfacing arthroplasty, *J Arthroplasty* Vol.26:198-208.

Antoniou, J., Zukor, D.J., Mwale, F., Minarik, W., Petit, A. & Huk, O.L. (2008). Metal ion levels in the blood of patients after hip resurfacing: a comparison between twenty-eight and thirty-six-millimeter-head metal-on-metal prostheses, *J Bone Joint Surg Am* Vol.90(Suppl. 3):142-8.

Aspenberg, P. & Herbertsson, P. (1996). Periprosthetic bone resorption. Particles versus movement, *J Bone Joint Surg Br* Vol.78:641–646.

Aspenberg, P. & Van der Vis, H. (1998). Fluid pressure may cause periprosthetic osteolysis. Particles are not the only thing, *Acta Orthop Scand* Vol.69(No.1):1-4.

Bai, X.C., Lu, D., Bai, J., Zheng, H., Ke, Z.Y., Li, X.M. & Luo, S.Q. (2004). Oxidative stress inhibits osteoblastic differentiation ofbone cells by ERK and NF-kB, *Biochem Biophys Res Commun* Vol.314:197–207.

Bai, X.C., Lu, D., Liu, A.L., Zhang, Z.M., Li, X.M., Zou, Z.P., Zeng, W.S., Cheng, B.L. & Luo, S.Q. (2005). Reactive oxygen species stimulates receptor activator of NF-kappaB ligand expression in osteoblast, *J Biol Chem* Vol.280:17497–17506.

Basu, S., Michaëlsson, K., Olofsson, H., Johansson, S. & Melhus, H. (2001). Association between oxidative stress and bone mineral density, *Biochem Biophys Res Commun* Vol.288(No.1):275-9.

Bechtold, J.E., Kubic, V. & Sobale, K. (2002). Bone ingrowth in the presence of particulate polyethylene, *Bone Joint Surg Br* Vol.84:915-919.

Bekker, P.J., Holloway, D.L., Rasmussen, A.S., Murphy, R., Martin, S.W., Leese, P.T., Holmes, G.B., Dunstan, C.R. & DePaoli, A.M. (2004). A single-dose placebo-controlled study of AMG 162, a fully human monoclonal antibody to RANKL, in postmenopausal women, *J Bone Miner Res* Vol.19(No.7):1059-66.

Bierbaum, B.E., Nairus, J., Kuesis, D., Morrison, J.C. & Ward, D. (2002). Ceramic-on-ceramic bearings in total hip arthroplasty, *Clin Orthop Relat Res* Vol.405:158-63.

Boutin, P. (1971). [Alumina and its use in surgery of the hip. (Experimental study)], *Presse Med;* Vol.79(No.14):639–640.

Boutin, P.& Blanquaert, D. (1981). A study of the mechanical properties of alumina-on-alumina total hip prosthesis, *Rev Chir Orthop Reparatrice Appar Mot* Vol.67(No.3):279-87.

Brooks, R.A., Wimhurst, J.A. & Rushton, N. (2002) Endotoxin contamination of particles produces misleading inflammatory cytokine responses from macrophages in vitro, *J Bone Joint Surg Br* Vol.84:295–299.

Campbell, D.G., Field, J.R. & Callary, S.A. (2010) Second-generation highly cross-linked X3™ polyethylene wear: a preliminary radiostereometric analysis study, *Clin Orthop Relat Res* Vol.468(No.10):2704-9.

Capello, W.N., Dantonio, J.A., Feinberg, J.R. & Manley, M.T. (2005). Alternative bearing surfaces: alumina ceramic bearings for total hip arthroplasty, *Instr Course Lect* Vol.54:171-6.

Catelas, I., Bobyn, J.D., Medley, J.B., Krygier, J.J., Zukor, D.J. & Huk, O.L. (2003). Size, shape, and composition of wear particles from metal-metal hip simulator testing: effects of alloy and number of loading cycles, *J Biomed Mater Res A* Vol.67: 312-327.

Charnley, J., Follacci, F.M. & Hammond, B.T. (1968). The long-term reaction of bone to self-curing acrylic cement, *J Bone Joint Surg Br* Vol.50:822–829.

Charnley, J. (1979). *Low Friction Arthroplasty of the hip,* Springer-Verlag, Berlin-Heidelberg-New York.

Chen, R.M., Lin, Y.L. & Chou, C.W. (2010). GATA 3 transduces survival signals in osteoblasts through upregulation of bcl-x(L) gene expression, *J Bone Miner Res* Vol.25(No.10):2193-204.

Cummings, S.R., San Martin, J., McClung, M.R., Siris, E.S., Eastell, R., Reid, I.R., Delmas, P., Zoog, H.B., Austin, M., Wang, A., Kutilek, S., Adami, S., Zanchetta, J., Libanati, C., Siddhanti, S. & Christiansen, C. (2009). FREEDOM Trial. Denosumab for prevention of fractures in postmenopausal women with osteoporosis, *N Engl J Med* Vol.361(No.8):756-65.

De Haan, R., Campbell, P.A., Su, E.P. & De Smet, K.A. (2008). Revision of metal-on-metal resurfacing arthroplasty of the hip: the influence of malpositioning of the components, *J Bone Joint Surg Br* Vol.90:1158-1163.

Doorn, P.F., Campbell, P. & Amstutz, H. (1999). Particle disease in metal-on-metal total hip replacements. *in*: Rieker, C.B., Windler, M. & Wyss, U. (eds.), *Metasul: A Metal-on-Metal Bearing,* Huber, Bern, pp. 113–119.

El-Warrak, A.O., Olmstead, M., Schneider, R., Meinel, L., Bettschart-Wolfisberger, R., Akens, M.K., Auer, J. & von Rechenberg, B. (2004). An experimental animal model of aseptic loosening of hip prostheses in sheep to study early biochemical changes at the interface membrane, *BMC Musculoskelet Disord* 5:7.

Engh, C.A., Massin, P. & Suthers, K.E. (1989). Roentgenographic assessment of the biologic fixation of porous-surfaced femoral components, *Clin Orthop Relat Res* Vol.257:107–128.

Fiorito, S., Goze, C., Adrey, J., Magrini, L., Goalard, C. & Bernier, P. (2001). Increase in free radicals on UHMWPE hip prostheses components due to inflamed synovial cell products, *J Biomed Mater Res* Vol.57:35–40.

Firkins, P.J., Tipper, J.L., Saadatzadeh, M.R., Ingham, E., Stone, M.H., Farrar, R. & Fisher, J. (2001). Quantitative analysis of wear and wear debris from metal-on-metal hip prostheses tested in a physiological hip joint simulator, *Biomed Mater Eng* Vol.11(No.2):143–157.

Fleury, C., Petit, A., Mwale, F., Antoniou, J., Zukor, D.J., Tabrizian, M. & Huk, O.L. (2006). Effect of cobalt and chromium ions on human MG-63 osteoblasts in vitro: morphology, cytotoxicity, and oxidative stress, *Biomaterials* Vol.27:3351-3360.

Friedl, G., Radl, R., Stihsen, C., Rehak, P., Aigner, R. & Windhager, R. (2009). The effect of a single infusion of zoledronic acid on early implant migration in total hip arthroplasty. A randomized, double-blind, controlled trial, *J Bone Joint Surg Am* Vol.91(No.2):274-81.

Goldring, S.R., Jasty, M., Roueke, C.M., Bringhurst, F.R. & Harris, W.H. (1986). Formation of a synovial-like membrane at the bone-cement interface. Its role in bone resorption and implant loosening after total hip replacement, *Arthritis Rheum* Vol.29(No.7):836–842.

Hallab, N., Merritt, K. & Jacobs, J.J. (2001). Metal sensitivity in patients with orthopaedic implants, *J Bone Joint Surg Am* Vol.83(No.3):428-36.

Hallab, N.J., Anderson, S., Stafford, T., Glant, T. & Jacobs, J.J. (2005). Lymphocyte responses in patients with total hip arthroplasty, *J Orthop Res* Vol.23(No.2):384-91.

Hamel, P., Abed, E., Brissette, L. & Moreau, R. (2008). Characterization of oxidized low-density lipoprotein-induced hormesis-like effects in osteoblastic cells, *Am J Physiol Cell Physiol* Vol.294(No.4):C1021-33.

Harris, W.H., Schiller, A.L., Scholler, J.M., Friberg, R.A. & Scott, R. (1976). Extensive localized bone resorption in the femur following total hip replacement, *J Bone Joint Surg Am* 58:612–618.

Harris, W.H. & Penenberg, B.L. (1987). Further follow-up on socket fixation using a metal-backed acetabular component for total hip replacement, *J Bone Joint Surg Am* Vol.69:1140–1143.

Hogg, N. (1998). Free Radicals in Disease, *Semin Reprod Endocrin* Vol.16:241-248.

Horowitzm S.M., Algan, S.A. & Purdon, M.A. (1996). Pharmacologic inhibition of particulate-induced bone resorption, *J Biomed Mater Res* Vol.31:91–96.

Jones, L.C. & Hungerford, D.S. (1987). Cement disease, *Clin Orthop Relat Res* Vol.225:192–206.

Kamikawa, K., Harada, Y., Nagata, K. & Moriya, H. (2001). Differential effects of oxidised and non-oxidised polyethylene particles on human monocyte/macrophages in vitro, *J Bone Joint Surg Br* Vol.83:593-7.

Keegan, G.M., Learmonth, I.D. & Case, C.P. (2007). Orthopaedic metals and their potential toxicity in the arthroplasty patient: A review of current knowledge and future strategies, *J Bone Joint Surg Br* Vol.89(No.5):567-73.

Khoschsorur, G.A., Winklhofer-Roob, B.M., Rabl, H., Auer, T., Peng, Z. & Schaur, R. J. (2000). Evaluation of a sensitive HPLC method for the determination of malondialdehyde, and application of the method different biological materials, *Chromatographia* Vol.52:181–184.

Kido, A., Pap, G., Nagler, D.K., Ziomek, E., Ménard, R., Neumann, H.W. & Roessner A. (2004). Protease expression in interface tissues around loose arthroplasties. *Clin Orthop Relat Res* Vol.425:230–236.

Kim, W.K., Meliton, V., Bourquard, N., Hahn, T.J. & Parhami, F. (2010). Hedgehog signaling and osteogenic differentiation in multipotent bone marrow stromal cells are inhibited by oxidative stress, *J Cell Biochem* Vol.111(No.5):1199-209.

Kinov, P., Leithner, A., Radl, R., Bodo, K., Khoschsorur, G. A., Schauenstein, K. & R. Windhager. (2006). Role of free radicals in aseptic loosening of hip arthroplasty, *J Orthop Res* Vol.24:55-62.

Kinov, P., Tivchev, P., Doukova, P. & Leithner, A. (2006). Effect of risedronate on bone metabolism after total hip arthroplasty: a prospective randomised study, *Acta Orthop Belg* Vol.72(No.1):44-50.

Kurtz, S.M. (2004). *The UHMWPE handbook: ultra-high molecular weight polyethylene in total joint replacement*, Elsevier, Boston.

Kurtz, S.M., Austin, M.S., Azzam, K., Sharkey, P.F., MacDonald, D.W., Medel, F.J. & Hozack, W.J. (2010). Mechanical properties, oxidation, and clinical performance of retrieved highly cross-linked crossfire liners after intermediate-term implantation, *J Arthroplasty* Vol.25(No.4):614-23.

Lam, J., Takeshita, S., Barker, J.E., Kanagawa, O., Ross, F.P. & Teitelbaum, S.L. (2000). TNF-alpha induces osteoclastogenesis by direct stimulation of macrophages exposed to permissive levels of RANK ligand, *J Clin Invest* Vol.106(No.12):1481-8.

Lean, J.M., Jagger, C.J., Kirstein, B., Fuller, K. & Chambers, T.J. (2005). Hydrogen peroxide is essential for estrogendeficiency bone loss and osteoclast formation, *Endocrinology* Vol.146:728 735.

Lee, M.C., Yoshino, F., Shoji, H., Takahashi, S., Todoki, K., Shimada, S. & Kuse-Barouch, K. (2005). Characterization by electron spin resonance spectroscopy of reactive oxygen species generated by titanium dioxide and hydrogen peroxide, *J Dent Res* Vol.84:178-82.

Li, M., Zhao, L., Liu, J., Liu, A.L., Zeng, W.S., Luo, S.Q. & Bai, X.C. (2009). Hydrogen peroxide induces G2 cell cycle arrest and inhibits cell proliferation in osteoblasts, *Anat Rec (Hoboken)* Vol.292(No.8):1107-13.

Lim, C.S. & Vaziri, N.D. (2004). Iron and oxidative stress in renal insufficiency, *Am J Nephrol* Vol.24:569–575.

Limbach, L.K., Wick, P., Manser, P., Grass, R.N., Bruinink, A. & Stark, W.J. (2007). Exposure of engineered nanoparticles to human lung epithelial cells: influence of chemical composition and catalytic activity on oxidative stress, *Environ Sci Technol* Vol.41(No.11):4158-63.

Lin, F. & Girotti, A.W. (1993). Photodynamic action of merocyanine 540 on leukemia cells: iron-stimulated lipid peroxidation and cell killing, *Arch Biochem Biophys* Vol.300(No.2):714-23.

Liu, H., Sun, J.C., Zhao, Z.T., Zhang, J.M., Xu, H. & Li, G.S. (2010). Fluoride-induced oxidative stress in three-dimensional culture of os732 cells and rats, *Biol Trace Elem Res* doi: 10.1007/s12011-010-8881-0 [Epub ahead of print]

Livermore, J., Ilstrup, D. & Morrey, B. (1990). Effect of femoral head size on wear of the polyethylene acetabular component, *J Bone Joint Surg Am* Vol.72:518–528.

Lubec, G. (1996). The hydroxyl radical: from chemistry to human disease, *J Investig Med* Vol.44(No.6):324-46.

Marmunti, M., Gavazza, M. & Catala, A. (2004). Nonenzymatic and enzymatic lipid peroxidation of microsomes and nuclei obtained from rat liver, *Mol Cell Biochem* Vol.265:1–9.

Mazière, C., Savitsky, V., Galmiche, A., Gomila, C., Massy, Z. & Mazière, J.C. (2010). Oxidized low density lipoprotein inhibits phosphate signaling and phosphate-induced mineralization in osteoblasts. Involvement of oxidative stress, *Biochim Biophys Acta* Vol.1802(No.11):1013-9.

McKay, G.C., Macnair, R., MacDonald, C. & Grant, M.H. (1996). Interactions of orthopaedic metals with an immortalized rat osteoblast cell line, *Biomaterials* Vol.17:1339-1344.

McKee, G.K. & Watson-Farrar, J. (1966). Replacement of arthritic hips by the McKee-Farrar prosthesis, *J Bone Joint Surg Br* Vol.48(No.2):245–259.

McKellop, H., Shen, F.-W., Lu, B., Campbell, P. & Salovey, R. (1999). Development of an extremely wear resistant ultra-high molecular weight polyethylene for total hip replacements, *J Orthop Res* Vol.17(No.2):157–167.

Millett, P.J., Allen, M.J. & Bostrom, M.P. (2002). Effects of alendronate on particle-induced osteolysis in a rat model, *J Bone Joint Surg Am* Vol.84:236-49.

Minotti, G. & Aust, S.D. (1992). Redox cycling of iron and lipid peroxidation, *Lipids* Vol.27(No.3):219-26.

Mirra, J.M., Amstutz, H.C., Matos, M. & Gold, R. (1976). The pathology of the joint tissues and its clinical relevance in prosthesis failure. *Clin Orthop Relat Res* Vol.117:221–240.

Mlakar, S.J., Osredkar, J., Prezelj, J. & Marc, J. (2010). The antioxidant enzyme GPX1 gene polymorphisms are associated with low BMD and increased bone turnover markers, *Dis Markers* Vol.29(No.2):71-80.

Mody, N., Parhami, F., Sarafian, T.A. & Demer, L.L. (2001). Oxidative stress modulates osteoblastic differentiation of vascular and bone cells, *Free Radic Biol Med* Vol.31:509–519.

Muratoglu, O.K., Bragdon, C.R., O'Connor, D.O., Jasty, M. & Harris, W.H. (2001). A novel method of crosslinking UHMWPE to improve wear, reduce oxidation and retain mechanical properties, *J Arthrop* Vol.16(No.2):149–160.

Muratoglu, O.K. & Kurtz, S.M. (2002). Alternate bearing surfaces in hip replacement, *in* Sinha, R.K. (ed.), *Hip replacement. Current trends and controversies,* Marcel Dekker, New York, pp. 1-46.

Ollivere, B., Darrah, C., Barker, T., Nolan, J. & Porteous, M.J. (2009). Early clinical failure of the Birmingham metal-onmetal hip resurfacing is associated with metallosis and softtissue necrosis, *J Bone Joint Surg Br* Vol.91:1025-1030.

Ozgocmen, S., Kaya, H., Fadillioglu, E., Aydogan, R. & Yilmaz, Z. (2007). Role of antioxidant systems, lipid peroxidation, and nitric oxide in postmenopausal osteoporosis, *Mol Cell Biochem* Vol.295(No.1-2):45-52.

Paprosky, W.G. & Burnett, R.S. (2002). Assessment and classification of bone stock deficiency in revision total hip arthroplasty, *Am J Orthop* Vol.31:459–464.

Park, S.K., Kim, J., Seomun, Y., Choi, J., Kim, D.H., Han, I.O., Lee, E.H., Chung, S.K. & Joo, C.K. (2001). Hydrogen peroxide is a novel inducer of connective tissue growth factor, *Biochem Biophys Res Comm* Vol.284:966–971.

Park, Y.S., Moon, Y.W., Lim, S.J., Yang, J.M., Ahn, G. & Choi, Y.L. (2005). Early osteolysis following second-generation metal-on-metal hip replacement, *J Bone Joint Surg Am* Vol.87:1515-1521.

Petit, A., Mwale, F., Tkaczyk, C., Antoniou, J., Zukor, D.J. & Huk O.L. (2005). Induction of protein oxidation by cobalt and chromium ions in human U937 macrophages, *Biomaterials* Vol.26:4416-4422.

Purdue, P.E., Koulouvaris, P., Nestor, B.J. & Sculco, T.P. (2006). The central role of wear debris in periprosthetic osteolysis, *HSS J* Vol.2(No.2):102-13.

Rached, M.T., Kode, A., Xu, L., Yoshikawa, Y., Paik, J.H., Depinho, R.A. & Kousteni, S. (2010). FoxO1 is a positive regulator of bone formation by favoring protein synthesis and resistance to oxidative stress in osteoblasts. *Cell Metab* Vol.11(No.2):147-60.

Reddy, G.K. & Enwemeka, C.S. (1996). A simplified method for the analysis of hydroxyproline in biological tissues, *Clin Biochem* Vol.29:225–229.

Riedle, B. & Kerjaschki, D. (1997). Reactive oxygen species cause direct damage of Engelbreth-Holm-Swarm matrix, *Am J Pathol* Vol.151:215–231.

Ring PA. (1967). Total hip replacement, *Proc R Soc Med* Vol.60(No.3):281-4.

Sabokbar, A., Fujikawa, Y., Neale, S., Murray, D.W. & Athanasou, N.A. (1997). Human arthroplasty derived macrophages differentiate into osteoclastic bone resorbing cells. *Ann Rheum Dis* Vol.56:414-420.

Sawyer, D.T. (1990). Iron induced activation of HOOH, *J Exp Pathol* Vol.31:116–131.

Schaich, K.M. (1992). Metals and lipid oxidation. Contemporary issues, *Lipids* Vol.27(No.3):209 18.

Schmalzried, T.P., Jasty, M. & Harris, W.H. (1992). Periprosthetic bone loss in total hip arthroplasty. Polyethylene wear debris and the concept of the effective joint space, *J Bone Joint Surg Am* Vol.74:849–863.

Shanbhag, A.S., Hasselman, C.T. & Rubash, H.E. (1997). Inhibition of wear debris mediated osteolysis in a canine total hip arthroplasty model, *Clin Orthop Relat Res* Vol.344:33-43.

Sieber, H.P., Rieker, C.B. & Köttig, P. (1999). Analysis of 118 second-generation metal-on-metal retrieved hip implants, *J Bone Joint Surg Br* Vol.81:46-50.

Tietze, F. (1969). Enzymic method for quantitative determination of nanogram amounts of total and oxidized glutathione: applications to mammalian blood and other tissues, *Anal Biochem* Vol.27:502–522.

Tkaczyk, C., Petit, A., Antoniou, J., Zukor, D.J., Tabrizian, M. & Huk, O.L. (2010). Significance of Elevated Blood Metal Ion Levels in Patients with Metal-on-Metal Prostheses: An Evaluation of Oxidative Stress Markers, *Open Orthop J* Vol.4:221-7.

Townsend, D.M., Tew, K.D. & Tapiero, H. (2003). The importance of glutathione in human disease, *Biomed Pharmacother* Vol.57(No.3-4):145-55.

Tsaryk, R. (2009). Effects of metal-induced oxidative stress on endothelial cells in vitro, *Dissertation*, Mainz.

Valko, M., Rhodes, C.J., Moncol, J., Izakovic, M. & Mazur, M. (2006). Free radicals, metals and antioxidants in oxidative stress-induced cancer, *Chem Biol Interact* Vol.160:1-40.

Van der Vis, H.M., Aspenberg, P., Marti, R.K., Tigchelaar, W. & Van Noorden, C.J. (1998). Fluid pressure causes bone resorption in a rabbit model of prosthetic loosening, *Clin Orthop Relat Res* Vol.350:201–208.

von Knoch, M., Wedemeyer, C. & Pingsmann, A. (2005). The decrease of particle-induced osteolysis after a single dose of bisphosphonates, *Biomaterials* Vol.26:1803–1808.

Wang, M.L., Hauschka, P.V., Tuan, R.S. & Steinbeck, M.J. (2002). Exposure to particles stimulates superoxide production by human THP-1 macrophages and avian HD-11EM osteoclasts activated by tumor necrosis factor-alpha and PMA, *J Arthroplasty* Vol.17:335–346.

Wei, X., Zhang, X., Flick, L.M., Drissi, H., Schwarz, E.M. & O'Keefe, R.J. (2009). Titanium particles stimulate COX-2 expression in synovial fibroblasts through an oxidative stress-induced, calpain-dependent, NF-kappaB pathway, *Am J Physiol Cell Physiol* Vol.297:C310-320.

Weitzmann, M.N. & Pacifici, R. (2006). Estrogen deficiency and bone loss: an inflammatory tale, *J Clin Invest* Vol.116:1186–1194.

Wiles, P. (1957). The surgery of the osteo-arthritic hip. *Br J Surg* Vol.45:488–497.

Willert, H.G., Semlitsch, M. (1977). Reactions of the articular capsule to wear products of artificial joint prostheses. *J Biomed Mater Res* Vol.11:157–164.

Willmann, G., (1998). Ceramics for total hip replacement—What a surgeon should know, Orthopedics Vol.21(No.2):173–177.

Windhager, R., Nemethova, M., Mutsaers, S., Lang, S., Kotz, R., Kitzmueller, E. & Lubec G. (1998). Evidence for the involvement of the hydroxyl radical in the pathogenesis of excessive connective tissue proliferation in patients with tumorendoprostheses, *Life Sci* Vol.62:1261–1269.

Witkiewicz-Kucharczyk, A. & Bal, W. (2006). Damage of zinc fingers in DNA repair proteins, a novel molecular mechanism in carcinogenesis, *Toxicol Lett* Vol.162:29-42.

Wolf, T., Kasemann, R. & Ottenwälder, H. (1989). Molecular interaction of different chromium species with nucleotides and nucleic acids, *Carcinogenesis* Vol.10:655-659.

Wynn-Jones, H., Macnair, R., Wimhurst, J., Chirodian, N., Derbyshire, B., Toms, A. & Cahir, J. (2011). Silent soft tissue pathology is common with a modern metal-on-metal hip arthroplasty, *Acta Orthop* Vol.82(No.3):301-7.

Yagi, K. (1982) Assay for serum lipid peroxide level and its clinical significance, *Biochem Med;* Vol.30: 223-241.

Yang, S.Y., Ren, W., Park, Y., Sieving, A., Hsu, S., Nasser, S. & Wooley, P.H. (2002). Diverse cellular and apoptotic responses to variant shapes of UHMWPE particles in a murine model of inflammation, *Biomaterials* Vol.23:3535–3543.

Yao, Z., Xing, L., Qin, C., Schwarz, E.M. & Boyce, B.F. (2008). Osteoclast precursor interaction with bone matrix induces osteoclast formation directly by an interleukin-1-mediated autocrine mechanism, *J Biol Chem* Vol.283(No.15):9917-24.

Zhang, X., Morham, S.G., Langenbach, R., Young, D.A., Xing, L., Boyce, B.F., Puzas, E.J., Rosier, R.N., O'Keefe, R.J. & Schwarz, E.M. (2001). Evidence for a direct role of cyclo-oxygenase 2 in implant wear debris-induced osteolysis, *J Bone Miner Res* Vol.16(No.4):660-70.

16

Aseptic Loosening of Total Hip Arthroplasty as a Result of Local Failure of Tissue Homeostasis

Jiri Gallo et al.*
Department of Orthopaedics, Palacky University, Teaching Hospital Olomouc, Czech Republic

1. Introduction *(Gallo)*

Total hip arthoplasty (THA) is the most effective and safest method for treating severe degenerative, post-traumatic and other diseases of the hip joint. It is estimated that more than 1,000,000 THAs are performed each year globally. The incidence of primary THA increased in the period 1990 to 2002 in the USA from 47/100,000 to 69/100,000 (Kurtz et al. 2007). A similar study in Denmark reported an increased rate of THAs from 101/100,000 to 131/100,000 during the period 1996 to 2002 (Pedersen et al. 2005). More importantly, modelled future projections expect further increase in the need for THAs.

It is believed that THA can reliably relieve pain and improve function in the majority of patients for a period of 15 to 20 years or more postoperatively. On this basis, with the extension of THAs to a younger and generally more active population, the expected time of service of THAs would be insufficient and the number of revision surgeries would therefore increase during this time. The Kaplan-Meier ten-year revision-free survival estimates for younger patients range from 72% (95%CI: 67-76) in Finland to 86% (95%CI: 84,5-88,2) in Sweden (Corbett et al. 2010). Hence, 14% to 28% of such patients on average did not achieve a 10-year THA functioning without revision.

The main reason for late failure of THA is *aseptic loosening accompanied by osteolysis* followed by infection and instability of the THA that compromise more the early postoperative

* Yrjö T. Konttinen[1], Stuart B. Goodman[2], Jacob P. Thyssen[3], Emmanuel Gibon[4], Jukka Pajarinen[1], Yuya Takakubo[5], Peter Schalock[6], Zygmunt Mackiewicz[7], Eemeli Jämsen[1], Martin Petrek[8], Rihard Trebse[9], Andrei Coer[10] and Michiaki Takagi[5]
[1]*Department of Medicine and Department of Anatomy, Helsinki University Central Hospital, ORTON Orthopaedic Hospital of the Invalid Foundation, COXA Hospital for Joint Replacement, Finland*
[2]*Department of Orthopaedic Surgery, Stanford University, USA*
[3]*Department of Dermato-Allergology Copenhagen University Hospital Gentofte, Denmark*
[4]*Department of Orthopaedic Surgery, Bichat Teaching Hospital, Paris School of Medicine, France*
[5]*Department of Orthopaedics, Yamagata University, Japan*
[6]*Department of Dermatology, Harvard Medical School, Massachusetts General Hospital, Boston, USA*
[7]*Department of Histology and Embryology, Medical University in Bialystok, Poland*
[8]*Department of Immunology, Palacky University Olomouc, Czech Republic*
[9]*Valdoltra Orthopaedic Hospital, Ankaran, Slovenia*
[10]*College of Health Care, University of Primorska, Izola, Slovenia*

period than the later one (Ulrich, Seyler et al. 2008). For this reason the above mentioned increase in rate of primary THAs is closely associated with increase in demand for revision THAs. The incidence of revision THAs in the USA increased from 9.5/100,000 to 15.2/100,000 between 1990 and 2002 and the projections by 2030 are even more impressive (Kurtz et al. 2007). With this in mind, research on the pathophysiology of aseptic loosening and osteolysis is of paramount importance and well justified.
This chapter provides a background on the current theory of aseptic loosening and osteolysis together with a brief overview of preventive measures.

2. Overview of the current theories on aseptic loosening and periprosthetic osteolysis *(Gallo, Goodman)*

The term "aseptic loosening" is closely related to the finding of *gross mechanical instability at the interface between the implant and bone bed* (Fig. 1). It is generally associated with pain and loss of function although it may also occur asymptomatically. Regarding the prevention the key question is what is the mechanism that first erodes the firm bond between implant and the bone bed.

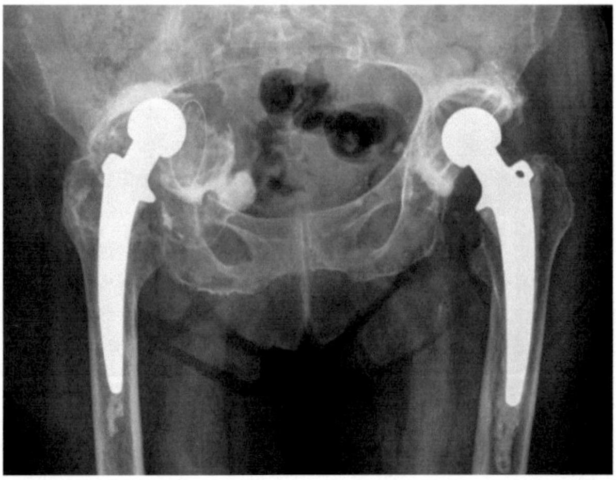

Fig. 1. Severe medial migration of the cemented cup at the right site in 86 year old female (17 yrs. postoperatively)

Aseptic loosening of total hip arthroplasty is hypothesised to be the *result of a harmful combination of mechanical and biological events destroying the bond between the implant and bone bed*. To date, a variety of host-, implant- and surgery-related factors have been delineated to explain the development of aseptic loosening and osteolysis. Some of these are accepted by the scientific community, others are the subject of intensive research, while yet others are only speculative having little or no clinical or research evidence.
There are specific factors that directly increase the risk of aseptic loosening while others induce conditions that increase the probability of developing aseptic loosening. A well acknowledged factor in preventing aseptic loosening is surgical experience and technique resulting in firm fixation and correct implant placement. Failure to achieve sound and long-term fixation of the implant to the bone bed is closely associated with premature aseptic loosening (Mjoberg 1994). Factors associated with the development of severe periprosthetic

osteolysis significantly influence the rate of aseptic loosening as it is believed that severe bone loss can facilitate the process of destabilisation of the implant regardless of its original sound placement (Gallo et al. 2010).

2.1 Mechanical theories on aseptic loosening

Proponents of mechanical theories explain aseptic loosening and periprosthetic osteolysis *to be the result of predominantly mechanical events* with stress and strain being the major drivers of the disease. These refer to the stresses and strains affecting the implant-bone interface during each step until they overwhelm the firmness of the interface. On this basis, Mjöberg stressed the importance of the quality of the initial fixation because he and others had revealed the close association between early migration of implant and risk of premature failure of THA due to aseptic loosening (Mjoberg 1994). Unfortunately, there is no agreed threshold of migration above which loosening can be predicted. Further it is not possible to compare directly the migration data of different studies (Derbyshire et al. 2009). In addition, it seems that the majority of cemented cups migrate during the first postoperative year and thus the revision rate is poorly predictable one year postoperatively even in cases with significant migration (Aspenberg et al. 2008). For this reason, the "mechanical theory" should be revised to include at least the distinction between stable, osseointegrated prostheses and those in which osseointegration has not developed after the first postoperative year and exhibit radiolucency around the implant, and continuous migration resulting in loosening.

2.2 Biological theories on aseptic loosening

According to biological theory, aseptic loosening is the *result of a series of predominantly biological processes*. Of these, the most important is the complex adverse host response to prosthetic particles and by-products which produce particle disease. Willert and Semlitsch were the first to introduce the concept of aseptic loosening as a result of periprosthetic tissue reaction to massive amounts of prosthetic microparticles (Willert and Semlitsch 1977). The key concept in particle disease is that *very small prosthetic particles* (the size of micrometers and less) *stimulate periprosthetic cells to express proinflammatory/ pro-osteoclastic cytokines and other substances that orchestrate increased accumulation/activity/survival of osteoclasts, and inhibit the osteogenic activity of osteoblasts*. As a result, osteoresorption predominates over osteogenesis at each bone multicellular unit on the bone surface around the implant leading eventually to macroscopically observed bone defects. The degree of bone loss according to this concept is a function of number and depth of deregulated resorption sites.

The expansion of particle disease across the joint is facilitated by joint fluid that is abundantly synthesized by synovial-like macrophages and fibroblasts. Joint fluid contributes to conversion of M0 on M1 macrophages (*Part 4.4*). In addition, it washes the prosthetic microparticles from the articulating surfaces, mediates signal molecules and enzymes and delivers them to the bone. For this reason, particle disease can recur at new sites, contributing in this way to overall weakening of the bone-implant interface.

A question remains as to what other biological factors underlie the destabilization of the implant associated with severity of bone defects. Of these, aging of the bone bed (senescence), stress-shielding, and cumulative fatigue changes at the bone-implant interface may contribute to weakening of the implant-bone fixation. Eventually, these separately or together lead to degradation of the fixation interface and increase the probability of aseptic loosening. The ultimate pathway of aseptic loosening is undoubtedly of mechanical origin. For this reason, a comprehensive theory of aseptic loosening has been proposed involving both biological and mechanical factors.

2.3 Comprehensive theory on aseptic loosening

A valid theory requires consideration of *both mechanical and biological factors in the pathophysiology of aseptic loosening and osteolysis* (Gallo et al. 2002). The micromotions arising at the bone-implant interface during normal gait cycles induce a bone resorption which occurs before any wear debris particles enter the system. Following a number of "empty spaces" at the implant-bone interface are quickly filled by fibrous membrane. Repeated "compression" (stress) of the membrane during each step can induce proliferation of fibroblasts that synthesize an abundant extracellular matrix to adapt to the mechanical stresses and strains around an implant. According to this concept, the process of aseptic loosening is about *sequential hypertrophy of the interface membrane* (biological reaction to mechanical strain; Fig. 2). At a later stage, the hypertrophic membrane facilitates the delivery of particles, cytokines, enzymes and other molecules from the joint space to the bone bed interconnecting mechanical and biological factors.

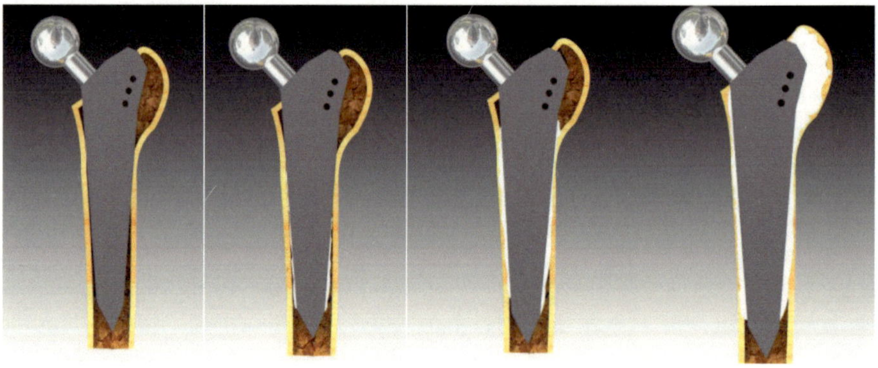

Fig. 2. Showing the process of gradual stem loosening as a result of hypertrophy of interface membrane (white) leading eventually to stem subsidence *(reproduced by courtesy of Jiri Lostak, MD)*

The mechanical environment can induce differentiation of mesenchymal stem cells via up-, down-regulation of mechano-sensitive genes and in this way it can influence tissue differentiation resulting for instance in excessive formation of fibrous tissue (Aspenberg et al. 2000). Interestingly, macrophages can be activated by cyclic pressure (0.138 MPa) alone. In fact, there is significant increase in their expression of TNF-α, IL-1β and IL-6 when treated jointly with polyethylene particles and pressure (McEvoy et al. 2002). Other studies have demonstrate the relative sensitivity of macrophages to simultaneous application of PMMA particles and mechanical strain (Jones et al. 2006). With this in mind, one may conclude that mechanical conditions can directly regulate the proliferation and expression capacity of a particular cell group. Another scenario is based on evidence that *high-pressure waves of the synovial joint fluid* can induce bone necrosis (Fahlgren et al. 2010). An abundance of joint fluid is synthesized by synovial-like macrophages and fibroblasts inside the artificial joint as a response to inflammatory and secretory signals produced by particle disease. The degree of intraarticular pressure depends in part on the volume of joint fluid, changes in position of the joint, and volume/draining capacity of the joint space assuming that high-volume and effectively drained joint space are associated with lower intraarticular pressures and vice versa. Other factors that may be important, but are not readily analysed include at least interactions between implant and its surroundings in terms of local tissue homeostasis maintenance/distortion, favourable composition of joint fluid, type of lubrication, individual motion/stress pattern, and genetic predisposition to aseptic loosening.

3. Local bone-soft tissue adaptations on an implant

3.1 What we know about the physiological reactions of the local tissues on the prosthesis and its waste products *(Konttinen, Pajarinen, Mackiewicz, Takagi, Jämsen, Takakubo, Gallo)*

A lot of research has been done on aseptic implant loosening, but there are few studies about the physiological, adaptive host responses to joint implants with a long and painless life-in-service. Loosened implants are surrounded by a fibrous implant capsule (Fig. 2). Contrary, well (physiologically) fixed implants are not characterized by fibrous implant capsule, synovial-membrane-like interface membrane (SLIM) or aggressive granulomatosis. They are characterized by some other features described below.

3.1.1 Physiological fixation of cemented implants

Cemented implants are fixed to bone with bone cement, polymethylmethacrylate (PMMA). Hip implant surgery damages descending metaphyseal arteries during the resection of the femoral head and the intramedullary nutritional artery during the implant bed preparation, which contribute to ischemia, lowering of pH and bone infarctions (Willert et al. 1974; Konttinen et al. 2001).

Willert and co-workers made a cadaver study of well-fixed implants to describe the physiological three-phase response of host bone to cement fixed implants. Toxic and lipolytic PMMA monomers and the exothermic polymerisation cause a marginal rim of necrosis of bone trabeculae at the cement-bone interface. After three weeks and up to two years postoperatively signs of repair of the implant bed are seen. This is perhaps in part stimulated by a local release of bone growth factors from the bone matrix and activated osteoclasts. Necrotic bone and bone fragments are resorbed by osteoclasts and macrophages. Newly produced or extended, irregularly orientated bone trabeculae grow as a lacework-like structure into the relatively smooth necrotic-fibrin clot-fatty-fibrotic bone-cement interface, which contains cement plugs, some of which protrude to reach direct contact with peri-implant bone. After two years bone repair is followed by remodelling of bone trabeculae, which are separated from the cement surface by a 0.1-1.5 mm thick fibrous membrane. This membrane grows into the empty spaces between the rough or cracked cement surface and contains some polyacrylamide pearls (from non-polymerized PMMA powder) close to the cement surface surrounded (isolated) by foreign-body giant cells and granulomas. Trabeculae of the already remodelled peri-implant bone were in the longitudinal sections orientated in parallel to the cement surface (Willert et al. 1974).

This work was nicely extended by Jasty and co-workers, who studied serial horizontal sections of the proximal femoral bone that enclosed the cemented femoral component still in place in the implant bed. They confirm that the bone is remodelled and disclose a curious pattern for this remodelling. The cement mantles of the well-fixed implants are surrounded by an inner, secondary dense neocortex. There is bone ingrowth from the neocortex into the undulating surface of the cement mantle. This neocortex is connected to the outer, primary femoral cortex by new trabecular bone struts. These authors reported very little fibrous tissue intervening between the host bone and cement mantle around well-fixed implants (Jasty et al. 1990). They also suggest that loosening of the implant from the cement mantle (debonding) and fractures and fragments of the cement mantle coupled with ingrowth of a fibrous tissue layer between the implant surface and cement mantle may trigger loosening (*Part 2.3*). Based on this, *stable, intact and firm cement mantle together with adaptive physiological bone remodelling response* around are associated with a well fixed symptomless cemented implant.

3.1.2 Physiological fixation of uncemented implants

A second mode of fixation is based on the use of special design features and surface technologies enabling bone interdigitating ingrowth to the porous surface of the implant (osteoconductive ingrowth surfaces). Biomaterials and coatings can modulate bone ingrowth. Finally, successful fixation of uncemented implants depends also on the remodelling of already existing bone.

The initial fixation of the porous-coated implants to bone depends on the shape of the implant (e.g. wedge fit, threaded design), and/or the tight micromechanical locking (press fit, friction fit, scratch fit, interference fit) of an implant to the bone bed. *The initial stability of the cementless implant is considered to be important for the secondary stabilization via bone ingrowth.* The rough implant surface destined to fix the implant to bone has to come in contact with bone because bone cannot bridge very large gaps, perhaps exceeding 1-2 millimetres between the implant surface and bone. The micromotion at the bone-implant interface is first larger but diminishes below ~40 μm as bone grows to the surface of the implant. According to cadaver studies bone ingrowth can reach up to 50% in well-fixed implant while further penetration of the porous spaces available at the contact surface can reach 80%. These values vary according to the quality of bone, type of implant/surface technology, and zone of implant (Engh et al. 1995).

Also this process is dependent on bone remodelling, i.e. formation of bone multicellular units (BMU) undergoing activation-reversal-formation (ARF) cycles, with net production of new cortical and trabecular bone. It is not quite certain, what is the micromotion at the bone-ingrowth surface area preventing bone ingrowth. In simulated stair climbing micromotion of cementless implants it is up to 280 μm (Burke et al. 1991) which is close to 100-400 μm pore size commonly used in the porous coated implants still allowing bone ingrowth. The best implant-bone contact (bone ingrowth) is achieved in contact with compact, cortical bone characterized by Haversian channels. In other areas the porous surface may be in contact with ingrown cancellous, medullary bone without Haversian channels interdigitating rough implant surface. By this way the implant surface is connected with the endosteal side of the cortex (Engh et al. 1995).

3.2 Does it exist something like long-term tolerance to an implant? (Takakubo, Pajarinen, Konttinen, Trebse, Coer, Mackiewicz, Takagi, Gallo)

Assume that an experienced surgeon places well and firmly an appropriate implant. During a functioning of such THA soluble and insoluble particles of prosthetic biomaterials are deliberated from the prosthetic joint surfaces and the implant-bone interface has to withstand mechanical stresses on levels of multiple body weight. The question is on the mechanisms preventing premature destabilization of such implants. Although aseptic loosening and osteolysis are of multifactorial origin and many factors cannot be included into the failure analysis we believe that there is some place for a concept of host long-term tolerance to implant. Biological and non-biological circumstances (factors) can be associated with long-term painless and stable THAs.

3.2.1 Genetic background of tolerance to an implant

Tolerance may be defined as a state of progressively decreased responsiveness to a wear and corrosion particles as well as other stresses related to implant functioning. It is reasonable to hypothesize that the genetic background (host responsiveness) of the implant patient plays a role in loosening of or tolerance to the implant. Technically the approach taken has been to look for eventual single-nucleotide polymorphisms (SNPs) in candidate genes. SNP refers to single nucleotide base changes in the coding DNA at a particular site (natural sequence variants, alleles). Candidates for this approach have been sought among molecules, which according to the current understanding play a role in the pathomechanism of loosening. These candidates form three main classes, namely *molecules regulating bone metabolism* (influencing the fixation of an implant and maintenance of it), *proteinases* involved in collagenous tissue destruction (size of the effective joint space), and *chemokines/ cytokines* regulating inflammatory response to wear debris (aggressive granulomatosis). These processes are at least in part genetically regulated which opens theoretically the opportunity to screen the population preoperatively for risk patients. Current status in this field is described in *part 4.7*.

In sensitized individuals even low local metal ion concentrations, such as cobalt and chrome, can cause T lymphocyte-mediated, *delayed-type hypersensitivity (DTH) reactions*. Metal ions can bind to self-peptides in the antigen presenting groove of the major histocompatibility complex (MHC) class II molecule altering self to altered-self, which is by the adaptive immune response recognized as non-self. Metal ions can bind to a protein altering its processing so that immunogenic cryptic (instead of tolerance-inducing dominant) epitopes are disclosed, causing DTH. They can modify MHC-II making it an immune-incompatible, "a foreign tissue-type antigen" (like in rejection of allogenic transplants) or they can activate the T-cell a bit like superantigens do. Tolerance to implant would require also immune tolerance against hapten-induced hypersensitivity reactions and in special cases it might be possible to test the implant patient-to-be pre-operatively for an eventual hypersensitivity with the help of epicutaneous patch or gamma-spot like tests (*Part 4.5*).

In a tolerant immunogenetic background wear particles are together with apoptotic bodies cleaned by M0 macrophages. *Some co-factors* may interfere with this tolerant host response to implant. Biomechanical loading (compression, tension, shear force) at the implant-bone interface may be one such cofactor. Occasional infections, microbial pathogen-associated molecular structures (PAMPs, e.g. lipopolysaccharide) and release of alarmins (e.g. high mobility group box 1) from damaged tissues (e.g. excessive biomechanical loading or ischemia) and necrotic or even activated cells can transform the M0 macrophage response into aggressive granulomatosis, which leads to peri-implant bone destruction. This in part, because both PAMPs and alarmins can opsonize wear particles. Various pattern recognizing receptors, such as Toll-like receptors (TLRs), mediate innate host responses and their SNPs may play a role here (Takagi et al. 2007; Pajarinen et al. 2010). In addition, primary and long-term fixation of the cemented and uncemented implants is dependent on the remodelling ability of the bone which is under genetic control. Peri-implant cells have to resorb damaged or necrotic peri-implant bone, repair it and then remodel it so that it maintains implant well fixed to the bone (*Part 3.1*). If fibrous interface and later synovial membrane-like interface or even foreign body-driven aggressive granulomatosus develop, activation-reversal-formation (ARF) cycles begin to dominate in bone multicellular units (BMUs) in peri-implant bone, contributing to the osteolysis and loosening of an implant.

3.2.2 Other contributors to long-term tolerance of total hip arthroplasty

Our knowledge on the factors associated with long-term functioning of a stable implant is in part based on comparison of tissues from patients with long-term survival of implant with tissues from those who suffer from loosening. In this line, it was for instance proposed that *successful patients*, in contrast to unsuccessful ones, could *effectively clear the joint space from the wear and other particles* and this way have diminished inflammatory stimulation (Zolotarevova et al. 2010). Also other patient-related factors, like *gender, age, body mass index or even particular chronic medication* (e.g. statins, bisphosphonates, nonsteroidal antiinflammatory drugs) could contribute to implant tolerance (Thillemann et al. 2010a; Thillemann et al. 2010b). Female gender seems to protect both the cemented and uncemented cups from early failure (Roder et al. 2010). Tolerance to implant seems to be improved with increasing age of the patients which could be explained not only by a decrease in activity level with no excessive cyclic loading in elderly patients but also a decreased responsiveness of the immune-inflammatory system might play some role (Ogino et al. 2008). Normal body mass index contributes to good implant tolerance at least in part via influencing bone remodelling around the implant and magnitude of mechanical stresses affecting bone-implant interface. A good general health and medication not adversely interfering with bone metabolism together with a good local quality of the bone could contribute to long-term maintenance of implant-bone fixation. In this line, it is advisable to check the health status and medication of particularly elderly patients to optimize bone metabolism and bone strength. Targeting the dizziness and an individualized training program (muscle strength, coordination, and balance) together with interventions to the physical living environment of the patient, e.g. carpets, handrails, bedrails, illumination, doorsteps and various technology-related aids, could protect the implant from excessive loads.

Implant fixation and loading are interrelated and should be in balance for implant tolerance (*Part 3.1*). The number (cyclic regular loading) and type (on a smooth or declining surface, stairs, squatting etc.) of steps taken and any accidental or traumatic overshoots (not considered in computer controlled implant simulation studies) play a role. The number of steps taken can vary from 395 to 17718 steps per day, corresponding from 144175 to 6467070 steps per year (Schmalzried et al. 1998). In this way, it has been emphasized that the occurrence of polyethylene wear is a function of use, not time in situ (Schmalzried et al. 2000). Peri-implant bone microfractures and even pathological interface mobility can develop around already well-fixed implants as a result of too high loading. This secondary loss of stability stimulates bone remodeling (Takagi et al. 2001), and increases a risk for formation of fibrous interface around the implant. Fibrous tissue can further transform to synovial like-lining as a result of contact with synovial fluid (*Part 2.2*). Fibrous tissue formation is also promoted by the inert and passive nature of the metallic and polymeric materials used in joint replacements. Apart of the deteriorating effects of cyclic and erratic loading on development of fibrous interface, biomechanical loading affects also fluid flow and pressure in the lacuno-canalicular system. Detailed dynamic morphometric studies have shown high-turnover periprosthetic bone remodeling, immature bone formation and high density of osteocyte canaliculi in low-mineralized areas around loosening implants (Takagi et al. 2001). This can expose cells in the 3D osteocytes-network to too high or low shear stress (drag force) leading to their apoptosis and aseptic necrosis. Osteocytes subjected to high pressures in peri-implant bone die a programmed cell death, apoptosis. Too low intracanalicular flow or obstruction of fluid inflow through surface pores by wear debris induces osteocyte apoptosis/bone necrosis. Taken together, patients should be strongly advised against extremely strenuous use of the implant to obtain good implant tolerance, but this is naturally also a patient and implant specific situation.

3.2.3 The effect of gliding pairs, implants and fixation

It is believed that the outcome of THA depends on optimal combination of patient, surgery and implant related factors. In this line, evidence-based implant surgery creates basic conditions for inducing an implant tolerance. Material and implant selections can also influence the conditions under which the tolerance to implant may develop. Regarding particle disease, key features are amount of particles together with their specific functional activity. Generally, ultra-high molecular weight polyethylene (UHMWPE) particles are considered more stimulating than ceramic particles. The amount of polyethylene wear debris has been significantly decreased by the development of highly cross-linked UHMWPE (HXLPE) even though concern on its specific functional activity remains. Wear rate was decreased by 50-95% by the 1st and 2nd generation HXLPE compared to conventional UHMWPE. As a result, the risk for osteolysis was diminished with 87% for the 1st generation of HXLPE liners compared to conventional UHMWPE liners (Kurtz et al. 2011).

In ceramic-on-ceramic (CoC) couples, with significant decrease of both the linear (5-300x) and the volumetric wear (30-2000x) in comparison to the metal on UHMWPE bearings (MoP), the risk for severe osteolysis is even lower. In metal on metal (MoM) articulations the linear wear is 5-150x less and the volumetric wear 30-1000 x less than in the conventional MoP (Jin et al 2006) but concerns remain regarding induction of both the delayed type hypersensitivity, e.g. **A**septic **L**ymphocyte-dominated **V**asculitis-**A**ssociated **L**esions (ALVAL). Taken together, if indeed a particle disease plays a significant role in loosening, these new materials might facilitate development of implant tolerance.

Information on the effects of specific implant design on tolerance to implant is obtained from finite element modeling (FEM), simulation, case-control cohort and arthroplasty register studies. FEM, experimentation *in silica*, has been used for implant design and testing, implant biomechanics and implant-induced responses, e.g. bone remodeling and stress shielding, but few studies have applied FEM to estimate the longevity of different implant designs, i.e. the long-term tolerance to implants (Korhonen et al. 2005). Another method suitable for implant testing is computer-controlled simulation of real implants (Lappalainen et al. 2003). Randomized controlled clinical trials are the best way to evaluate specific implants in clinical practice. Unfortunately, they are rare. More frequent small and medium size observational cohort studies performed in a single center or geographical area can be biased. In that case, the most reliable information on the performance of different implants can be obtained using arthroplasty registers. Such registry studies also support the practice involving combination of antibiotics in the bone cement and systemically to decrease the risk of revision, i.e. improve implant tolerance (Engesaeter et al. 2003). Implant register studies can also be used to help to identify the ideal patient to maximize implant tolerance.

4. Local host response to prosthetic wear debris

4.1 Hierarchy of immune reactions to prosthetic wear particles *(Gallo)*

Aseptic loosening and osteolysis can be understood to be the result of chronic high-grade inflammatory disease induced by exposure of local tissue to massive quantities of prosthetic particles. For this reason predominantly investigated is the role of the immune system in its pathophysiology. Currently, there is a large body of evidence supporting the concept of the immune system acting major influence on particle disease. In this section, we will focus on the role of the different parts of the immune system in the process of aseptic loosening and osteolysis.

Basically the immune system consists of two tightly associated segments: *the innate immune system and the adaptive immune system.* The former consists of a set of pattern-recognition receptors (PRRs) that evolved to recognize pathogen-associated molecular patterns (PAMPs), triggering rapid and robust response to invading pathogens following their recognition. The adaptive immune system evolved to produce a highly specific response to unique antigen presentation after innate instructions are conveyed to the second line of host-immunity associated in particular with T and B cells. A distinction should be made between at least the *inflammatory T_H1 response* inducing and perpetuating inflammation via expression of IFN-γ, IL-2, TNF-alpha and activation of macrophages, NK cells, cytotoxic lymphocytes, and *anti-inflammatory T_H2 and T_H3 responses* associated characteristically with expression of IL-4, IL-5 and TGF-β and IL-10 cytokines, respectively (Matzinger 2007). From a functional point of view we can distinguish *cells/pathways/molecules that trigger the immune response to wear debris and those that regulate host response,* assuming the latter may play an important role in resolving inflammation and prevention of tissue damage.

The immune response is triggered after recognition of special surface motifs on invading pathogen (PAMPs) by PRRs. Intact pathogens can be composed of a number of PAMPs which induce activation of multiple PRRs simultaneously and, vice versa, different PRRs can recognize the same PAMP (Kumar et al. 2011). Currently, there is growing evidence that activation of PRRs is an important part of host adverse reaction against prosthetic particles (Lahdeoja et al. 2010). This could be explained by adherence of immunoreactive substances (lipopolysaccharides, lipoteichoic acid, fragments of bacteria, components of complement etc.) on wear debris particles. Some researchers have demonstrated that i) *PAMPs adhere to the particles;* ii) *adherent PAMPs increase significantly the biological response to the particles;* iii) *PAMPs do this by activating their PRRs* (Greenfield et al. 2010). In addition, particles deliberated from THA are coated immediately with serum proteins creating *a protein-particle complex* that may result in a damage/danger-associated molecular pattern picture *irrespective of endotoxin* (Sun et al. 2003). Engagement of TLRs leads to activation of the NF-κβ signalling pathway with subsequent expression of pro-inflammatory cytokines, strongly boosting the immune response (Pearl et al. 2011). In the same way also other receptors (e.g. NOD-like receptor proteins) may participate in activation of the immune response to wear debris (St Pierre et al. 2010). Some of these are structurally involved in the cytosolic multi-protein complex known as the "inflammasome" which is considered a critical part of the inflammatory response. After appropriate stimulus, IL-1β and IL-18 convert from their inactive precursor molecules (pro-1β and pro-IL-18) into biologically active molecules that are then released from inflammasomes (Caicedo et al. 2009). From the clinical viewpoint, lipopolysaccharide has been detected in periprosthetic tissues without any other signs of infection in patients (Nalepka, Lee et al. 2006). In addition, some patients who underwent revision arthroplasty due to aseptic loosening had positive culture and/or PCR detected

bacteria (Dempsey et al. 2007). In one recent study, it was even found that the extension of osteolysis correlated with proportion of positive sonication cultures (Sierra et al. 2011).
Participation of the adaptive immune system in host response to prosthetic wear debris is still a subject of controversy despite the fact that several reports have described lymphocytes in periprosthetic tissues, retrieved from patients with aseptically failed metal-on-metal (MoM) or non-MoM implants (Fujishiro et al. 2011; Ng et al. 2011). One recent study revealed increased serum concentration of cobalt and chromium in patients with MoM THA which positively correlated with increased proportion of HLA DR+ CD8+ T-cells in these patients (Hailer et al. 2011). In the same study, it was proposed that macrophages around THA could create haptenic metal ions in the context of self peptides (metal ion-altered self) as antigens in combination with MHC class II molecules, leading to T-cell priming. Weyand et al proposed antigen-recognition events when they characterised T cells in periprosthetic membranes (Weyand et al. 1998). They found identical T-cell receptor sequences suggesting identical antigen specificity and in addition, transcription of IL-2 and IFN-γ, indicating functional activity of at least some lymphocytes. Moreover, in this study, IFN-γ transcription correlated with extension of bone loss. Sensitization to various heavy metals after THA is described elsewhere in this chapter (*Part 4.5*).

4.2 Chemokines and cellular chemotaxis during the inflammatory response to wear particles from orthopaedic implants *(Gibon, Goodman, Gallo)*

The biological reaction to polymers, ceramics and metallic wear particles is *a non-specific foreign body and chronic inflammatory response*. A type IV lymphocyte-driven hypersensitivity reaction involving a specific antigen has been found for a small percentage of cases with predominantly metal-on-metal bearing surfaces (*Part 4.5*). This section will focus on the inflammatory processes associated with wear particles from orthopaedic implants, emphasizing local and systemic cell signaling mediated by chemotactic cytokines called chemokines.

4.2.1 The inflammatory reaction to wear particles

Resident macrophages are amongst the first cells involved in particle-associated inflammation and initiate cell recruitment via the release of chemokines. Macrophage activation may occur with or without phagocytosis, by cell membrane contact with particles (Goldstein et al. 1975). Several receptors in the outer membrane of macrophages (e.g. CD11b, CD14, Toll-like Receptors and others) are involved in the activation of macrophages after contact with particulate debris. These receptors act through transmembrane proteins and different intracellular pathways and result in the release of cytokines, chemokines and other substances that induce cell recruitment. One of the most important intracellular pathways involved in signal transduction is the *mitogen-activated protein kinase (MAP-Kinase) pathway*. The MAP-kinase pathway then activates transcription factors such as the Nuclear Factor Kappa B (NFκB), which activates a cluster of genes for the production of pro-inflammatory cytokines, chemokines and related substances (Tuan et al. 2008). Besides macrophages, other resident cells are involved in the inflammatory process including fibroblasts, mesenchymal stem cells, osteoblasts, lymphocytes and others. Retrieval studies demonstrated that the periprosthetic cells produced high levels of pro-inflammatory cytokines and other factors including TNFα, IL-1, IL-6, M-CSF, RANKL, and others (*Part 4.3*).

4.2.2 Accumulation of chemokines

In addition to pro-inflammatory cytokines, chemo-attractive cytokines are also produced by different cell types involved in the inflammatory response at the bone-implant interface including: polymorphonuclear leukocytes, monocytes, macrophages, osteoblasts, fibroblasts and synovial cells. Monocyte chemoattractant protein-1 (MCP-1) is one of the most abundantly released chemokines and is an immediate early stress-responsive factor (Tuan et al. 2008). Macrophage inhibitory protein-1 (MIP-1 or CCL2) and interleukin 8 (IL-8) are also involved in these events.

MCP-1 is a C-C chemokine (γ chemokine subfamily) and its gene location in humans is 17q11.2. MCP-1 is primarily secreted by monocytes, macrophages and dendritic cells. With regards to bone, MCP-1 is also expressed by osteoblasts and osteoclasts. MCP-1 can bind to several receptors (CCR2, CCR4, CCR5) but binds preferentially to the CCR2. CCR2 has two isoforms: CCR2A and CCR2B; the expression of the different isoforms is restricted to specific cell types. Mononuclear cells and vascular smooth muscle cells express CCR2A whereas CCR2B is mainly expressed by monocytes and activated NK cells (Deshmane et al. 2009). MCP-1 regulates the migration and infiltration of monocytes, dendritic cells, memory T-lymphocytes and NK cells. Production of MCP-1 is under the direct control of the transcription factor NFκB.

MIP-1 belongs to the same subfamily of chemokines as MCP-1 (the C-C chemokine family), and is secreted primarily by activated macrophages and T-lymphocytes. Other cells may also secrete MIP-1. MIP-1 has two main isoforms: MIP-1α (CCL3) and MIP-1β (CCL4). In mice, MIP-1α and MIP-1β are encoded by one gene each, however in humans, MIP-1α is encoded by at least three genes and MIP-1β by two, all located in chromosome 17 (Menten et al. 2002). Inducers of MIP-1 release are IL-1, IL-7, LPS and specific adhesion molecules (e.g. intercellular adhesion molecule-1, ICAM-1). High levels of MIP-1α have been observed when macrophages from retrieved periprosthetic tissues have been challenged with titanium alloy and polymethylmethacrylate particles (Nakashima et al. 1999). The release of MIP-1α increases the systemic recruitment of macrophages and has a paracrine effect enhancing IL-1 and IL-6 release (Cook 1996; Menten et al. 2002). Although MCP-1 has a specific receptor (CCR2), MIP-1 acts through several receptors (CCR1, CCR5), (Proudfoot 2002).

Interleukin-8 (IL-8) is a member of the CXC chemokine family, and also has the designation CXCL8. It is an early stress responsive chemokine and the main cellular sources are: macrophages, endothelial cells, epithelial cells, and cells of the mesenchymal lineage such as mesenchymal stem cells and osteoblasts. IL-8 is a potent chemokine that induces the chemotaxis of neutrophils and monocytes/macrophages, and increases the mobility of osteoclasts (Baggiolini and Clark-Lewis 1992). Il-8 is also an angiogenic factor. IL-8 does not have a specific receptor but acts through the coupled G protein receptors CXCR1 and CXCR2, which are receptors for other chemokines (e.g. GCP-2, NAP-2, Gro-α and others), (Proudfoot 2002). When osteoblasts are challenged with phagocytosable titanium particles, the IL-8 peak in gene expression occurs within 1-2 hours after particle exposure (Fritz et al. 2002). The biological mechanism of IL-8 expression involves first a protein tyrosine phosphorylation after contact with Ti particles and then activation of the pro-inflammatory NF-κB through two subunits, p50 (NF-κB1) and p65 (RelA) to bind the IL-8 gene promoter.

4.2.3 Accumulation of cells

Under the influence of chemotactic and other immunoregulatory signals, many different inflammatory and reparative cells migrate through local tissues regionally and systemically through the blood stream to the areas of particle generation. Recent murine studies involving continuous intra-osseous infusion of ultra high molecular weight polyethylene (UHMWPE) particles have demonstrated an increase in the systemic trafficking of reporter macrophages to the particle infusion site using non-invasive imaging (bioluminescence) and immunofluorescence microscopy (Ren et al. 2010). Furthermore, a decrease in bone mineral density has been observed within the UHMWPE particle-infused femora (Ren et al. 2011). This suggests that wear particles stimulate a systemic response, mediated by chemokines released locally. Recent unpublished studies in our laboratory have demonstrated that inhibition of the MCP-1-CCR2 chemokine-receptor axis can mitigate this response, including reversing in part, particle-induced bone loss.

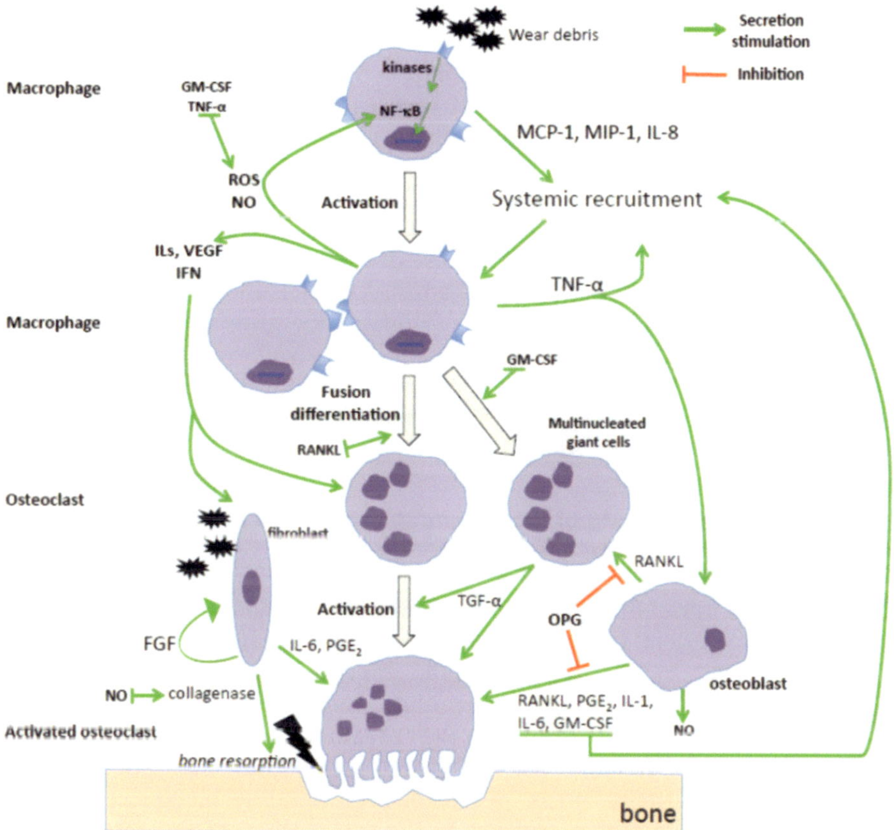

Fig. 3. Biologic reaction induced by orthopaedic wear particles on host cells; note the complex interaction of different cell types and factors to the presence of wear particles. Chemokines play a central role in cell recruitment. This diagram does not include the type 4 immune reaction to metallic wear particles.
IL = interleukin, TNFα = tumor necrosis factor α, GM-CSF = granulocyte macrophage colony-stimulating factor, MCP-1 = monocyte chemoattractant protein-1, MIP-1 = macrophage inhibitory protein-1, ROS = reactive oxygen species, NO = nitric oxide, VEGF = vascular endothelial growth factor, NF-κB = nuclear factor κ B, IFN = interferon, RANKL = receptor activator of nuclear factor κ B ligand, TLR = toll-like receptor, FGF = fibroblast growth factor, OPG = osteoprotegerin, TGFα = transforming growth factor α, PGE_2 = prostaglandin E2

After systemic and local cell trafficking to the inflammatory site, mononuclear macrophages may undergo a process called *macrophage fusion*. This results in polykaryons known as multinucleated "foreign body" giant cells which can be small (and contain 3-6 nuclei) or large (7-50 nuclei). Macrophage fusion is complex and requires the presence of specific cytokines and other factors (*Part 4.4*). The presence of foreign body giant cells has been widely demonstrated within the bone-implant interface (Goodman et al. 1989). Multinucleated giant cells have the capability to strongly express transforming growth factor-α (TGF α) as shown by Al-Saffar et al in their tissue retrieval study (Al-Saffar and Revell 2000). TGF-α is a key factor involved in angiogenesis, neovascularization and has been shown to impact both osteoclastic bone resorption and osteoclast-like cell growth and differentiation (Takahashi et al. 1986).
In vitro studies using murine bone marrow macrophages have shown that polymethylmethacrylate (PMMA) particles stimulate both RANKL expression, increase the number of osteoclasts and induce the formation of multinucleated giant cells (Clohisy et al. 2003). The authors also observed that PMMA particles activate the NF-κB and c-jun/AP-1 transcription factors, both of which mediate the osteoclastogenic effect of RANKL. Thus, *after contact with orthopaedic wear debris, resident macrophages become activated and release pro-inflammatory cytokines, chemokines and other factors*. MCP-1, MIP-1 and IL-8 release evokes the systemic recruitment of macrophages to the site of inflammation. Macrophage accumulation maintains the inflammatory process with release of pro-inflammatory cytokines that have paracrine and autocrine functions. Macrophage fusion induces the local release of TGF-α by multinucleated foreign body giant cells that facilitates the growth and differentiation of osteoclasts. Further cytokine release (TNF-α, IL-1, RANKL and others) by resident macrophages, fibroblasts, and cells of the osteoprogenitor cell line maintains a heightened inflammatory state and promotes the growth and differentiation of osteoclasts. These interlinked pathways are summarized in figure 3.

4.3 Cytokines and orchestrating of local adverse reaction to prosthetic particles *(Pajarinen, Takakubo, Mackiewicz, Takagi, Konttinen)*

Cytokines are small (15-25 kd) protein or glycoprotein messenger molecules that mediate intercellular (or even intracellular) communication and modulate immune reactions. They are produced, to some extent, by virtually all types of cells but by cells of the epithelial and hematopoietic origin as well as the cells of the immune system in particular. Typically cytokines are, after cell activation, secreted as soluble mediators into the extracellular space where they exert their function by binding to their specific high-affinity receptors located on the target cell membrane. Cytokine binding to its receptors induces receptor conformational changes and receptor dimerization or polymerization, binding of co-receptors in some instances and binding of adaptor proteins to the cytoplasmic tails, which leads to the activation of intracellular signalling cascades, activation or inactivation of specific transcriptional factors and finally up- or down regulation of gene expression. Some cytokines are not secreted but act in an intracrine (inside the cell) or juxtacrine (bound to cell membrane and requiring a direct cell-to-cell contact) mode of action while others are confined to the extracellular matrix (ECM) and released only when ECM proteins are degraded or damaged.
Cytokines control a very wide variety of different cell functions including cell growth, differentiation, migration, activation and survival. They are essentially involved into the development of blood cells (hematopoiesis) and not only in to the development and coordination of innate immune reaction and initial acute inflammation reaction but also to

the activation and proper polarization of adaptive immunity, development of chronic inflammation as well as tissue regeneration and healing.

4.3.1 Functional classification of cytokines

Currently already more than 200 different cytokines are known. Cytokines can be classified into several broad categories by their functional properties. Such classification is at best a simplification as the biological functions of specific cytokines vary considerably depending on the context. For example, cell type and cells activation state as well as the presence of other activating or inhibiting signals derived from e.g. cell-to-cell and cell-to-ECM contacts and other cytokines can alter the final outcome of the cytokine signalling. This phenomenon is known as *cytokine pleiotropy*: one cytokine typically has multiple functions. Considerable *redundancy* exists in cytokine signaling, different cytokines can activate very similar intracellular signalling pathways and transcription factors and thus have very similar effects on the target cell. Cytokines can have *synergy* so that they enhance each other's signalling and the net sum of the effect is far greater than their additive effects. As cytokines typically regulate the secretion of other cytokines and the expression of each other's receptors, a complex and integrated network of cytokine functions is formed.

At the beginning of the inflammation reaction resident tissue macrophages are activated by exo- or endogenous danger signals recognized by different pattern recognition receptors (e.g. TLRs) to produce *pro-inflammatory cytokines* e.g. tumor necrosis factor alpha (TNFα), Il-1β and IL-6. These cytokines activate and enhance the innate immune response, induce the secretion of anti-microbial molecules and other cytokines that refine the immune response, evoke systemic inflammatory response discussed above and importantly induce the expression of adhesion molecules in local microvascular beds in the process known as endothelial activation. Activated endothelium of post-capillary venules expresses selectin and integrin ligands, namely adhesion molecules (e.g. glycam-1, VCAM-1, ICAM-1), to which circulating and marginalized leukocytes effectively stick (capture and rolling), adhere and finally transmigrate from vascular compartment into the inflamed tissue. In unison with the pro-inflammatory cytokine production, macrophages, activated endothelial cells and other cells start to produce *chemokines* that further guide and activate transmigrated leukocytes to the site of inflammation along their increasing concentration gradient. The chemokines are discussed in more detail in *part 4.2* of this chapter. Also *interferons* are secreted by the cells of the innate immunity at the early stages of innate immune reaction. They are traditionally classified in two groups having very distinct functions. Type I interferons ("anti-viral interferons"), including IFNα (13 subtypes), IFNβ and IFNω (3 subtypes), are produced by macrophages after e.g. TLR recognition of viral structures (double stranded RNA or DNA). IFNγ, the only member of type II interferons ("immune interferon"), is secreted to some extend by macrophages and in greater magnitude by activated Th1 and NK-cells and is an important activating signal for macrophages which enhances their ability to secrete pro-inflammatory cytokines and kill phagocytosed bacteria.

The initial strong pro-inflammatory response must be well regulated and typically pro-inflammatory cytokines are rapidly degraded, their actions are inhibited by soluble or solubilised receptor proteins (e.g. IL-1RA) and further counterbalanced by production of *anti-inflammatory cytokines* e.g. IL-4, IL-10, transforming growth factor-β (TGF-β), which efficiently inhibit the production of pro-inflammatory cytokines and function of innate immunity. After the initial inflammatory reaction is resolved the tissue regenerative processes are rapidly engaged. *Growth factors* represent a diverse group of cytokines that regulate these tissue regenerative processes by modulating the growth and differentiation, of various cell types and tissues. Colony stimulating factors (CSF) typically control the myeloid development of monocytes and granulocytes, while epidermal growth factor (EGF), vascular endothelial growth factor (VEGF) and fibroblast growth factor (FGF) are secreted by macrophages and fibroblasts during regeneration of various tissues and they control e.g. formation of granulation tissue.

If the initial activation of innate immunity does not rapidly lead to the resolution of inflammation, the adaptive immune system is gradually activated by in particular professional antigen capturing, processing and presenting dendritic cells and macrophages that present MHC II-bound antigenic epitopes to the T-cell receptors (TCRs) of naïve CD4+ T-helper (Th) cells. The cytokine milieu that accompanies the antigen presentation process crucially determines the nature of the *developing immune response* (Th type 1, 2, 17, Treg). It is in the field of bone biology useful to distinguish a group of cytokines that control the formation, activation and survival of bone resorbing cells, osteoclasts. The complete list of cytokines that have been shown to *support osteoclastogenesis* or their bone resorptive activity is quite extensive and includes e.g. TNFα, IL-1, IL-6, IL-7, macrophage-CSF (M-CSF), IL-11, IL-17, MIP-1α/β, IFN-γ-induced protein-10 (IP-10) and monokine induced by IFN-γ (MIG), bone (or body) morphogenic proteins 2 and 7 (BMP2, 7) and VEGF among others. Cytokines that *inhibit osteoclastogenesis* include IFNγ, IFNβ, IL-4, IL-10, IL-13 and IL-18. Yet some cytokines play a dual role: low concentrations of TGF-β stimulate osteoclast formation and high concentrations inhibit it. However, none of the above-mentioned cytokines seems to be absolutely necessary for osteoclast development (Theill et al. 2002). The most important cytokine system controlling the osteoclast formation and function is the *RANKL/ RANK/OPG system* (Boyle et al. 2003). Mesenchymal cells, e.g. osteoblasts, mesenchymal stromal cells and fibroblasts as well as activated T cells tightly control osteoclastogenesis by producing receptor activator of nuclear factor kappa B ligand RANKL, which is produced in both cell membrane-bound and solubilized forms. Binding of RANKL to its receptor RANK expressed on osteoclast progenitors or macrophages in the presence of M-CSF, leads to cell fusion and formation of mature bone resorbing osteoclasts. In addition mesencymal cells produce osteoprotegerin (OPG) which is a soluble decoy receptor for RANKL and acts to limit and regulate its function. A high RANKL/OPG ratio is thus considered to drive osteoclastogenesis. RANKL/RANK/OPG system seems to represent the final common pathway in osteoclastogenesis, and many of the above-mentioned cytokines that drive or inhibit osteoclastogensis act by regulating RANKL or OPG levels. In the presence of low levels of M-CSF, RANKL seems to both sufficient and necessary for the complete differentiation of osteoclast precursors into mature osteoclasts.

4.3.2 Cytokines in aseptic loosening

As the monocyte/macrophage and foreign body giant cells (FBGCs) are by far the most dominant cell type in the periprosthetic tissue, the wear particle activated macrophage has long been considered to *play a pivotal role in the development of aseptic loosening*.

Several studies over the years have demonstrated that monocyte/macrophages challenged *in vitro* with wear particles are activated to produce a wide variety of pro-inflammatory cytokines, chemokines and growth factors, including TNFα, IL-1β, IL-6, IL-8, MCP-1 and MIP-1α/β, VEGF, M-CSF, GM-CSF and even more so if particles are contaminated with bacterial products (Holt et al. 2007; Purdue et al. 2007; Goodman and Ma 2010). Also the shape, size, number, and biomaterial composition of wear particles seem to have an effect on the quantity and quality of the cytokines produced. This wear particle induced macrophage activation is possibly mediated by various types of cell surface pattern recognition receptors e.g. Toll-like receptors (Takagi et al. 2007; Tamaki et al. 2009) and likely involves the activation and action of transcription factor NF-kB (Lahdeoja et al. 2010; Pearl et al. 2011).

The mere wear particle stimulation of pure monocyte/macrophage cultures is not sufficient to drive osteoclastogeneis or foreign body giant cell formation, most likely due to lack of RANKL signalling. Further *in vitro* studies using other relevant cell types of the periprosthetic tissue have demonstrated that, to some extent, wear particles as such and especially pro-inflammatory cytokines effectively *up-regulate RANKL production* from periprosthetic tissue fibroblasts and osteoblasts as well as suppress osteoblast formation and function (Vermes et al. 2001; Mandelin et al. 2005a).

Consistent with *in vitro* findings, numerous studies of the explanted periprosthetic tissues and pseudosynovial fluid have demonstrated increased production of vast array pro-inflammatory cytokines, chemokines and growth factors including e.g. TNFα, IL-1β, IL-6, IL-8, M-CSF, GM-CSF, MCP-1, MIP-1α as well as increased RANKL/OPG ratio favouring osteoclast formation (Mandelin et al. 2003; Holt et al. 2007; Purdue et al. 2007; Goodman and Ma 2010). Pseudosynovial fluid from aseptically loosened implants effectively induces formation of osteoclasts in cell culture conditions and OPG diminished this effect (Kim et al. 2001; Mandelin et al. 2005b). It should be noted however, that there is some discrepancy in these findings and, for example, the strong pro-inflammatory cytokines TNFα and IL-1β are not detected so consistently as e.g. IL-6, IL-8 or MCP-1, MIP-1α/β or RANKL possibly reflecting individual variations or different stages of the disease progression (Purdue et al. 2007). Because systemic inflammation reaction (e.g. fever, fatigue, cachexia) is not typically observed in patients with aseptic osteolysis, the observed low levels of TNFα and IL-1 might actually represent poorly understood aspects of particle induced chronic inflammation.

Studies conducted in animal models have further elaborated the role of pro-inflammatory cytokines and RANKL in the aseptic osteolysis. Several of these models have shown that implanted wear particles of various nature cause inflammation and *increase RANKL/OPG ratio and osteolysis* (Purdue et al. 2007). This reaction can be prevented or reduced by inhibiting TNFα signalling by using TNFα neutralizing antibody or by deleting TNF receptor (Childs et al. 2001). Similarly blocking of RANK signalling by RANK antagonist or OPG, or using mice genetically lacking RANK prevented experimental osteolysis in murine model of particle induced osteolysis (Childs et al. 2002; Ulrich-Vinther et al. 2002). Contradicting *in vivo* findings do also exist e.g. Taki et al. could not observe decrease in osteolysis in IL-1r and IL-6 or TNF double knock-out mice but concluded that osteolysis was likely mediated by other pro-inflammatory cytokines (Taki et al. 2007).

Taken together, following speculations can be made based on the detected cytokine profile of periprosthetic tissue. *First,* the definite majority of the cytokines detected are pro-inflammatory cytokines or chemokines secreted primary by cells of the innate immunity, which supports the essential role of activated macrophages in the process of aseptic loosening. *Second,* RANKL seems to be the most important end-point cytokine driving the osteoclast formation and loosening. *Third,* if only the cytokine profile of peri-implant tissues is considered, the role of adaptive immunity seems unlikely as both Th1 and Th2 signature and effector cytokines IFNγ and IL-4 are not generally detected from the peri-implant tissues. Furthermore both IFNγ and IL-4 effectively suppress the formation of osteoclasts. In this regard the possible role of Th 17 cells in the aseptic osteolysis seems an interesting line of further research as their signature cytokine IL-17 has been shown to favour osteoclastogenesis. *Fourth,* the nature of FBGCs remains somewhat elusive as morphologically sound FBGCs can be made in cell culture conditions using long term IL-4 stimulation, but as stated the IL-4 is not present in the periprosthetic tissue in any considerable amounts.

Based on the *in vitro* cell stimulation experiments and explanted tissue analysis, a following sequence of events can be postulated: wear particles activate macrophages, even more so if particles are coated by microbial products or alarmins. TLRs and other pattern recognition receptors of the innate immunity might mediate this wear particle induced cell activation. Activated macrophages produce pro-inflammatory chemokines, cytokines and growth factors which cause, via local endothelial activation and chemotaxis, further recruitment of monocytes and osteoclast precursors to the periprosthetic tissue. Pro-inflammatory cytokines, and to some extend also wear particles directly, drive the production of RANKL from mesenchymal cells and at the same time suppress the production of OPG and bone formation. Together with the pro-inflammatory cytokines they create an environment which favours ostoclastogenesis, bone resorption and finally prosthesis loosening. As the RANK/RANKL/OPG system seems represent the final common pathway in the pro-inflammatory cytokine mediated osteolysis, inhibition of RANKL might seem as a rational means to prevent aseptic osteolysis.

4.4 Key cell players – macrophages, fibroblasts, lymphocytes, osteoblasts, osteoclasts *(Gallo, Goodman)*

Histological and immunohistochemical studies of retrieved tissues have shown that when loosening is associated with osteolysis, the cellular profile is dependent on the method of prosthesis fixation (cemented or uncemented). Indeed, in the cemented group, tissue was more plentiful and often composed of highly vascularized fibrous tissue with a preponderance of macrophages and, to a lesser degree, T lymphocytes. With uncemented implants, tissue was less abundant and less cellular and more fibrous in nature. In addition to large numbers of fibroblasts, macrophages were also abundant but with increased numbers of all T-lymphocyte subgroups (Goodman et al. 1998).

Macrophages

Macrophages comprise a *heterogeneous group of cells* that play an important role in both the activation of the immune response and tissue homeostasis. They are *derived from monocytes which arise from myeloid progenitor cells in the bone marrow.* After maturation in bone marrow, monocytes are released into the circulation, then enter the tissues and differentiate into *tissue macrophages (M0)* that can survive for several months. Here, they can be activated by microbial/non-microbial agents (proinflammatory *M1 macrophage activation*), by IL-4, IL-13 etc. produced locally by mast cells and/or TREG lymphocytes (*M2 antiinflammatory tissue-remodelling macrophages*), or by other signals (*M2-like immunoregulatory macrophages*). Suppression of cytokine signalling 1 (SOCS1) is a key determinant of differential macrophage activation and function influencing the overall macrophage balance in tissues together with other factors (Ma et al. 2003; Whyte et al. 2011).

Macrophages are considered *the most potent phagocytic cells* in tissues around the THA and there are believed to be able to phagocytise even non-opsonized particles, e.g. polyethylene, metal or polymethylmethacrylate. After phagocytosis of the wear particles (the "fuel of the particle disease"), the macrophages have to become activated to produce pro-inflammatory cytokines and orchestrate their microenvironment towards increased osteoclast differentiation and osteolysis. The mechanism by which macrophages recognize particles and become activated as a result is not fully understood. In this context it is interesting to speculate if perhaps excessive biomechanical loading, mast cell activation and/or tissue necrosis can release alarmins which could initiate expression of polarizing cytokines. Another option is that microbes or microbe-derived pathogen-associated molecular patterns could provide the danger signal initiating polarization of M0 to other macrophage subtypes (Tamaki et al. 2009). In fact, early in the adaptation process, tissue macrophages exhibit traits specific for the tissue in which they reside and, in the resolution phase of inflammation, they induce original tissue repair or fibrosis. It has been postulated that during initial or middle phases of tissue response on wear particle load M1 macrophage activation pattern could play a key role while end-stage of aseptic loosening could be associated with alternatively activated macrophages expressing predominantly chemokines such as CHIT1 and CCL18 (Koulouvaris et al. 2008).

Macrophages have their own weak bone-resorptive capacity but more importantly they are the *cell reservoir for the generation of multinucleated giant cells* (MGCs). Of these the multinuclear bone resorbing osteoclast derived from M0 macrophages is the most important consumer of bone. Induction of monocyte/macrophage-derived multinucleated giant cells has been demonstrated in response to hematopoietic growth factors (e.g. IL-3, granulocyte macrophage colony stimulating factor, GM-CSF), and IL-4. The role of adhesion molecules in polykaryon cell formation has also been reported, and mainly involves intercellular adhesion molecule-1 (ICAM-1/CD54) and the receptor CR3 (CD11b/CD18) expressed by multinucleated giant cells (Anderson et al. 2008). Furthermore, immunohistochemical analysis of tissues retrieved from aseptic loosened total hip and knee replacements has shown high levels of ICAM-1 and its receptor CD11b expressed by giant cells and phagocytic cells containing metal and polyethylene particles.

Fibroblasts/ Fibrocytes

Fibrocytes are *mesenchymal cells that arise from monocyte precursors derived from blood.* They express features of both macrophages and fibroblasts dependent on local factors participating in acute response to injury/surgery and also play an important role in regulation/ resolution of chronic inflammation (Reilkoff et al. 2011). Their increased occurrence in periprosthetic tissues long after the healing phase could be associated with disturbance of local tissue homeostasis.

About 30% of periprosthetic membrane is composed of fibroblasts and these cells exhibit a very high proliferation rate pointing on their activation state (Koreny et al. 2006). Fibroblasts are *tissue resident cells* that have the capacity to synthesize and remodel extracellular matrix. In this way they create the local tissue architecture and also develop a milieu in which particular homeostatic regulation (e.g. inflammation, repair) can occur (Buckley 2011). Thus, they could significantly influence the fate of a prosthesis because they govern the switch to resolving postoperative inflammation and formation of fibrous capsule (repair) during the initial postsurgery period (Anderson 2009). In fact, fibroblasts and fibrocytes residing in surface layers of the periprosthetic capsule are the first cell types that come into contact with prosthetic particles. Later, a series of interactions between immune cells (esp. macrophages) and fibroblasts could determine the overall adaptative capacity of periprosthetic tissues for wear debris. For this reason, fibroblasts in concert with other cells greatly influence the grade of periprosthetic inflammation.

Aberrant expression of adhesion molecules, chemokines, cytokines, and their receptors could increase the inflammatory status, and vice-versa.

Lymphocytes

Local perivascular infiltrates of lymphocytes and even diffuse lymphocytes have been identified in specimens of periprosthetic tissue from both MoM and non-MoM implants (Fujishiro et al. 2011). *Lymphocytes are a kind of leukocyte circulating in the blood.* Precursors of both T and B cells are cloned in bone marrow but T cells require in addition, maturation in the thymus. The surface of each T cell displays thousands of identical T cell receptors and according to the presence of one or the other of two surface glycoproteins, they are designated as CD4 and CD8 T lymphocytes. The recruitment of lymphocytes into peripheral tissues where there is inflammation and/or damage is mediated by chemokines and adhesion molecules. In tissues, each B and T cell develops a specific response for a particular antigen interplaying complexly with innate immunity. As a result, different classes of pathogens stimulate differentiation of $CD4^+$ T cells into effector T cells (Th1, Th2, Th17 subsets). The aim is to induce the best response to a particular danger signal without vast tissue damage. Therefore, an important role is played by the activity of regulatory T (Treg) cells which suppress inappropriate adaptive immune response via several regulatory mechanisms (e.g. TGF-β, IL-10).

T lymphocytes are key players in the process of local and systemic bone loss associated with inflammation (Djaafar et al. 2010). Importantly, direct cell-to-cell contact between activated T cells and pre-osteoclasts is critical for their maturation in osteoclasts via RANKL and other pro-inflammatory cytokines pathways. Natural killer cells (lymphocytes of the innate immune system) have been shown to be a principal tissue-infiltrating lymphocyte subset in patients with particle-mediated inflammation (Huss et al. 2010). However, despite the above-mentioned consequences, the role of the specific immune system in particle disease remains controversial.

Osteoblasts

The osteoblast is a *mesenchymal cell with a primary role in bone formation and remodelling*. To do this, they come in contact with other cell groups of different origins (including osteoclasts, macrophages, lymphocytes, bone marrow cells) and synthesize a variety of cytokines and chemokines. Such interactions likely play an important role under both physiologic and pathological conditions.

Given the problem is increased bone resorption around the implant, the interplay between osteoblasts and other cell groups likely creates an environment favouring increased osteoclast maturation and/or suppressed osteoblast activity. Investigated have been the following possible explanations. First, some types of prosthetic particles could be toxic to osteoprogenitor cells leading to slowing of their maturation. Second, wear debris could suppress the function of mature osteoblasts inhibiting their osteogenic capacity. Third, osteoblasts could phagocytose prosthetic particles and express pro-inflammatory and pro-osteoclastogenic molecules on their surface, contributing in this way to the severity of bone resorption. The same can be achieved by chronic inflammatory microenvironment that up-regulates osteoblast synthesis of pro-osteoclastogenic molecules (Granchi et al. 2005; Fujii et al. 2011). Osteoblasts can contribute to the predominance of bone resorption at implant-bone interface also by specific interaction between them and T cells. Osteoblasts can express immunoreactive structures on their surfaces (superantigens) which directly stimulate T cells in their surroundings (Stanley et al. 2006). Activated T cells could express RANKL and M-

CSF, required for maturation of osteoclasts and also for formation of other giant cells having potentially important implications for periprosthetic osteolysis and aseptic loosening.

Osteoclasts

Osteoclasts are *multinucleated bone-resorbing cells* that together with osteoblasts, play a pivotal role in bone homeostasis and bone remodeling. Osteoclast precursors *derive from bone marrow as M0 macrophages* circulating in blood until penetrating tissues and binding to the bone surface utilizing cell-specific signalling pathways. The mechanism of recognition of a particular place on the bone surface is not known. On the other hand, the integrins mediating the bonding of pre-osteoclast to the bone site are well described (e.g. $\alpha_v\beta_3$). At the bone site, pre-osteoclasts fuse into multinucleated cells under the influence of fusion factors (e.g. dendritic cell-specific transmembrane protein; DC-STAMP) and then maturate in a particular milieu with the help at least of macrophage colony-stimulating factor (M-CSF) and receptor activator of nuclear factor kappa B ligand (RANKL), (Fig. 3). TNF-α and IL-1 potentiate this process, whereas a soluble RANKL neutralizer osteoprotegerin (OPG) inhibits it (Anderson et al. 2008). Indeed, RANKL/OPG ratio is considered a key regulator of osteoclastogenesis although *in vivo,* the RANKL-RANK interaction may occur in a direct cell-cell contact, e.g. between mesenchymal stromal cells and osteoclast progenitors or osteoblasts and pre-osteoclasts. A few giant osteoclasts form the cutting cone at basic multicellular units (BMU) in osteons (compact bone) and hemi-osteons (trabecular bone) that undergo resorption over a few weeks. The resorption space (lacuna) in healthy bone is filled in a few months by the closing cone composed of osteoblasts. However, under pathological conditions such as particle-mediated inflammation, the distortion of the coupling mechanism prevents closure of cone by osteoblasts. Hence, increased osteoclast bone resorption along with other mechanisms continues to create larger bone defects.

4.5 Contribution of allergic and other metal ion mediated responses to loosening of a total hip arthroplasty *(Thyssen, Schalock)*

Allergy and sensitization are frequently used terms, but their definitions should be clarified. Sensitization may be defined as "the process in which exposure to an antigen results in the development of hypersensitivity" whereas a definition of allergy could be "an altered body reaction, usually hypersensitivity, as a response to exposure to a specific substance". It is generally accepted that all metal prostheses release metal debris following wear and corrosion. This has been shown by measuring significantly elevated level of metal ions in hip arthroplasty patients; e.g capsular and periprosthetic tissues, the liver, spleen and lymph nodes, serum and urine (Hallab and Jacobs 2009). Metal ions may potentially activate the immune system, a response that is mainly adaptive rather than innate (Hallab et al. 2008). Typically, large particulate wear debris particles (more than 150 nm to 10 µm) are phagocytosed by cells including macrophages, which present antigens to circulating T-lymphocytes resulting in delayed type hypersensitivity reactions (Hallab and Jacobs 2009). Allergic complications following insertion of metallic orthopaedic implants are plenty and summarized in table 1. In this section, we will discuss the possible association between metal allergy and loosening of hip arthroplasties.

Immune reactions described adjacent to metal implants *include T-cell mediated type IV reactions but likely are multifactorial*. Peri-implant reactions seem to be Th1 dominant. Hence, increased levels of IFN-γ and IL-6 in metal hypersensitive joint arthroplasty patients (Hallab et al. 2008) as well as low IFN-γ and elevated levels of IL-17 in nickel allergic patients with symptomatic joint implants but not in Ni allergic patients with well-functioning joint implants (Summer et al. 2010) have been reported. Tissues near metal devices in those with metal hypersensitivity may have elevated immune cells/markers including: CD3þ T-lymphocytes, CD4þ cells, CD11cþ macrophages/dendritic cells, and cells with abundant MHC class II (HLA-DR) expression (dendritic cells), (Cadosch et al. 2009). Foreign body giant cell formation is often noted when phagocytosis of foreign particles by macrophages, including metals. Ingesting macrophages then secrete the proinflammatory cytokines TNF-α, IL-6 and IL1-α and β (Cadosch et al. 2009). At high concentrations, Ti and V cause production of superoxide anions in neutrophils and nickel ions break down neutrophil cell membranes at high levels (Kumazawa et al. 2002).

A novel mechanism for aseptic loosening of metal implants was suggested recently (Cadosch et al. 2010a). Osteoclasts mature and grow on titanium metals, leading to degradation, uptake and eventual release of the metal ions by the osteoclasts. This might explain increases in metal ion in systemic circulation, increased recruitment of osteoclast precursors via synthesis of specific chemokines, and also it can contribute to osteoclast differentiation. CCL17/TARC, CCL22/MDC, RANK-L, M-CSF and pro-inflammatory cytokines (CCR4) are elevated in the peri-implant environment (Cadosch et al. 2010b). This leads to loosening of the device as supporting surrounding bone is resorbed. In addition to being present in joint loosening, CCR4 is involved in the inflammatory reaction in cutaneous allergic contact dermatitis reactions (Vocanson et al. 2009). The link between cutaneous dermatitis and CCR4 is not proven, but is an area for further inquiry. While this evidence specifically address Ti metal, these same mechanisms could be relevant for other metal ions as well. Below, a description of the epidemiology of metal allergy and recommendation for clinical practice will be provided.

Reactions	
Cutaneous:	**Extra-cutaneous:**
Localized allergic (contact) dermatitis	Implant loosening
Systemic allergic (contact) dermatitis	Pain
Urticaria	Swelling/tumor formation
Bullous reactions	Chronic inflammation
Vasculitis	
Impaired wound healing	

Table 1. Selected clinical manifestations of delayed type hypersensitivity reactions

4.5.1 Epidemiology

Metal allergy, as defined by a positive patch reaction to a given metal, is frequent in the general population since up to 17% of adult women and 3% of adult men are nickel sensitized (Thyssen et al. 2007). Chromium and cobalt allergy are less frequent and occur in about 1-2%. Other prevalent causes of metal allergy include gold and palladium resulting in positive patch test reactions in about 10% of dermatitis patients albeit these are rarely clinically relevant (Faurschou et al. 2011). The prevalence of other metals, e.g. titanium, platinum, molybdenum, manganese and other has not yet been evaluated in general populations and are general infrequent in dermatitis patients.

It has often been debated whether metal allergy increases the risk of developing delayed type hypersensitivity reactions, e.g. loosening of THA. The literature was recently reviewed and it was concluded that metal allergy might in a minority increase the risk of complications caused by a delayed type hypersensitivity reaction (Thyssen et al. 2011a). Also, we do not know how to identify the subgroups of metal contact allergic patients with a potentially increased risk of complications following insertion of a metal implant. However, it seems to be certain that insertion of metal bearings increase the prevalence of metal allergy as a review showed it was 25% among patients with well-functioning hip arthroplasties and 60% among patients with a failed or a poorly functioning implants (Hallab et al. 2001); considerably higher frequencies than general population estimates (Thyssen et al. 2007). Despite the higher prevalence in the latter patient group, it remains unknown whether the higher prevalence is caused by implant loosening or whether metal hypersensitivity results in loosening.

4.5.2 Metal exposure

In addition to metallic devices and prostheses, metal exposure is also related to intake of food and water, dental work, tattooing, and prolonged skin contact with metal objects. These exposures may all result in metal sensitization although oral intake sometimes may lead to tolerance. Oral intake of food and water as well as implantation seems rarely to result in allergic complications or clinical disease. However, skin contact with metal objects e.g. jewellery often results in skin sensitization and dermatitis at the site of skin contact. Several field studies have recently demonstrated that nickel release in concentrations that result in sensitization and dermatitis remains common in Europe and the United States (Thyssen and Menne 2010; Thyssen et al. 2011b).

4.5.3 Patch testing

Patch testing is widely used to establish a diagnosis of delayed type hypersensitivity to metals. The reproducibility of the patch test is high but allergen dependent (Brasch et al. 1994). Patch tests are typically applied to the upper back and occluded for 48 hr. Readings should be performed at least on day 3 or 4 and if possible on more than one occasion (Wahlberg 2006). Patch test studies have suggested that 24-34.5% of positive patch test reactions potentially are missed when readings are not performed beyond day 2 (Uter et al. 1996). Ready-to-use test systems such as the Thin-layer Rapid Use Epicutaneous (TRUE) test® generally have a good concordance with conventional patch test systems using e.g. Finn Chambers®, except for cobalt (Lazarov et al. 2007). Patch testing intends to identify contact sensitized subjects by distinguishing between negative, irritant and allergic reactions. Thus, a valid positive patch test reaction typically requires a trained and experienced person that adheres to a set of valid criteria. Currently, the recommendations from the International Contact Dermatitis Research Group (ICDRG) dictate that homogeneous redness and infiltration in the entire test area is scored as a 1+ reaction, homogeneous redness, infiltration, and vesicles in the test area are scored as a 2+ reaction, and homogeneous redness, infiltration, and coalescing vesicles in the test area as a 3+ reaction (Wilkinson et al. 1970). 1+, 2+, or 3+ readings should be interpreted as positive responses indicating contact sensitization whereas irritant responses, doubtful (+?) responses, or negative readings should be interpreted as negative responses (Fig. 4). Clinicians should be aware that false positive and negative reactions may be encountered

(Wahlberg 2006). Albeit there is raising concern that the patch test mainly measures cutaneous metal allergy rather than allergic reactions caused and effectuated by systemic immune cells, the patch test has worked well to establish an association between metal ion concentrations in the blood and urine, metal allergy and loosening of 1st generation metal-on-metal hip implants. It is clear that a system test, e.g. the lymphocyte transformation test that measures immune reactivity in bone near structures or the blood may have a higher sensitivity and it is therefore warranted. However, no such test system is currently available for allergist and surgeons in most centres and countries.

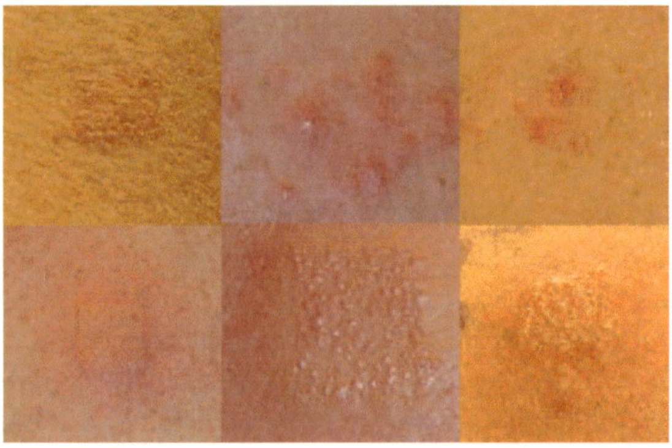

Fig. 4. Patch test reactions following 48 hours of occluded 5% nickel sulphate exposure. Upper line from left to right: irritative reaction, doubtful reaction (+?), and doubtful reaction (+?). Lower line from left to right: weak positive (1+), moderate positive (2+), and strong positive (3+) allergic reactions.

4.5.4 Other tests available

In vitro tests such as the macrophage migration test, the lymphocyte blastic transformation test and the lymphocyte transformation test have mostly been used in research projects (Rasanen and Tuomi 1992; Bordignon et al. 2008). None of these have become routine analyses in the clinical setting, even when 2 or 3 methods have been combined. The lymphocyte transformation test measures proliferation of lymphocytes from peripheral blood in the presence and absence of a potential allergen after incubation for 7 days. The result is reported as a stimulation index (SI) and is therefore quantitative. The little use of such *in vitro* test is mainly explained by an overall limited availability, a small number of allergens that can be tested, and the need for fast examination of lymphocytes after sampling since they rapidly become incapable of proliferating. Nevertheless, the lymphocyte proliferation test has been claimed to better reflect immune reactions within the body whereas the patch test mainly rather reflect cutaneous reactivity. Thus, a linear correlation was identified between serum metal ion levels and lymphocyte reactivity suggesting that *in vivo* metal release is directly associated with metal contact allergy (Hallab et al. 2004).

4.5.5 Clinical work-up

It is difficult to make general principles for good clinical practice before and after surgery regarding delayed type hypersensitivity reactions to orthopaedic implants. Allergic reactions to metal ions released from implants are rare and at the same time metal allergy remains very frequent. This obviously makes it difficult to identify the few allergic subjects at risk before developing implant failure. Although it is a matter of controversy, it seems sensible to refrain from routine patch testing/allergy testing prior to surgery unless the patient has already had implant surgery with complications suspected to be allergic or a history of clinical metal intolerance of sufficient magnitude to be of concern to the patient or a health provider (Thyssen et al. 2011a). If a patient is strongly allergic to e.g. nickel or cobalt, one should consider inserting titanium based alloys. To demonstrate causal relationship between delayed type of hypersensitivity and aseptic loosening strict criteria (Tab. 2) should be followed (Thyssen et al. 2011a).

Criteria	Description
1.	Histology consistent with a delayed type hypersensitivity reaction.
2.	Positive patch test reaction to a metal used in the implant (often strong reactions).
3.	Positive in vitro test to metals, e.g. the lymphocyte transformation test.
4.	Complete recovery following removal of the offending implant material.

Table 2. Objective criteria that support a causative association between metal release from the implant, metal allergy and delayed type hypersensitivity reactions such as implant loosening, malfunction, pain or chronic inflammation (from Thyssen et al. 2011a)

4.6 Aseptic loosening as a result of local failure of tissue homeostasis *(Gallo)*

The term "homeostasis" was coined by Claude Bernard in 1865 to describe the constancy of the internal environment as a condition of health. Metchnikoff has introduced the concept into immunology together with the term physiological inflammation to mean active maintenance of tissue harmony, tissue harmony (Medzhitov 2010). Given that the majority of patients profit from THA, it appears that low-grade periprosthetic inflammation occurring around "healthy" THA may be a normal adaptive response to the continual burden of prosthetic particles and mechanical stresses associated with implant use. For this reason, processes leading to osteolysis and aseptic loosening can be investigated as a problem of maladaptation.

In reality, no one knows what are the histological and immunological parameters associated with long-term "physiological" tissue homeostasis around THA, a baseline for true understanding of periprosthetic pathology. We can only translate data from models of THA (animal *in vivo* or *in vitro*) to the human situation (El-Warrak et al. 2004; Ma et al. 2009) and compare these with analyses of tissues from failed THAs. Unfortunately, tissues retrieved during revision surgery reflect late stages of the process when local homeostasis has long failed in the majority of cases.

What parameters are typical for physiological equilibrium between implant derived signals and healthy status of periprosthetic tissues in terms of maintenance of at least their architecture and function? The first and inevitable condition is *stable interface between implant and bone* which protects tissues from the deleterious effects of mechanical stimuli (stable equilibrium of implant-bone interface). The ideal condition is when the bone around the implant is protected from excessive mechanical stresses and strains and at the same time can undergo bone remodelling. The next critical step is *the ability to resolve inflammation induced by surgical trauma together with prevention of biofilm formation* on the prosthetic surface. Both the inability to achieve a steady very low-inflammatory status as early as possible and the

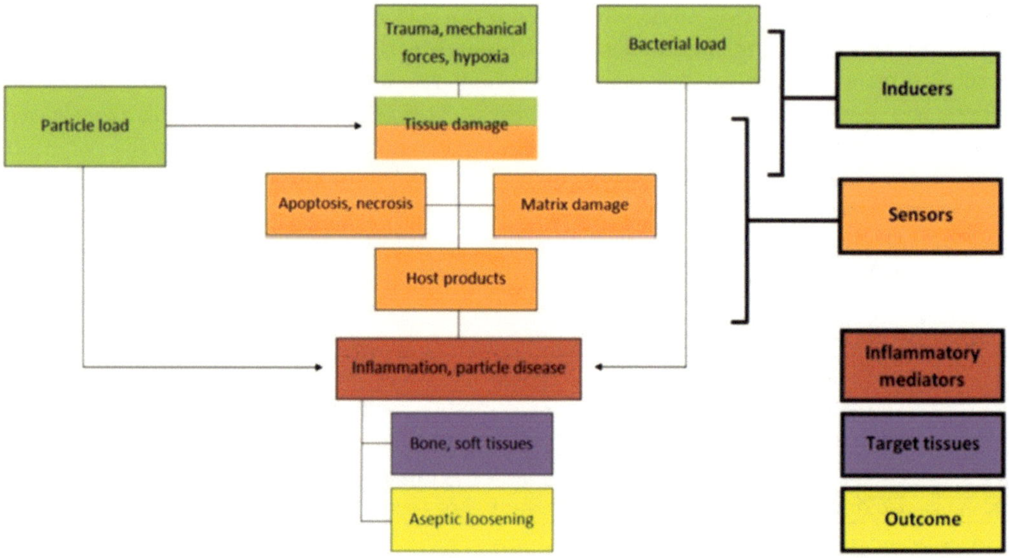

Fig. 5. Components of inflammatory response to a potential set of biological and physical insults associated with total hip arthroplasty (inducers of inflammation); host sensors detect the occurrence of inducers at tissues and their recognizing triggers expression of inflammatory mediators that affect the tissues where the inducers occur (according to Medzhitov 2010)

occurrence of microbial biofilm in the joint can maintain chronic inflammation which seriously compromises the local tissue homeostasis. The third critical step is the ability of tissues *to counteract the continual delivery of soluble (ionic) and insoluble (particles) debris* liberated from the prosthetic surfaces without increased inflammation and tissue damage. Prosthetic debris can induce a multitude of interactions which greatly increase the probability of chronic inflammation and predominance of osteoclasts over the osteoblasts at the bone-implant interface (*Part 2.2*). To avoid developing particle disease, there has to be much stronger regulation ability to overcome the above inflammatory and destructive processes. If these regulatory factors were known, new preventative and regulative measures could be proposed. The fourth critical step is the *regenerative potential of the periprosthetic tissues* that can restore tissue damage regardless whether this is of mechanical, biological or combined origin. Recently for instance, it has been proposed that a part of the inter-individual variance in the risk of early prosthetic migration (i.e. late aseptic loosening development) could be explained by patient-specific differences in the regeneration processes around the implant early post-operatively (Aspenberg et al. 2008). Taken together, when these steps concur, the probability of aseptic loosening is reduced and mutatis mutandis, if any of these steps is disturbed the route to aseptic loosening is open.

Normal tissue homeostasis is regulated by *complex cross-talk between stem cells, their differentiated cells, the local microenvironment, and the whole organism* (Perez-Losada and Balmain 2003). Basically, this depends on the right cell being in the right place at the right time (Buckley 2011). In periprosthetic reality this means, having sufficient number of functional macrophages, osteoblasts, fibrocytes-fibroblasts, and lymphocytes in a configuration that prevents development of chronic inflammation, fluid oversecretion, and increased accumulation of osteoclasts around the implant. The number of terminally differentiated cells is regulated by the mitotic activity of the stem cells in a poorly understood feedback interaction with local and systemic factors.

A very important role is also played by the local microenvironment which may favour development a particular cell line (Konttinen et al. 2005). In the case of THA, the inducers of inflammation can never be completely eliminated thus the tissues are under permanent activation load not only by mechanical stresses and particles but also by cytokines/ chemokines produced by cells previously activated by particles and/or microbial remnants. In fact, even under such conditions, the majority of periprosthetic tissues (patients) develop a steady state for a long time postoperatively. How is this possible? Can the tissues of successful patients develop something akin to "tolerance" (decreased responsiveness to the prosthesis-related stimuli)? Generally, to keep tissues in low-inflammatory steady state *require as low load of inducers as possible and also very fine tuning of sensors together with strict control of the quantity and activities of effector molecules/cells* (Fig. 5). On the other hand, the inability to resolve chronic high-grade inflammation can lead to irreversible tissue damage with restoration of different tissues (fibrous tissue instead of bone, formation of granulomas etc.).

4.6.1 Control of prosthesis-related inducers

Regarding the control of prosthesis-related inducers, most important appears to be *reduction of the particle loads* either using hard bearings or modern technologies of prosthetic surface treatment (*Part 5.1*). Of biological inflammation inducers, the most important roles are played by *cell necrosis, extracellular matrix damage* (both deliberating damage-associated molecular patterns, DAMPs), *reactive oxygen species (ROS), hypoxia, and activation of PRRs.*

Cell necrosis can affect both macrophages and other cell groups. It can be a result of strong foreign particle load (particles are *per se* undigestable, cytotoxic, genotoxic), hypoxia, ROS or unfavourable mechanical conditions. These stimuli can lead separately or combined to irreparable DNA damage and eventually cell death. Molecules released from dying cells together with breakdown products of the extracelullar matrix are considered important inducers of inflammation. In contrast, ingestion of apoptotic cells is associated with release of inflammation-resolving cytokines IL-10 and TGF-β (Nathan and Ding 2010). From this, it follows that the ratio of necrotic cells to apoptotic cells around the implant could play a significant role in relation to periprosthetic homeostasis (Landgraeber et al. 2009).

Hypoxia seems to be a common feature in aseptic loosening. Bone-implant interface membranes can suffer from hypoxia because it is hypovascular, due to chronic hypoxia-reperfusion injury of the interface membrane which is caused by implant loading. There is also increased oxygen consumption by local inflammatory cells (Santavirta et al. 1999). A hypoxic environment induces the expression of hypoxia-inducible factors (HIF-1α, HIF-2α) and some heat shock proteins that adapt the gene expression to oxygen availability within the hypoxic tissue. For this reason, decreased profileration is a fundamental physiological response to hypoxia in many cell types (Hubbi et al. 2011). Proliferation of progenitor cells is controlled by the hypoxia-sensitive Notch signalling pathway which maintains them in an undifferentiated state (Hilton et al. 2008). On the other hand, tissue macrophages are relatively well adapted to hypoxic conditions. This could at least partially explain their massive presence in periprosthetic membranes. Monocytes continue to differentiate into tissue macrophages even under severe hypoxia (0.2% O_2) and macrophages increase significantly their expression of HIF-1α mRNA and pro-angiogenic cytokine vascular endothelial growth factor (VEGF) as a response to chronic hypoxia. Hypoxia stimulates osteoclast differentiation, viability and activity, the latter predominantly via increased activity of hydrolytic enzymes including cathepsin K and in this way it could directly contribute to the extension of bone resorption around the THA. On the other hand, this effect depends on time and O_2 concentration with reduction in number and activity of osteoclasts as a function of longevity and severity of hypoxia (Knowles and Athanasou 2009). Osteoblastic cell lines can exhibit decreased growth, differentiation and mineralization capacity under hypoxic conditions. Moreover, these cells predominantly induce angiogenesis via increased secretion of VEGF (Knowles and Athanasou 2009). An important role in the transduction of hypoxic signal to bone-implant interface may be played by osteocytes via increased expression of HIF and osteopontin leading eventually to osteocyte-induced osteoclastic bone resorption (Gross et al. 2005).

Activation of PRRs by occurrence of PAMPs in periprosthetic tissues can distort local tissue homeostasis at any time postoperatively (Greenfield et al. 2010). PRRs have a strong potential to trigger inflammation via several pathways including differentiation of more aggressive M1 and M17 macrophages, multinuclear foreign body giant cells, osteoclasts and granulomas (Anderson et al. 2008). In addition, it has been shown that polymeric alkane structures released during UHMWPE breakdown can directly activate PRRs (TLR-1, 2 signalling pathway) while UHMWPE particles phagocytosed by periprosthetic cells induce endosomal destabilization and inflammasome activation (Maitra et al. 2009).

4.6.2 Tuning of inflammatory sensors and their response to prosthetic-related stimuli

Currently there is no evidence supporting the concept of "adaptation of inflammatory sensors" to chronic stimuli associated with prosthesis. The following is therefore simply translated from knowledge of the response of macrophages to microbial stimuli (Medzhitov and Horng 2009).

After several hours or days of prosthetic-related stimulation, the expression of several hundreds of genes could be induced by macrophages, fibroblasts and other cell groups. These gene expressions determine cell response to the stimuli. Simultaneously, a set of regulators is co-activated to control intensity and extension of the local inflammatory response (negative regulators of inflammation). These can be distinguished as *signal-specific regulators and gene-specific regulators.* The first category consists of regulators that inhibit signal transduction by PRRs and other inflammatory pathways (e.g. IL-1R-associated kinase M, IRAKM; suppressor of cytokine signalling, SOCS – proteins). The second category comprises transcriptional repressors (basal repressors and inducible repressors) or other negative regulators that modulate gene expression (e.g. microRNAs, long-non coding RNAs). Although there is no evidence that currently supports the existence of "adaptors" on prosthetic stimuli, we believe they must exist. Assuming their role, it may be postulated that in the absence of a key part of the negative feedback loop the proinflammatory cytokines/chemokines develop severe inflammatory microenvironment associated especially with the predominance of activated osteoclasts over functional osteoblasts , and vice versa, effective negative regulation of sensors could protect from development of osteolysis and aseptic loosening (*Parts 4.2, 4.3*).

4.6.3 Control of the effectors

Generally, macrophages lie at the centre of the process called particle disease. Therefore there is a question *whether activated macrophages can be deactivated* and what are the mechanisms underlying the tolerance to chronic unsolvable signalling. Theoretically, there are at least two ways leading to deactivation of macrophages. The first is associated with decrease in stimulation signalling level (e.g. interferon gamma and other cytokines, lipopolysaccharides and other bacterial stimuli). The second could be associated with activity of tissue-resident cells inducing negative modulation of macrophage pro-inflammatory activities and macrophage apoptosis (Valledor et al. 2010).

Activated fibroblasts perpetuate inflammation via inappropriate expression of survival molecules leading to the retention of activated cells in affected tissues or ectopic secretion of chemokines supporting recruitment of new cells as a fuel for continuation of inflammation (Buckley 2011). They also express several bone-resorbing metalloproteinases and "osteoclastogenic" cytokines in periprosthetic membranes including M-CSF, VEGF or RANKL contributing together with suppression of osteoblast function, to functional predominance of bone resorption over osteogenesis (Koreny et al. 2006). Based on these observations, it seems inevitable that deactivated and quiescent fibroblasts can, like macrophages significantly contribute to the resolution of particle-induced inflammation. Recent studies have revealed that inflammation is not generic but contextual. Therefore, *tissue-resident fibroblasts are able to switch the inflammation to the resolution.* In this connection, it is important to know which mechanisms induce fibroblast anti-inflammatory and regeneration activities. Firstly, fibroblasts could act as a source of anti-inflammatory and regenerative cytokines such as IL-4, IL-10, FGF and several others. Secondly, fibroblasts can provide anti-inflammatory stromal microenvironment in the periprosthetic interface membrane involving a plethora of cell-to-cell and perhaps also paracrine interactions (Buckley 2011).

Lymphocytes together with other cells enhance osteoclast differentiation; stimulate formation of foreign body giant cells and exhibit many other activities contributing to tissue damage. On the other hand, they have several pathways by which they *can "shift" the immune response in favour of T_H2 and T_H3* instead of T_H1 and T_H17 responses or delayed type of hypersensitivity (Matzinger and Kamala 2011).

Until now, we have assumed that the immune system alone dictates the direction and fate of periprosthetic tissues after stimulation by prosthetic derivates. However, this concept does not reflect the reality of the situation. Currently discussed is the concept of *tissue-appropriate immunity*, stressing the role of tissues in control of the effector mechanisms that prevent self-destruction (Matzinger and Kamala 2011). On this basis, tissue-resident cells might influence the response to stimulus in order to maintain the health of affected tissues by modifying cell activities and via soluble anti-inflammatory factors. Unfortunately, no such strategy is available currently in clinical practice to modify the above processes and induce/maintain localized tissue homeostasis around THA.

4.7 Individual susceptibility to aseptic loosening/ development of periprosthetic osteolysis *(Gallo, Petrek)*

High variability in survival of THAs, aseptic loosening/size of periprosthetic osteolysis has been observed between individuals with similar polyethylene wear rates. For this reason, the question is how to explain such a degree of inter-patient variability? This could be caused for example, by differences in implants (e.g. type of bearing material, sterilisation method, shape of prosthesis, surface technology etc.), variations in surgical technique (orientation of implants, final quality of bone-implant interface, protection of bone bed from joint fluid etc.), and variations due to patient-related factors (e.g. age, co-morbidities, level of activity and differences in mechanical loading). In addition, genetic factors can contribute to the risk for aseptic loosening (Fig. 6). Engh et al estimated that both wear and patient propensity to osteolysis might together account for 53% of the variance in total area of osteolysis (Engh et al. 2011).

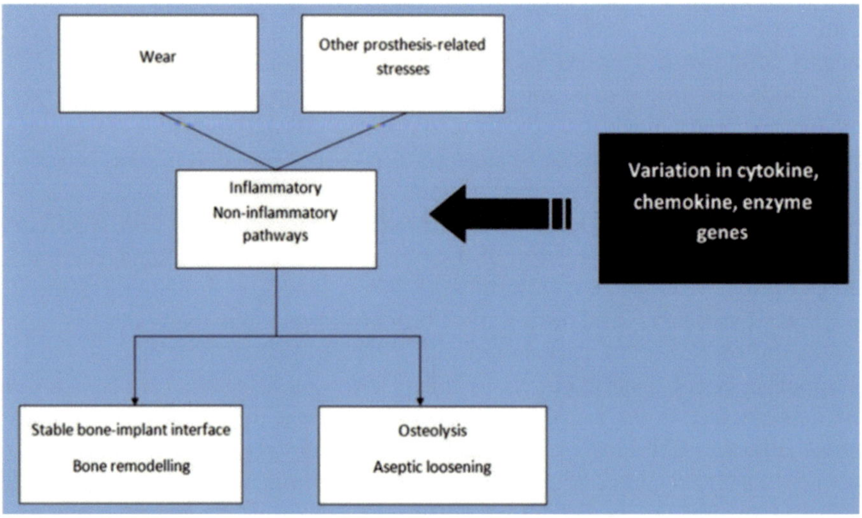

Fig. 6. Functional variation in genes for cytokines (other molecules) could influence the rate of aseptic loosening via contribution to severity of bone resorption around the implant

4.7.1 Methods for investigating genetic susceptibility to aseptic loosening/ periprosthetic osteolysis

The question is which genes (genotype) could influence the fate of implant in terms of premature aseptic loosening/ periprosthetic osteolysis (phenotype). A gene is traditionally defined as a segment of DNA encoding a protein. Single nucleotide polymorphism (SNP) is a common form of variation in the human genome implicating that a single base change in the DNA sequence could influence the amount/functionality of secreted proteins. With the sequencing of the human genome, it has been recognized that SNPs occur about once every 1000 base pairs (Dupuis and O'Donnell 2007). The key problem is *how to distinguish the gold (functional polymorphisms) from fool´s gold (unimportant variants).* By genotyping a large number of SNPs in a large number of patients there is a good chance of detecting those that are significantly associated with the target disease. Unfortunately, epigenetic factors and further DNA sequence variants such as copy number variants create other sources of variation between individuals. In addition, there are several non-coding small regulatory molecules (e.g. miRNAs, siRNAs) that significantly influence the process of translation of genes into effector proteins.

According to the number of genes participating in the pathophysiology of a disease and the size of their effect, *polygenic predisposition* assuming small/ marginal effects of many genes fits much better to the model of THA failure than the oligogenic model with two or more major gene (locus) effects. In this line, the odds ratios of 1.2 to 1.6 are required for differentiating true effects of individual genetic variants on a complex disease from the potential impact of bias (Ioannidis et al. 2006). Studies reporting weaker individual size effects are unlikely to be used for predicting a target condition; on the other hand, a combination of several even weaker genetic variants (especially at multiple loci) can increase the chance for reasonable prediction.

Genetic variation in patient-specific response to THA can be determined by several methods. For example, *genetic association studies* investigate possible association between the occurrences of phenotypic traits and candidate genetic variants using special rules and computational algorithms. In the case of *genome-wide association studies* the effects of up to 500,000 SNPs are analysed simultaneously, giving rise to an initial set of promising susceptibility genes that are further tested in a separate replication study.
When dealing with a genetic - environmental interaction it is necessary *to test simultaneously cases, controls exposed to the same key pathogenetic factors as the cases but do not exhibit the risk phenotype, and the population control.* In the case of aseptic loosening/osteolysis it is however rather difficult to recruit completely comparable cases and controls making it hard to address the question of individual susceptibility to these complications. In addition, identifying and characterizing the targets (mechanisms/molecules) for a genetic-association study is a key prerequisite for genetic investigation, and vice versa, inaccuracy in understanding the true pathophysiology of aseptic loosening/osteolysis compromises their outcomes. Therefore, the initial step of any genetic-association study should be *choice of potentially valuable candidate genes* followed by their validation in a candidate-gene study (Chanock et al. 2007).

4.7.2 Current status of the research

Wilkinson et al were the first to publish a study on the association between polymorphisms in the gene encoding for TNF alpha and risk of periprosthetic osteolysis in THA (Wilkinson et al. 2003). After this introductory work several papers were published nominating other molecules as candidates involved in the processes of aseptic loosening/ osteolysis. Structurally and functionally, these include receptors, intracellular mediators, enzymes, cytokines and other proteins. A recently published systematic review on genetically determined susceptibility to aseptic loosening of THA, revealed several areas of potential agreement (SNPs of TNF-238A allele, IL1RA +2018C allele, polymorphisms in genes for IL-6, MMP-1 etc.), but also several sources of heterogeneity between studies, showing the need for large multi-centre prospective studies that should provide stronger evidence for genetic predisposition to THA premature failure (Del Buono et al. 2011). As a result, further progress in the field of genetic risk of aseptic loosening/ osteolysis will require both sophisticated research strategy and statistics (e.g. improved risk-analysis models) to overcome a series of challenges. Fortunately, as experience accumulates, there is increased interest of orthopaedic specialty in the outcomes of such research.

5. Prevention of aseptic loosening/ periprosthetic osteolysis *(Gallo, Goodman, Konttinen)*

5.1 Biomaterial solutions

Based on the pathophysiology of periprosthetic osteolysis and aseptic loosening, there is clear that advances in biomaterials can improve at least partially the survival of THA by reducing the extension and intensity of particle disease. Here we focus only on bearing surfaces, although the material of implant and surface technology also influence the resistance against osteolytic membrane and joint fluid expansion.

5.1.1 Advances in polyethylene

The wear of ultra high molecular weight polyethylene (UHMWPE) is a major contributor to premature failure of THAs. For this reason, a number of years ago, it was questioned whether this material should be retained or withdrawn (Amis 1996). Fortunately, over the recent decades, several processing techniques have been developed to improve the mechanical and tribological performance of UHMWPE. More recent technologies involving high degree cross-linkage of the linear chains of UHMWPE (highly-cross linked polyethylene, HXLPE) have been incorporated into clinical practice for several years. These also differ from company to company according to method used for the elimination of residual free radicals that could lead to oxidative degradation of bearing surface (heating, infiltration of vitamin E etc.). In comparison to ceramic-on-ceramic (CoC) THA, the advantage of HXLPE is greater variety in terms of head sizes and offset. Also the cost of HXLPE is substantially lower than that for hard bearing surfaces. On the other hand, there remains a concern about the risk of fatigue fracture of acetabular liners even though the cases reported were made predominantly of first generation HXLPE (Furmanski et al. 2009). Little is known on the biological activity of HXLPE particles. It was demonstrated moderately increased specific biological activity in comparison to particles of conventional polyethylene (Illgen et al. 2009). Despite that, there is growing evidence that the use of modern HXLPE bearings decrease significantly wear rate and by this way may reduce the risk of premature osteolysis development although the majority of studies report outcomes with less than 10 years follow-up (Kurtz et al. 2011).

5.1.2 Advances in ceramic bearings

The amount of prosthetic particles can be significantly reduced using CoC bearings in THA. Ceramics, in general are very hard materials with excellent biocompatibility. In addition, use of third generation ceramic bearings, reduces the predicted risk for fracture of ceramic bearings to approaching nil. Currently there is enough evidence supporting the further use of CoC bearings in the case of THA (Hannouche et al. 2011). Concerns remain about the "squeaking" of ceramic implants, impingement of the femoral neck on the edge of ceramic liner and microseparations of ceramic surfaces.

Oxinium is a Zr-2.5 Nb alloy that has been oxidized at elevated temperature to grow a zirconium oxide ceramic layer on the surface of the implant. Such surface treatment increases the wear resistance of the implant. However, there is only limited clinical experience with Oxinium™ femoral heads in THA.

5.1.3 Advances in metal

Bearing surfaces made of cobalt, chromium and molybdenum alloys are currently a subject of controversy because of their biological consideration. The main reason is that metallic wear particles can induce implant hypersensitivity, ALVAL (*Part 3.2.2*), may contribute to tissue necrosis and also to induction and perpetuation of periprosthetic particle disease (Watters et al. 2010; Basko-Plluska et al. 2011). In addition, the levels of metal ions in serum and urine also can be elevated for a long time in patients with stable and functional implants in comparison to controls without metallic implants. Although long-term data are not available, the International Agency for Research on Cancer (IARC) has classified implanted foreign bodies consisting of metallic cobalt, nickel and chromium in Group 2B defined as possibly carcinogenic in humans (McGregor et al. 2000). The main concern is that exposure of human cells to cobalt and chromium may induce chromosomal aberrations and damage DNA, potentially leading to carcinoma (Beyersmann and Hartwig 2008). From a purely epidemiological view, the current evidence for clinical carcinogenetic effects of metal-on-metal THAs is limited and rigorous long-term studies are needed to answer the above question. Taken together, above potential consequences from the clinical usage of bearing surfaces made of cobalt, chromium, molybdenum alloy should be discussed with the patient prior to his/her surgical procedure.

5.2 Design solutions

THA has to withstand repetitive mechanical loading and long term exposure in the human body without compromising the integrity of either implant or bone-implant interface (Tarala et al. 2011). Engineers can help to prevent, at least partially, the development of periprosthetic osteolysis and aseptic loosening by creating a design and surface characteristics that increase the resistance of implant-bone interface to osteolytic granulomas and preventing access of joint fluid to the bone bed. The current evidence is in favour of bone remodeling being responsible for long-term bone-implant fixation. In this line, more biologically active prosthetic surfaces have been introduced into clinical practice (e.g. porous metals, hydroxyapatite coating etc.). Currently, multifunctional surfaces are tested with the aim of improving osseointegration and preventing the formation of biofilm. Recently, attempts have been made to coat implants with mesenchymal stromal (stem) cells (MSCs). The hypothesis is that such cells could enhance bone formation and subsequent implant fixation via intramembranous or endochondral ossification. However, the eventual role and fate of endogenously mobilized or exogenously delivered MSCs in implant fixation is still poorly known.

5.3 Patient selection

The final outcome of THA depends on a large number of factors including the design of the implant, surgical technique, and patient selection. Currently there are no scientifically proven criteria for matching individuals to particular implant. At the time of surgery, the decision should involve the *age of the patient, his/her local bone status and overall health condition* enabling rough estimation of time in use for the THA. Based on current best evidence, younger more active patients have several options to minimize wear, loosening and osteolysis, and thereby optimize implant longevity. These alternatives include ceramic-on-ceramic bearings or ceramic head or highly polished cobalt-chrome femoral heads articulating with highly-cross linked polyethylene.
Another concern relates to *primary diagnosis* and the expecting of worse prognosis especially in patients with osteoarthritis after developmental dysplasia in comparison with those with idiopathic osteoarthritis. This may be associated at least partially with severity of dysplasia (Chougle et al. 2005). In fact, experienced surgeon and choice of implant could also play a role. Recent analysis from the Danish Hip Arthroplasty Registry failed to reveal substantial differences in revision risk between the above groups with follow-up of from 0.5 to 12 years postoperatively (Thillemann et al. 2008). Low revision rate has been observed in both cemented and cementless THA (Sochart and Porter 1997; Rozkydal et al. 2005). Rheumatoid arthritis does not require a special approach even in young patients. Regarding the choice of implant in these patients, a higher risk of revision was found for THAs with uncemented cups and cemented stems according in the Finnish Arthroplasty Registry (Eskelinen et al. 2006). However, the difference in survivorship between cemented and uncemented THAs disappeared in patients older than 55 years old (Makela et al. 2011).

5.4 Operative procedures

Surgically-related variables are those related to wear rate and those that influence the strength of implant-bone fixation. Wear rate can be influenced primarily by *appropriate choice of implant and experienced surgical technique* especially in terms of positioning of the cup and stem, assuming both the inappropriate bearing surfaces and/or incorrect positioning of the implants contribute to increased wear rate and risk of osteolysis development (Little et al. 2009). Surgical technique can also influence the strength of implant-bone interface. In this connection, any mistake during cementation can increase the risk of premature failure (Barrack, Mulroy et al. 1992). In support, it seems that high-volume surgeons can achieve lower revision rates than low-volume surgeons especially during the early period after the surgery (Losina et al. 2004).

5.5 Life with total hip arthroplasty

Charnley believed that THA is appropriate for older people with limited physical expectations (Charnley and Feagin 1973). Later on, younger and more active patients were indicated for prosthetic hip surgery and the expectations of these patients have increased continually. In fact, younger patients who are treated by THA wish to return to recreational and even competitive sports activity. At the same time, patient activity is considered one of the most important factors in the risk of failure especially via increased wear-rate of bearing surfaces (Schmalzried et al. 2000). By this way, *those who experience high-levels of activity are at increased risk for failure due to aseptic loosening and osteolysis*, and vice versa, lower impact activities are less likely to create conditions appropriate to loosening (Kilgus et al. 1991; Lubbeke et al. 2011). Regarding the stability of bone-implant interface, there may be a concern about cracks followed by fracture of the cement mantle in association with high-impact load. Surgeons should advise patients with THA that all high-impact activities could compromise the durability of their implant, especially in terms of accelerated wear and premature aseptic loosening. Another possible concern is risk of fall and direct contact during these sport activities that could lead to catastrophic failure, periprosthetic fracture or dislocation of THA. In addition, patients should know that return to a high-load level is not possible without achieving a very good muscle condition and also appropriate skills in their coordination beforehand as muscles can share the forces traversing an artificial joint and thus could prevent its damage. On the other hand, regular repetitive physical activities positively affect both the bone (in accordance with Wolff´s law) and muscles near the artificial joint (Clifford and Mallon 2005; Wilson and Villar 2011).

6. Conclusions *(Gallo)*

Aseptic loosening is the leading cause of THA failure in the intermediate and long-term postoperative period. Causally it is associated with rapid wear rate inducing adverse host reaction to wear debris and to repetitive mechanical stresses and strains of the bone-implant interface. Here, we introduced the concept of failure of local tissue homeostasis as underlying the majority of processes leading to aseptic loosening. Given that the implant is stable in the second postoperative year and no gross pathology of bone-implant interface is seen on x-ray, then the fate of implant depends on the ability of host tissues (both, bone and soft tissues) to maintain homeostasis with minimum inflammation despite the occurrence of chronic mechanical and particle load. In this connection, the problem is the inability to maintain the balance at bone-implant interface and resolve inflammation in the periprosthetic tissues that can induce the excessive bone resorption around the implant (osteolysis) leading eventually to aseptic loosening. The increased knowledge of the mechanisms regulating the balance in periprosthetic tissues might open new avenues to prevent aseptic loosening and periprosthetic osteolysis.

7. List of abbreviations used in the chapter

ALVAL	Aseptic Lymphocyte-dominated Vasculitis-Associated Lesions
ARF	Activation-Reversal-Formation cycles (bone remodelation)
BMP	Bone Morphogenetic Protein
BMU	Bone Multicellular Unit
CD	Cluster of Differentiation
CoC	Ceramic on Ceramic
DTH	Delayed-Type Hypersensitivity
ECM	ExtraCellular Matrix
FBGCs	Foreign Body Giant Cells
FGF	Fibroblast Growth Factor
GM-CSF	Granulocyte Macrophage Colony Stimulating Factor
HIF	Hypoxia-Induced Factor
HLA	Human Leukocyte Antigen (HLA DR+ is a MHC II class II cell surface receptor)
HXLPE	Highly Cross-Linked PolyEthylene
ICAM	InterCellular Adhesion Molecule
IFN-γ	Interferon gama
IL-1β, 2 ..	Interleukins
IRAK	Interleukin-1-Receptor-Associated Kinase
LPS	LipoPolySaccharide
MCP-1	Monocyte Chemoattractant Protein-1
M-CSF	Macrophage Colony-Stimulating Factor
MHC	Major Histocompatibility Complex
MIP	Macrophage Inhibitory Protein
MoM	Metal on Metal
MoP	Metal on Polyethylene
MPa	Megapascal (pressure unit)
MSCs	Mesenchymal Stromal/Stem Cells
NF-κβ	Nuclear Factor kappa beta
NK cells	Natural Killer cells
OPG	Osteoprotegerin
PAMPs	Pathogen-Associated Molecular Patterns
PMMA	PolyMethylMethAcrylate (bone cement)
PRRs	Pattern-Recognition Receptors
RANK	Receptor Activator of Nuclear factor Kappa beta
RANKL	Receptor Activator of Nuclear factor Kappa beta Ligand
ROS	Reactive Oxygen Species
SLIM	Synovial membrane-Like Interface Membrane
SNP	Single-Nucleotide Polymorphism
SOCS	Suppressor Of Cytokine Signalling
TGF	Transforming Growth Factor
THA	Total Hip arthroplasty
TLRs	Toll-Like Receptors
TNF-α	Tumor Necrosis Factor alpha
TREG	T-REGulatory lymphocytes
UHMWPE	Ultra-High Molecular Weight PolyEthylene
VCAM	Vascular Cell Adhesion Molecule
VEGF	Vascular Endothelial Growth Factor

8. Acknowledgements

This study was supported by Internal Grant Agency Ministry of Health, Czech Republic (NT/11049-5), the Sigrid Juselius Foundation, by the Helsinki University Central Hospital evo-funds, Finska Läkaresällskapet, Wilhelm och Else Stockmanns Stiftelse, ORTON Orthopaedic Hospital of the Invalid Foundation, National Doctoral Programme of Musculoskeletal Disorders and Biomaterials, Danish Council for Strategic Research, European Science Foundation "Regenerative Medicine" RNP, and by Grant 1R01AR055650-04 from the National Institute of Health and the French Granting Agency E.F.M.C. N°1.
We apologize to all authors whose work could not be cited due to space limitations.

9. References

Al-Saffar, N. and P. A. Revell (2000). "Differential expression of transforming growth factor-alpha and macrophage colony-stimulating factor/colony-stimulating factor-1R (c-fins) by multinucleated giant cells involved in pathological bone resorption at the site of orthopaedic implants." J Orthop Res 18(5): 800-7.

Amis, A. A. (1996). "Is polyethylene still the best prosthetic bearing surface?" J Bone Joint Surg Br 78(3): 345-8.

Anderson, J. M. (2009). In vitro and in vivo monocyte, macrophage, foreign body giant cell, and lymphocyte interactions with biomaterials. In: Biological interactions on material surfaces. Eds. D. A. Puleo, Bizios, R. Dordrecht, Springer: 225-244.

Anderson, J. M., A. Rodriguez, et al. (2008). "Foreign body reaction to biomaterials." Seminars in Immunology 20(2): 86-100.

Aspenberg, P., N. Basic, et al. (2000). "Reduced expression of BMP-3 due to mechanical loading: a link between mechanical stimuli and tissue differentiation." Acta Orthop Scand 71(6): 558-62.

Aspenberg, P., P. Wagner, et al. (2008). "Fixed or loose? Dichotomy in RSA data for cemented cups." Acta Orthop 79(4): 467-73.

Baggiolini, M. and I. Clark-Lewis (1992). "Interleukin-8, a chemotactic and inflammatory cytokine." FEBS Lett 307(1): 97-101.

Barrack, R. L., R. D. Mulroy, Jr., et al. (1992). "Improved cementing techniques and femoral component loosening in young patients with hip arthroplasty. A 12-year radiographic review." J Bone Joint Surg Br 74(3): 385-9.

Basko-Plluska, J. L., J. P. Thyssen, et al. (2011). "Cutaneous and systemic hypersensitivity reactions to metallic implants." Dermatitis 22(2): 65-79.

Beyersmann, D. and A. Hartwig (2008). "Carcinogenic metal compounds: recent insight into molecular and cellular mechanisms." Arch Toxicol 82(8): 493-512.

Bordignon, V., F. Palamara, et al. (2008). "Nickel, palladium and rhodium induced IFN-gamma and IL-10 production as assessed by in vitro ELISpot-analysis in contact dermatitis patients." BMC Immunol 9: 19.

Boyle, W. J., W. S. Simonet, et al. (2003). "Osteoclast differentiation and activation." Nature 423(6937): 337-42.

Brasch, J., T. Henseler, et al. (1994). "Reproducibility of patch tests. A multicenter study of synchronous left-versus right-sided patch tests by the German Contact Dermatitis Research Group." J Am Acad Dermatol 31(4): 584-91.

Buckley, C. D. (2011). "Why does chronic inflammation persist: An unexpected role for fibroblasts." Immunol Lett 138(1): 12-4.

Burke, D. W., D. O. O'Connor, et al. (1991). "Micromotion of cemented and uncemented femoral components." J Bone Joint Surg Br 73(1): 33-7.

Cadosch, D., M. S. Al-Mushaiqri, et al. (2010a). "Biocorrosion and uptake of titanium by human osteoclasts." J Biomed Mater Res A 95(4): 1004-10.

Cadosch, D., O. P. Gautschi, et al. (2010b). "Titanium induced production of chemokines CCL17/TARC and CCL22/MDC in human osteoclasts and osteoblasts." J Biomed Mater Res A 92(2): 475-83.

Cadosch, D., E. Chan, et al. (2009). "Metal is not inert: role of metal ions released by biocorrosion in aseptic loosening--current concepts." J Biomed Mater Res A 91(4): 1252-62.

Caicedo, M. S., R. Desai, et al. (2009). "Soluble and particulate Co-Cr-Mo alloy implant metals activate the inflammasome danger signaling pathway in human macrophages: a novel mechanism for implant debris reactivity." J Orthop Res 27(7): 847-54.

Clifford, P. E. and W. J. Mallon (2005). "Sports after total joint replacement." Clin Sports Med 24(1): 175-86.

Clohisy, J. C., E. Frazier, et al. (2003). "RANKL is an essential cytokine mediator of polymethylmethacrylate particle-induced osteoclastogenesis." J Orthop Res 21(2): 202-12.

Cook, D. N. (1996). "The role of MIP-1 alpha in inflammation and hematopoiesis." J Leukoc Biol 59(1): 61-6.

Corbett, K. L., E. Losina, et al. (2010). "Population-based rates of revision of primary total hip arthroplasty: a systematic review." PLoS One 5(10): e13520.

Del Buono, A., V. Denaro, et al. (2011). "Genetic susceptibility to aseptic loosening following total hip arthroplasty: a systematic review." Br Med Bull. Epub ahead of print Jun 7.

Dempsey, K. E., M. P. Riggio, et al. (2007). "Identification of bacteria on the surface of clinically infected and non-infected prosthetic hip joints removed during revision arthroplasties by 16S rRNA gene sequencing and by microbiological culture." Arthritis Res Ther 9(3): R46.

Derbyshire, B., R. J. Prescott, et al. (2009). "Notes on the use and interpretation of radiostereometric analysis." Acta Orthop 80(1): 124-30.

Deshmane, S. L., S. Kremlev, et al. (2009). "Monocyte chemoattractant protein-1 (MCP-1): an overview." J Interferon Cytokine Res 29(6): 313-26.

Djaafar, S., D. D. Pierroz, et al. (2010). "Inhibition of T cell-dependent and RANKL-dependent osteoclastogenic processes associated with high levels of bone mass in interleukin-15 receptor-deficient mice." Arthritis Rheum 62(11): 3300-10.

Dupuis, J. and C. J. O'Donnell (2007). "Interpreting results of large-scale genetic association studies: separating gold from fool's gold." JAMA 297(5): 529-31.

El-Warrak, A. O., M. Olmstead, et al. (2004). "An experimental animal model of aseptic loosening of hip prostheses in sheep to study early biochemical changes at the interface membrane." BMC Musculoskelet Disord 5: 7.

Engesaeter, L. B., S. A. Lie, et al. (2003). "Antibiotic prophylaxis in total hip arthroplasty: effects of antibiotic prophylaxis systemically and in bone cement on the revision

rate of 22,170 primary hip replacements followed 0-14 years in the Norwegian Arthroplasty Register." Acta Orthop Scand 74(6): 644-51.
Engh, C. A., H. Ho, et al. (2011). "Osteolysis propensity among bilateral total hip arthroplasty patients." J Arthroplasty 26(4): 555-61.
Engh, C. A., J. P. Hooten, Jr., et al. (1995). "Evaluation of bone ingrowth in proximally and extensively porous-coated anatomic medullary locking prostheses retrieved at autopsy." J Bone Joint Surg Am 77(6): 903-10.
Eskelinen, A., P. Paavolainen, et al. (2006). "Total hip arthroplasty for rheumatoid arthritis in younger patients: 2,557 replacements in the Finnish Arthroplasty Register followed for 0-24 years." Acta Orthop 77(6): 853-65.
Fahlgren, A., M. P. Bostrom, et al. (2010). "Fluid pressure and flow as a cause of bone resorption." Acta Orthop 81(4): 508-16.
Faurschou, A., T. Menne, et al. (2011). "Metal allergen of the 21st century--a review on exposure, epidemiology and clinical manifestations of palladium allergy." Contact Dermatitis 64(4): 185-95.
Fritz, E. A., T. T. Glant, et al. (2002). "Titanium particles induce the immediate early stress responsive chemokines IL-8 and MCP-1 in osteoblasts." J Orthop Res 20(3): 490-8.
Fujii, J., Y. Yasunaga, et al. (2011). "Wear debris stimulates bone-resorbing factor expression in the fibroblasts and osteoblasts." Hip Int.
Fujishiro, T., D. J. Moojen, et al. (2011). "Perivascular and diffuse lymphocytic inflammation are not specific for failed metal-on-metal hip implants." Clin Orthop Relat Res 469(4): 1127-33.
Furmanski, J., M. Anderson, et al. (2009). "Clinical fracture of cross-linked UHMWPE acetabular liners." Biomaterials 30(29): 5572-82.
Gallo, J., V. Havranek, et al. (2010). "Male gender, Charnley class C, and severity of bone defects predict the risk for aseptic loosening in the cup of ABG I hip arthroplasty." BMC Musculoskelet Disord 11: 243.
Gallo, J., P. Kaminek, et al. (2002). "Particle disease. A comprehensive theory of periprosthetic osteolysis: a review." Biomed Pap Med Fac Univ Palacky Olomouc Czech Repub 146(2): 21-8.
Goldstein, I. M., D. Roos, et al. (1975). "Complement and immunoglobulins stimulate superoxide production by human leukocytes independently of phagocytosis." J Clin Invest 56(5): 1155-63.
Goodman, S. B., P. Huie, et al. (1998). "Cellular profile and cytokine production at prosthetic interfaces. Study of tissues retrieved from revised hip and knee replacements." J Bone Joint Surg Br 80(3): 531-9.
Goodman, S. B., R. C. Chin, et al. (1989). "A clinical-pathologic-biochemical study of the membrane surrounding loosened and nonloosened total hip arthroplasties." Clin Orthop Relat Res(244): 182-7.
Goodman, S. B. and T. Ma (2010). "Cellular chemotaxis induced by wear particles from joint replacements." Biomaterials 31(19): 5045-50.
Granchi, D., I. Amato, et al. (2005). "Molecular basis of osteoclastogenesis induced by osteoblasts exposed to wear particles." Biomaterials 26(15): 2371-9.
Greenfield, E. M., M. A. Beidelschies, et al. (2010). "Bacterial pathogen-associated molecular patterns stimulate biological activity of orthopaedic wear particles by activating cognate Toll-like receptors." J Biol Chem 285(42): 32378-84.

Gross, T. S., K. A. King, et al. (2005). "Upregulation of osteopontin by osteocytes deprived of mechanical loading or oxygen." J Bone Miner Res 20(2): 250-6.

Hailer, N. P., R. A. Blaheta, et al. (2011). "Elevation of circulating HLA DR(+) CD8(+) T-cells and correlation with chromium and cobalt concentrations 6 years after metal-on-metal hip arthroplasty." Acta Orthop 82(1): 6-12.

Hailer, N. P., G. Garellick, et al. (2010). "Uncemented and cemented primary total hip arthroplasty in the Swedish Hip Arthroplasty Register." Acta Orthop 81(1): 34-41.

Hallab, N., K. Merritt, et al. (2001). "Metal sensitivity in patients with orthopaedic implants." J Bone Joint Surg Am 83-A(3): 428-36.

Hallab, N. J., S. Anderson, et al. (2004). "Immune responses correlate with serum-metal in metal-on-metal hip arthroplasty." J Arthroplasty 19(8 Suppl 3): 88-93.

Hallab, N. J., M. Caicedo, et al. (2008). "Th1 type lymphocyte reactivity to metals in patients with total hip arthroplasty." J Orthop Surg Res 3: 6.

Hallab, N. J. and J. J. Jacobs (2009). "Biologic effects of implant debris." Bull NYU Hosp Jt Dis 67(2): 182-8.

Hannouche, D., A. Zaoui, et al. (2011). "Thirty years of experience with alumina-on-alumina bearings in total hip arthroplasty." Int Orthop 35(2): 207-13.

Hilton, M. J., X. Tu, et al. (2008). "Notch signaling maintains bone marrow mesenchymal progenitors by suppressing osteoblast differentiation." Nat Med 14(3): 306-14.

Holt, G., C. Murnaghan, et al. (2007). "The Biology of Aseptic Osteolysis." Clin Orthop Relat Res 460: 240-252.

Hubbi, M. E., W. Luo, et al. (2011). "MCM Proteins Are Negative Regulators of Hypoxia-Inducible Factor 1." Mol Cell 42(5): 700-12.

Huss, R. S., J. I. Huddleston, et al. (2010). "Synovial tissue-infiltrating natural killer cells in osteoarthritis and periprosthetic inflammation." Arthritis Rheum 62(12): 3799-805.

Chanock, S. J., T. Manolio, et al. (2007). "Replicating genotype-phenotype associations." Nature 447(7145): 655-60.

Charnley, J. and J. A. Feagin (1973). "Low-friction arthroplasty in congenital subluxation of the hip." Clin Orthop Relat Res(91): 98-113.

Childs, L. M., J. J. Goater, et al. (2001). "Efficacy of etanercept for wear debris-induced osteolysis." J Bone Miner Res 16(2): 338-47.

Childs, L. M., E. P. Paschalis, et al. (2002). "In vivo RANK signaling blockade using the receptor activator of NF-kappaB:Fc effectively prevents and ameliorates wear debris-induced osteolysis via osteoclast depletion without inhibiting osteogenesis." J Bone Miner Res 17(2): 192-9

Chougle, A., M. V. Hemmady, et al. (2005). "Severity of hip dysplasia and loosening of the socket in cemented total hip replacement. A long-term follow-up." J Bone Joint Surg Br 87(1): 16-20.

Illgen, R. L., 2nd, L. M. Bauer, et al. (2009). "Highly crosslinked vs conventional polyethylene particles: relative in vivo inflammatory response." J Arthroplasty 24(1): 117-24.

Ioannidis, J. P., T. A. Trikalinos, et al. (2006). "Implications of small effect sizes of individual genetic variants on the design and interpretation of genetic association studies of complex diseases." Am J Epidemiol 164(7): 609-14.

Jasty, M., W. J. Maloney, et al. (1990). "Histomorphological studies of the long-term skeletal responses to well fixed cemented femoral components." J Bone Joint Surg Am 72(8): 1220-9.

Jin, Z. M., Fischer, J., Ingham E. (2006). Biotribology: material design, lubrication, and wear in artificial hip joints. In: Handbook of Lubrication and Tribology. Volume I Application and Maintenance. Ed. G. E. Totten. Boca Raton, FL, CRC Press.

Jones, L. C., M. Tucci, et al. (2006). "Macrophages and fibroblasts respond differently to PMMA particles and mechanical strain." Biomed Sci Instrum 42: 223-30.

Kilgus, D. J., F. J. Dorey, et al. (1991). "Patient activity, sports participation, and impact loading on the durability of cemented total hip replacements." Clin Orthop Relat Res(269): 25-31.

Kim, K. J., S. Kotake, et al. (2001). "Osteoprotegerin inhibits in vitro mouse osteoclast formation induced by joint fluid from failed total hip arthroplasty." J Biomed Mater Res 58(4): 393-400.

Knowles, H. J. and N. A. Athanasou (2009). "Acute hypoxia and osteoclast activity: a balance between enhanced resorption and increased apoptosis." J Pathol 218(2): 256-64.

Konttinen, Y. T., M. Takagi, et al. (2001). "Acid attack and cathepsin K in bone resorption around total hip replacement prosthesis." J Bone Miner Res 16(10): 1780-6.

Konttinen, Y. T., D. Zhao, et al. (2005). "The microenvironment around total hip replacement prostheses." Clin Orthop Relat Res(430): 28-38.

Koreny, T., M. Tunyogi-Csapo, et al. (2006). "The role of fibroblasts and fibroblast-derived factors in periprosthetic osteolysis." Arthritis Rheum 54(10): 3221-32.

Korhonen, R. K., A. Koistinen, et al. (2005). "The effect of geometry and abduction angle on the stresses in cemented UHMWPE acetabular cups--finite element simulations and experimental tests." Biomed Eng Online 4(1): 32.

Koulouvaris, P., K. Ly, et al. (2008). "Expression profiling reveals alternative macrophage activation and impaired osteogenesis in periprosthetic osteolysis." J Orthop Res 26(1): 106-16.

Kumar, H., T. Kawai, et al. (2011). "Pathogen recognition by the innate immune system." Int Rev Immunol 30(1): 16-34.

Kumazawa, R., F. Watari, et al. (2002). "Effects of Ti ions and particles on neutrophil function and morphology." Biomaterials 23(17): 3757-64.

Kurtz, S., K. Ong, et al. (2007). "Projections of primary and revision hip and knee arthroplasty in the United States from 2005 to 2030." J Bone Joint Surg Am 89(4): 780-5.

Kurtz, S. M., H. A. Gawel, et al. (2011). "History and Systematic Review of Wear and Osteolysis Outcomes for First-generation Highly Crosslinked Polyethylene." Clin Orthop Relat Res (469): 2262-77.

Lahdeoja, T., J. Pajarinen, et al. (2010). "Toll-like receptors and aseptic loosening of hip endoprosthesis-a potential to respond against danger signals?" J Orthop Res 28(2): 184-90.

Landgraeber, S., S. Jaeckel, et al. (2009). "Pan-caspase inhibition suppresses polyethylene particle-induced osteolysis." Apoptosis 14(2): 173-81.

Lappalainen, R., M. Selenius, et al. (2003). "Reduction of wear in total hip replacement prostheses by amorphous diamond coatings." J Biomed Mater Res B Appl Biomater 66(1): 410-3.

Lazarov, A., M. David, et al. (2007). "Comparison of reactivity to allergens using the TRUE Test and IQ chamber system." Contact Dermatitis 56(3): 140-5.

Little, N. J., C. A. Busch, et al. (2009). "Acetabular polyethylene wear and acetabular inclination and femoral offset." Clin Orthop Relat Res 467(11): 2895-900.

Losina, E., J. Barrett, et al. (2004). "Early failures of total hip replacement: effect of surgeon volume." Arthritis Rheum 50(4): 1338-43.
Lubbeke, A., G. Garavaglia, et al. (2011). "Influence of patient activity on femoral osteolysis at five and ten years following hybrid total hip replacement." J Bone Joint Surg Br 93(4): 456-63.
Ma, J., T. Chen, et al. (2003). "Regulation of macrophage activation." Cell Mol Life Sci 60(11): 2334-46.
Ma, T., S. G. Ortiz, et al. (2009). "In vivo murine model of continuous intramedullary infusion of particles--a preliminary study." J Biomed Mater Res B Appl Biomater 88(1): 250-3.
Maitra, R., C. C. Clement, et al. (2009). "Endosomal damage and TLR2 mediated inflammasome activation by alkane particles in the generation of aseptic osteolysis." Mol Immunol 47(2-3): 175-84.
Makela, K. T., A. Eskelinen, et al. (2011). "Cemented versus cementless total hip replacements in patients fifty-five years of age or older with rheumatoid arthritis." J Bone Joint Surg Am 93(2): 178-86.
Mandelin, J., T. F. Li, et al. (2005a). "Interface tissue fibroblasts from loose total hip replacement prosthesis produce receptor activator of nuclear factor-kappaB ligand, osteoprotegerin, and cathepsin K." J Rheumatol 32(4): 713-20.
Mandelin, J., T. F. Li, et al. (2003). "Imbalance of RANKL/RANK/OPG system in interface tissue in loosening of total hip replacement." J Bone Joint Surg Br 85(8): 1196-201.
Mandelin, J., M. Liljestrom, et al. (2005b). "Pseudosynovial fluid from loosened total hip prosthesis induces osteoclast formation." J Biomed Mater Res B Appl Biomater 74(1): 582-8.
Matzinger, P. (2007). "Friendly and dangerous signals: is the tissue in control?" Nat Immunol 8(1): 11-3.
Matzinger, P. and T. Kamala (2011). "Tissue-based class control: the other side of tolerance." Nat Rev Immunol 11(3): 221-30.
McEvoy, A., M. Jeyam, et al. (2002). "Synergistic effect of particles and cyclic pressure on cytokine production in human monocyte/macrophages: proposed role in periprosthetic osteolysis." Bone 30(1): 171-7.
McGregor, D. B., R. A. Baan, et al. (2000). "Evaluation of the carcinogenic risks to humans associated with surgical implants and other foreign bodies - a report of an IARC Monographs Programme Meeting. International Agency for Research on Cancer." Eur J Cancer 36(3): 307-13.
Medzhitov, R. (2010). "Inflammation 2010: new adventures of an old flame." Cell 140(6): 771-6.
Medzhitov, R. and T. Horng (2009). "Transcriptional control of the inflammatory response." Nat Rev Immunol 9(10): 692-703.
Menten, P., A. Wuyts, et al. (2002). "Macrophage inflammatory protein-1." Cytokine Growth Factor Rev 13(6): 455-81.
Mjoberg, B. (1994). "Theories of wear and loosening in hip prostheses. Wear-induced loosening vs loosening-induced wear--a review." Acta Orthop Scand 65(3): 361-71.
Nakashima, Y., D. H. Sun, et al. (1999). "Induction of macrophage C-C chemokine expression by titanium alloy and bone cement particles." J Bone Joint Surg Br 81(1): 155-62.
Nalepka, J. L., M. J. Lee, et al. (2006). "Lipopolysaccharide found in aseptic loosening of patients with inflammatory arthritis." Clin Orthop Relat Res 451: 229-35.

Nathan, C. and A. Ding (2010). "Nonresolving inflammation." Cell 140(6): 871-82.
Ng, V. Y., A. V. Lombardi, Jr., et al. (2011). "Perivascular lymphocytic infiltration is not limited to metal-on-metal bearings." Clin Orthop Relat Res 469(2): 523-9.
Ogino, D., H. Kawaji, et al. (2008). "Total hip replacement in patients eighty years of age and older." J Bone Joint Surg Am 90(9): 1884-90.
Pajarinen, J., E. Cenni, et al. (2010). "Profile of toll-like receptor-positive cells in septic and aseptic loosening of total hip arthroplasty implants." J Biomed Mater Res A 94(1): 84-92.
Pearl, J. I., T. Ma, et al. (2011). "Role of the Toll-like receptor pathway in the recognition of orthopedic implant wear-debris particles." Biomaterials 32(24): 5535-42.
Pedersen, A. B., S. P. Johnsen, et al. (2005). "Total hip arthroplasty in Denmark: incidence of primary operations and revisions during 1996-2002 and estimated future demands." Acta Orthop 76(2): 182-9.
Perez-Losada, J. and A. Balmain (2003). "Stem-cell hierarchy in skin cancer." Nat Rev Cancer 3(6): 434-43.
Proudfoot, A. E. (2002). "Chemokine receptors: multifaceted therapeutic targets." Nat Rev Immunol 2(2): 106-15.
Purdue, P. E., P. Koulouvaris, et al. (2007). "The cellular and molecular biology of periprosthetic osteolysis." Clin Orthop Relat Res 454: 251-61.
Rasanen, L. and M. L. Tuomi (1992). "Diagnostic value of the lymphocyte proliferation test in nickel contact allergy and provocation in occupational coin dermatitis." Contact Dermatitis 27(4): 250-4.
Reilkoff, R. A., R. Bucala, et al. (2011). "Fibrocytes: emerging effector cells in chronic inflammation." Nat Rev Immunol 11(6): 427-35.
Ren, P. G., Z. Huang, et al. (2010). "Surveillance of systemic trafficking of macrophages induced by UHMWPE particles in nude mice by noninvasive imaging." J Biomed Mater Res A 94(3): 706-11.
Ren, P. G., A. Irani, et al. (2011). "Continuous infusion of UHMWPE particles induces increased bone macrophages and osteolysis." Clin Orthop Relat Res 469(1): 113-22.
Roder, C., B. Bach, et al. (2010). "Obesity, age, sex, diagnosis, and fixation mode differently affect early cup failure in total hip arthroplasty: a matched case-control study of 4420 patients." J Bone Joint Surg Am 92(10): 1954-63.
Rozkydal, Z., P. Janicek, et al. (2005). "Total hip replacement with the CLS expansion shell and a structural femoral head autograft for patients with congenital hip disease." J Bone Joint Surg Am 87(4): 801-7.
Santavirta, S., Takagi, M., Gomez-Barrena, E., Nevalainen, J., Lassus, M., Salo, J., Konttinen, Y.T. (1999). "Studies of host response to orthopedic implants and biomaterials." J Long Term Eff Med Implants 9: 67-76.
Schmalzried, T. P., E. F. Shepherd, et al. (2000). "The John Charnley Award. Wear is a function of use, not time." Clin Orthop Relat Res(381): 36-46.
Schmalzried, T. P., E. S. Szuszczewicz, et al. (1998). "Quantitative assessment of walking activity after total hip or knee replacement." J Bone Joint Surg Am 80(1): 54-9.
Sierra, J. M., S. Garcia, et al. (2011). "Relationship between the degree of osteolysis and cultures obtained by sonication of the prostheses in patients with aseptic loosening of a hip or knee arthroplasty." Arch Orthop Trauma Surg. Epub ahead of print May 11.

Sochart, D. H. and M. L. Porter (1997). "The long-term results of Charnley low-friction arthroplasty in young patients who have congenital dislocation, degenerative osteoarthrosis, or rheumatoid arthritis." J Bone Joint Surg Am 79(11): 1599-617.

St Pierre, C. A., M. Chan, et al. (2010). "Periprosthetic osteolysis: characterizing the innate immune response to titanium wear-particles." J Orthop Res 28(11): 1418-24.

Stanley, K. T., C. VanDort, et al. (2006). "Immunocompetent properties of human osteoblasts: interactions with T lymphocytes." J Bone Miner Res 21(1): 29-36.

Summer, B., C. Paul, et al. (2010). "Nickel (Ni) allergic patients with complications to Ni containing joint replacement show preferential IL-17 type reactivity to Ni." Contact Dermatitis 63(1): 15-22.

Sun, D. H., M. C. Trindade, et al. (2003). "Human serum opsonization of orthopedic biomaterial particles: protein-binding and monocyte/macrophage activation in vitro." J Biomed Mater Res A 65(2): 290-8.

Takagi, M., S. Santavirta, et al. (2001). "High-turnover periprosthetic bone remodeling and immature bone formation around loose cemented total hip joints." J Bone Miner Res 16(1): 79-88.

Takagi, M., Y. Tamaki, et al. (2007). "Toll-like receptors in the interface membrane around loosening total hip replacement implants." J Biomed Mater Res A 81(4): 1017-26.

Takahashi, N., B. R. MacDonald, et al. (1986). "Recombinant human transforming growth factor-alpha stimulates the formation of osteoclast-like cells in long-term human marrow cultures." J Clin Invest 78(4): 894-8.

Taki, N., J. M. Tatro, et al. (2007). "Comparison of the roles of IL-1, IL-6, and TNFalpha in cell culture and murine models of aseptic loosening." Bone 40(5): 1276-83.

Tamaki, Y., Y. Takakubo, et al. (2009). "Increased expression of toll-like receptors in aseptic loose periprosthetic tissues and septic synovial membranes around total hip implants." J Rheumatol 36(3): 598-608.

Tarala, M., D. Janssen, et al. (2011). "Balancing incompatible endoprosthetic design goals: a combined ingrowth and bone remodeling simulation." Med Eng Phys 33(3): 374-80.

Theill, L. E., W. J. Boyle, et al. (2002). "RANK-L and RANK: T cells, bone loss, and mammalian evolution." Annu Rev Immunol 20: 795-823.

Thillemann, T. M., A. B. Pedersen, et al. (2008). "Implant survival after primary total hip arthroplasty due to childhood hip disorders: results from the Danish Hip Arthroplasty Registry." Acta Orthop 79(6): 769-76.

Thillemann, T. M., A. B. Pedersen, et al. (2010a). "Postoperative use of bisphosphonates and risk of revision after primary total hip arthroplasty: a nationwide population-based study." Bone 46(4): 946-51.

Thillemann, T. M., A. B. Pedersen, et al. (2010b). "The risk of revision after primary total hip arthroplasty among statin users: a nationwide population-based nested case-control study." J Bone Joint Surg Am 92(5): 1063-72.

Thyssen, J. P., A. Linneberg, et al. (2007). "The epidemiology of contact allergy in the general population--prevalence and main findings." Contact Dermatitis 57(5): 287-99.

Thyssen, J. P. and T. Menne (2010). "Metal allergy--a review on exposures, penetration, genetics, prevalence, and clinical implications." Chem Res Toxicol 23(2): 309-18.

Thyssen, J. P., T. Menne, et al. (2011a). "Pragmatic approach to the clinical work-up of patients with putative allergic disease to metallic orthopaedic implants before and after surgery." Br J Dermatol 164(3): 473-8.

Thyssen, J. P., W. Uter, et al. (2011b). "The EU Nickel Directive revisited--future steps towards better protection against nickel allergy." Contact Dermatitis 64(3): 121-5.

Tuan, R. S., F. Y. Lee, et al. (2008). "What are the local and systemic biologic reactions and mediators to wear debris, and what host factors determine or modulate the biologic response to wear particles?" J Am Acad Orthop Surg 16 Suppl 1: S42-8.

Ulrich-Vinther, M., E. E. Carmody, et al. (2002). "Recombinant adeno-associated virus-mediated osteoprotegerin gene therapy inhibits wear debris-induced osteolysis." J Bone Joint Surg Am 84-A(8): 1405-12.

Ulrich, S. D., T. M. Seyler, et al. (2008). "Total hip arthroplasties: What are the reasons for revision?" Int Orthop 32(5): 597-604.

Uter, W. J., J. Geier, et al. (1996). "Good clinical practice in patch testing: readings beyond day 2 are necessary: a confirmatory analysis. Members of the Information Network of Departments of Dermatology." Am J Contact Dermat 7(4): 231-7.

Valledor, A. F., M. Comalada, et al. (2010). "Macrophage proinflammatory activation and deactivation: a question of balance." Adv Immunol 108: 1-20.

Vermes, C., R. Chandrasekaran, et al. (2001). "The effects of particulate wear debris, cytokines, and growth factors on the functions of MG-63 osteoblasts." J Bone Joint Surg Am 83-A(2): 201-11.

Vocanson, M., A. Hennino, et al. (2009). "Effector and regulatory mechanisms in allergic contact dermatitis." Allergy 64(12): 1699-714.

Wahlberg, J. E., Lindberg, M. (2006). Patch test. Contact Dermatitis. P. J. Frosch, Menne, T., Lepoittevin, J-P. Berlin, Springer.

Watters, T. S., D. M. Cardona, et al. (2010). "Aseptic lymphocyte-dominated vasculitis-associated lesion: a clinicopathologic review of an underrecognized cause of prosthetic failure." Am J Clin Pathol 134(6): 886-93.

Weyand, C. M., A. Geisler, et al. (1998). "Oligoclonal T-cell proliferation and interferon-gamma production in periprosthetic inflammation." Lab Invest 78(6): 677-85.

Whyte, C. S., E. T. Bishop, et al. (2011). "Suppressor of cytokine signaling (SOCS)1 is a key determinant of differential macrophage activation and function." J Leukoc Biol. Epub ahead of print May 31.

Wilkinson, D. S., S. Fregert, et al. (1970). "Terminology of contact dermatitis." Acta Derm Venereol 50(4): 287-92.

Wilkinson, J. M., A. G. Wilson, et al. (2003). "Variation in the TNF gene promoter and risk of osteolysis after total hip arthroplasty." J Bone Miner Res 18(11): 1995-2001.

Willert, H. G., J. Ludwig, et al. (1974). "Reaction of bone to methacrylate after hip arthroplasty: a long-term gross, light microscopic, and scanning electron microscopic study." J Bone Joint Surg Am 56(7): 1368-82.

Willert, H. G. and M. Semlitsch (1977). "Reactions of the articular capsule to wear products of artificial joint prostheses." J Biomed Mater Res 11(2): 157-64.

Wilson, M. J. and R. N. Villar (2011). "Hip replacement in the athlete: is there a role?" Knee Surg Sports Traumatol Arthrosc 19(9): 1524-30.

Zolotarevova, E., G. Entlicher, et al. (2010). "Distribution of polyethylene wear particles and bone fragments in periprosthetic tissue around total hip joint replacements." Acta Biomater 6(9): 3595-600.

17

Current Possibilities for Detection of Loosening of Total Hip Replacements and How Intelligent Implants Could Improve Diagnostic Accuracy

Cathérine Ruther et al.*
Department of Orthopaedics, University of Rostock
Germany

1. Introduction

Where pain is experienced following a total hip replacement (THR), there needs to be clarification as to whether the cause is due to an infected or mechanically loose THR. The major complication after implantation of a THR is aseptic loosening, caused by stress shielding and wear-particle induced osteolysis with an incidence of 75 % (Malchau et al., 2002). A further prevalent reason for implant loosening is a sepsis due to infection of the periprosthetic membrane.

The optimal management in case of hip pain is an often discussed controversy. Currently, several diagnostic methods are used to identify the loosening status of the THR and to establish a basis for revision management. All these techniques are based on imaging methods. An overview of the main imaging methods used is given in figure 1. Although the devices and technology are highly developed, a 100 % diagnostic accuracy is not available (Temmerman et al., 2005). Plain radiographs are mainly used to identify the loosening status of a THR and most decisions on how to treat disorders after THR can be made (Ostlere & Soin, 2003). The time period between e.g. the onset of an infection and the possibility to identify any changes within the THR can be very long (Itasaka et al., 2001). Hence, in early loosening diagnosis, identifying radiolucent lines or increased uptake in radionuclide scanning can be very complex owing to the difficulty with excluding loosening (Love et al., 2001; Udomkiat et al., 2001). Therefore, surgeons cannot verify the actual loosening status accurately until the point of surgical intervention. Thus, the surgeon carries the risk of revising a sufficiently integrated THR. A major clinical problem in diagnosing loosening of a THR is to identify the moment where revision surgery is required. Loosening of THR should be diagnosed precisely and early in order to avoid massive osteolysis of the femur.

---

* Ulrich Timm[2], Hartmut Ewald[2], Wolfram Mittelmeier[1], Rainer Bader[1], Rico Schmelter[3], Armin Lohrengel[3] and Daniel Kluess[1]
[1]*Department of Orthopaedics, University of Rostock, Germany*
[2]*Department of General Electrics, University of Rostock, Germany*
[3]*Institute of Mechanical Engineering, University of Technology Clausthal-Zellerfeld, Germany*

In this article, a review of diagnostic possibilities to detect the loosening status of a THR is given. In general, diagnostic methods can be divided into imaging and implant integrated sensors (Fig. 1). The most important research activities were conducted in the field of vibrometry with the use of accelerometers (Marschner et al., 2009). Moreover, new research topics which link sensors to THR are described. Finally, we propose a new excitation method for detection of total hip stem loosening using vibrometry.

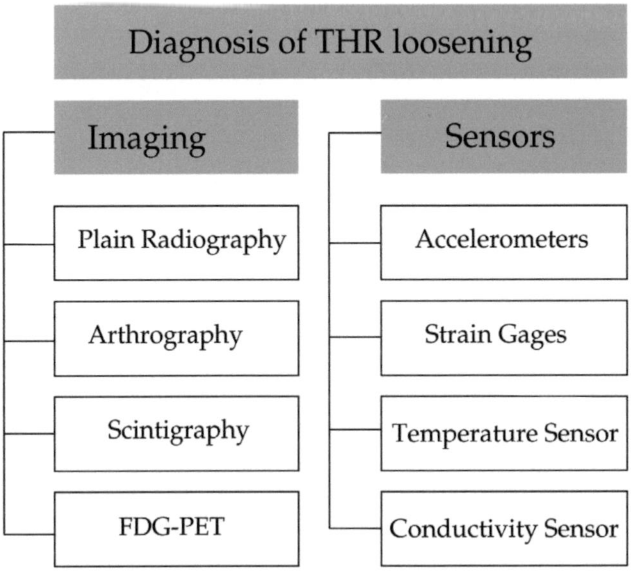

Fig. 1. Overview of the modalities which can be used to diagnose loosening of the THR

2. Conventional diagnostic investigation of disorders after THR

2.1 Plain radiography

Plain radiography is an imaging modality, which is less cost-intensive than other imaging techniques and therefore the first method used to determine the osseointegration of a THR (Nilsson et al., 1994). Diagnosis of THR loosening typically requires a plain radiograph - in the optimal case it can be compared with an immediate post operative radiograph - and clinical symptomatic like hip pain. In order to achieve an accurate interpretation of the radiography, the observer needs adequate clinical expertise regarding the surgical techniques applied in THR (Cuckler, 2010). Two different views are usually taken into account: the anteroposterior view of the hip and pelvis and the lateral view (supine position) to investigate the affected femoral stem (Temmerman et al., 2005).
The radiographic criteria vary between the type and operative technique of the THR (Ostlere & Soin, 2003). Different radiographic criteria for the identification of loosening were reported (DeLee & Charnley, 1976; Dihlmann et al., 1991; Gruen et al., 1979, Johnston et al., 1990). The appearance of radiolucent lines around the endoprosthetic components as distinctive periprosthetic membrane is one criteria (Paterson et al. 1986), when the width of the radiolucency is more than 2 mm (Fig. 2) (Böhler et al. 1994).

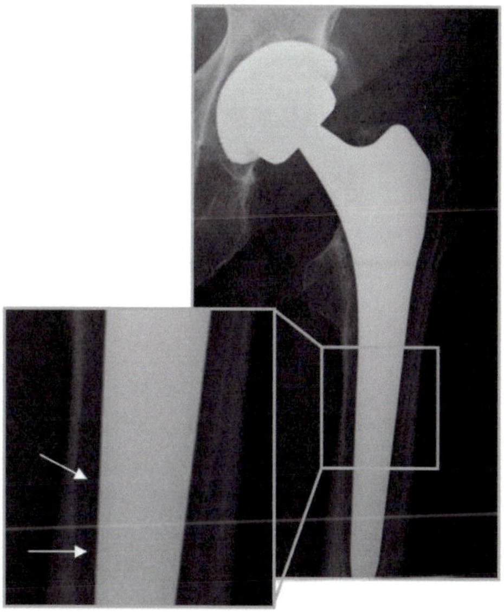

Fig. 2. Radiograph of an uncemented THR with a clearly visible radiolucent line at the interface of the femoral component

Cemented components can be identified by radiolucency between bone and cement (Sarmiento et al., 1990), while in the uncemented case, radiolucent lines occur between the implant and bone. However, some radiolucency can be observed e.g. in the proximal part of the uncemented Zweymueller design hip stem, though the THR is well osseointegrated (Suckel et al., 2009). This example impedes a precise interpretation of the THR with plain radiographs, because these findings can be associated with loose as well as well fixed THR. The ambiguity in diagnosing loosening can be compensated by comparing the current radiograph with a previous post-operative reference (Wroblewski, 1991). Additional radiographic criteria refer to the tilt of any component. Another feature indicating impeding failure in both cemented and uncemented prostheses is focal osteolysis, due to the particle response of the tissue. Osteolysis is usually seen as decrease of osseointegration at the femoral site or bone destruction beneath the acetabular component (Keogh et al., 2003). Migration of the THR, particularly the femoral component, is the most significant and certain criteria to differentiate between a loosened and a fixed implant. If the location of the implant in the bone stock determined in the radiographs has changed over a distance of more than 4 mm in the postoperative follow-up the implant can be identified as loosened.
Plain radiography is the imaging of choice to assess osseointegration of THRs since in the standard clinical follow-up this is mainly the only imaging required (Ostlere & Soin, 2003). Radiography has been consistently reported to be an accurate technique to assess cemented and uncemented THR loosening. However, in some cases, especially in the observation of infectious THR other methods like e.g. scintigraphy have to be adducted since differentiation between aseptic and septic loosening using radiographs may not be possible. Many studies evaluating the sensitivity and specificity of radiographs in diagnosing loosening of the THR have been published (Fig. 3). Despite radiography and radiographic criteria being highly developed, an accuracy of 100 % in diagnosing loosening can not yet be achieved (Miniaci et al., 1990; Ovesen et al., 2003; Pfahler et al., 1998).

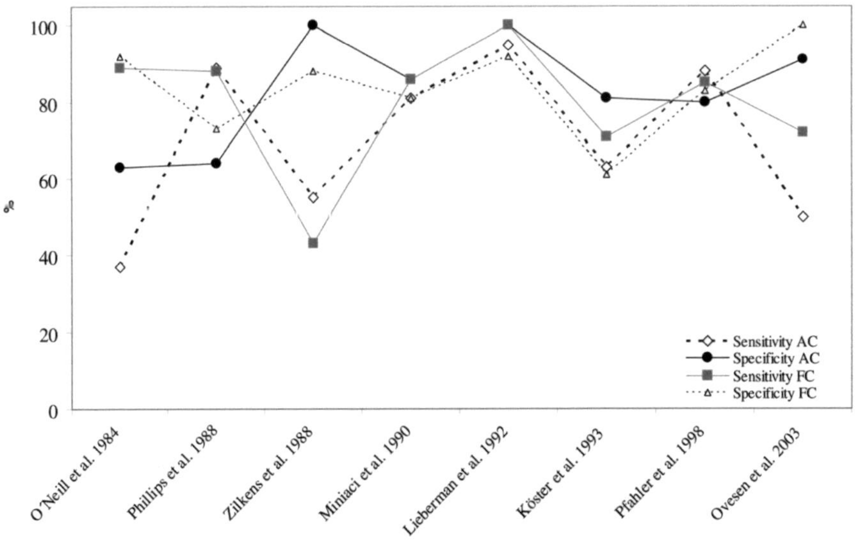

Fig. 3. Literature comparison of selected results determining sensitivity and specificity of loosening diagnosis of the femoral component (FC) and the acetabular component (AC) using plain radiography

The highest accuracy in diagnosing loosening of femoral (98 %) and acetabular components (97 %) was documented by Lieberman et al. (Lieberman et al., 1993). These data show the lowest accuracy of 76 % for femoral components (Köster et al., 1993) and 66 % for acetabular components (Ovesen et al., 2003) and demonstrate that the loosening status of the THR cannot be verified precisely (Lyons et al., 1985). In this context it is important to mention that not every author differentiates between investigating the acetabular and the femoral component (Gelman et al., 1976; Barentsz et al., 1986; Tehranzadeh et al., 1981).

2.2 Arthrography

Arthrography is an imaging method which is mainly used in addition to plain radiography in case of unresolved pain of the artificial joint (Newberg & Wetzner 1985). Contrast agents are injected into the joint for the visualization of the periprosthetic membrane around the THR and the cement-bone interface, in order to increase the accuracy and therefore specificity and sensitivity in loosening diagnosis (Hendrix et al. 1983). Several methods to perform arthrography of the hip joint are applied: Conventional arthrography is performed using x-ray examination under fluoroscopic guidance, in which anterolateral puncture of the hip joint is often applied (Hendrix et al., 1983). Anteroposterior and lateral views are normally the views which are obtained during the examination of the THR. Additionally, arthrography can be executed by using magnetic resonance imaging (MRI) or computed tomography (CT).

Arthrographic criteria for loosening are based on the infiltration of the injected contrast agents into the periprosthetic membrane or into the cement-bone interface (Ovesen et al., 2003) (Fig. 4). The THR and the contrast medium have similar radiographic densities. For that reason, the small width of the periprosthetic membrane cannot be clearly visualized by conventional arthrography. Therefore, digital subtraction arthrography (DSA) has been introduced, in which subtracted images can be made during injection of the contrast agents. Joint motion can reduce the resolution of the arthrogram and for this reason a pixel shift is applied to reduce motion artefacts (Apple et al., 1986; Ginai et al., 1996).

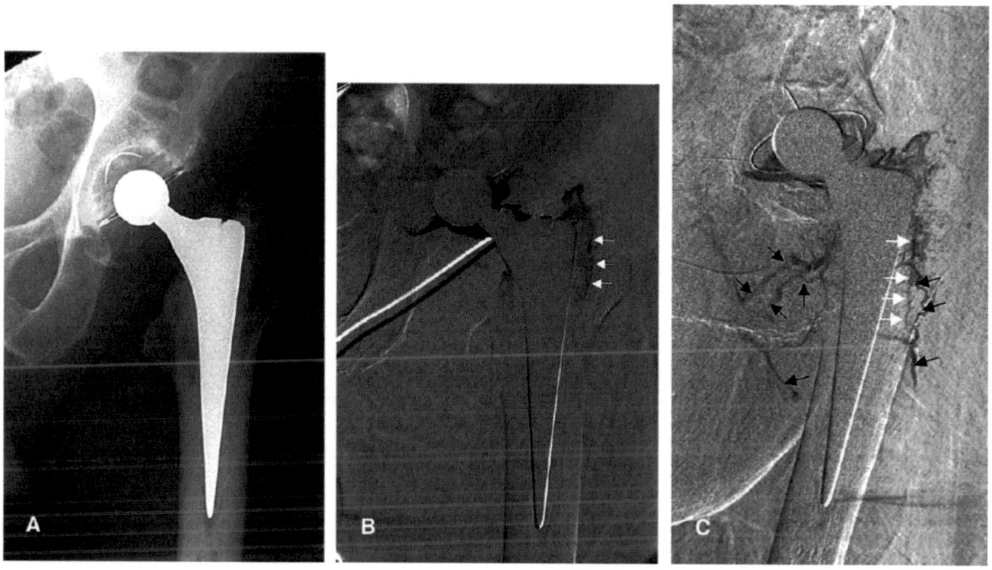

Fig. 4. (A) Cemented painful total hip arthroplasty in 60-year-old man with no signs of loosening on plain radiographs. The patient also had a history of spinal stenosis. (B) interoposterior and (C) 45° oblique DSA clearly show a thin contrast leakage at the bone-cement interface in zones 1 and 2. White arrow indicates contrast in the interface; black arrow indicates filling of the lymphatic system. At repeat surgery, loosening of the femoral component was confirmed (Ovesen et al. 2003)

Increasing the injected amount of contrast media into the hip joint can be helpful to improve the expressiveness of the achieved arthrogram (Palestro, 2003). One arthrographic criterion for loosening is the contrast leakage in the interface distal to the intertrochanteric line (Ovesen et al., 2003). For the acetabular component, contrast leakage in three zones around the implant has to be considered (DeLee & Charnley, 1976).

Digital subtraction techniques can be used to increase the sensitivity. Temmerman et al. found an increased sensitivity of 15 % compared to conventional nuclear arthrography for the examination of the acetabular component (Temmerman et al., 2004). In contrast to this optimization, arthrography is identified to be non specific for the acetabular component (Köster et al., 1993). This result is based on the overall sensitivity of nuclear arthrography for acetabular components, which was determined to 57 %, whereas the value of specificity lies at 67 % (Temmerman et al., 2005). However, there is a discrepancy of the benefit of arthrography. Several researchers present the arthrogram as the only picture revealing contrast leakage and therefore loosening of the THR (Hardy et al., 1988; O`Neill & Harris, 1986). Other studies conclude that the selection of patients for revision was influenced by the results of the arthrography (Phillips & Kattapuram, 1982). Ovesen et al. reported a sensitivity and specificity for the femoral component of 93 % and 92 % respectively (Ovesen et al. 2003). They concluded that digital subtraction arthrography is a useful technique for further diagnosis of loosened THR (Fig. 5). The minimum sensitivity of nuclear arthrography was found by Miniaci et al. (Miniaci et al., 1990), whereas the minimum specificity of nuclear arthrography was determined to be 75 % (Herzwurm et al. 1991). Studies using arthrography often do not discriminate between cemented or uncemented components (Maus et al., 1987). The mentioned results are summarized in Fig. 5.

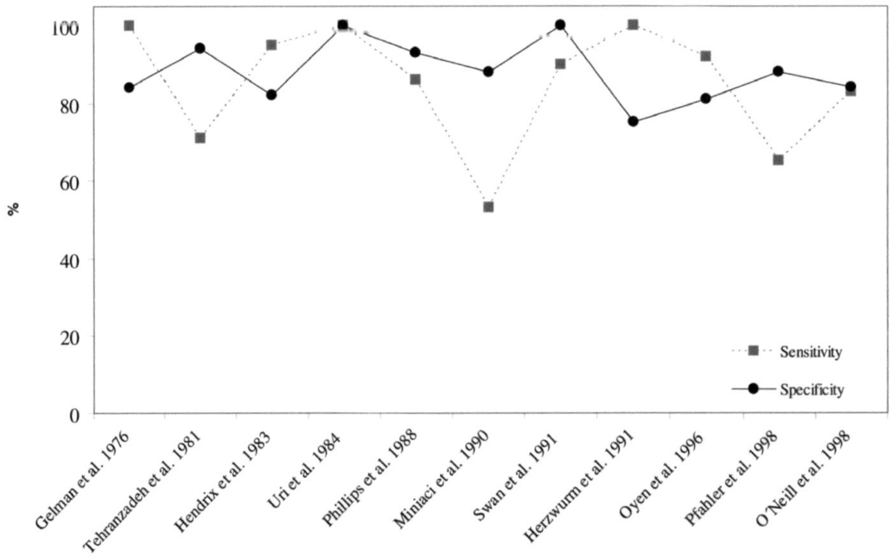

Fig. 5. Literature comparison of the results determining sensitivity and specificity of loosening diagnosis of the femoral component of the THR using nuclear arthrography

Temmermann et al. evaluated the mean sensitivity/specificity of several studies with nuclear arthrography (85 %/83 %) and subtraction arthrography (86 %/85 %) (Temmerman et al., 2005). Hence, these results show only a 4 % higher sensitivity/specificity than plain radiographs. For this reason arthrography does not add a significant benefit to the plain radiography results for the THR. Arthrography gets more and more abandoned, because of the risk of infection and the absent additional benefit, in case of aseptic loosening.

2.3 Scintigraphy

Examination of an infected THR can be performed by using scintigraphy, which is often combined with white blood cell imaging (Larikka et al., 2001). Scintigraphy uses radioisotopes as body radiation source by producing a two-dimensional picture using a gamma-camera for the detection of the radiation (Katz et al., 1986; Zilkens et al. 1988) (Fig. 6). Usually, a two-phase or triple-phase bone scan is generated (Segura et al., 2004). The triple-phase bone scan is an enhancement with a reputation of high sensitivity (Reinartz 2009) and uses gallium scans to improve its specificity (Kraemer et al., 1993). However the data in the literature about its diagnostic efficiency show a considerable variability. This inconsistency is caused by the use of highly differing scan interpretation criteria.
Scintigraphic criteria are based on the suggestion of Wilson et al. (Wilson et al., 1997). Mechanical loosening of the femoral component should show a significant pathological uptake of radioisotopes in the distal part of the THR at the tip and increased periprosthetic

uptake. A second substantial lesion in the region of the lesser trochanter is a further sign for loosening and supports the first presumption.

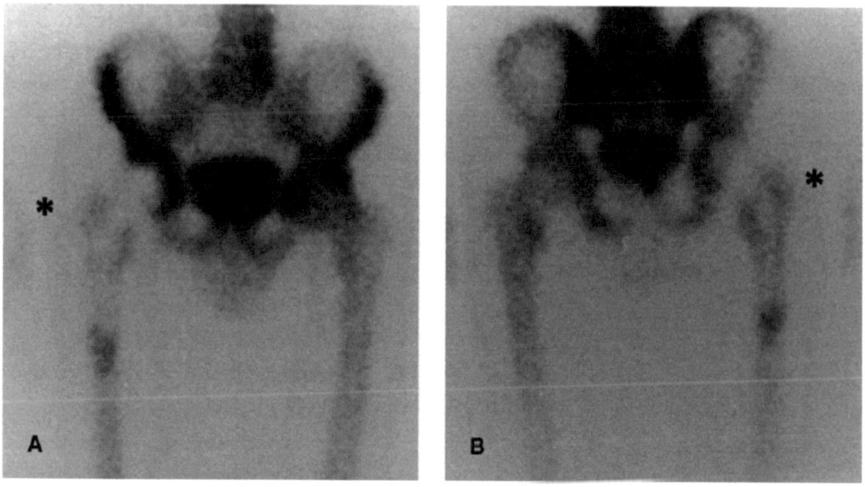

Fig. 6. 99mTc bone scan with normal anterior and posterior image of the prosthesis, without signs of loosening or infection (Kisielinski et al., 2003)

A continuous pathological uptake at the cup-bone-interface is a sign of loosening of the acetabular component. Finally, for diagnosing infection the blood pool images need to show a substantial lesion in the region of the lesser trochanter. A loosening of the acetabular cup is diagnosed in cases with a continuous pathological uptake in the cup-bone interface. In the case that a pathological uptake around the THR can be found in the additional blood pool

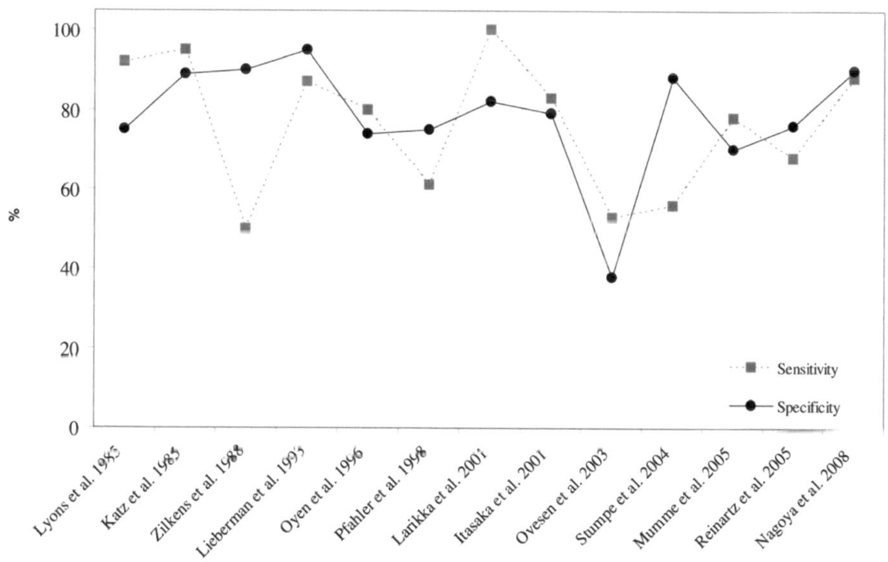

Fig. 7. Literature comparison of the results determining sensitivity and specificity of loosening diagnosis of THR using bone scintigraphy

image the diagnosis of infection and septic loosening is positive. Due to a normal bone scan, the existence of a sepsis can be excluded and an additional white blood cell imaging should be taken into account.
Mean sensitivity and specificity of scintigraphy are at 85 % and 72 % (Temmermann et al. 2005) (Fig. 7). Reinartz found a mean sensitivity/specificity of 78 % /84 % for diagnosing THR loosening with triple-phase bone scans (Reinartz 2009). It was also concluded, that bone scans of THR's are highly sensitive but not specific (Segura et al., 2004). The lowest sensitivity was found by Zilkens et al. with a value of 50 % (Zilkens et al., 1988), while the lowest specificity was 38 %(Ovesen et al., 2003).

2.4 FDG-PET

Based on the principle of scintigraphy, fluorodeoxyglucose-positron emission tomography (FDG-PET) uses radionuclides (FDG) which visualize the transport and metabolic rate of

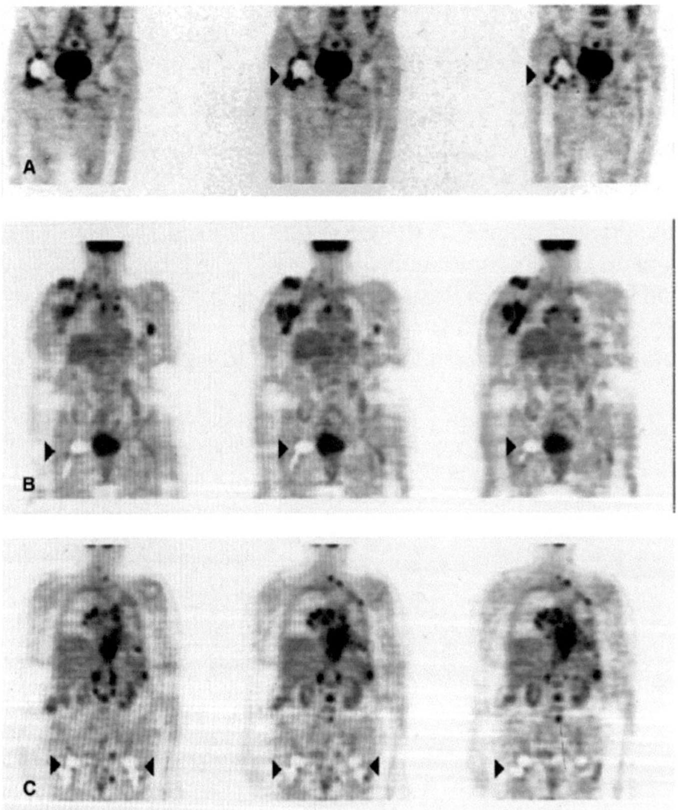

Fig. 8. (A) 18F-FDG-PET coronary slices 7 mm thick showing right-sided artificial hip joint in the patient. Increased glucose metabolism particularly around prosthesis neck and polyethylene inlay (arrowheads) is seen. (B) 18FFDG-PET of a patient with a clinically inconspicuous right-sided hip prosthesis without suggestive signs concerning the implant. (C) 18F- DGPET showing bilateral hip joint implants of a patient without any clinical discomforts of the hips. There are no signs of enhanced glucose consumption in the joint capsules as well as around both prostheses (Kisielinski et al., 2003)

glucose by emitting positrons for the generation of cross-sections (Fig. 8). FDG-PET is one of the most expensive imaging modalities and has already been documented to be a precise method to diagnose infection particularly (Chryssikos et al., 2008). Active cells like leukocytes and macrophages show a higher energy demand compared to other cells and therefore preferred ingest the FDG (Reinartz, 2009). Due to this fact, infected tissue with a high number of active cells revealed an increased uptake of FDG, which leads to a positive finding in the PET scan (Stumpe & Strobel, 2006). Furthermore, higher FDG uptake in patients with aseptic loosening of the THR can be explained by wear debris and the development of granulomatous tissue in the periprosthetic membrane around the THR (DeHeer et al., 2001; Kadoya et al., 1998).
The criteria for the interpretation of a PET scan differ between different studies (Reinartz et al., 2005). In the area of the femoral component an increased uptake of FDG can be interpreted as loosening or infection, while an increased uptake at the femoral head and neck cannot be determined as loosening or unspecific (Zhuang et al., 2007). In contrast the increased uptake of FDG at the distal tip of the stem is unspecific. Furthermore, a high uptake at the implant-bone interface of the acetabular component can be identified as a pathologic process or a sign of loosening (Mayer-Wagner et al., 2009).
Based on the great variety of interpretation criteria to analyse PET scans, sensitivities of PET to implant loosening differ from 33 % (Stumpe et al., 2004) to 100 % (Zhuang et al., 2002), while specificity varies from 78 % (Vanquickenborne et al., 2003) to 100 % (Zhuang et al., 2002) with an average of 85 %/90 % and an accuracy of 89 % (Reinartz, 2009) (Fig. 9).

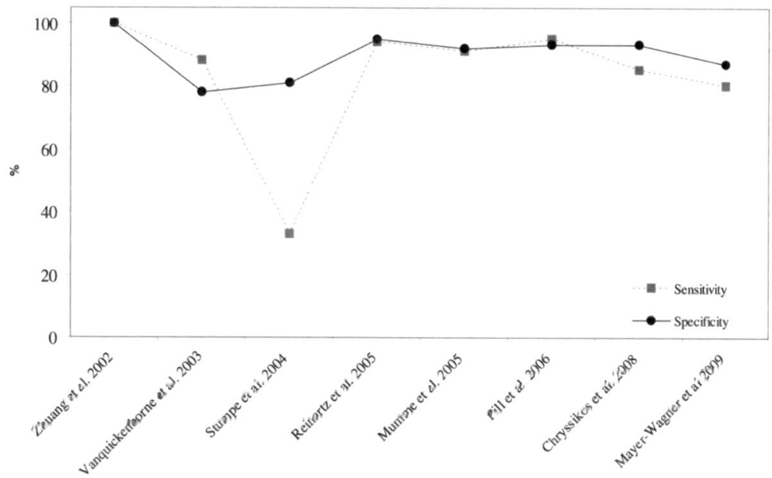

Fig. 9. Literature comparison of the results determining sensitivity and specificity of loosening diagnosis of THR using FDG-PET

2.5 Summary of actual loosening diagnostics using imaging techniques

Figure 10 shows the comparison of the mean sensitivities and specificities of the presented imaging methods to diagnose loosening of the THR. FDG-PET has both, the highest sensitivity and specificity and therefore is the most accurate method to diagnose loosening exactly. Although the high accuracy, FDG-PET is highly cost-intensive, for that reason it has not reached the status of a standard examination.

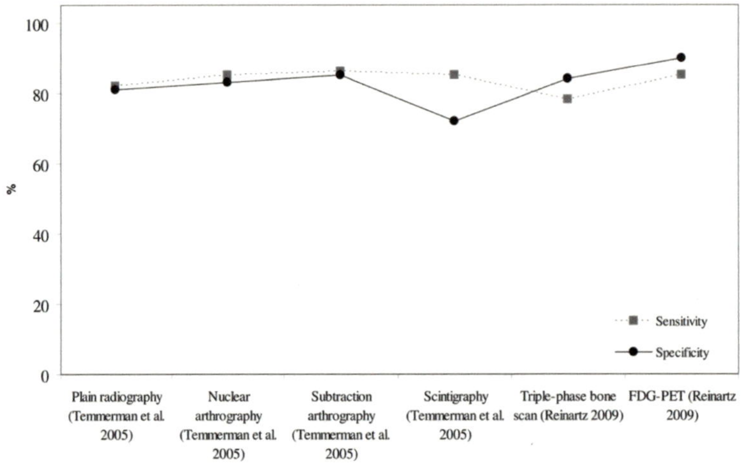

Fig. 10. Comparison of different diagnostic imaging methods with regard to sensitivity and specificity of loosening diagnosis of the femoral component of THRs

These results prove that, considering the background of up to one million total hip replacements conducted worldwide every year, an advanced method for diagnosing implant loosening is needed. Intelligent implants with integrated sensors have the potential to revolve the diagnostic methods to raise sensitivity and specificity of loosening diagnostics to a higher level.

3. New diagnostic techniques under research – intelligent implants

3.1 Sensors for characterization of the implant-bone interface

Intelligent implants are highly complex systems incorporating sensors, actuators and signal procession and have potential for advanced therapy or diagnosis. A main issue of intelligent implants is miniaturization. Smaller implants and sensors have lower area of influence to their ambient environment. Referring to the femoral component of THRs, it could be equipped with small batteries and a wireless signal transmission and power consumption. Common sensors exhibit at least one sensing unit, a processing unit, a transceiver unit and an energy unit. In the field of microsystems some diagnostic systems reached the status of implantable passive and telemetric prototypes (Bergmann et al., 2001, Marschner et al., 2009). Most notably the application of strain gages used in fracture healing implants are the system of the highest development status compared to other orthopaedic and trauma implants (Wilson et al., 2009). In case of THR, sensors are subject to stringent clinical requirements, like gamma sterilization, which may affect the functionality of the sensors inside the implant. Other requirements are the stability of the sensor and the electronic equipment during impaction of the THR and at least the same lifetime than the THR has. There are different working principles to realize a sensor, which can be used to characterize the implant-bone interface to detect loosening of the THR (Fig. 11).

The preferred detected properties, which were mainly considered, are the acoustical in combination with mechanical properties. The detection of micromotion with an in vivo sensor unit at the distal femoral component was proposed by Hao et al. (Hao et al., 2010). The differential variable reluctance transducer is mounted in the bone cavity and has no direct contact with the THR. The resistance inductance bridge based technique enables small axial displacements of a rod to be measured about a pre-determined zero reference point. Detection of acoustical properties includes measuring of the resonance frequency which correlates with the stiffness of the implant-bone interface (Li et al., 1996). Resonance frequency and dampening are the most frequently measured properties and reached the highest development status compared to other detection methods using in vivo sensors. This method is called vibrometry. Measuring the biological properties e.g. the temperature at the border of the implant, can only be used in cases of infection and is even more a parameter for additional reference measurements.

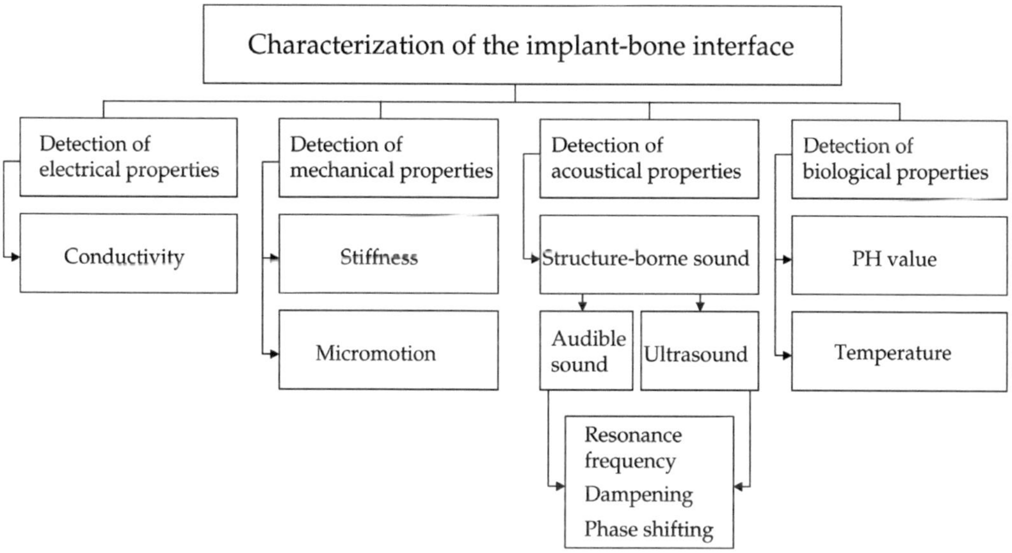

Fig. 11. Overview of the possible parameters which can be detected in order to identify the status of loosening of the THR

3.2 Vibrometry

Diagnostic investigation involving measuring the resonance frequencies of implants has its roots in the field of dentistry (Glauser et al., 2003; Huang et al., 2003). This field of research extended to determining the primary stability of THR during surgery (Lannocca et al., 2007). The eigenfrequency present the governing nature of the vibration motion of a structure. A disturbed structure vibrates in a way that is determined by the structures mass, cross sections, geometric relationships in its assembly, Young's modulus of its components and dampening factors.

The THR integrated in the femoral bone can be described as a system which vibrates in its multiple axial, lateral, and torsional eigenmodes after excitation (Qi et al., 2003). These eigenmodes change with the loosening state and the localization of loosening of the THR. Different eigenmodes are associated with the corresponding eigenfrequency. The changing of the eigenfrequencies of the THR-femur-system due to the loosening state can be measured as vibrations or structure-borne sound in a resonance frequency analysis. By means of a finite-element analysis, Qi et al. determined which minimal sensitivity of an in vivo accelerometer is required in order to detect differences in eigenfrequencies. Therefore, they considered three different situations: distal loosening, proximal loosening and central loosening. Because soft tissue dampening and connections to the upper/ lower joints will absorb acoustic energy, sensitivity of the sensors may have to be higher to acquire the signals for further processing. On the other hand, high sensitivity sensors have a greater chance to be affected by various noises.

A milestone in the linking of sensors to THR was reached by Rosenstein (Rosenstein et al. 1989), who introduced analysis of resonance frequencies involving an accelerometer. By inducing a sinusoidal signal at the femoral condyles with an electrodynamic shaker, the implant bone interface was excited. The shaker was placed perpendicular to the femur in order to induce bending eigenmodes of the THR-femur-system. Bending modes have the maximum influence on the sound emission into the adjacent soft tissue. The accelerometer is placed at the major trochanter for detection of the resulting vibrations. Applying this technology, Li et al. suggest that a well fixed THR behaves linear, while a loosened THR shows a non-linear acoustic behaviour (Li et al., 1996). In general, the signal amplitude decreases as the interface failure increases due to the decreasing structural stiffness of the implant-bone-compound (Qi et al., 2003).

Puers et al. instrumented the THR with a miniaturized accelerometer placed in the ball-head of the THR. They were the first research group who developed an implantable telemetry unit for the monitoring of the vibration output signal (Puers et al., 1999) (Fig. 12). In cadaver experiments they chose an excitation frequency between 100-200 Hz, which has to be considered critical in view of the findings, that the sensitive frequency band begins at 1.5 kHz (Qi et al., 2003). Further performances of the cadaver experiments are not described.

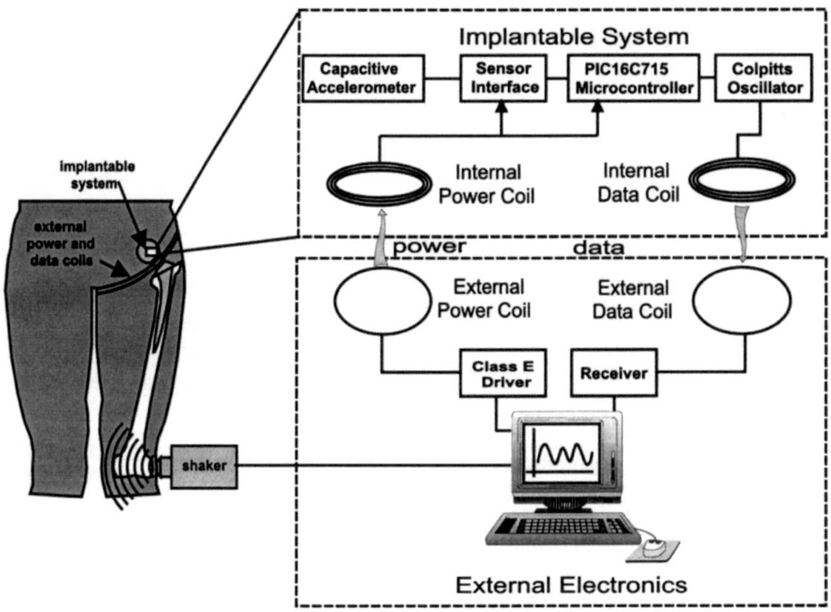

Fig. 12. Total system for the detection of hip prosthesis loosening

One problem of the vibration analysis with in vivo accelerometer was the low signal-to-noise ratio of available accelerometers. In a further study this principle was continued by Marschner et al. (Marschner et al., 2010). Wireless lock-in measurement was introduced and the THR was instrumented with a coil, amplifier, microcontroller and telemetry unit in the distal end of the hip stem. The lock-in amplifier separates the measurement signal from noise.

The availability of results which compare different loosening states of the THR and therefore sensitivity of the proposed sensor systems is rare. Indeed, the presented devices are available, but only few results verify the possibility to detect a difference between a loose and a well fixed implant. Currently sensitivity and specificity of vibration analysis in THR can only be estimated. Georgiou et al. stated a 20 % higher sensitivity measured with vibration analysis (80 %) than with radiographs (60 %) (Georgiou et al., 2001). The finite element analysis of Qi et al. showed that a loose THR can be identified reliable if 1/3 of the femoral component has no direct bone contact (Qi et al., 2003). One of the main problems of the resonance frequency analysis of THR is the soft tissue damping of the output vibration signal. Furthermore, connection to the tibia and the pelvis can decrease the energy rate of the acoustic sound waves.

In another in vitro study the accelerometer was replaced by a blood flow ultrasound probe which enabled consistent detection of the vibrations for a loose and a fixed THR (Rowlands et al., 2008). The ultrasound probe lead to increased amplitudes of the output vibrations compared to the accelerometer signal. Dahl et al. applied ultrasound to detect osseous integration of the total ankle replacement (Dahl et al., 2010). The cadaveric testing demonstrated that the ultrasound technique could distinguish between loose and fixed implant components. In a further study, a trans-femoral implant was measured with accelerometers. It could be shown that the eigenfrequency increases with the weight bearing rehabilitation time (Shao et al., 2007).

Paech et al investigated the natural frequency of four different types of THR and determined these sound patterns in further cadaver tests with bovine and human bone (Paech et al., 2007). The excitation of the THR was reached by using an acoustically neutral steel ball of 120 g as activating impact for sound emission. However, this is not reproducible for application in clinical studies.

Besides problems in signal analysis and soft tissue dampening, functional sustainment of the integrated electronics during sterilization and impaction of the THR seems to be a significant challenge. Nevertheless detailed research into simulation of different loosening states and significant test results are expected. Furthermore the excitation has to be optimized in order to avoid pressure pain induced by the electrodynamic shaker (Georgiou et al., 2001).

3.3 A new excitation method to detect aseptic loosening

3.3.1 Principle of the novel excitation concept

In the proposed concept, an oscillator integrated in the THR is used. The oscillator consists of a magnetic body which is fixed on a flat steel spring (Ruther et al., 2010) (Fig 13). This oscillator is excited by a coil placed outside the patient. The oscillator impinges inside the THR and excites the THR to vibrate in its eigenfrequency. This can be considered as an alternative to the electrodynamic shaker, which was used by different research groups. The excitation in the implant bending modes leads to a sound emission to the surrounding bone and soft tissue. The sound waves can be detected by a vibration sensor, which is applied outside the patient's hip opposite to the excitation coil.

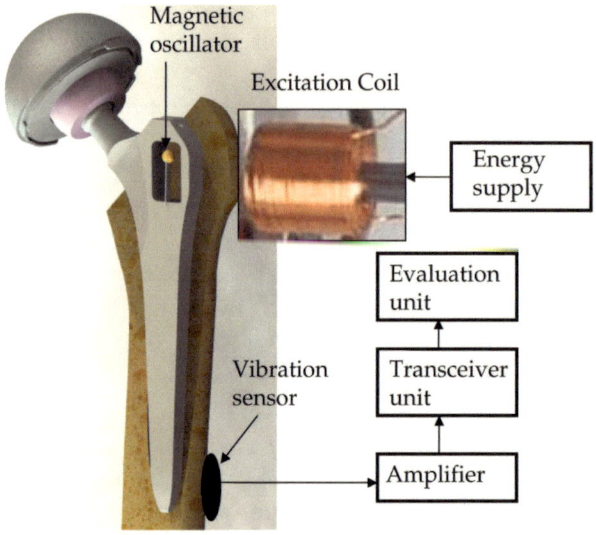

Fig. 13. Functional principle of the novel in vivo excitation method inside the femoral component of the THR

3.3.2 Material and methods

For testing of the new in vivo excitation principle a custom straight total hip stem with an integrated oscillator in the proximal part of the implant was used (Fig. 14). By embedding a femoral component of a present THR system (CBH Schaft Size 3, MATHYS European Orthopaedics AG, Bettlach, Switzerland) in epoxide resin with different embedding heights, the differences in resonance frequency were recorded. The experimental set up was placed in a water reservoir, which was the first simulation of soft tissue. This was performed according to the procedure of Paech et al. (Paech et al., 2007). The excitation was realized by a coil outside the water reservoir with a distance of 50 mm to the oscillator. The coil excited the oscillator in its first eigenfrequency of 70 Hz. A piezoelectric vibration sensor for broadband measurements between 1 and 24 kHz (Metra, Radebeul, Germany) with a high sensitivity of 100 mV/g was fixed outside the water reservoir to detect the transmitted oscillations.

In order to determine how the eigenfrequency changes with different embedding heights, we conducted a modal analysis using the finite-element method. Therefore, a model of the femoral component was constructed with a gap in the proximal part where the oscillator is placed. The FE-solver Abaqus V6.9 (Dassault Systémes, Simulia, Providence, RI, USA) was used to calculate the eigenfrequencies of the components with the given material data in table 1.

Material	Young's modulus (MPa)	Poisson ratio	Density (g/cm^3)
Ti6Al4V	114000	0.342	4.432

Table 1. Material properties of the straight CBH femoral component used in the numerical simulation

The material data of the components in terms of density, Young's modulus and Poisson ratio were collected from the manufacturer information. All components were modelled as linear-elastic materials.

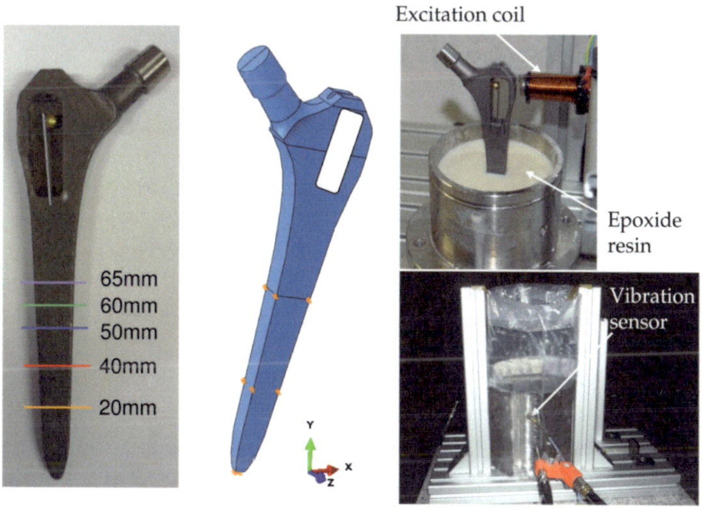

Fig. 14. Left: Prototype of a femoral component with the embedding heights tested in a cylindrical setup with epoxide resin. Middle: Model of the femoral component for finite-element analysis exemplarily with an embedded height of 65 mm. Right: Experimental setup with embedded hip stem and the applied water reservoir with external vibration sensor.

For post-mortem investigation of a porcine leg, a small cuboid-formed implant prototype was manufactured (Fig. 15). This implant may be applied for animal experiments in further studies.

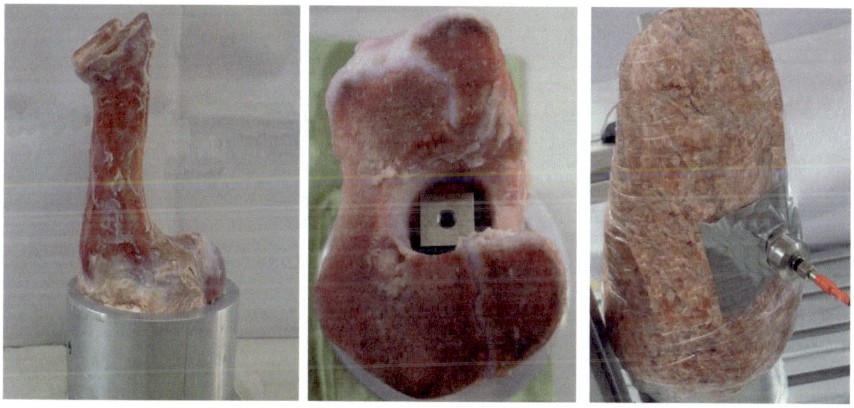

Fig. 15. Left: Porcine femur embedded within epoxide resin. Middle: Experimental prototype for the feasibility study in porcine bone, implanted in the femoral condyle. Right: Experimental setup with ground porcine muscle tissue around the porcine femur with the coupled accelerometer

In a first experimental in vitro set-up, the implant was inserted in the femoral condyles with press fit fixation. In order to simulate an advanced loosening the bore whole was reamed, filled with water and then the implant was reinserted. For simulation of soft tissue, ground porcine muscle tissue was arranged around the femur. The vibration sensor was placed perpendicular to the femur to detect bending eigenfrequencies.

3.3.3 Results and discussion

The results of the numerical modal analysis show that the higher the embedding height of the femoral component, the higher the eigenfrequency due to an increased system stiffness (Fig. 16). According to Qi et al., the highly sensitive frequency band is over 2.5 kHz due to higher differences between the eigenfrequencies (Qi et al., 2002).
Characteristic progressions of the structure borne sound are shown in figure 17 exemplarily in case of the 65 mm embedding height (well fixed THR) and the 20 mm embedding representative for a loose THR. The signal of the 65 mm embedded THR resulted in a higher dampening than the 20 mm embedded component simulating loosening. As a result the time in which the vibration signal achieved the complete deactivation of the excited state varies. The well fixed femoral component resulted in an oscillation time of 1.6 ms. In contrast to the stable component, the THR with an unstable seating (20 mm) showed an oscillation time of 3.3 ms. After Fast Fourier Transformation (FFT), frequency shifts and dampening of the spectral amplitude were evaluated. In the frequency spectrum the system with the loose THR had its first eigenfrequency at 328 Hz, while the first eigenfrequency of the system with the well fixed THR was at 926 Hz. The amplitudes in the frequency graph are dampened by about 75 % by increasing the embedding height from 20 to 65 mm.

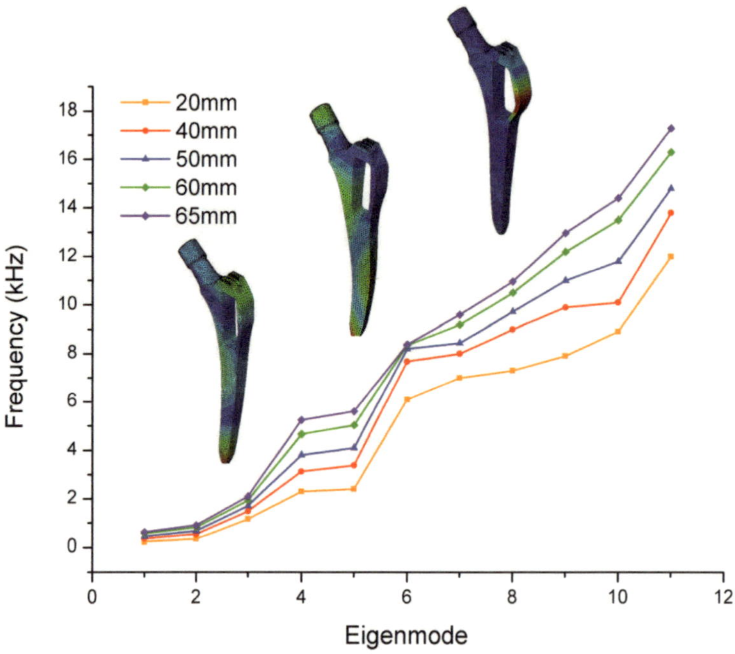

Fig. 16. Results of the eigenfrequencies with increasing embedding height of the CBH femoral component using finite-element-analysis

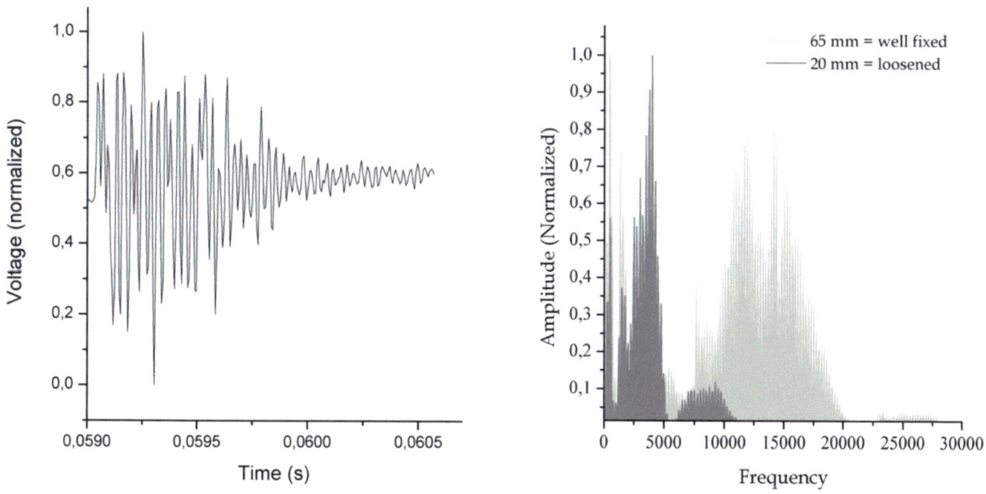

Fig. 17. Left: Characteristic voltage signal of the produced structure-borne sound of the 65 mm embedded CBH hip stem proportional to acceleration recorded by the detection coil. Right: Frequency spectrum using Fast Fourier Transformation. Comparison between 20 mm and 65 mm embedded hip stem.

The characteristic progression of the small cuboid-formed prototype is presented in figure 18. As seen in the experiments with the femoral component, the fixed prototype reveals a higher dampening of the sensor signal compared to the simulation of complete loosening. The displacement of the balance point in the area of lower frequency in case of advanced loosening is obvious.

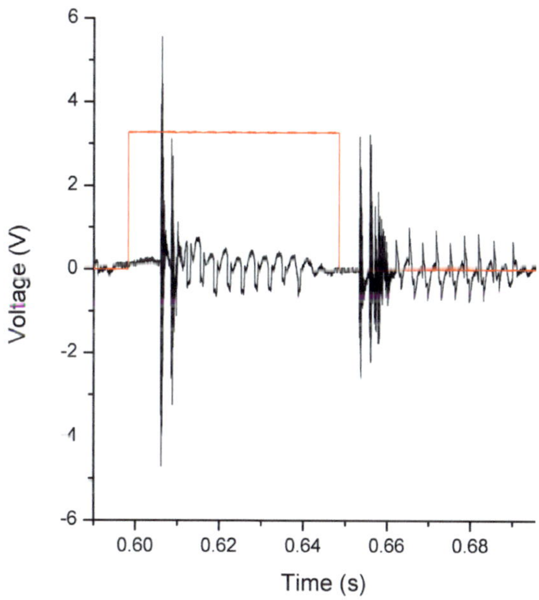

Fig. 18. Characteristic voltage signal of the produced structure-borne sound in the press fitted implant prototype proportional to acceleration.

These first test results demonstrate differences between two different states of fixation of both the femoral component and a prototype for latter animal experiments. Hence, this confirms the potential usability of the novel non-invasive approach for detecting implant loosening. In further tests, the influence of the femur-tibia and the femur-pelvis connection has to be investigated. Additionally, the femoral component will be integrated in a human cadaveric femur and measured with defined loosening zones. Moreover, the oscillators could be used in animal studies in order to determine the quality of osseointegration e.g. of new implant coatings and materials.

4. Conclusion

In loosening diagnostics of THR using imaging, an accuracy of 100 % is currently not available. This fact raises the demand for a new system to diagnose loosening exactly. Different approaches have been taken into consideration. Vibrometry, where accelerometers are used to detect resonance frequencies in vivo, seems to be a promising approach. Due to the disadvantage of the excitation with an electrodynamic shaker, we proposed a small mechanical oscillator as novel excitation approach for vibrometry. In the experiments with a Zweymueller femoral component a higher dampening coefficient could be identified in case of a fixed implant. Furthermore, within in vitro experiments using an implant inserted in the porcine femur the same promising results could be achieved.

5. Acknowledgment

This research project was funded by the Deutsche Forschungsgemeinschaft (DFG - German Research Foundation) under Reg. No. KL 2327/1.
Reprinted from Publication "The diagnostic value of digital subtraction arthrography and radionuclide bone scan in revision hip arthroplasty, Vol.18, No.6, pp. 735–740, Ovesen, O., Riegels-Nielsen, P., Lindequist, S., Jensen, I., Munkner, T., Torfing, T., et al. (2003), *Journal of Arthroplasty,*" and "Fluordeoxyglucose positron emission tomography detection of inflammatory reactions due to polyethylene wear in total hip arthroplasty, Vol.18, No.4, pp. 528–532, Kisielinski, K., Cremerius, U., Reinartz, P., & Niethard, F. U. (2003), *Journal of Arthroplasty*" and "A telemetry system for the detection of hip prosthesis loosening by vibration analysis, Vol.85, No.1-3, pp. 42-47, Puers, R., Catrysse, M., Vandevoorde, G., Collier, R. J., Louridas, E., Burny, F., Donkerwolcke, M., Moulart, F., (2000)., *Sensors and Actuators A: Physical,* " with permission from Elsevier.

6. References

Apple, J. S., Roberts, L. J., Gamba, J., Martinez, S., Khoury, M., & Ford, K. (1986). Digital subtraction arthrography of the prosthetic hip. *Southern Medical Journal*, Vol.79, No.7, pp. 808–810, ISSN 0038-4348

Barentsz, J. O., Lemmens, J. M., & Slooff, T. J. (1986). The use of subtraction arthrography in total hip arthroplasties. *Roefo*, Vol.144, No.4, pp. 440–446, ISSN 1438-9010

Bergmann G, Deuretzbacher G, Heller M, Graichen F, Rohlmann A, Strauss J, Duda GN (2001). Hip contact forces and gait patterns from routine activities. *Journal of Biomechanics*, Vol.34, No.7, pp. 859-871, ISSN 1435-2443

Böhler, M., Knahr, K., Riegler, M., & Salzer, M. (1994). Ten-year results of cemented Weller-type total hip arthroplasties. Analysis using different definitions of failure. *Archives of Orthopaedic and Trauma Surgery*, Vol.113, No.2, pp. 57–60, ISSN 0936-8051

Chryssikos, T., Parvizi, J., Ghanem, E., Newberg, A., Zhuang, H., & Alavi, A. (2008). FDG-PET imaging can diagnose periprosthetic infection of the hip, *Clinical Orthopaedics and Related Research*, Vol. 466, No.6, pp.1338-1342, ISSN 0009-921X

Cuckler, J. M. (2010). Unexplained pain after THR: what should i do? *Orthopedics*, Vol.33, No.9, p.648, ISSN 0147-7447

Dahl, M. C., Kramer, P. A., Reinhall, P. G., Benirschke, S. K., Hansen, S. T., & Ching, R. P. (2010). The efficacy of using vibrometry to detect osteointegration of the Agility total ankle. *Journal of Biomechanics*, Vol.43, No.9, pp. 1840–1843, ISSN 0021-9290

DeHeer, D. H., Engels, J. A., DeVries, A. S., Knapp, R. H., & Beebe, J. D. (2001). In situ complement activation by polyethylene wear debris. *Journal of Biomedical Materials Research*, Vol.54, No.1, pp. 12–19, ISSN 0021-9304

DeLee, J. G., & Charnley, J. (1976). Radiological demarcation of cemented sockets in total hip replacement. *Clinical Orthopaedics and Related Research*, No.121, pp. 20–32, ISSN 0009-921X

Dihlmann, W., Dihlmann, S. W., & Hering, L. (1991). Alloarthroplasty of the hip joint. Radiologic diagnosis of loosening and infection in cemented total endoprostheses. *Radiologe*, Vol.31, No.10, pp. 496–505, ISSN 0033-832X

Gelman, M. I., Coleman, R. E., Stevens, P. M., & Davey, B. W. (1978). Radiography, radionuclide imaging, and arthrography in the evaluation of total hip and knee replacement. *Radiology*, Vol.128, No.3, pp. 677–682, ISSN 0033-8419

Georgiou, A. P., & Cunningham, J. L. (2001). Accurate diagnosis of hip prosthesis loosening using a vibrational technique. *Clinical Biomechanics*, Vol.16, No.4, pp. 315–323, ISSN 0268-0033

Ginai, A. Z., van Biezen, F. C., Kint, P. A., Oei, H. Y., & Hop, W. C. (1996). Digital subtraction arthrography in preoperative evaluation of painful total hip arthroplasty. *Skeletal Radiology*, Vol.25, No.4, pp. 357–363, ISSN 0364-2348

Glauser, R., Sennerby, L., Meredith, N., Ree, A., Lundgren, A. K., Gottlow, J., et al. (2004). Resonance frequency analysis of implants subjected to immediate or early functional occlusal loading. Successful vs. failing implants. *Clinical Oral Implants Research*, Vol.15, No.4, pp. 428–434, ISSN 0905-7161

Gruen, T. A., McNeice, G. M., & Amstutz, H. C. (1979). "Modes of failure" of cemented stem-type femoral components: a radiographic analysis of loosening. *Clinical Orthopaedics and Related Research*, No.141, pp. 17–27, ISSN 0009-921X

Hardy, D. C., Reinus, W. R., Totty, W. G., & Keyser, C. K. (1988). Arthrography after total hip arthroplasty: utility of postambulation radiographs. *Skeletal Radiology*, Vol.17, No.1, pp. 20–23, ISSN 0364-2348

Hendrix, R. W., Wixson, R. L., Rana, N. A., & Rogers, L. F. (1983). Arthrography after total hip arthroplasty: a modified technique used in the diagnosis of pain. *Radiology*, Vol.148, No.3, pp. 647–652, ISSN 0033-8419

Huang, H. - M., Chiu, C. - L., Yeh, C. - Y., Lin, C. - T., Lin, L. - H., & Lee, S. - Y. (2003). Early detection of implant healing process using resonance frequency analysis. *Clin Oral Implants Res*, Vol.14, No.4, pp. 437–443, ISSN 0905-7161

Itasaka, T., Kawai, A., Sato, T., Mitani, S., & Inoue, H. (2001). Diagnosis of infection after total hip arthroplasty. *Journal of Orthopaedic Science*, Vol.6, No 4, pp. 320–326, ISSN 0949-2658

Kadoya, Y., Kobayashi, A., & Ohashi, H. (1998). Wear and osteolysis in total joint replacements. *Acta Orthopaedica Scandinavica Supplementum*, Vol.278, pp. 1–16, ISSN 0300-8827

Katz, G., Morscher, E., Fridrich, R., & Kentsch, A. (1986). [Evaluation of scintigraphic procedures for clarifying pain conditions in hip joint prostheses]. *Schweizerische Medizinische Wochenschrift*, Vol.116, No.21, pp. 703–707, ISSN 0036-7672

Keogh, C. F., Munk, P. L., Gee, R., Chan, L. P., & Marchinkow, L. O. (2003). Imaging of the painful hip arthroplasty. *American Journal of Roentgenolgy*, Vol.180, No.1, pp. 115–120, ISSN 0361-803X

Kisielinski, K., Cremerius, U., Reinartz, P., & Niethard, F. U. (2003). Fluordeoxyglucose positron emission tomography detection of inflammatory reactions due to polyethylene wear in total hip arthroplasty. *Journal of Arthroplasty*, Vol.18, No.4, pp. 528–532, ISSN 0883-5403

Koster, G., Munz, D. L., & Kohler, H. P. (1993). Clinical value of combined contrast and radionuclide arthrography in suspected loosening of hip prostheses. *Archives of Orthopaedic and Trauma Surgery*, Vol.112, No.5, pp. 247–254, ISSN 0936-8051

Kraemer, W. J., Saplys, R., Waddell, J. P., & Morton, J. (1993). Bone scan, gallium scan, and hip aspiration in the diagnosis of infected total hip arthroplasty. *Journal of Arthroplasty*, Vol.8, No.6, pp. 611–616, ISSN 0883-5403

Lannocca, M., Varini, E., Cappello, A., Cristofolini, L., & Bialoblocka, E. (2007). Intra-operative evaluation of cementless hip implant stability: a prototype device based on vibration analysis. *Medical Engineering and Physics*, Vol.29, No.8, pp. 886–894, ISSN 1350-4533

Larikka, M. J., Ahonen, A. K., Junila, J. A., Niemela, O., Hamalainen, M. M., & Syrjala, H. P. (2001). Extended combined 99mTc-white blood cell and bone imaging improves the diagnostic accuracy in the detection of hip replacement infections. *European Journal of Nuclear Medicine*, Vol.28, No.3, pp. 288–293, ISSN 0340-6997

Li, P. L., Jones, N. B., & Gregg, P. J. (1996). Vibration analysis in the detection of total hip prosthetic loosening. *Medical Engineering and Physics*, Vol.*18;No.*7, pp. 596–600, ISSN 1350-4533

Lieberman, J. R., Huo, M. H., Schneider, R., Salvati, E. A., & Rodi, S. (1993). Evaluation of painful hip arthroplasties. Are technetium bone scans necessary? *Journal of Bone and Joint Surgergy*, Vol.75, No.3, pp. 475–478, ISSN 0301-620X

Love, C., Tomas, M. B., Marwin, S. E., Pugliese, P. V., & Palestro, C. J. (2001). Role of nuclear medicine in diagnosis of the infected joint replacement. *Radiographics*, Vol.21, No.5, pp. 1229–1238, ISSN 0271-5333

Lyons, C. W., Berquist, T. H., Lyons, J. C., Rand, J. A., & Brown, M. L. (1985). Evaluation of radiographic findings in painful hip arthroplasties. *Clinical Orthopaedics and Related Research*, No.195, pp. 239–251, ISSN 0009-921X

Malchau, H., Herberts, P., Eisler, T., Garellick, G., & Soderman, P. (2002). The Swedish Total Hip Replacement Register. *Journal of Bone and Joint Surgergy Am*, Vol.84-A Suppl 2, pp. 2–20, ISSN 0021-9355

Maus, T. P., Berquist, T. H., Bender, C. E., & Rand, J. A. (1987). Arthrographic study of painful total hip arthroplasty: refined criteria. *Radiology*, Vol.162, No.3, pp. 721–727 ISSN 0033-8419

Mayer-Wagner, S., Mayer, W., Maegerlein, S., Linke, R., Jansson, V., & Muller, P. E. (2010). Use of 18F-FDG-PET in the diagnosis of endoprosthetic loosening of knee and hip implants. *Archives of Orthopaedics and Trauma Surgery*, Vol.130, No.10, pp. 1231–1238, ISSN 0936-8051

Miniaci, A., Bailey, W. H., Bourne, R. B., McLaren, A. C., & Rorabeck, C. H. (1990). Analysis of radionuclide arthrograms, radiographic arthrograms, and sequential plain radiographs in the assessment of painful hip arthroplasty. *Journal of Arthroplasty*, Vol.5, No.2, pp. 143–149, ISSN 0883-5403

Mumme, T., Reinartz, P., Alfer, J., Muller-Rath, R., Buell, U., & Wirtz, D. C. (2005). Diagnostic values of positron emission tomography versus triple-phase bone scan in hip arthroplasty loosening. *Archives of Orthopaedic and Trauma Surgery*, Vol.125, No.5, 322–329, ISSN 0936-8051

Nagoya, S., Kaya, M., Sasaki, M., Tateda, K., & Yamashita, T. (2008). Diagnosis of peri-prosthetic infection at the hip using triple-phase bone scintigraphy. *Journal of Bone and Joint Surgergy Br*, Vol.90, No.2, pp. 140–144, ISSN 0301-620X

Newberg, A. H., & Wetzner, S. M. (1985). Digital subtraction arthrography. *Radiology*, Vol.*154, No.*1, pp. 238–239, ISSN 0033-8419

Nilsson, L. T., Frazen, H., Carlsson, A. S., & Onnerfalt, R. (1994). Early radiographic loosening impairs the function of a total hip replacement. The Nottingham Health Profile of 49 patients at five years. *Journal of Bone and Joint Surgergy Br*, Vol.76, No.2, pp. 235–239, ISSN 0301-620X

O'Neill, D. A., & Harris, W. H. (1984). Failed total hip replacement: assessment by plain radiographs, arthrograms, and aspiration of the hip joint. *Journal of Bone and Joint Surgergy Am*, Vol.66, No.4, pp. 540–546, ISSN 0021-9355

Ovesen, O., Riegels-Nielsen, P., Lindequist, S., Jensen, I., Munkner, T., Torfing, T., et al. (2003). The diagnostic value of digital subtraction arthrography and radionuclide bone scan in revision hip arthroplasty. *Journal of Arthroplasty*, Vol.18, No.6, pp. 735–740, ISSN 0883-5403

Oyen, W. J., Lemmens, J. A., Claessens, R. A., van Horn, J. R., Slooff, T. J., & Corstens, F. H. (1996). Nuclear arthrography: combined scintigraphic and radiographic procedure for diagnosis of total hip prosthesis loosening. *Journal of Nuclear Medicine*, Vol.37, No.1, pp. 62–70, ISSN 0161-5505

Palestro, C. J. (2003). Nuclear medicine, the painful prosthetic joint, and orthopedic infection. *Journal of Nuclear Medicine*, Vol.44, No.6, pp 927–929, ISSN 0161-5505

Paterson, M., Fulford, P., & Denham, R. (1986). Loosening of the femoral component after total hip replacement. The thin black line and the sinking hip. *Journal of Bone and Joint Surgergy Br*, Vol.68, No.3, pp. 392–397, ISSN 0301-620X

Pfahler, M., Schidlo, C., & Refior, H. J. (1998). Evaluation of imaging in loosening of hip arthroplasty in 326 consecutive cases. *Archives of Orthopaedic and Trauma Surgery*, Vol.117, No.4-5, pp. 205–207, ISSN 0936-8051

Phillips, W. C., & Kattapuram, S. V. (1982). Prosthetic hip replacements: plain films and arthrography for component loosening. *American Journal of Roentgenology*, Vol.138, No.4, 677–682, ISSN 0361-803X

Puers, R., Catrysse, M., Vandevoorde, G., Collier, R. J., Louridas, E., Burny, F., Donkerwolcke, M., Moulart, F., (2000). A telemetry system for the detection of hip prosthesis loosening by vibration analysis, *Sensors and Actuators A: Physical,* Vol.85, No.1-3, pp. 42-47, ISSN 0924-4247

Qi, G., Mouchon, W. P., & Tan, T. E. (2003). How much can a vibrational diagnostic tool reveal in total hip arthroplasty loosening? *Clinical Biomechanics (Bristol, Avon),* Vol.18, No.5, pp. 444–458, ISSN 0268-0033

Reinartz, P. (2009). FDG-PET in patients with painful hip and knee arthroplasty: technical breakthrough or just more of the same. *Quaterly Journal of Nuclear Medicine and Molecular Imaging,* Vol.53, No.1, pp. 41–50, ISSN 1824-4785

Reinartz, P., Mumme, T., Hermanns, B., Cremerius, U., Wirtz, D. C., Schaefer, W. M., et al. (2005). Radionuclide imaging of the painful hip arthroplasty: positron-emission tomography versus triplephase bone scanning. *Journal of Bone and Joint Surgergy Br,* Vol.87, No.4, pp. 465–470, ISSN 0301-620X

Rosenstein A.D., McCoy G.F., Bulstrode C.J., McLardy-Smith P.D., Cunningham J.L., Turner-Smith A.R (1989). The differentiation of loose and secure femoral implants in total hip replacement using a vibrational technique: an anatomical and pilot clinical study. *Proceedings of Institute of Mechanical Engineering,* Vol.203, No.2, pp. 77-81, ISSN 0954-4119

Rowlands, A., Duck, F. A., & Cunningham, J. L. (2008). Bone vibration measurement using ultrasound: application to detection of hip prosthesis loosening. *Medical Engineering and Physics,* Vol.30, No.3, pp. 278–284, ISSN 1350-4533

Ruther, C., Ruther, C., Biemann, A., Nierath, H., Ewald, H., Mittelmeier, W., Bader, R., Kluess, D., (2010). A new concept for non-invasive radiation-free detection of implant loosening, 56th Annual Meeting of the Orthopaedic Research Society, New Orleans, Louisiana, USA, March 6-9, 2010, pp. 2413.

Sarmiento, A., Ebramzadeh, E., Gogan, W. J., & McKellop, H. A. (1990). Total hip arthroplasty with cement. A long-term radiographic analysis in patients who are older than fifty and younger than fifty years. *Journal of Bone and Joint Surgergy Am,* Vol.72, No.10, 1470–1476, ISSN 0021-9355

Segura, A. B., Munoz, A., Brulles, Y. R., Hernandez Hermoso, J. A., Diaz, M. C., Bajen Lazaro, M. T., et al. (2004). What is the role of bone scintigraphy in the diagnosis of infected joint prostheses? *Nuclear Medicine Communications,* Vol.25, No.5, pp. 527–532, ISSN 0143-3636

Shao F. Xu W., Crocombe A., Ewins D. (2007). Natural frequency analysis of osseointegration for trans-femoral implant. *Annals of Biomedical Engineering,* Vol.35, No.5, pp. 817-824, ISSN 0090-6964

Stumpe, K. D. M., & Strobel, K. (2006). 18F FDG-PET imaging in musculoskeletal infection. *Quaterly Journal of Nuclear Medicine and Molecular Imaging,* Vol.50, No.2, pp. 131–142, ISSN 0033-8419

Stumpe, K. D. M., Notzli, H. P., Zanetti, M., Kamel, E. M., Hany, T. F., Gorres, G. W., et al. (2004). FDG PET for differentiation of infection and aseptic loosening in total hip replacements: comparison with conventional radiography and three-phase bone scintigraphy. *Radiology*, Vol.231, No.2, pp. 333–341, ISSN 1824-4785

Suckel, A., Geiger, F., Kinzl, L., Wulker, N., & Garbrecht, M. (2009). Long-term results for the uncemented Zweymuller/Alloclassic hip endoprosthesis. A 15-year minimum follow-up of 320 hip operations. *Journal of Arthroplasty*, Vol.24, No.6, pp. 846–853, ISSN 0883-5403

Tehranzadeh, J., Schneider, R., & Freiberger, R. H. (1981). Radiological evaluation of painful total hip replacement. *Radiology*, Vol.141, No.2, pp. 355–362, ISSN 0033-8419

Temmerman, O. P. P., Raijmakers, P. G. H. M., Berkhof, J., David, E. F. L., Pijpers, R., Molenaar, M. A., et al. (2006). Diagnostic accuracy and interobserver variability of plain radiography, subtraction arthrography, nuclear arthrography, and bone scintigraphy in the assessment of aseptic femoral component loosening. *Archives of Orthopaedic and Trauma Surgery*, Vol.126, No.5, pp. 316–323, ISSN 0936-8051

Temmerman, O. P. P., Raijmakers, P. G. H. M., Berkhof, J., Hoekstra, O. S., Teule, G. J. J., & Heyligers, I. C. (2005). Accuracy of diagnostic imaging techniques in the diagnosis of aseptic loosening of the femoral component of a hip prosthesis: a meta-analysis. *Journal of Bone and Joint Surgergy Br*, Vol.87, No.6, pp. 781–785, ISSN 0301-620X

Temmerman, O. P. P., Raijmakers, P. G. H. M., David, E. F. L., Pijpers, R., Molenaar, M. A., Hoekstra, O. S., et al. (2004). A comparison of radiographic and scintigraphic techniques to assess aseptic loosening of the acetabular component in a total hip replacement. *Journal of Bone and Joint Surgergy Br*, Vol.86-A, No.11, pp. 2456–2463, ISSN 0021-9355

Udomkiat, P., Wan, Z., & Dorr, L. D. (2001). Comparison of preoperative radiographs and intraoperative findings of fixation of hemispheric porous-coated sockets. *Journal of Bone and Joint Surgergy Br*, Vol.83-A, No.12, pp. 1865–1870, ISSN 0021-9355

Uri, G., Wellman, H., Capello, W., Robb, J., & Greenman, G. (1984). Scintigraphic and X-ray arthrographic diagnosis of femoral prosthesis loosening: concise communication. *Journal of Nuclear Medicine*, Vol.25, No.6, pp. 661–663, ISSN 0161-5505

Vanquickenborne, B., Maes, A., Nuyts, J., Van Acker, F., Stuyck, J., Mulier, M., et al. (2003). The value of (18)FDG-PET for the detection of infected hip prosthesis. *European Journal of Nuclear Medicine Molecular Imaging*, Vol.30, No.5, pp. 705–715, ISSN 1619-7070

Walker, C. W., FitzRandolph, R. L., Collins, D. N., & Dalrymple, G. V. (1991). Arthrography of painful hips following arthroplasty: digital versus plain film subtraction. *Skeletal Radiology*, Vol.20, No.6, pp. 403–407, ISSN 0364-2348

Wilson, D. J., Morgan, R. L., Hesselden, K. L., Dodd, J. R., Janna, S. W., & Fagan, M. J. (2009). A single-channel telemetric intramedullary nail for in vivo measurement of fracture healing. *Journal of Orthopaedics and Trauma*, Vol.23, No.10, pp. 702–709, ISSN 0890-5339

Wroblewski, B. M. (1991). Clinical and radiographic evaluation of total hip replacement. A standard system of terminology for reporting results. *Journal of Bone and Joint Surgery Am*, Vol.73, No.6, p. 948, ISSN 0021-9355

Zhuang, H., Yang, H., & Alavi, A. (2007). Critical role of 18F-labeled fluorodeoxyglucose PET in the management of patients with arthroplasty. *Radiologic Clinics of North America*, Vol.45, No.4, pp. 711–8, vii, ISSN 0033-8389

Zilkens, K. W., Wicke, A., Zilkens, J., & Bull, U. (1988). Nuclear imaging in loosening of hip-joint endoprostheses. *Archives of Orthopaedic and Trauma Surgery*, Vol.107, No.5, pp. 288–292, ISSN 0344-8444

18

Management of Bone Loss in Primary and Revision Knee Replacement Surgery

Matteo Fosco[1], Rida Ben Ayad[1], Luca Amendola[1],
Dante Dallari[1] and Domenico Tigani[2]
[1]*First Ward of Orthopaedic Surgery, University of Bologna, Rizzoli Orthopaedic Institute, Bologna*
[2]*Department of Orthopaedic Surgery, Santa Maria alle Scotte Hospital ,Siena*
Italy

1. Introduction

Total knee arthroplasty (TKA) often deal with bone defect localized in areas corresponding to tibial and femoral articular surfaces, a condition that is often observed in revision knee prosthetic surgery but occasionally in primary arthroplasty of the knee too. Such intraoperative situation, could create a main problem in maintaining proper alignment of the implant components and in establishing sufficient bone stock to achieve a stable bone-implant interface. The surgeon must assess the degree of complexity preoperatively and intraoperatively and have a broad armamentarium available during surgery.

Multiple surgical options are available to repair or reconstruct the loss of bone, these include: bone cement, bone grafts, metal augments and custom-made implants.

Principles to consider in bone loss management are knee-related (particularly defect size and location, ligament stability, limb alignment) and patient-related (age, body mass index, activity level, life expectancy).

2. Primary TKA

Bone loss observed during primary arthroplasty of the knee is less frequent than during revision surgery. In primary implants causes of bone defect include:

- Osteonecrosis;
- Sequelae of fracture of tibial plateau or femoral condyles;
- Bone cysts;
- Previous tibial osteotomies;
- Inflammatory arthropathies.

However final cause is always represented by bone erosion, secondary to varus or valgus deformity of the knee; the consequent overload of medial or lateral compartment bring to collapse of the subchondral bone (Tigani et al., 2004).

Typically, in varus knee bone defect contribute to collapse of the medial tibial plateau, firstly in the posteromedial site. Instead, in valgus knee, bone defect may involve the tibia (with a contained central defect) and the external femoral condyle, that is defective in the distal and posterior sites (Insall & Easley, 2001) (Fig. 1).

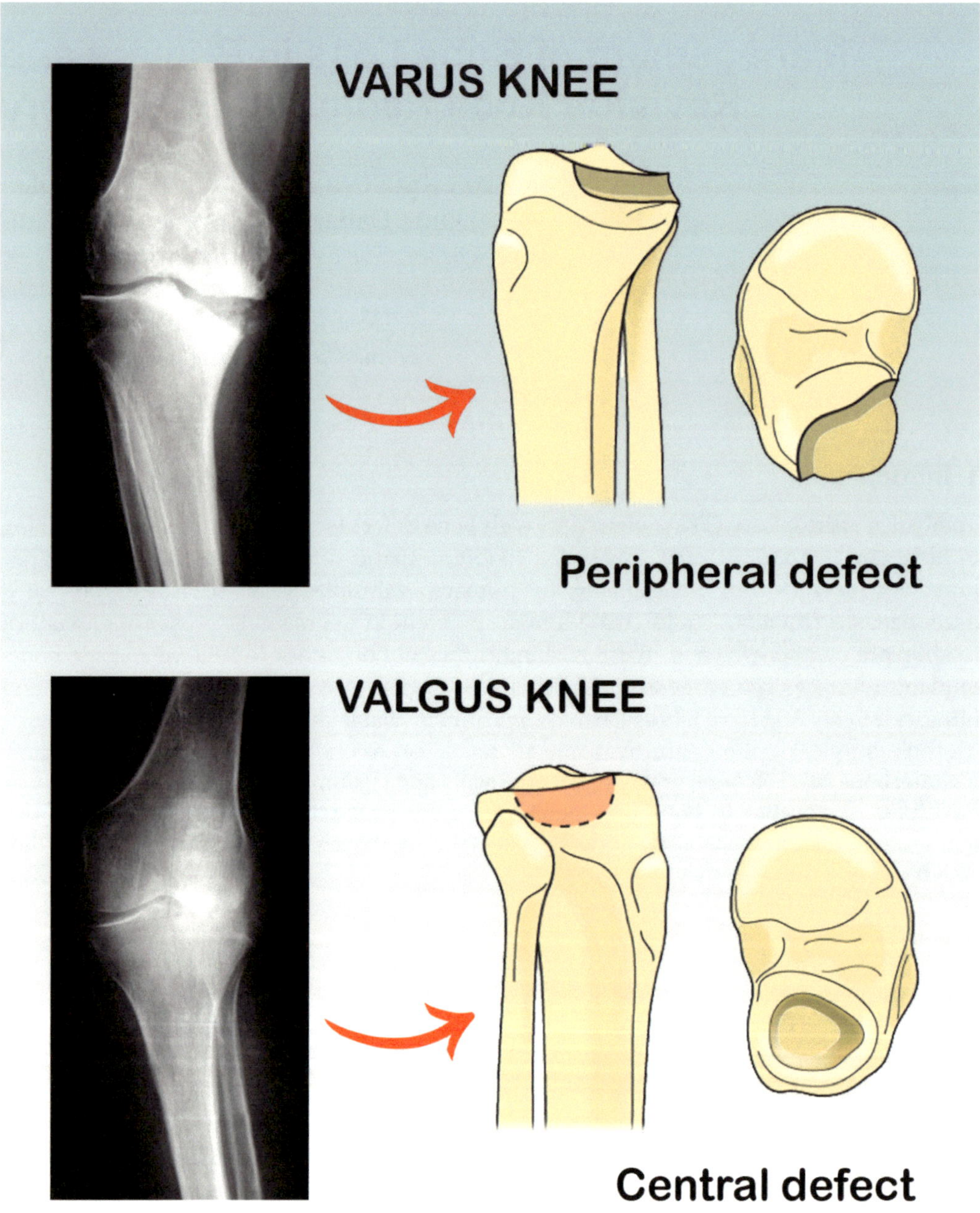

Fig. 1. Usually varus knee appears with bone defect in posteromedial site of tibial plateau. Instead, in valgus knee bone defect usually involves the central part of lateral tibial hemiplateau and the external femoral condyle.

Type	*Single condylar/hemiplate involvement (%)*	*Depth(mm)*
I *(a/b)*	minimal < 50%	< 5
II *(a/b)*	> 50 < 70%	5-10
III *(a/b)*	> 70% < 90%	> 10
IV *(a/b)*	> 90%	> 10

a) Intact peripheral rim
b) Deficient peripheral rim

Table 1. Rand classification of bone loss (modified from Rand JA, 1991).

First classification of bone defects thus consists on distinction between central forms (with defect confined within the peripheral bone cortex), and peripheral forms (characterized by involvement of the peripheral cortex). In 1991 Rand proposed a classification that considers the percentage extent of the defect into the tibial plateau or femoral condyle, distinguishing between four grades of increasing severity of the lesion (Rand, 1991) (Table 1).
The most common defect is observed in the presence of a varus knee, with defect located in the posteromedial region of the tibia; the lesion is characterized by the presence of an important sclerosis of the subchondral bone and its depth usually doesn't exceed 8 to 10mm. In such simple cases, resection of the tibial plateau allow to completely remove the defect, without requiring further procedures.
Instead, in deeper and more severe lesions, tibial resection of more than 12 mm, could lead to sacrifice important ligamentous structures and has been observed to considerably alters bone quality, thus requiring other options (Laskin, 1989).

3. Revision TKA

Bone loss in revision TKA could always be considered as a consequence of the previous arthroplasty. In these cases, on preoperative radiographs bone loss is often underestimated relative to the true bone loss found during revision surgery. In a retrospective analysis of 31 patients with symptomatic TKAs who had osteolytic lesions confirmed by computed tomography, plain radiography detected only 17% of the osteolytic lesions (Reish et al, 2004).
The final evaluation of bone loss is made more accurately during surgery, after component removal; so that various classification systems used are mainly based on the size and type of the defect found intraoperatively.
Clatworthy and Gross firstly classified defects as contained central forms, and uncontained peripheral forms (with involvement of the peripheral cortical rim), then further distinguishing between intact metaphyseal bone or not (Clatworthy & Gross, 2003). The most practical system is the Anderson Orthopedic Research Institute (AORI) classification described by Engh, that considers bone loss from the tibia and femur independently (T and F) (Engh & Ammeen, 1999); distinction is then made depending on involvement of 1 condyle/plateau (A) or 2 (B) (Table 2,3).

Femoral defect			
F1	F2a	F2b	F3
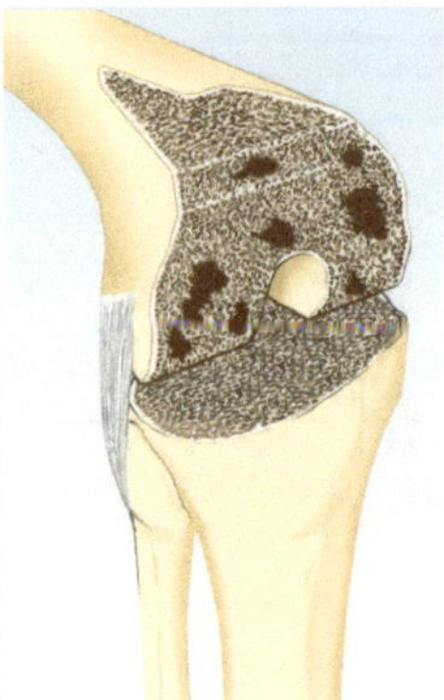	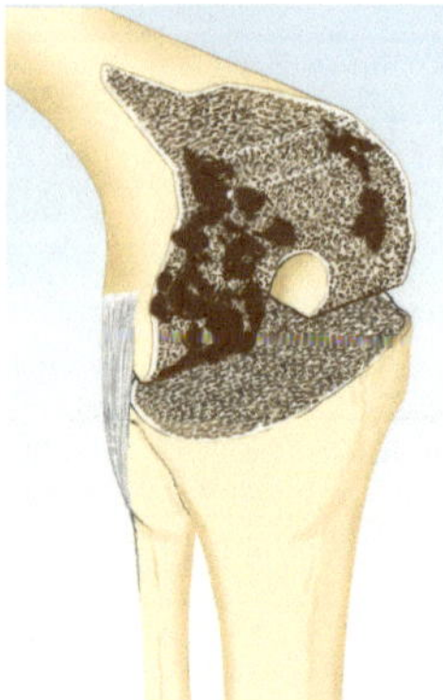	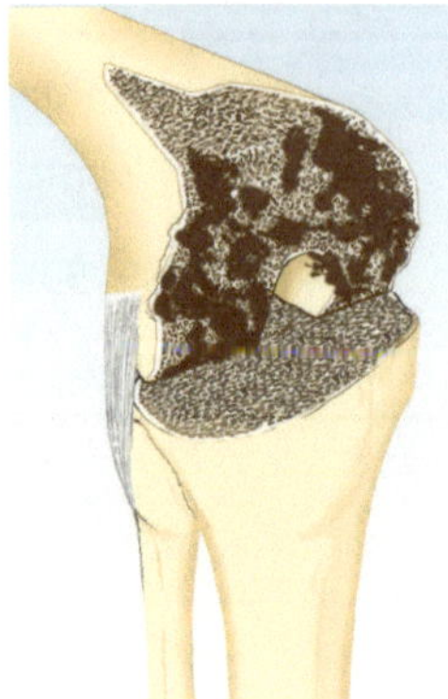	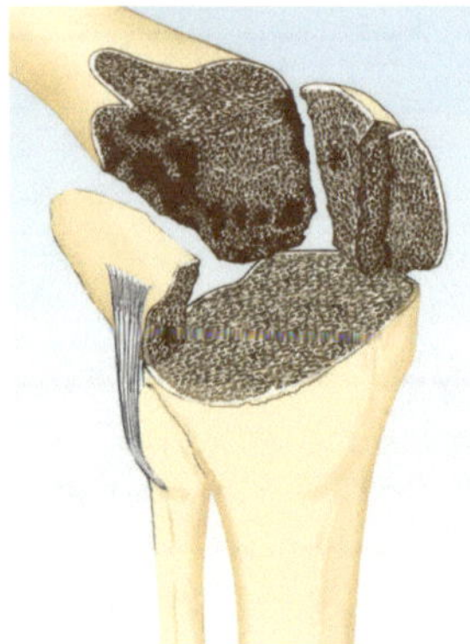
Small amounts of bone loss not compromising component stability (contained, minor defects)	Damaged unicondylar structural bone (noncontained)	Damaged bicondylar structural bone (noncontained)	Significant bone loss compromising a major portion of the condyles with ligamentous instability (noncontained)

Table 2. Classification of femoral defect (modified from Engh & Ammeen, 1999). Contained defect is considered as a loss of metaphyseal cancellous bone with a significant loss of surrounding cortical support

Tibial defect			
T1	T2a	T2b	T3
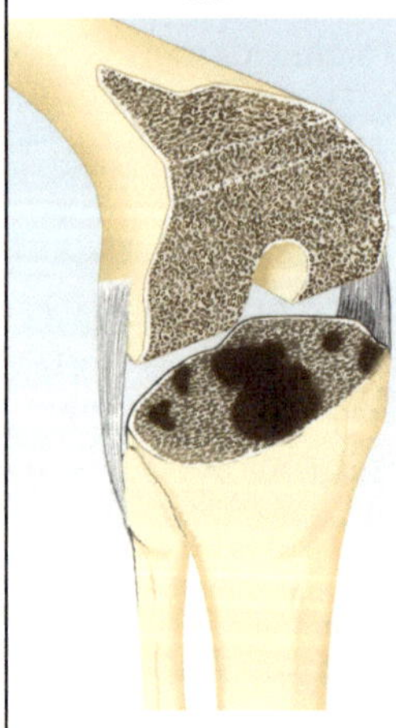	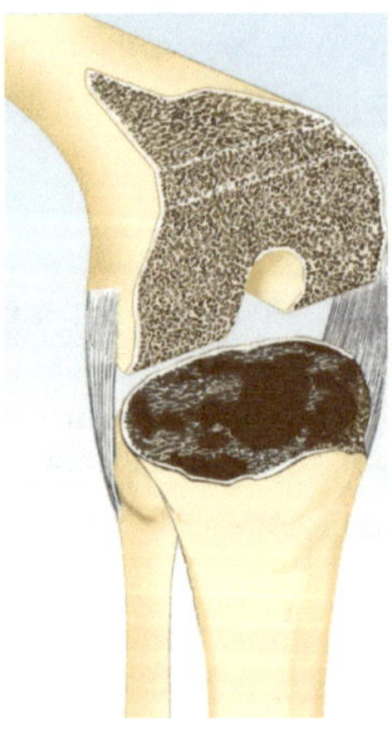	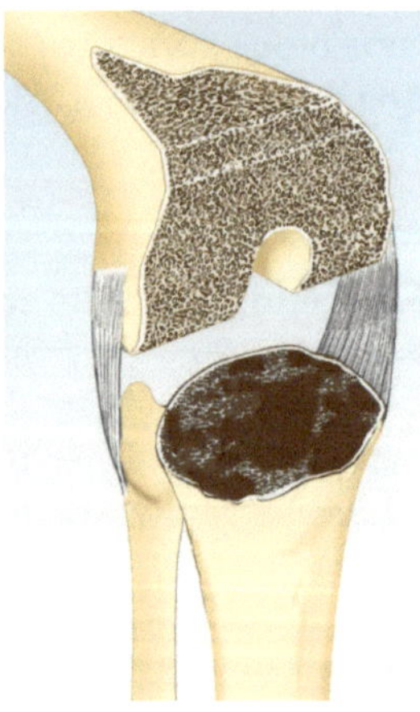	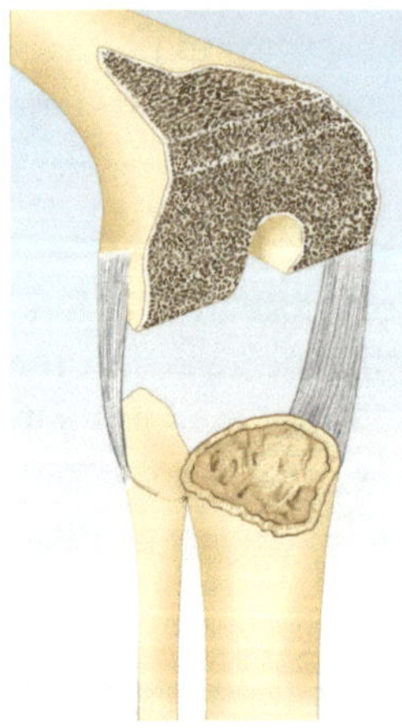
Small amounts of bone loss not compromising component stability (contained)	Damaged unilateral metaphyseal bone needing augmentation to maintain joint line (noncontained)	Damaged bilateral metaphyseal bone needing augmentation to maintain joint line (noncontained)	Significant bone loss compromising a major portion of the plateau, that may involve detachment of the patellar tendon (noncontained)

Table 3. Classification of tibial defect (modified from Engh & Ammeen, 1999).

Main causes of bone loss during revision arthroplasty are stress shielding, wear debris and implant loosening; these factors may be interrelated (Lombardi et al, 2010):

- Stress shielding causes an "osteopenic" type of bone loss behind the prosthetic components, due to pressure shielded by the implant and redistributed to the bone-cement-implant interface;
- Wear debris of polyethylene, cement and metal particles; in contrast to the less common osteopenic type of bone loss seen in stress shielding, wear causes an "osteolytic" type of bone loss, around apparently stable implants (Van Loon et al, 1999). Osteolysis is defined as the periprosthetic replacement of bone by chronic inflammatory tissue without evidence of loosening. This type of osteolysis is more common in young, male, overweight patients with osteoarthritis;
- Implant aseptic loosening resulting in direct mechanical bone loss at the cement-bone interface;
- Implant septic loosening;
- Iatrogenic damage resulting directly from implant removal, thus representing an important factor in preserving bone stock during revision TKA. Removal of components with no loosening or with an intercondylar box or stems will create large bone defects. Cement should be removed using small sagittal saw and flexible osteotomes, avoiding levering which could cause a fracture.

The objectives of revision surgery include reestablishment of the anatomic joint line, long-term joint stability, and restoration of bone stock with a fast return to full weight-bearing and function.

So that, implant selection should be based not only on the status of the ligamentous and soft tissue stabilizing structures, but also on the severity and type of bone loss.

4. Management of bone defects

Various options exist to manage bone defects, available in both primary and revision surgery. Indication to whether option to use, depends on knee-related and patient-related factors.

4.1 Translating the prosthetic component away from the bone defect

This option is useful when marginal bony defect exist particularly at the tibial side. Nevertheless smaller tibial tray determines lesser contact surface and greater load concentration (Figure 2).

4.2 Cement filling

The use of cement seems to be applicable in knee arthroplasty, either alone or in combination with screws, but only in cases of relatively small defects (Figure 3). Some authors (Lotke et al., 1991; Ritter et al., 1993) have observed good medium or long term results, while others (Brooks et al., 1984; Freeman et al., 1982; Insall & Ealsey, 2001) had obtained poor ones. Moreover these studies showed that weak biomechanical characters of cement do not improve in resistance of the implant with use of support screws.

So that we currently suggest cement only for peripheral small defects with defect extension of less than 50% of bone surface and less than 5mm of depth. In larger lesions, alone or in combination with support screws, it is not recommended.

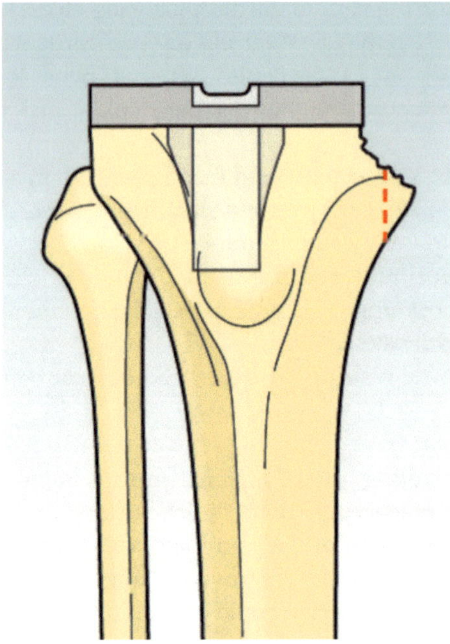

Fig. 2. Translating tibial component could be a viable option for very small defect; this technique should not be used in angular deformity due to abnormal concentration of load forces.

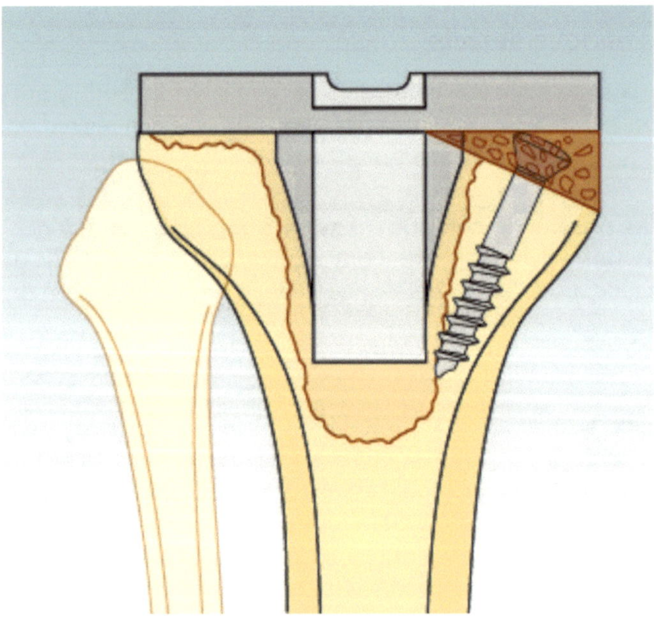

Fig. 3. Cement filling could be used with or without screws (modified from Brooks et al.,1984).

4.3 Bone grafting

Recently, grafting constitutes a frequent option used for the treatment of bone defect in knee arthroplasty. The rationale in using bone grafts consisted in the possibility of a new formation of vital bone, through a process of osteoinduction and/or osteoconduction. Autoplastic bone grafts are likely to be used for limited defects, while structural allograft could be necessary in cases of larger lesions.

Bone grafts, both homoplastic and autoplastic, are to be preferred in younger patients because they allow for bone regeneration that represents an essential condition in case of reintervention.

4.3.1 Autologous bone grafting

In primary TKA, the resected femoral condyles or tibial plateau sometimes can be used as a source of autograft for tibial defects; morcelized bone obtained from the tibia and femoral resections can be used as autograft in contained defects.

Its use have been advocated by various authors (Dorr et al., 1986; Scuderi et al., 1989), constituting a viable option due to excellent osteoinductive, osteoconductive and osteogenic properties (Fig. 4).

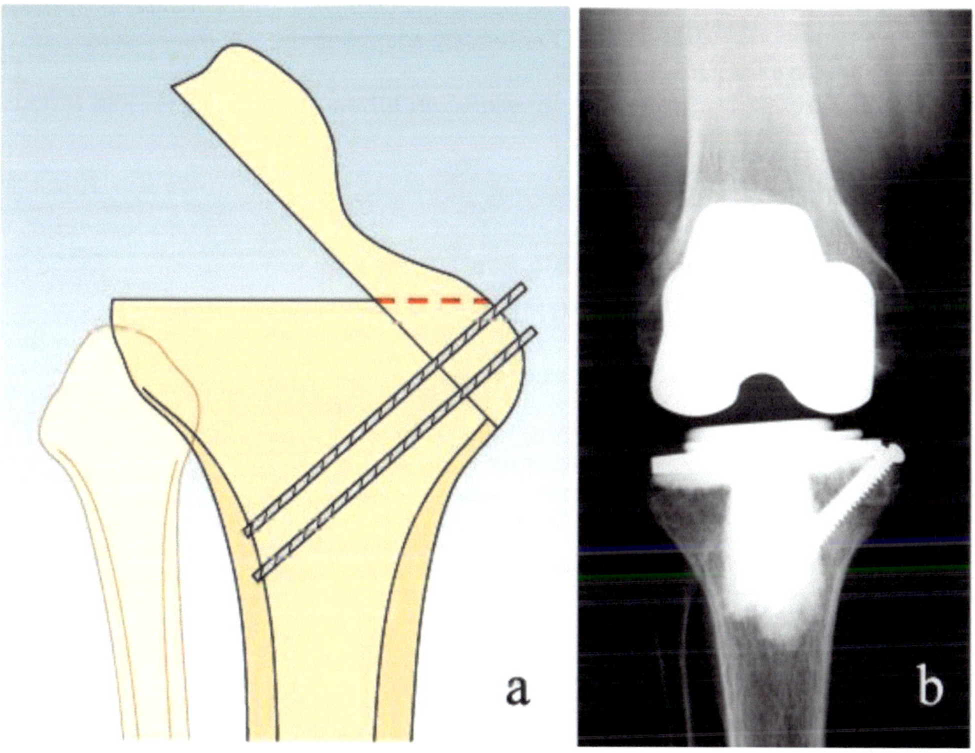

Fig. 4. An oblique planar cancellous surface is created on the recipient side, and coaptation of proximal tibia autograft surface is ensured to this recipient bed by screw or wire fixation. (courtesy of Dr. E.A. Martucci)

Nevertheless Laskin in a series of 26 patients with severe tibial bone loss treated by TKA using autogenic bone graft into the defect, observed 4 cases of grafts fragmentation with

implant subsidence within the first year (Laskin, 1989). Moreover needle biopsy in 9 cases in which the graft had not fragmented, revealed osteocytes in the lacunae in only 4 grafts. In each of four knees, there was a complete radiolucency between the graft and the tibial host bone. The final author's conclusion is to reevaluate the use of modular prostheses in large fragment defects but to continue using bone graft for smaller, circumscribed defects.
Possible reason of autoplastic graft failure have been ipothetised:

- Varus alignment of the leg.
- Avascular host bed for the graft
- Insufficient graft press-fit.
- Incomplete coverage of the graft by the tibial component.
- Extravasation of the cement between graft and host.

Currently there are insufficient clinical data to state with certainty that bone stock restoration with autogenic bone graft will in fact aid future revisions when necessary.

4.3.2 Allogeneic bone grafting

The limited availability of autologous graft may not be enough to compensate an extensive bone defect and use of homoplastic bone could be indicated (Fig. 5).
Cancellous or structured bone allograft could be used but always have to be considered some rules:

- The graft have to be modeled, thus to precisely adapt it to the defect;
- The graft have to be perfectly stabilized;
- The graft have to be "protected" by use of an intramedullary stems, able to reduce mechanical stress forces.

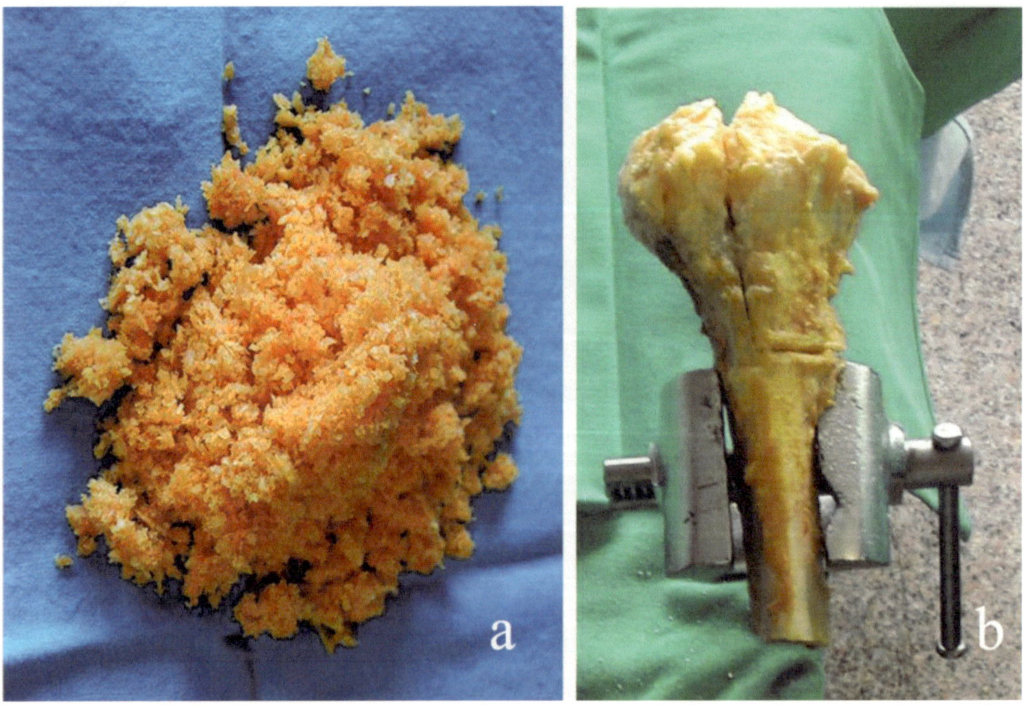

Fig. 5. (a) Cancellous bone allograft, added with antibiotic. (b) Structural bone allograft molded intraoperatively before implanting.

Nevertheless difficulties using bone homologous grafts consisted on:

- Need of a bone bank support;
- Grafts resorbtion;
- Increased risk of infection;
- Disease transmission.

4.3.3 Structural massive bone allograft

Structural bone allograft offers numerous advantages, including biocompatibility, bone stock restoration and potential for ligaments reattachment. Regarding their versatility it is possible to treat a wide range of bone deficiency allowing the surgeon to shape the allograft to fit the bone defect and avoid unnecessary removal of host bone. Finally allograft is relatively cost-effective if compared to the high cost of custom-made implants.

The goals of structural allograft reconstruction are to maximize the stability of the graft-host bone contact and provide a stable platform for fixation of the implant. The first step is to remove all the nonviable bone and soft tissue from in and around the defect, the presence of viable bone is absolutely necessary to maximize the likelihood of graft incorporation. Conversion of the oblique peripheral defects into rectangular space with vertical and horizontal surfaces has been demonstrate to improve stability for components fixation. The angular patterns have also a biological advantage since it allows improving the contact area of the host-graft construct maximizing the probability of graft incorporation. Regarding the choice of the graft it is important to shape the allograft similarly in order to fit the defect precisely. Graft fixation too is an important step to be taken in consideration: mainly used are partially or fully threaded cancellous screws.

In the literature there are various papers reporting about the use of allograft to restore bone defect during revision knee arthroplasty, especially for uncontained defects. In some cases with circumferential segmental bone defect of tibial plateau, have been demonstrated about 25% of allograft failure (De Long et al., 2007; Engh & Ammeen, 2007). Engh & Ammeen, whose have reviewed the results of 49 knees with severe tibial bone loss, found only four cases of failure for reasons not-directly related to collapse or resorption of the graft; most of patients had contained defect and ten presented an uncontained deficiency of which only four cases were restored with full segment allograft. Recently Backstein D, et al have reported 85.2% of success rate at an average follow-up of 5.4 years in a series of 68 revision that required a structural allograft for the treatment of uncontained defect (Backstein et al., 2006).

Even if a variability of result are present in the literature, due to the significant difference of the lesion treated, all authors agree on affirm that the use of a intramedullary stem with a sufficient length to engage diaphyseal bone is mandatory to decrease axial and shear loads to the structural allograft in accordance with previously data emerging from the laboratory (Mounasamy et al, 2006).

We have experienced reconstruction with massive structural allograft during primary total knee replacement for severe segmental medial post-traumatic tibial plateau defect in arthritic knee (Tigani et al., 2011); neither acute nor chronic complications were observed, and radiological examination referred no signs of prosthetic loosening or secondary resorption, with good grafting integration to host bone (Fig. 6).

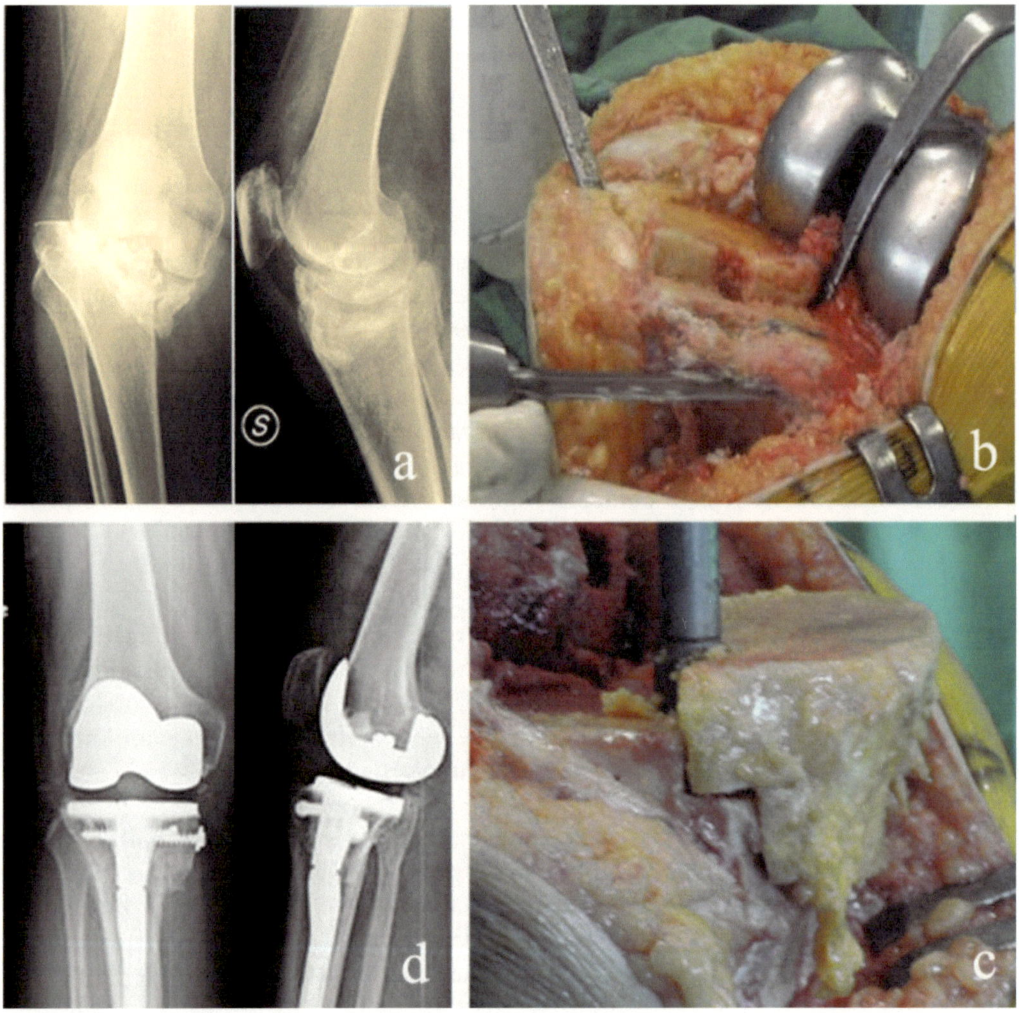

Fig. 6. (a) Pre-operative plain radiographs showing post-traumatic severe depressed medial bone stock loss; (b) preparation of tibial plateau, in a way to convert oblique defect to rectangular stepped one; (c) Fitting the allograft into the defect; (d) last follow-up plain radiographs, 12 months after the surgery.

4.4 Modular components (metal augments)

The use of metal augments for bone deficiencies has become quite popular since mid Eighties, after the work of Brooks et al which indicated that biomechanically the modular augments are equivalent to a custom implant (Brooks et al., 1984). In last decades a new biomaterial is largely used in knee prosthetic surgery: porous tantalum, in its trabecular form (trabecular metal, TM; Zimmer, Warsaw, Ind, US). TM show excellent mechanical characteristics compared to conventional implant materials (i.e. titanium and cobalt chromium): good biocompatibility, high porosity, low modulus of elasticity (Levine et al., 2007). Moreover biological advantages of TM include its negative charge and interconnective pores, which form a scaffolding and surface for osteoblast-mediated bone ingrowth (Bobyn et al., 1999). These unique material properties of porous trabecular metal allow it to achieve immediate structural support, together with early bony ingrowth and late restoration of bone stock.

TM is available in many shapes and forms (Fig. 7): porous or solid, rectangular or wedge shaped, and can be attached with the use of cement or screws. It can be applied quickly, allow intraoperative custom fabrication, supply excellent biomechanical properties, and require minimal bone resection as the augments attach on the residual bone.

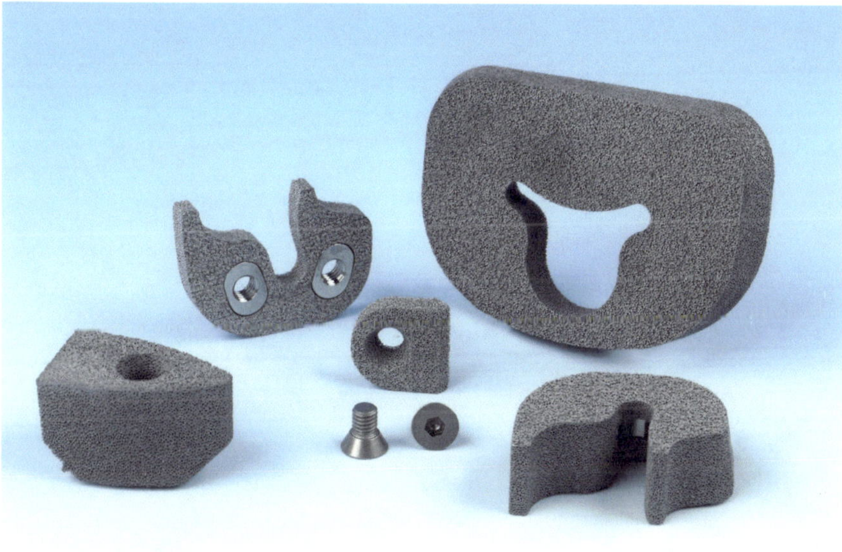

Fig. 7. TM modular augments (courtesy of Zimmer, Warsaw, Ind, US).

Preference between wedges and blocks should be accorded to the augmentation that most closely fills the defect (Fig. 8). The exception to this may be when a constrained insert is necessary; in this instance block may have some advantage because of its ability to directly transmit torsional loads as a result of geometric interlock. Even this, blocks avoid shear stress but necessitate removal of some intact host bone.

On the tibial side, multiple sizes of metal wedges and blocks are available, up to full tibial block for defects of entire plateau, thus maintaining balanced flexion and extension spaces. Femoral defects can be reconstructed with metal blocks in increments of 5 mm; because bone loss in femur is most often on the posterior and distal surfaces, augments fixed to the distal and posterior femoral condyles are used.

Surgical advantages of metal augments with respect to bone graft are:

- Possibility to customize the implant intraoperatively;
- Need not be incorporated into host bone;
- Do not carry a risk of nonunion or collapse.

Despite the versatility and a wide geometry of augments, including hemi-wedges, full wedges, and symmetric spacers, these materials can manage only a limited defect, up to 20 mm of deep.

In our practice we prefer to use cement and a step cut technique for Engh type 1 defects of less than 5 mm depth, and metal augmentation for type 2 defects of more than 5–10 mm.

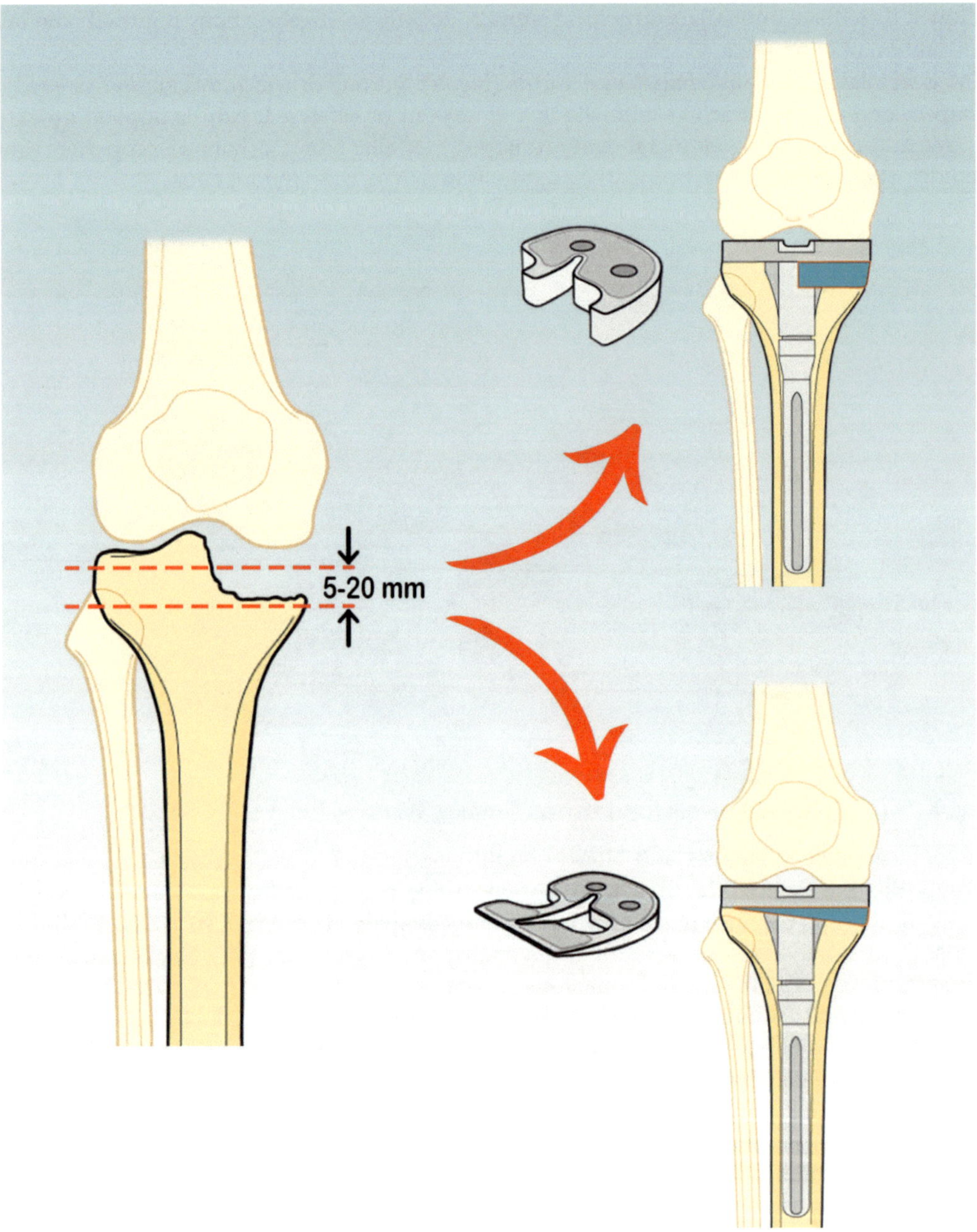

Fig. 8. TM augments in tibia are available in a rectangular or wedge fashion

The success rates in the literature using these augments range from 84–98% good or excellent results (Lucey et al., 2000; Radnay & Scuderi, 2006; Rand, 1991). Nevertheless, we think like others, that metal augmentation should be reserved to elderly patients in reason of secondary implant failure and low resistance with the time.

4.5 Metaphyseal bone loss

Familiarity with the rationale and strategies for metaphyseal fixation in revision TKA is a valuable addition to the armamentarium of the revision surgeon. In the revision setting, reliance on metaphyseal area fixation is important to carry a portion of the axial load and protecting epiphyseal ingrowth (Haidukewych et al., 2011). Metaphyseal bone loss have historically required any one or numerous of the following: cement, impaction grafting with mesh containment, metal augmentation (TM cones or metaphyseal sleeves), structural bulking grafts, custom-made or hinged/tumor-like prostheses.

Porous tantalum structural cones (Fig. 9), which are a new modern extension among the family of metal augments, have been introduced in attempt to achieve a real structural and biomechanical reconstruction of such important metaphyseal bone defects. They are useful when there are significant bone defects, or if there is cortical deficiency or fracture. Tibial tantalum cones could be used with cemented or cementeless technique while femoral tantalum cones must be cemented to the bone in the United States and may be used with or without cement elsewhere.

Tantalum cones along with offset stems, increase contact area between the implant, cone, and host bone, thus serving as a mechanical platform and as support for the revision implants with less stress shielding and disuse atrophy of the surrounding bone. In addition, tantalum's low modulus of elasticity is optimal to load transfer without stress shielding problems (Radnay & Scuderi, 2006). The modular nature of the cones allows to closely fill the defect addressing to both cancellous bone loss and cortical defects. Moreover the unique material properties of porous trabecular metal allow it to achieve rapid bony ingrowth with the potential for long-term biologic fixation and restoration of bone stock. During our experience with 12 femoral and tibial tantalum cones, we registered no cases of aseptic loosening or migration, with good osteointegration to surrounding bone, in both cemented and cementless cases. Therefore we think these implants may eliminate the need for extensive bone grafting that have historically been necessary in the presence of large defects.

Recently modular porous coated press fit metaphyseal sleeves have been developed as modular prosthetic adjunctive (DePuy, Warsaw, Ind, US) to obtain fixation in the metaphyseal region. Sleeves have gained initial popularity because of possibility of acting as IM cutting guide. Moreover the interface between metaphyseal sleeves and the implant is created by a Morse tapered junction, while is cemented between TM cones and the implant. However theoretical failure of the junction between metaphyseal sleeves and articular component may occur during impaction or over time and unlike TM cones, sleeves cannot be customized with a burr and cannot be used in more severe uncontained defects (Haidukewych et al., 2011). Pagnotto et al. presented early results with porous-coated metaphyseal sleeves to fill Engh type 2 and 3 defects in revision total knee replacement (53 tibial and 32 femoral sleeves). After 2 years mean of follow-up he reported revision of five sleeves (three for infection and two for loosening); all 80 of the remaining 80 sleeves showed radiographic evidence of ingrowth (Pagnotto et al., 2011).

We agree with other authors that although promising results of metaphyseal metal implants, concerns still exist regarding stress shielding and difficulty of their removal. Particularly literature is lacking of long-term follow-up studies to determine the durability of these constructs and studies are needed to compare TM cones or metaphyseal sleeves to alternative reconstructive techniques.

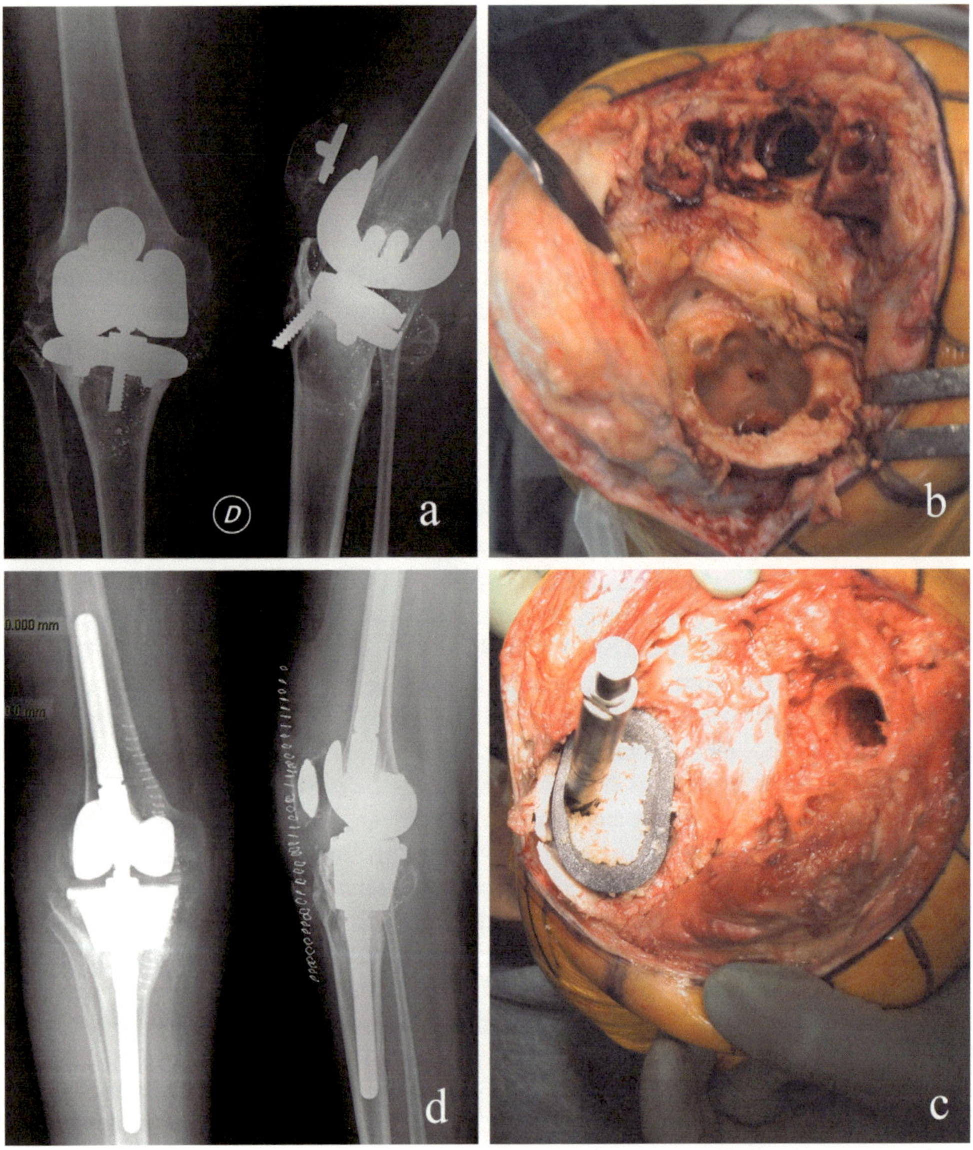

Fig. 9. (a) Aseptic knee prosthesis failure in a 58 years old patient. (b) Intraoperatively a severe confined cavitary deficiency of the medial and lateral tibial plateau was found. (c) The defect was filled with TMT cone and cancellous allograft. (d) Postoperative radiological result.

4.6 Custom-made prostheses

Custom-made prostheses represent an excellent biomechanical solution; nevertheless they show some disadvantages:

- High costs.
- Delay until the implant is available.
- Poor versatility during surgery.

Custom-made implants are currently being indicated for treatment of complex bone loss and for peripheral defects exceeding 15 mm in depth (Fig. 9). Use of custom implants have been reduced with the advent of modular prosthesis.

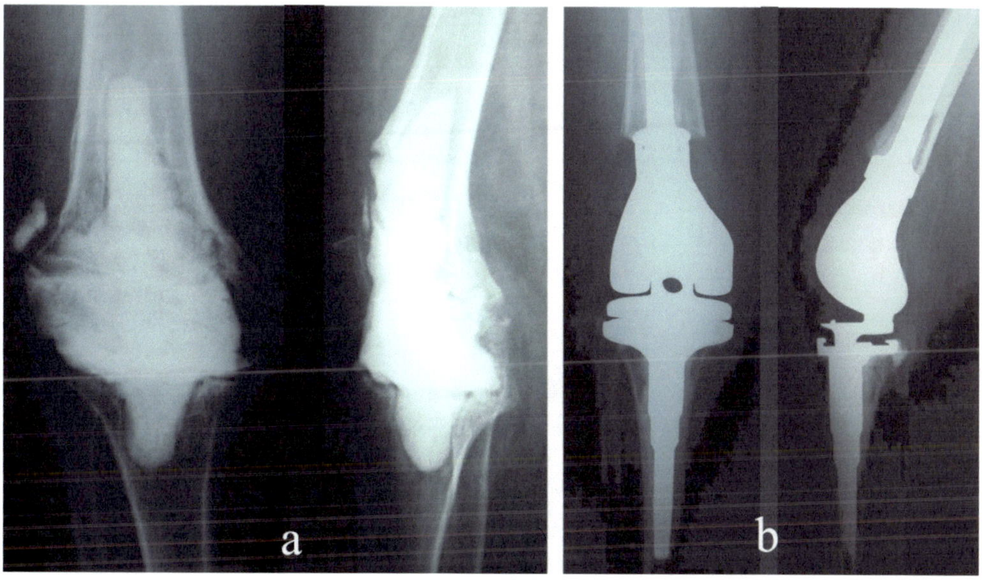

Fig. 10. (a) Severe bone defect caused by septic mobilisation and treated with two-staged revision. (b) Reconstruction was made with custom-made hinged prosthesis.

5. Surgical management

Whatever classification used to determine best treatment and whatever any surgical option is available (Table 4), always have to be considered some rules.

Careful component removal is critical to preserve bone stock; the cancellous bone is much weaker away from the native articular surface.

We prefer the use of a small sagittal saw and flexible osteotomes to loosen the components and their fixation interfaces. After careful and successful exposure and component removal, the surgeon assesses the bone defects and begins the reconstruction.

Tibia influences the flexion and extension spaces and establishes a platform for the subsequent arthroplasty. The surgeon must recognize severe proximal tibial bone loss, and recreate the appropriate height to allow for proper component placement and gap balancing. With contained defects, the goal is to obtain firm seating of the tibial tray on a rim of viable bone along with rigid press fixation of an intramedullary stem. Likewise, femoral condyle bone loss can influence femoral component's size and sagittal position. The joint line is an average of 25 mm from the lateral epicondyle and 30 mm from the medial epicondyle; the distance from the epicondyles to the posterior joint line is similar to the distal joint line and is helpful in confirming the correct femoral component size.

Adjustments to ensure correct femoral component rotation usually require augmentation of the posterolateral condyle; additional modification to the position and size of the femoral component may be needed as the flexion and extension gaps are balanced. Once the gaps are equal and stable, the tibial polyethylene is correctly sized.

If there is functional loss of the medial or lateral collateral ligaments, soft tissue instability, inability to balance the flexion and extension spaces, or a severe valgus deformity, then a constrained condylar prosthesis is necessary.

Defect Type			Treatment Options
Clatworthy classification	*Engh classification*	*Rand classification*	
Contained, undamaged metaphysis	1	<5 mm depth, <50% unicondylar/plateau involvement	Prosthetic component translation, PMMA fill, morcelized allograft, autograft
Contained undamaged metaphysis	2a	5-10 mm depth, >50% unilateral condylar/plateau involvement	Morcelized allograft or metal augments
Contained undamaged metaphysis	2a	10-20 mm depth, unicondylar/plateau involvement	Metal augments, metaphyseal sleeves, structural allografts
Contained undamaged metaphysis	2b	<20mm depth, bicondylar/plateau involvement	Metal augments (full block in tibia), metaphyseal sleeves, structural allografts
Uncontained damaged metaphysis	2b	<20mm depth, bicondylar/plateau involvement	TM cones, structural allografts, custom-made prostheses
Uncontained damaged metaphysis	3	>20 mm depth	Structural allografts, megaprostheses, custom-made prostheses, TM cones

Table 4. Surgical algorithm according to bone defect size.

6. Patellar bone loss

Compromised patellar bone stock poses significant technical problems in primary and revision knee arthroplasty. In revision knee surgery bone deficiency is normally secondary to loosening of the patellar button and osteolysis that affects severely the patella. In primary cases it is rare that the patella has been so eroded that resurfacing is not possible.

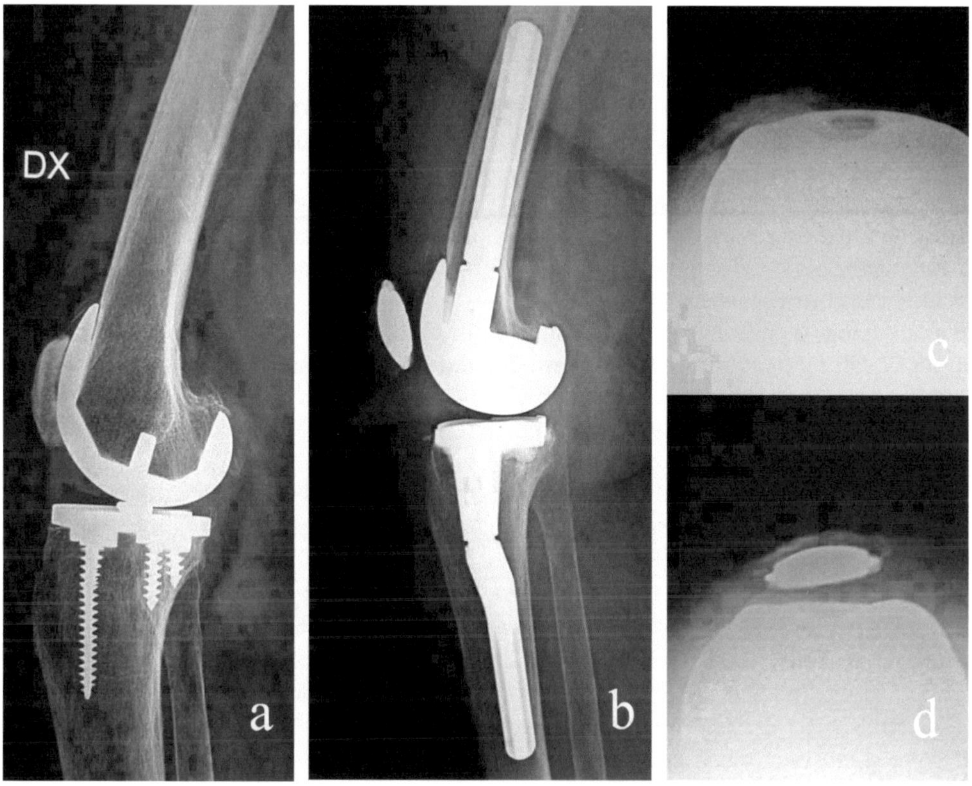

Fig. 11. (a,b) Lateral radiographs of total knee prosthesis revision, with patella extremely dug out, long and thin on preoperative. (c) Note lateral patella subluxation, and reestablishment of correct balancing after TMT patella prosthesis implantation.

This happens in severe patello-femoral arthritis or inflammatory arthropathy, when the patella may be thin and track laterally before and during arthroplasty. Treatment depends on the quality of the remaining bone stock and options include non-resurfacing, retention of the remaining thin patellar shell or total patellectomy (Pagnano et al., 1998). Nevertheless these solutions have been associated with lower functional results compared with resurfaced patella. A patellar bone grafting procedure has been described to provide patellar bone for possible future revision (Hassen, 2001). The "gull wing" patellar osteotomy (Kelly et al., 2002) has also been proposed in case of low demand patients, whereas in some cases it is possible to rebuild a damaged patella with K-wires in a reinforcing configuration to support the pegs of the patellar implant using the so called "rebar" technique (Tigani et al, 2009). Trabecular metal patella represents a viable therapeutic option for severe damaged patella; we experienced use with this technique (Tigani et al., 2009) in revision cases with more than 50% amount of residual bone, obtaining reliable bony fixation despite the quality of residual bone (Fig. 11).

We therefore exclude TM patella in cases of previous patellectomy, where soft tissue have to be used for fixation of the TM implant, because of reported migration and loosening of the implant in these difficult cases.

7. Intramedullary stems

In revision total knee arthroplasty, the mechanical stability of the femoral and tibial components is increased by the addition of intramedullary stems. Whatever solution is indicating to compensate bone loss, the use of an extended femoral and tibial stems reduce the stress forces on the metaphyseal region and bone-implant interface. Stem extensions, with or without offset, can supplement fixation, decrease stress at the bone-implant interface, and help address asymmetric bone defects. Offset stems can assist with implant alignment on the metaphysis, reducing the incidence of coronal or sagittal components malalignment and helping balance the flexion and extension spaces by effectively translating the components.

The stem ability to protect the proximal tibia or distal femur has been demonstrated in a laboratory setting using finite element model and cadaver models. Brooks et al used stems in conjunction with various bone augmentation techniques for defect in the proximal tibia: they suggested that a 70-mm stem carried from 23% to 38% of the axial load (Brooks et al., 1984).

A finite element analysis has revealed that the predicted bone loss is even greater in stemmed components compared to stemless ones; this may have consequences to discouraged routine use of stems in revision TKA (van Lenthe et al., 2002). Nevertheless Stern and Insall (Stern & Insall, 1992) advocates routine use of stemmed components in revision TKA. Engh et al used femoral stems mainly to protect large structural grafts in revision TKA (Engh et al., 1997). Meneghini et al. advise the use of cemented stemmed extension to maximize early implant fixation and allow for successful biologic ingrowth of the TM cones into the remaining part of the bone (Meneghini et al., 2008). We recommend to add stem extensions when using metal augments to decrease stress at the bone-implant interface.

Cemented stems allow for intraoperative adjustment with unusual anatomy and achieve fixation in large canals and osteopenic bone (Murray et al., 1994). The main disadvantages are that they are difficult to remove if revision is necessary and since they are not canal filling, they do not guarantee alignment (Parsley et al., 2003). Cementless press-fit stem extensions are easy to use and facilitate component alignment, and diaphyseal engaging stems ensure fixation (Radnay & Scuderi, 2006). In our practice with stemmed components of TKA, we prefer to use hybrid fixation in both femur and tibia, with proximal cementation just in the metaphyseal area as usual. In fact, Jazrawi et al. demonstrated in a cadaveric study that a press-fit modular cementless stem could achieve equivalent stability than a somewhat shorter fully cemented stem (Jazrawi et al., 2001), whereas Albrektsson et al. showed with radiostereogrammetic analysis that a long cementless stem provide optional stability (Albrektsson et al., 1990).

8. Future perspectives

We verified that treatment of bone defects associated with knee prosthetic surgery include many different surgical techniques and options, each with specific disadvantages and complications. Generally, in the elderly bone loss should be accomplished using artificial materials, while in younger patients, therapy should be addressed to regeneration of new bone as a foundation for future revision procedures. So that, an ideal bone substitute should possesses osteogenic, osteoinductive and osteoconductive potential.

The "osteogenic" potential of the graft corresponds to capacity of cells living within the donor graft to survive during transplantation, then proliferate and differentiate to osteblasts and eventually to osteocytes. "Osteoinduction" on the other hand is the stimulation and activation of host mesenchymal stem cells from the surrounding tissue, which differentiate into bone-forming osteoblasts. This process is mediated by a cascade of signals and the activations of several extra and intracellular receptors the most important of which belong to the TGF-beta family (Cypher & Grossman, 1996). "Osteoconduction" describes the facilitation and orientation of blood-vessel and the creation of the new Haversian systems into the bone scaffold. Finally these three properties together allow "osteointegration" between the host bone and the grafting material surfaces (Giannoudis et al., 2005).

The gold standard for regeneration of new bone is autologous bone graft, which contains a scaffold, osteoblasts, and the necessary signalling proteins and molecules. However, autograft is of limited availability and may be insufficient due to poor quality (eg, osteoporosis). Furthermore, it may fail in clinical practice as most of the cellular (osteogenic) elements do not survive transplantion (Sandhu et al., 1999).

Thus alternatives to autograft bone have emerged. Perhaps the most common bone substitute is cancellous allograft, which is osteoconductive only, and rely on a viable vascularized bone bed for incorporation. Moreover bone graft provided by musculoskeletal tissue bank could provoke immune response and transmission of viral disease; the processing of allograft tissue lowers this risk but can significantly weaken the biologic and mechanical properties initially present in the bone tissue (Giannoudis et al., 2005).

Bone substitutes could be used to replenish lost bone stock during total knee arthroplasty. A bone-graft substitute to be useful should be: osteoconductive, osteoinductive, biocompatible, bio-resorbable, structurally similar to bone, easy to use, and cost-effective (Giannoudis et al., 2005).

Recombinant growth factors such as bone morphogenetic proteins (BMPs) have osteoinductive capacity (Greenwald et al., 2001). Nevertheless because they are powerful in small amounts, and they are expensive, their indication in knee prosthetic surgery is still limited. Contrary platelet rich plasma (PRP) is largely available as it is prepared from centrifugation of autologous blood; it is an osteopromotive adjunct with the ability to enhance natural bone formation by stimulatory signals. Both BMPs and PRP need a scaffold to support their bone regeneration properties.

Demineralized bone matrix (DBM) corresponds to portion of bone without the mineral phases, extracted by strong acids (Peterson et al., 2004). The demineralization process leaves behind the growth factors, the noncollagenous proteins and collagen, and therefore DBM is osteoconductive and osteoinductive. However, few prospective, randomized clinical studies delineate the efficacy of DBM, and the material can be costly.

Nowadays many synthetic substitutes are available, used either alone or in combination with other biologic adjuncts. Synthetic bone graft materials available include calcium sulphates, special glass ceramics (bioactive glasses) and calcium phosphates. Calcium phosphate-based implants have the most similar composition to human bone, in particular those made of hydroxyapatite (HA) (Paderni et al., 2009). HA-based substitutes provide an osteoconductive scaffold to which mesenchymal stem cells and osteoinductive growth factors can migrate and differentiate into functioning osteoblasts (Fujishiro et al., 2005). These materials can be sterilized and are moldable, but generally do not have sufficient mechanical properties to support full immediate weight bearing.

Despite of being osteoconductive, the HA is not osteoinductive: in order to achieve a satisfying bone ingrowth, further factors could be added, such as multipotential stromal stem cells or PRP growth factors (Boyde et al., 1999), in order to favour and accelerate bone regeneration. Nowadays, combination of mature stromal cells and HA-based scaffolds represent an useful tissue regeneration approach to be used in a clinical setting: unfortunately, only few papers describe the clinical use of massive graft made of HA-based scaffolds (Marcacci et al., 2007) and long-term comparative studies are needed to evaluate their clinical effectiveness (Table 5).

Material		Osteoconduction	Osteoinduction	Osteogenesis	Notes
Bone autograft		+++	++	++	Gold standard: all elements for bone regeneration
Bone allograft	Structural	+++	\	\	Fresh frozen allografts show better mechanical properties than freeze-dried ones.
	Morcelised	+	\	\	
Bone morphogenetic proteins (BMPs)		\	+++	+	Potentially limited availability. Scaffold is needed
Platelet-rich plasma (PRP)		\	++	++	Large availability. Scaffold is needed
Demineralized bone matrix (DBM)		++	+	\	High cost
Hydroxyapatite (HA)		++	\	\	Immediate structural support
Composite grafts: BMPs+HA		+++	+++	+++	Good perspective in the future

Table 5. Different materials available as bone substitutes and their respective biologic properties.

9. Conclusions

As the incidence of primary and revision total knee arthroplasty will continue to increase, proper management of femoral and tibial bone loss represents a common situation that have to be faced by the orthopedic surgeon. The choice between different surgical options depends on dimension and characteristics of bone defect but are also patient-related.

Whatever technique is used in the management of bone loss during knee arthroplasty, certain fundamentals must be applied and the remaining bone structure will guide treatment. For treatment of any periarticular defect requiring more than a minimal prosthetic augment, it is imperative to use stemmed components to transfer stress away from the joint line. Reestablishment of well-aligned and stable implants is necessary for successful reconstruction, but this can't be accomplished without a sufficient restoration of an eventual bone loss.

10. Acknowledgment

We thank Mrs Mariapia Cumani for graphical support.
The authors did not receive any outside funding or grants in support of their research or for preparation of this work.

11. References

Albrektsson, B.E.; Ryd, L.; Carlsson, L.V.; Freeman, M.A.; Herberts, P.; Regnér, L. & Selvik, G. (1990). The effect of a stem on the tibial component of knee arthroplasty. A roentgen stereophotogrammetric study of uncemented tibial components in the Freeman-Samuelson knee arthroplasty. *J Bone Joint Surg Br*, Vol.72, No.2, (March 1990), pp. 252-8, ISSN 0301-620X

Backstein, D.; Safir, O. & Gross, A. (2006). Management of bone loss: structural grafts in revision total knee arthroplasty. *Clin Orthop Relat Res*, Vol.446, (May 2006), pp.104-12, ISSN 1528-1132

Bobyn, J.D.; Stackpool, G.J.; Hacking, S.A.; Tanzer, M. & Krygier, J.J. (1999). Characteristics of bone ingrowth and interface mechanics of a new porous tantalum biomaterial. *J Bone Joint Surg Br*, Vol.81, No.5, (September 1999), pp.907-14, ISSN 0301-620X

Boyde, A.; Corsi, A.; Quarto, R.; Cancedda, R. & Bianco, P. (1999). Osteoconduction in large macroporous hydroxyapatite ceramic implants: evidence for a complementary integration and disintegration mechanism. *Bone*, Vol.24, No.6, (June 1999), pp.579–89, ISSN 1873-2763

Brooks, P.J., Walker, P.S. & Scott, R.D. (1984). Tibial component fixation in deficient tibial bone stock. *Clin Orthop Relat Res*, Vol.184, (April 1984), pp.302-8, ISSN 1528-1132

Clatworthy, M. & Gross, A.E. (2003). Management of bony defects in revision total knee arthroplasty. In: *The Adult Knee*, JJ Callaghan, AG Rosenberg, HE Rubash, PT Simonian, TL Wickiewicz, (Eds.), 1455-64, Lippincott Williams & Wilkins, ISBN 0-7817-3247-6, Philadelphia, PA

Cypher, T.J. & Grossman, J.P. (1996). Biological principles of bone graft healing. *J Foot Ankle Surg*, Vol.35, No.5, (September-October 1996), pp.413-7, ISSN 0449-2544

De Long, W.G. Jr; Einhorn, T.A.; Koval, K.; McKee, M.; Smith, W.; Sanders, R. & Watson, T. (2007). Bone grafts and bone graft substitutes in orthopaedic trauma surgery. A critical analysis. *J Bone Joint Surg Am*, Vol.89, No.3, (March 2007), pp.649-58, ISSN 1535-1386

Dorr, L.D.; Ranawat, C.S.; Sculco, T.A.; McKaskill, B. & Orisek, B.S. (1986). Bone graft for tibial defects in total knee arthroplasty. *Clin Orthop Relat Res* Vol.205, (April 1986), pp.153-65, ISSN 1528-1132

Engh, G.A. & Ammeen, D.J. (1999). Bone loss with revision total knee arthroplasty: defect classification and alternatives for reconstruction. *Instr Course Lect, Vol.*48, (1999), pp.167-75, ISSN 0065-6895

Engh, G.A. & Ammeen, D.J. (2007). Uses of structural allograft in revision total knee arthroplasty in knees with sever tibial bone loss. *J Bone Joint Surg Am,* Vol.89, No.12, (December 2007), pp.2640-7, ISSN 1535-1386

Engh, G.A.; Herzwurm, P.J. & Parks, N.L. (1997).Treatment of major defects of bone with bulk allografts and stemmed components during total knee arthroplasty.*JBone JointSurg Am,*Vol.79,No.7,(July 1997),pp.1030-9,ISSN 1535-1386

Freeman, M.A.; Bradley, G.W. & Revell, P.A. (1982). Observations upon the interface between bone and polymethylmethacrylate cement. *J Bone Joint Surg Br,* Vol.64, No.4, (1982), pp.489-93, ISSN 0301-620X

Fujishiro, T.; Nishikawa, T.; Niikura, T.; Takikawa, S.; Nishiyama, T.; Mizuno, K.; Yoshiya, S. & Kurosaka, M. (2005). Impaction bone grafting with hydroxyapatite: increased femoral component stability in experiments using Sawbones. *Acta Orthop,* Vol.76, No.4, (August 2005), pp.550–4, ISSN 1745-3682

Giannoudis, P.V.; Dinopoulos, H. & Tsiridis, E. (2005). Bone substitutes: an update. *Injury,* Vol.36, Suppl 3, (November 2005), pp.20-7, ISSN 1879-0267

Greenwald, A.S.; Boden, S.D.; Goldberg, V.M.; Khan, Y.; Laurencin, C.T. & Rosier, R.N. (2001). Bone-graft substitutes: facts, fictions and application. *J Bone Joint Surg Am.* Vol.83, Suppl 2 Pt 2, (2001), pp.98-103, ISSN 1535-1386

Haidukewych, G.J.; Hanssen, A. & Jones, R.D. (2011). Metaphyseal fixation in revision total knee arthroplasty: indications and techniques. *J Am Acad Orthop Surg.* Vol.19, No.6, (June 2011), pp.311-8, ISSN 1067-151X

Hassen, A. (2001). Bone-grafting for severe patellar bone loss during revision knee arthroplasty. *J Bone J Surg Am,* Vol.83, No.2, (February 2001), pp.171–6, ISSN 1535-1386

Insall, J.N. & Easley, M.E. (2001). Surgical techniques and instrumentation in total knee arthroplasty. In: *Surgery of the knee,* JN Insall, WN Scott (Eds.), ISBN 978-0-443-06682-5, Churchill-Livingstone, New York

Jazrawi, L.M.; Bai, B.; Kummer, F.J.; Hiebert, R. & Stuchin, S.A. (2001). The effect of stem modularity and mode of fixation on tibial component stability in revision total knee arthroplasty. *J Arthroplasty,* Vol.16, No.6, (September 2001), pp.759-67, ISSN 1532-8406

Kelly, M.A. (2004). Extensor mechanism complications in total knee arthroplasty. *Instr Course Lect,* Vol.53, (2004), pp.193-9, ISSN 0065-6895

Laskin, R.S. (1989). Total knee arthroplasty in the presence of bony defects of the tibia and marked knee instability. *Clin Orthop Relat Res,* Vol.248, (November 1989), pp.66-70, ISSN 1528-1132

Levine, B.; Sporer, S.; Della Valle, C.J.; Jacobs, J.J. & Paprosky, W. (2007). Porous tantalum in reconstructive surgery of the knee: a review. *J Knee Surg,* Vol.20, No.3, (July 2007), pp.185-94, ISSN 1938-2480

Lombardi, A.V.; Berend, K.R. & Adams, J.B. (2010). Management of bone loss in revision TKA: it's a changing world. *Orthopedics,* Vol.33, No.9, (September 2010), pp.662, ISSN 1938-2367

Lotke, P.A.; Wong, R.Y.& Ecker, M.L. (1991). The use of methylmethacrylate in primary total knee replacements with large tibial defects. *Clin Orthop Relat Res,* Vol.270, (September 2001), pp.288-94, ISSN 1528-1132

Lucey, S.D.; Scuderi, G.R.; Kelly, M.A. & Insall, J.N. (2000). A practical approach to dealing with bone loss in revision total knee arthroplasty. *Orthopedics*, Vol.23, No.10, (October 2000), pp.1036–41, ISSN 1938-2367

Marcacci, M.; Kon, E.; Mukhacev, V.; Lavroukov, A.; Kutepov, S.; Quarto, R.; Mastrogiacomo, M. & Cancedda, R. (2007). Stem cells associated with macroporous bioceramics for long bone repair: 6 to 7-year outcome of a pilot clinical study. *Tissue Eng.* Vol.13, No.5, (May 2007), pp.947–955, ISSN 1557-8690

Meneghini, R.M.; Lewallen, D.G.& Hanssen, A.D. (2008). Use of porous tantalum metaphyseal cones for severe tibial bone loss during revision total knee replacement. *J Bone Joint Surg Am*, Vol.9, No. 1, Januay 2008, pp.78-84, ISSN 1535-1386

Mounasamy, V.; Ma, S.Y.; Schoderbek, R.J.; Mihalko, W.M.; Saleh, K.J. & Brown, T.E. (2006). Primary total knee arthroplasty with condylar allograft and MCL reconstruction for a comminuted medial condyle fracture in an arthritic knee-a case report. *Knee*, Vol.13, No.5, (October 2006), pp.400-3, ISSN 1873-5800

Murray, P.B.; Rand, J.A. & Hanssen, A.D. (1994). Cemented long-stem revision total knee arthroplasty. *Clin Orthop Relat Res*, Vol.309, (December 1994), pp.116-23, ISSN 1528-1132

Paderni, S.; Terzi, S. & Amendola, L. (2009). Major bone defect treatment with an osteoconductive bone substitute. *Chir Organi Mov*, Vol.93, No.2, (September 2009), pp.89-96, ISSN 1973-2538

Pagnano, M.W.; Scuderi, G.R. & Insall, J.N. (1998). Patellar component resection in revision and reimplantation TKA. *Clin Orthop Relat Res*, Vol.356, (November 1998), pp.134–8, ISSN 1528-1132

Pagnotto, M.; Fedorka, C.J.; McGough, R.L.; Crossett, L.S. & Klatt, B.A. (2011). Revision total knee replacement with porous-coated metaphyseal sleeves. Paper. In: *AAOS 2011 Annual Meeting*, San Diego, February 2011

Parsley, B.S.; Sugano, N.; Bertolusso, R. & Conditt, M.A. (2003). Mechanical alignment of tibial stems in revision total knee arthroplasty. *J Arthroplasty*. Vol.18, Suppl 1, (October 2003), pp.33–6, ISSN 1532-8406

Peterson, B.; Whang, P.G.; Iglesias, R.; Wang, J.C. & Lieberman, J.R. (2004). Osteoconductivity of commercially available demineralized bone matrix. *J Bone Joint Surg Am*. Vol.86, No.10, (October 2004), pp.2243-50, ISSN 1535-1386

Radnay, C.S. & Scuderi, G.R. (2006). Management of bone loss: augments, cones, offset stems. *Clin Orthop Relat Res*, Vol.446, (May 2006), pp.83-92, ISSN 1528-1132

Rand, J.A. (1991). Bone deficiency in total knee arthroplasty. Use of metal wedge augmentation. *Clin Orthop Relat Res*, Vol.271, (October 1991), pp.63-71, ISSN 1528-1132

Rand, J.A. (1998). Modular augments in revision total knee arthroplasty. *Orthop Clin North Am*, Vol. 29, No.2, (April 1998), pp.347–53, ISSN 1558-1373

Reish, T.G.; Clarke, H.D.; Scuderi, G.R.; Math, K.R. & Scott, W.N. (2006). Use of multi-detector computed tomography for the detection of periprosthetic osteolysis in total knee arthroplasty. *J Knee Surg*, Vol.19, No.4, (October 2006), pp.259-64, ISSN 1938-2480

Ritter, M.A.; Keating, E.M.& Faris, P.M. (1993). Screw and cement fixation of large defects in total knee arthroplasty. A sequel. *J Arthroplasty*, Vol.8, No.1, (February 1993), pp.63-5, ISSN 1532-8406

Sandhu, H.S.; Grewal, H.S. & Parvataneni, H. (1999). Bone grafting for spinal fusion. *Orthop Clin North Am*, Vol.30, No.4, (October 1999), pp.685-98, ISSN 1558-1373

Scuderi, G.R.; Insall, J.N. & HaasSB. (1989). Inlay autogenic bone grafting of tibial defects in primary total knee arthroplasty *Clin Orthop Relat Res*, Vol.248, (November 1989), pp.93-7

Stern, S.H. & Insall, J.N. (1992). Posterior stabilized prosthesis. Results after follow-up of nine to twelve years. *J Bone Joint Surg Am*, Vol.74, No.7, (August 1992), pp.980-6, ISSN 1535-1386

Tigani, D.; Dallari, D.; Coppola, C.; Ben Ayad, R.; Sabbioni, G. & Fosco, M. (2011). Total knee arthroplasty for post-traumatic proximal tibial bone defect: three cases report. *Open Orthop J*, Vol.14,No.5,(April 2011),pp.143-50,ISSN 1874-3250

Tigani, D.; Trentani, P.; Trentani, F.; Andreoli, I.; Sabbioni, G. & Del Piccolo, N. (2009). Trabecular metal patella in total knee arthroplasty with patella bone deficiency. *Knee*, Vol.16, No.1, (January 2009), pp.46-9, ISSN 1873-5800

Tigani, D.; Trentani, P.; Trentani, F.; Marinelli, A.; Bianchi, G. & Fravisini, M. (2004). The treatment of bone defects in primary arthroplasty of the knee. *Chir Organi Mov*, Vol.89, No.1, (January-March 2004),pp.29-33, ISSN 1973-2538

van Lenthe, G.H.; Willems, M.M.; Verdonschot, N.; de Waal Malefijt, M.C. & Huiskes, R. (2002). Stemmed femoral knee prostheses: effects of prosthetic design and fixation on bone loss. *Acta Orthop Scand*, Vol.73, No.6, (December 2002), pp.630-7, ISSN 0001-6470

Van Loon, C.J.; de Waal Malefijt, M.C.; Buma, P.; Verdonschot, N. & Veth, R.P. (1999). Femoral bone loss in total knee arthroplasty. A review. *Acta Orthop Belg*, Vol.65, No.2, (June 1999), pp.154-63, ISSN 0001-6462

Part 4

Infection

19

Infection in Primary Hip and Knee Arthroplasty

Michelle M. Dowsey, Trisha N. Peel and Peter F.M. Choong
University of Melbourne, Department of Surgery, St. Vincent's Hospital Melbourne
Department of Orthopaedics, St. Vincent's Hospital Melbourne
Australia

1. Introduction

Since the advent of prosthetic joint replacement, patients suffering from bone and joint pathology have benefited from significant improvements in mobility and pain relief. In Australia 39,200 hip replacements and 39,500 knee replacements were performed in 2009 (Australian Orthopaedic Association National Joint Replacement Registry [AOA NJRR]) (Graves, et al. 2010). With an ageing population, the number of patients undergoing these procedures is projected to increase significantly over time. Data from the United States of America predicts that by 2030, the number of patients undergoing primary hip and knee replacement will increase by 174% and 673% respectively (Kurtz, et al. 2007). The major complication of such techniques is infection of the prosthetic device, which is associated with significant costs to individual patients and to the public health system. Significant morbidity is associated with prosthetic joint infections including the need for further operative procedures, long-term antibiotic therapy, and prolonged hospitalisation. Thereafter, the mortality rate from prosthetic joint infection is estimated to be between 1.0 to 2.7 procent (Ahnfelt, et al. 1990, Zimmerli 2006, Zimmerli, et al. 2004). Aside from the effects on the individual patient, the financial cost to the health system is considerable. The estimated hospital costs is $ 96 166 (US) per patient requiring revision arthroplasty for infection, which is 4.8 times the cost of a primary arthroplasty(Bozic & Ries 2005).
This chapter examines the underlying epidemiology, diagnosis, treatment and challenges in managing this problem.

2. Epidemiology

2.1 Incidence

Identification of prosthetic joint infection currently relies on diagnostic criteria, which include: histopathologic evidence of acute inflammation of periprosthetic tissue, presence of a sinus tract, macroscopic purulence surrounding the prosthesis observed intraoperatively or two or more positive microbiological cultures with the same organism isolated from the prosthetic joint fluid or tissue(Berbari, et al. 1998). We report a rate of prosthetic joint infection between 1.0 – 2.0% in primary lower limb arthroplasty and this is congruent with current literature (Dowsey & Choong 2008, 2009, Swan, et al. 2011). In the United States the rate of infection in knee and hip arthroplasty was 0.92% and 0.88% respectively in a recent review of Medicare data. (Kurtz, et al. 2008). The majority of arthroplasty infections occur in the two years following prosthetic joint surgery. The incidence of knee arthroplasty infection within 2 years was 1.55% decreasing to 0.46% in the subsequent 8 years. Corresponding data in the hip arthroplasty population showed an incidence of 1.63% within 2 years and 0.59% between two to ten years (Kurtz, et al. 2010, Ong, et al. 2009)

2.2 Risk factors

A number of preoperative risk factors for prosthetic joint infection have been identified and these include pre-existing patient co-morbidities such as obesity, diabetes mellitus, rheumatoid arthritis and a history of prior malignancy. Body mass index (BMI) greater than $40kg/m^2$ has been associated with a 9 fold increased risk of knee infection in our series (Dowsey & Choong 2009). Similar studies have shown that for every 1 kg/m^2 increase in body mass index, there was an associated 8% increase in the risk of deep prosthetic joint infection. The association between obesity and deep prosthetic infections is particularly marked in the hip arthroplasty population with the risk of infection increasing from 0.9% in patients within the normal weight range, to 9.1% in morbidly obese(Choong, et al. 2007, Dowsey & Choong 2008). Diabetes mellitus also predisposes patients to deep prosthetic joint infection with 5.3% of diabetic patients developing a prosthetic joint infection in one study (Dowsey & Choong 2009, Yang, et al. 2001). Postulated mechanisms for the increased risk include impaired leucocyte function and impaired wound healing in diabetic patients. Rheumatoid arthritis has been associated with a higher risk of deep prosthetic joint infections. Patients with rheumatoid arthritis have been reported to have a greater than 2.5 fold increase in the risk of arthroplasty infection compared to patients with osteoarthritis (Bengtson & Knutson 1991, Poss, et al. 1984). Whether this is due to impaired immunity secondary to the underlying disease or whether it is a reflection of the increased use of immunosuppressive medications in this cohort remains unclear (Berbari, et al. 2006b). A diagnosis of malignancy not involving the index joint has been identified as a risk factor for the subsequent development of prosthetic joint infection(Berbari, et al. 1998).

Operative risk factors associated with deep prosthetic joint infection include higher American Society of Anaesthesiologist's (ASA) and National Nosocomial Infections Surveillance (NNIS) scores, bilateral surgery, knee arthroplasty, arthroplasty type and operating room conditions. Berbari et al showed that increasing NNIS score was associated with increasing risk of deep prosthetic joint infection; NNIS score 1 was associated with a 1.7 fold increase, increasing to 3.9 with a NNIS score of 2 (Berbari, et al. 1998). The ASA score, a component of the NNIS score, was also associated with an increased risk of arthroplasty infections (Pulido, et al. 2008). Pulido et al identified close to a six-fold increase in risk of prosthetic joint infection in patients undergoing simultaneous bilateral arthroplasty surgery. In the same study, knee arthroplasty, when compared to hip arthroplasty, was independently associated with a higher risk of developing deep prosthetic joint infection (Pulido, et al. 2008). The type of prosthesis used also appears to influence the risk of infection. A 20-fold increased risk of infection with metal hinged prosthetic knee joints compared to metal-to-plastic prostheses has been reported (Poss, et al. 1984).

A number of postoperative risk factors for prosthetic joint infection have also been identified. The most important of these appears to be postoperative wound complications including the presence of superficial infection and/or wound discharge (Bengtson & Knutson 1991, Surin, et al. 1983, Wymenga, et al. 1992). Superficial infection, occurs within 30 days of the operative procedure, only involves the superficial structures and additionally includes one of the following features: purulent discharge, isolation of micro-organisms through aseptic sampling techniques or clinical features of infection (Horan, et al. 1992). Applying this definition, patients with a postoperative surgical site infection had around a 36 fold increase in the risk of the subsequent development of a deep prosthetic wound in one study(Berbari, et al. 1998). Similarly, in another study examining patients with deep prosthetic infections acquired in the perioperative period, 25 of the 26 patients described preceding wound complications, which included; the persistent drainage of fluid from the wound, development of a haematoma under the wound, a superficial infection or a stitch abscesses (Poss, et al. 1984). Of note we have demonstrated that the use of closed suction drainage in total knee arthroplasty is protective of prosthetic knee infection and this may be due the role of a drainage tube in minimizing haematoma formation (Dowsey & Choong 2009). Early post-operative persistent discharge of fluid from the wound has been associated with a 3.2 times higher risk of deep prosthetic joint infection. Often in these cases the same pathogenic organisms isolated from the discharging fluid is later recovered at time of reoperation on the infected hip (Surin, et al. 1983).

Postoperative medical complications including atrial fibrillation and myocardial infarction have also been implicated as risk factors for deep prosthetic joint infection, with a 6-fold and 20-fold respective increase reported (Pulido, et al. 2008). One postulated mechanism to account for this association is that standard management of these medical conditions includes anticoagulation. In the postoperative period this may increase the risk of bleeding and haematoma formation near the wound, which in itself may increase the risk of infection. Secondly, these medical complications may necessitate longer inpatient hospital stay, which may be associated with nosocomial acquisition of infection. Allogenic blood transfusion was also identified as conferring a twofold increased risk of prosthetic infection, again the risk may be via an association with bleeding and haematoma formation near the wound, or possibly as a marker of complications and prolonged hospitalisation (Pulido, et al. 2008).

Nosocomial infections, particularly urinary tract infections have also been identified as risk factors for deep prosthetic joint infections. Surin et al demonstrated that patients with remote infections in the postoperative period were three times more likely to develop deep infections. Over three quarters of these infections were urinary tract infections. Interestingly however, there was no correlation between causative agents of the nosocomial infection and the micro-organism ultimately isolated from the infected prosthesis (Surin, et al. 1983). These results have been confirmed by other studies (Pulido, et al. 2008, Wilson, et al. 1990). Bengston et al highlighted the significance of skin infections in haematogenous seeding of the prosthesis. One third of patients with haematogenous seeding in this cohort had concurrent or preceding skin infections that were identified as the probable primary focus for the bacteraemia(Bengtson & Knutson 1991).

2.3 Microbiology

Staphylococcus species account for approximately half of all prosthetic joint infections; this includes *Staphylococcus aureus* and coagulase negative Staphylococcus species, both methicillin sensitive and resistant. Gram-negative bacilli infections and polymicrobial infections are the two next most common groups of pathogens described. Other gram-positive bacteria such as Streptococcus and Enterococcus species occur less commonly (Bengtson & Knutson 1991, Berbari, et al. 1998, Fitzgerald, et al. 1977, Moran, et al. 2007, Pandey, et al. 2000, Pulido, et al. 2008, Steckelberg & Osmon 2000). Importantly, in all series, a small number of cases meet the definition for prosthetic joint infection, and yet remain culture negative on standard microbiologic techniques.

Reference	1	2	3	4	5	6	7	8	9	
Total number of isolates	***112***	***248***	***81***	***578***	***63***	***462***	***357***	***42***	***112***	
Coagulase negative Staphylococcus	13	31	48	30	21	19	17	24	33	**27.3**
Staphylococcus aureus	23	21	14	23	38	22	42	19	17	**23.8**
Streptococcus spp	5	7	10	9	13	9	6	12	10.7	**9.4**
Enterococcus spp	3	6	7	3	0	1	3	10	6.3	**4.6**
Diptheroids	2	4	4	0.5	2	0.6	1	0	5.4	**2.6**
Gram-negative bacilli	6	28	0	6	11	8	5	29	16.1	**12.7**
Propionibacterium	0	0.4	3	1.5	0	0	0.3	2	0.9	**0.9**
Polymicrobial	33	0	12	12	6	19	15	0	0	**9.7**
Anaerobes	3	2	0	2	0	6	2	2	6.3	**3.0**
Other	1	4	0	2	0	3	0.3	19	2.7	**3.5**
Culture negative	5	0	0	11	10	12	8	2	1.8	**5.2**

1. (Moran, et al. 2007), 2. (Sharma, et al. 2008), 3. (Pandey, et al. 2000), 4. (Steckelberg & Osmon 2000), 5. (Pulido, et al. 2008), 6. (Berbari, et al. 1998), 7. (Bengtson & Knutson 1991), 8. (Fitzgerald, et al. 1977), 9. (McDonald, et al. 1989)

Table 1. Microbiological isolates in reported literature (percent)

3. Pathogenesis

3.1 Acquisition of infection

Acquisition of prosthetic joint infection occurs by two mechanisms: direct inoculation and haematogenous seeding. Direct inoculation of the prosthesis may occur at the time of implantation or with manipulation of the arthroplasty and is thought to be the predominant mechanism of infection. In a study by Southwood et al the 50% infective dose (ID_{50}) of *Staphylococcus aureus* required to induce infection with direct inoculation of the prosthesis was just 50 organisms. This compared to an intravenous inoculum dose of 100 000 organisms at the time of operation for bacteraemic seeding and infection of the prosthesis to occur. Southwood also demonstrated that three weeks after implantation of the prosthesis, the likelihood of bacteraemic seeding of the prosthesis was significantly reduced. In fact, in the rabbit model, the inoculum of intravenous bacteria required was near to the lethal dose(Southwood, et al. 1985). Nevertheless, haematogenous seeding remains an important cause of arthroplasty infections and it has been reported that up to 34% of patients with prosthetic joints in-situ developed deep infection of that prosthesis following an intercurrent episode of *Staphylococcus aureus* bacteraemia (Murdoch, et al. 2001).

Whilst theoretically distinct, clinically there is significant overlap between both mechanisms of infection. The simplified view is that infection resulting from inoculation occurs within the first year of implantation whilst haematogenous infections occur later. However the clinical presentation of prosthetic joint infections acquired during the original operation may be much more delayed, particularly with low virulence organisms such as coagulase negative staphylococcus species (Steckelberg & Osmon 2000). Furthermore, up to 50% of suspected prosthetic joint infections of haematogenous origin present within the first two years (Deacon, et al. 1996). However it is important to note that distinguishing between whether an episode of bacteraemia led to haematogenous seeding of a prosthetic joint or whether the primary source of the bacteraemia was a subclinical prosthetic joint infection can be problematic.

3.2 The role of biofilms

The pathogenesis of prosthetic joint infections is intimately connected to the property of biofilm formation by microorganisms. The presence of this biofilm can have a critical effect on the likely success of treatment for a number of reasons. Bacteria can exist in two unique forms; the free living or planktonic forms characterised by rapid cellular division, and the stationary or sessile forms characterised by slower cellular division (Costerton 1999, Costerton, et al. 1995).

The sessile bacteria secrete an extracellular matrix or slime. Together the microorganisms and this matrix comprise what is known as 'the biofilm'. The abiotic matrix performs a number of functions including provision of anchorage onto structures to support the sessile colonies(Donlan & Costerton 2002). It also facilitates communication between bacteria within the biofilm. This communication termed 'quorum sensing', is analogous to the paracrine signalling in multicellular organisms and enables the bacteria to regulate their gene synthesis(Gristina & Costerton 2009). Importantly, the matrix can provide bacteria with protection from antimicrobial chemicals and from host defense mechanisms. This impairment of host defense mechanisms has been demonstrated in a number of in vitro models. For example, the extracellular slime produced by *Staphylococcus epidermidis* can inhibit the phagocytic activity of neutrophils(Shiau & Wu 1998).

The concentration of antibiotic required to inhibit the growth of bacteria in biofilms is higher than that required to kill free living bacteria. The mean inhibitory concentration (MIC) of many antibiotics is higher with the sessile forms than corresponding planktonic forms. Studies have demonstrated up to a 1000 fold increase in the MIC to particular antibiotics for bacteria moving from the planktonic to the sessile phenotype (Amorena, et al. 1999, Jones, et al. 2001, Rose & Poppens 2009, Schwank, et al. 1998, Souli & Giamarellou 1998, Stewart & Costerton 2001). This poses a major challenge for clinicians interpreting the reported antibiotic susceptibility results of bacteria, as our standard laboratory antibiotic susceptibility testing uses only the planktonic forms of bacteria. Newer technologies including the Calgary Biofilm Device can enable antibiotic susceptibility testing of the sessile phenotype of bacteria, but at present these are limited to a research setting and are not widely available(Ceri, et al. 1999).

There are a number of postulated mechanisms for the apparent resistance of biofilm residing bacteria to the effects of antibiotics. Firstly, the antibiotic may be deactivated at the surface of the biofilm. Secondly, the altered nutritional and biochemical environment within the biofilm may alter the activity of the antibiotics. Thirdly, antibiotics, particular cell wall active antibiotics such as betalactam antibiotics, rely on rapid growth and reproduction of the microorganism for their effect. These antibiotics are effective against the planktonic phenotype but have limited efficacy against the sessile phenotype as cellular turnover is greatly reduced. Finally the sessile forms act as 'spore-like' structures, which may act as a

nidus for later relapse of infection (Costerton 1999, Stewart & Costerton 2001, Trampuz, et al. 2003, Zimmerli 2006).
The properties of the biofilm alter with time; with age many biofilms become increasingly resistant to antibiotics. Monzon et al demonstrated the efficacy of vancomycin against *Staphylococcus epidermidis* decreased as a biofilm aged. This phenomenon was not consistent with all antibiotics; the activity of rifampicin and tetracyclines was not altered (Monzon, et al. 2002). Using Ribosomal RNA Fluorescence In Situ Hybridization studies, Poulson et al assessed the growth rate of biofilms and demonstrated that the cellular turnover was significantly higher in younger biofilms compared to established biofilms (Poulsen, et al. 1993). This finding could account for the difference to antimicrobial susceptibility observed.
Implant factors are also recognised to play a role in the pathogenesis of infection. Biochemical properties of prosthetic material influences bacterial adhesion and may impair host immune responses. For example, methyl methacrylate cement has been shown to inhibit complement and lymphocyte activity (Panush & Petty 1978, Petty 1978).

4. Diagnosis

4.1 Clinical features

The clinical diagnosis of prosthetic joints is challenging. Many typical symptoms of infection are often absent. Pain is the predominant symptom of prosthetic joint infections and is present in 90 to 100% of patients. The presence of fever is variable with 9 to 43% of patients in most case series having documented elevated temperatures (Canner, et al. 1984, Inman, et al. 1984, McDonald, et al. 1989, Miley, et al. 1982, Morrey, et al. 1989, Windsor, et al. 1990). In acute infections, erythema and swelling of the joint are often present, but are less common in more chronic infections (Del Pozo & Patel 2009, Miley, et al. 1982, Zimmerli, et al. 2004). A discharging sinus is associated with chronic, indolent presentations (Del Pozo & Patel 2009).
Zimmerli et al classifies arthroplasty infections as: Early (developing in the first three months after surgery), Delayed (occurring three to 24 months after surgery) and Late (greater than 24 months). This classification roughly correlates to important observed differences in the causative pathogens; with virulent organisms such as *Staphylococcus aureus* characteristically presenting earlier and more indolent pathogens such as coagulase negative Staphylococcus usually presenting later (Zimmerli, et al. 2004).

4.2 Laboratory studies

Peripheral blood leucocytosis is a poor predictor of infected arthroplasty; less than 10% of patients with an infected prosthesis have an elevated white cell count in most series (Canner, et al. 1984, Inman, et al. 1984, Zimmerli, et al. 2004). Other biochemical tests, such as the erythrocyte sedimentation rate (ESR) and C-reactive protein (CRP) are more useful diagnostic tests for these infections. For patients with proven infection of knee or hip arthroplasty, the ESR had a sensitivity of 81-92% and a specificity of 90-96%, while the CRP had a sensitivity of 84-89% and a specificity of 83-96% (Bottner, et al. 2007, Spangehl, et al. 1999). There are however, limitations to the diagnostic utility of the ESR and CRP. These markers are normally elevated after primary uncomplicated arthroplasty; the ESR peaks in the first week and may remain elevated for up to a year, while the CRP peaks at day 2 and may remain elevated for 3 weeks (Aalto, et al. 1984, Larsson, et al. 1992, Shih, et al. 1987).

The search for other biochemical markers of infection has included interleukin 6 (Il-6), tumour necrosis factor α (TNF-α) and procalcitonin C. Il-6 and TNF-α are cytokines released by monocytes and macrophages in the setting of infection (Bottner, et al. 2007). Procalcitonin is a precursor of calcitonin, and has been shown to be a specific marker of bacterial sepsis (Fernandez Lopez, et al. 2003). In a review by Bottner et al of 78 patients undergoing revision arthroplasties Il-6, TNF-α and procalcitonin were all significantly elevated in patients with confirmed septic loosening. The sensitivity and specificity respectively of Il-6 was 95% and 87%, TNF-α 43% and 94% and procalcitonin 33% and 98%. (Bottner, et al. 2007). Il-6 is elevated in the post-operative period for primary arthroplasty however, in a study by Shah et al, Il-6 was shown to return to normal levels within 2 days of the operation. Therefore there is potential diagnostic utility of Il-6 over CRP and ESR in the early post-operative period if infection is suspected, particularly in the first 21 days (Shah, et al. 2009).

Synovial fluid characteristics can be used to assist in diagnosis of prosthetic joint infections. In a study by Trampuz and colleagues, the leucocyte count was significantly higher in patients with prosthetic joint infection with a median of 18.9 x $10^3/\mu L$ (range, 0.3 to 178 x $10^3/\mu L$) compared to a median leucocyte count of 0.3 x $10^3/\mu L$ (range, 0.1 to 16 x $10^3/\mu L$) in patients with aseptic loosening. Using receiver operating characteristic (ROC) curves the authors found a synovial total white cell count 1.7 x $10^3/\mu L$ and a leucocyte differential of greater than 65% neutrophils had a sensitivity and specificity of 94%, 88% and 97%, 98% respectively (Trampuz, et al. 2004).

4.3 Radiological studies

Plain radiographs lack sensitivity and specificity in diagnosing septic arthroplasty. Findings such as lucency around the prosthesis can be noted in both septic and aseptic loosening situations (Figure 1 A-D). In early infection plain radiographs are frequently normal (Miller 2005).

Technetium-Methylene Diphosphonate (MDP) bone scintigraphy is a sensitive test for prosthetic joint infection (Figure 1 E-G), but lacks specificity, as it does not differentiate between aseptic and septic loosening(Ghanem, et al. 2009). The bone scan can also remain positive for a year following primary arthroplasty. Bone scan does have a high negative predictive value therefore bone scans potentially can be used to exclude infection in the setting of a painful prosthetic joint (Smith, et al. 2001). Similar findings have been documented with newer modalities such as ^{18}F-Fluoro-deoxyglucose positron emission tomography (FDG-PET) (Delank, et al. 2006, Zoccali, et al. 2009). A recent meta-analysis of FDG-PET reported a sensitivity of 82.1% and specificity of 86.6% for the presence of prosthetic joint infection, and hence this may be a useful test if available(Kwee, et al. 2008).

Computer tomography (CT) and magnetic resonance imaging are not considered useful imaging modalities due to artefact from the metal prosthesis interfering with interpretation of imaging findings. However newer CT scanners can minimise this effect and may be useful in detecting abnormalities of the soft tissues in periprosthetic infections (Figure 2 A-E) but do not diagnose periprosthetic bone abnormalities well (Cyteval, et al. 2002)

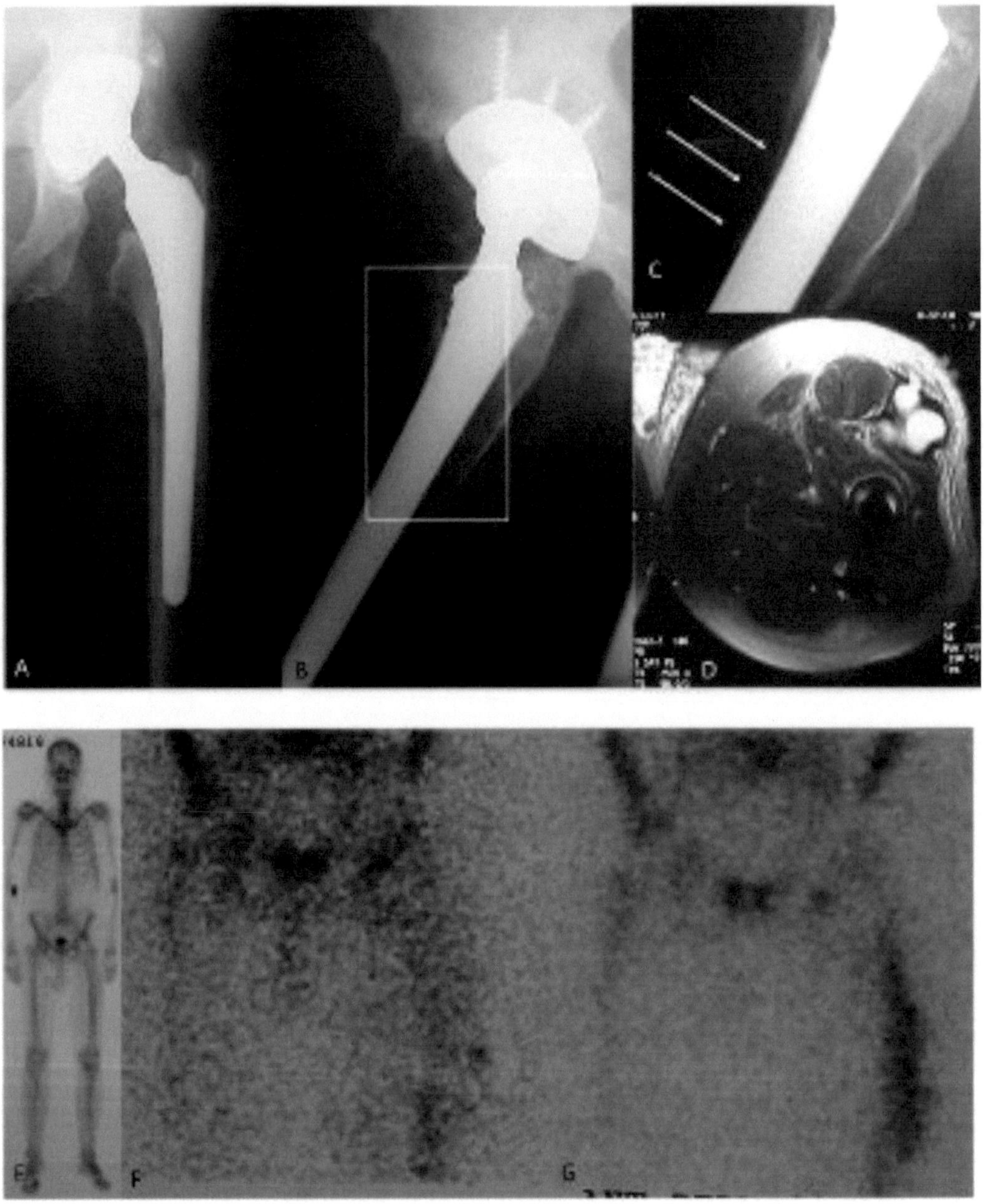

Fig. 1. (A) Painful (left) cementless hip prosthesis in situ. (B) Note extrinsic scalloping of anterior cortex of femoral diaphysis (box). (C) Magnified image of anterior femoral cortex with extrinsic scalloping (arrows) caused by soft tissue abscess (D). (E) Nuclear bone scan (TcMDP) demonstrating mild uptake over left proximal femur. Indium white cell scan at (F) 4 hours and (G) showing marked retention of nuclear tracer at 20 hours.

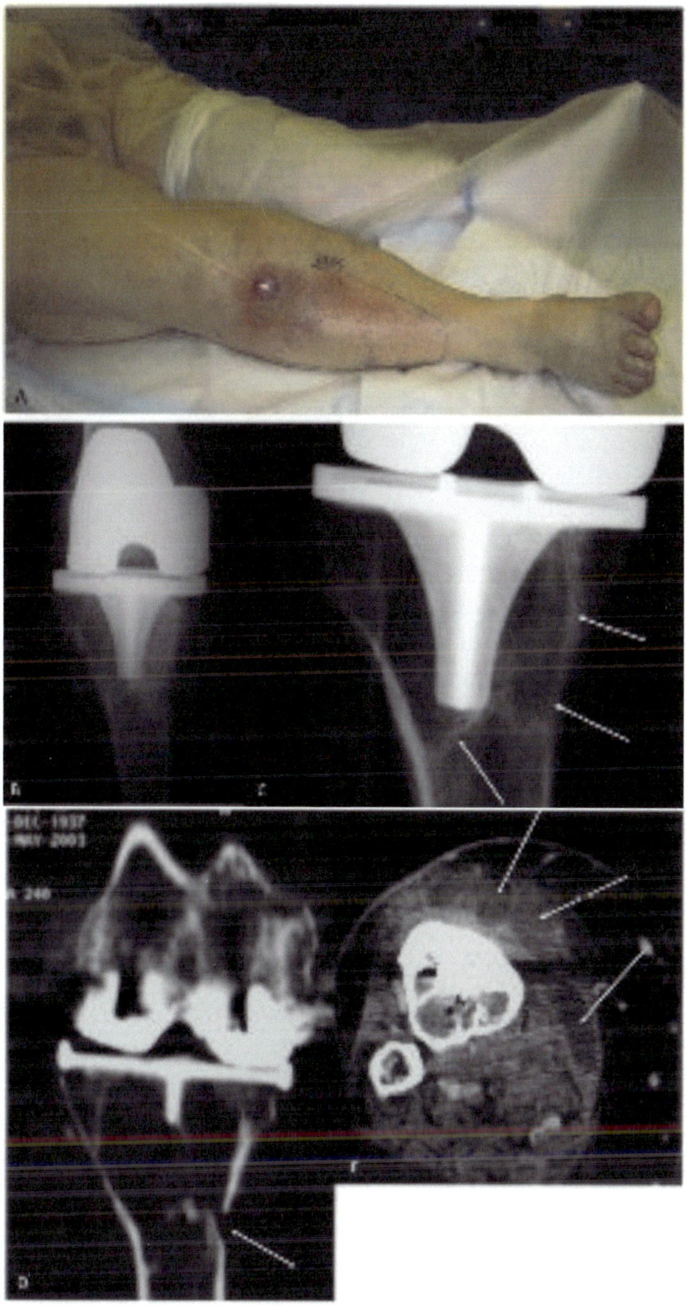

Fig. 2. (A) Localised infective sinus at the centre of incision used for total knee joint replacement. (B) plain radiograph showing periprosthetic sclerosis and lysis under the tibial component. (C) Magnified image showing obvious periprosthetic lysis (arrows). (D) Computer tomogram showing lysis under tibial component extending through medial cortex as cloaca (arrow). (E) Computer tomogram demonstrating soft tissue abscess formation (arrows) in continuity with intramedullary suppuration.

4.4 Histopathology diagnosis

Intraoperative frozen section histopathologic studies of periprosthetic tissue can be used as an adjunctive test for the diagnosis of prosthetic joint infections. An early paper showed a correlation between the polymorphonuclear leucocyte (PMN) count in tissue on histopathologic examination and the diagnosis of infection (Mirra, et al. 1976). Subsequent studies using frozen section histopathology for revision arthroplasty (using a PMN count of five to ten cells per high power field to diagnose infection) had a sensitivity of 50-93% and sensitivity of 77-100% (Bori, et al. 2006, Frances Borrego, et al. 2007, Ko, et al. 2005, Nunez, et al. 2007). It should be noted that inflammatory conditions such as rheumatoid arthritis may also cause a high PMN count, hence lowering specificity (Mirra, et al. 1976).

4.5 Microbiology diagnosis

The identification of the causative pathogen in a prosthetic device infection is of paramount importance. It allows for the institution of appropriate management strategies for infection including selection of the most appropriate antibiotic to target the pathogen, while minimising unnecessary antibiotic overuse, thus decreasing the incidence of drug toxicity and generally permitting simpler drug regimens to improve patient adherence.

It has earlier been noted that culture negative prosthetic joint infections continue to occur. Recent studies have focused on methods to increase the sensitivity of microbiological diagnostic techniques to address this problem. In a prospective study, which aimed to establish microbiological criteria for the diagnosis of prosthetic joint infection in revision arthroplasty, Atkins et al found that the isolation of indistinguishable microorganisms from three or more periprosthetic tissue samples has a sensitivity of 65% and a specificity of 99.6% for prosthetic joint infection. Utilising mathematical modelling the authors recommended that five to six intraoperative specimens of periprosthetic tissue be obtained to optimise the likelihood of a microbiologic diagnosis in prosthetic joint infection. They also noted that routine gram staining of periprosthetic tissue at revision arthroplasty had a very low sensitivity (12%) and the authors recommended that gram stain should be abandoned in revision arthroplasty cases, instead relying on culture (Atkins, et al. 1998).

Prolonged cultures may also help to improve the diagnostic yield. An increase in positive culture results of 24.6% when culture incubation of periprosthetic tissue samples was increased from 3 to fourteen days has been reported and in particular the isolation of fastidious organisms, such as Propionibacterium species was increased (Schafer, et al. 2008).

A number of techniques have been developed in an attempt to disrupt the biofilm and increase the yield of microbiological cultures. One such technique is ultrasonification whereby the explanted prosthesis is placed in a sterile polyethylene bag then in a sterile anaerobic jar, Ringer's solution is added and sonification is performed. The sonicate fluid is cultured aerobically and anaerobically. One study comparing sonification to standard tissue culture involving 331 patients of whom 79 had prosthetic joint infections; sonification yielded an additional 14 microbiological diagnosis with a reported sensitivity of 78.5% and specificity of 98.8%. The authors noted that sonification was particularly useful in cases where patients had received antibiotics perioperatively (Trampuz, et al. 2007).

4.6 Molecular techniques

Newer molecular techniques have been applied to prosthetic joint infections to increase the diagnostic yield including polymerase chain reaction (PCR), fluorescent in situ hybridization (FISH) and immunofluorescent microscopy (IFM). Both PCR and FISH target specific regions of bacterial genetic material, commonly bacterial ribosomal RNA (rRNA). The advantage of using rRNA is that it is highly conserved in bacterial species compared to most protein encoding genes. Both methods can use broad range oligonucleotide primers or more targeted primers including genus and species specific primers (Amann & Fuchs 2008).

A number of studies investigating the role of bacterial 16s rRNA PCR have been performed. Sensitivities of this technique ranged from 63-100% in detecting bacteria involved in prosthetic joint infection (De Man, et al. 2009, Hoeffel, et al. 1999, Mariani, et al. 1996, Moojen, et al. 2007). In a study by Mariani et al 50 patients with symptoms following total knee arthroplasty underwent synovial fluid and intraoperative tissue sampling for culture and PCR; cultures were positive in fifteen specimens compared to 32 specimens when PCR was applied (Mariani, et al. 1996). Likewise Tunney et al used PCR in a study of 120 patients undergoing prosthetic hip joint revision. The explanted prosthesis underwent ultrasonification and this fluid was cultured and underwent 16s DNA PCR. Standard microbiologic cultures were positive in 22% of patients, compared to 72% of patients with positive results from PCR (Tunney, et al. 1999). The limitation of these studies was a paucity of correlation with clinical or histological features of infection. In a review of 34 patients with confirmed prosthetic joint infection Vandercam et al found that PCR was positive in 31 of 34 patients (91.2%), compared to positive microbiological culture in 22 of 34 patients (64.7%). Of import, eight of the nine patients with positive PCR but negative culture results had received antibiotic therapy in the prior ten days (Vandercam, et al. 2008). Despite these promising results, the weakness of 16s ribosomal RNA PCR techniques is the low specificity and high false positive rate. In a study by Clarke et al 29% of the patients without septic arthritis (on the basis of clinical, radiological, biochemical, intraoperative findings, culture and histology) had positive PCR results, this was particularly pronounced in the cohort undergoing revision arthroplasty for aseptic loosening where 46% of patients had positive PCR (Clarke, et al. 2004). The high false positive rate may be due to a number of factors including contamination of specimen or the reagents and detection of necrotic bacterial DNA (Bauer, et al. 2006). Importantly though, many patients labelled as having aseptic loosening may in fact have had low grade chronic infection contributing to prosthesis loosening. Given that there is no gold standard to define prosthetic joint infection, the specificity of PCR remains difficult to judge.

FISH is a technique that uses labelled oligonucleotide probes that hybridise to specific genetic regions on bacteria and are subsequently visualised using fluorescent microscopy or flow cytometry (Amann & Fuchs 2008, Moter & Gobel 2000). Probes to detect bacterial rRNA or other genetic targets are available and these include species specific probes, therefore allowing identification and simultaneous observation of the different bacteria. FISH also allows an appreciation of the architectural arrangement of the organisms within the biofilm which can assist in differentiating true infections from contamination (McDowell & Patrick 2005, Moter & Gobel 2000). In orthopaedic infections it has been demonstrated that *Staphylococcus aureus* and *Staphylococcus epidermidis* could be visualised and differentiated in an experimental biofilm. Additionally, in a clinical case of septic loosening of a hip prosthesis, *Staphylococcus epidermidis* was visualised using FISH techniques in periprosthetic tissue samples(Krimmer, et al. 1999). FISH has otherwise not yet been widely applied to prosthetic joint infections in a clinical setting.

Immunofluorescence microscopy (IFM) is another novel nonculture technique for diagnosing prosthetic joint infections. In immunofluorescence microscopy, samples are mixed with monoclonal antibodies (MAb) to specific antigens on bacterial cell walls. Samples are then incubated with a second antibody conjugated with a fluorescent dye. The bacteria are then visualised using fluorescence microscopy(Tunney, et al. 1999). As with FISH, IFM can be used to assess the biofilm structure and can detect multiple pathogens (McDowell & Patrick 2005, Tunney, et al. 1999). In the study by Tunney et al IFM was performed on the sonicate fluid from explanted prostheses using Mab for both Propionibacterium and Staphylococcus species. (Tunney, et al. 1999).

5. Treatment

5.1 Treatment goal

Optimal treatment of prosthetic joint infections involves the eradication of infection whilst maintaining function of the joint and patient quality of life (Zimmerli, et al. 2004). However there are no large, multi-centred, randomised prospective studies of treatment strategies to guide recommendations. The successful treatment of prosthetic joints is contingent on the elimination of the biofilm dwelling microorganism. The two mainstay methods of achieving this are through either surgical removal of the prosthesis or through use of biofilm active antibiotics in conjunction with surgical debridement and retention of the prosthesis.

The surgical strategies used to treat arthroplasty infections include: resection arthroplasty, one-stage or two-stage exchange procedures, amputation and debridement and retention. Resection arthroplasty entails the removal of all foreign material including cement, resection of devitalised tissue and bone and may or may not involve arthrodesis. Exchange procedures involve resection arthroplasty with reimplantation of a new joint prosthesis performed at the time of removal of the infected prosthesis (one-stage exchange); or delayed by a variable period of time while antibiotic therapy is administered (two-stage exchange). Debridement and retention of the prosthesis usually involves open arthrotomy, removal of all infected and necrotic bone, exchange of liners and lavage of the joint (Giulieri, et al. 2004, Matthews, et al. 2009, Rand, et al. 1986, Steckelberg & Osmon 2000, Trampuz & Zimmerli 2008, Zimmerli, et al. 2004).

A number of factors influence the surgical approach selected for an individual patient, these include a patient's general health and fitness for anaesthesia, condition of the prosthesis and bone stock, the causative agent, the timing of the infection relative to the prosthesis insertion, the availability of effective antibiotics and clinicians' and patient preference.

5.2 Systemic antibiotic therapy without surgical debridement

Administration of antibiotic therapy without surgical management is not routinely recommended, as it is rarely associated with successful cure. Early studies of antibiotic therapy alone for prosthetic joint infections had disappointing results with successful outcomes in as little as 8-15% of patients (Bengtson, et al. 1989, Canner, et al. 1984). The confounding factor when analysing these poor results is that biofilm active antibiotics, were not used. Treatment with biofilm active antibiotics alone including rifampicin and ciprofloxacin for three to six months has yielded successful outcomes in highly selected patients; those presenting with early infections (less than one year following implant), infection due to *Staphylococcus aureus*, absence of implant loosening and strict adherence to treatment (Trebse, et al. 2005). However, antibiotic suppression alone is generally reserved for patients with significant comorbidities in whom surgery is contraindicated, who are without evidence of systemic infection and where tolerable oral antibiotics are available. Given the low likelihood of cure, many clinicians view this as long term, often lifelong suppressive therapy, embarked upon without curative intent (Steckelberg & Osmon 2000, Zimmerli, et al. 2004).

5.3 Exchange arthroplasty

Interpretation of the current literature describing the outcomes of patients having one- and two-stage exchange procedures is challenging owing to the heterogeneity of the patient populations, the causative organisms and the surgical techniques (including use of antibiotic impregnated cement), the differences in the duration of patient follow up and probable publication bias. The greatest concern with one-stage exchange procedures is the implantation of the prosthesis into an infected field with subsequent reinfection of the revised arthroplasty. In one-stage exchange, reported success rates range from 38-100%; but there is significant variability in the definition of success which includes freedom from infection, freedom from pain or simply the presence of a functional joint (Callaghan, et al. 1999, Jamsen, et al. 2009, Steckelberg & Osman 2000). In examination of the outcomes of one-stage exchange revision hip arthroplasty, 80% (range 57-92%) of patients have been reported to remain infection free after one-stage exchange without the use of antibiotic cement (Steckelberg & Osman 2000). When antibiotic impregnated cement was used, 88% (range 76-100%) of patients have been reported to remain infection free at follow up (Callaghan, et al. 1999, Jackson & Schmalzried 2000, Langlais 2003, Steckelberg & Osman 2000). Results for one-stage exchange in knee arthroplasty revision are in general worse than for hips, with only 65% (range 57-100%) of patients remaining free of recurrence of infection at follow up (Steckelberg & Osmon 2000). On the basis of these results, one-stage exchange of an infected prosthesis is rarely advised for prosthetic knee infections(Trampuz & Zimmerli 2008, Zimmerli, et al. 2004). There are, however some advantages with one-stage exchange; patients undergo a single operation and generally require a shorter period of hospitalisation in total.

Consensus recommendations for one-stage exchange suggest that it should only be considered where there is minimal soft tissue damage and where less virulent organisms are involved (Hirakawa, et al. 1998, Jackson & Schmalzried 2000, Miley, et al. 1982, Trampuz & Zimmerli 2008, Zimmerli, et al. 2004). The presence of sinus tract is considered a relative contraindication for one-stage exchange. Ideally the causative agent should be known prior to resection arthroplasty and treatment commenced preoperatively(Zimmerli, et al. 2004).

In two-stage exchange procedures, reimplantation is delayed for a variable length of time from 2 weeks to several months. Spacers impregnated with antibiotic are commonly inserted to maintain limb length and improve patient mobility during that interval (Leunig, et al. 1998). Antibiotics with activity against the isolated pathogen are administered for at least 6 weeks. Tissue samples are often routinely taken from the periprosthetic tissue at the time of reimplantation for microbiological culture to assess the efficacy of the interim treatment (Insall, et al. 1983, Wilson, et al. 1990, Windsor, et al. 1990). In infections with

difficult-to-treat micro-organisms such as MRSA, resistant enterococci and fungi, current consensus guidelines recommends prolonged interval between removal and reimplantation without the use of a spacer (Trampuz & Zimmerli 2008, Zimmerli, et al. 2004)
Two-stage exchange, in general, has a higher success rate compared to one-stage with rates of 63-100% (Colyer & Capello 1994, Haleem, et al. 2004, Jamsen, et al. 2009, Woods, et al. 1983). In hip arthroplasty two-stage exchange without the use of antibiotic impregnated cement, 81% of patients (range 53-100%) remain free of recurrent infection increasing to 93% (73-100%) when antibiotic cement is used (Laffer, et al. 2006, Langlais, et al. 2006, Steckelberg & Osman 2000). In knee arthroplasty infections, 84% (38-100%) of patients in whom antibiotic cement is not used, and 88% (63-100%) of patients in whom antibiotic impregnated cement is used remain infection free following two stage exchange (Bengtson, et al. 1989, Grogan, et al. 1986, Hanssen, et al. 1994, Insall, et al. 1983, Morrey, et al. 1989, Rand, et al. 1986, Wang & Chen 1997, Wasielewski, et al. 1996, Wilson, et al. 1990, Windsor, et al. 1990, Woods, et al. 1983).
A number of factors potentially influence treatment outcomes in two-stage exchange procedures. Polymicrobial infection, infection with virulent organisms including *Staphylococcus aureus* and methicillin resistant coagulase negative Staphylococcus species, the presence of rheumatoid arthritis and a history of prior multiple revisions have all been shown to associated with lower rates of success in two-stage exchanges (Hirakawa, et al. 1998, Lim, et al. 2009, Mittal, et al. 2007). Current consensus guidelines recommend two-stage exchange in chronic infections with moderately or severely damaged tissue or if a sinus tract is present (Trampuz & Zimmerli 2008, Zimmerli, et al. 2004).

5.4 Resection arthroplasty

Resection arthroplasty and amputation are generally reserved for patients with refractory infections particularly where there is severe loss of bone stock or where functional improvement following revision is unlikely (Trampuz & Zimmerli 2008, Zimmerli, et al. 2004). Whilst rates of recurrence of infection are low, patients have worse functional outcomes and up to 80% of patients report residual pain following resection (Morrey, et al. 1989).

5.5 Debridement and retention of the prosthesis

Debridement and retention of the prosthesis is an attractive treatment option for many patients given that it is the least invasive, with a lower surgical morbidity, and is generally associated with good functional outcomes (Trampuz & Zimmerli 2008, Zimmerli, et al. 2004). Open arthrotomy and debridement is recommended when attempting retention of the prosthesis as poorer results are reported with arthroscopic 'washout' compared to open 'washout'(Laffer, et al. 2006). Following debridement, patients should receive biofilm active antibiotics generally for a longer duration than with surgical exchange or resection.
Early studies of debridement and prosthesis retention strategies to treat prosthetic joint infection were disappointing with recurrence of infection at 2 years reported in 69% of patients (Brandt, et al. 1997). Poor outcomes have been reported when symptoms are present greater than 8 days, when a sinus tract is present and with late chronic infections; In some instances all patients with late infection experienced treatment failure (Berbari, et al.

2006a, Crockarell, et al. 1998, Marculescu, et al. 2006b). High failure rates have also observed with specific organisms, only 12% of patients with *Staphylococcus aureus* infection experiencing successful treatment outcomes (Deirmengian, et al. 2003, Marculescu, et al. 2006a). Gram-negative infections, polymicrobial infections and culture negative prosthetic joint infections were also associated with higher rates of recurrence of infection following debridement and retention (Berbari, et al. 2007, Hsieh, et al. 2009a, Marculescu & Cantey 2008). However, successful outcomes have been reported in the setting of early or haematogenous infections (Morrey, et al. 1989, Wasielewski, et al. 1996). Tsuyakama et al reported a successful outcome in 71% of patients with early infections treated with debridement of the prosthetic joint followed by four weeks of parenteral antibiotics with an average follow up of 3.8 years (Tsukayama, et al. 1996).

Newer treatment strategies evolved as understanding of the role of biofilm in the pathogenesis of prosthetic joint infections increased. In vivo studies using guinea pig tissue-cage animal model by Widmer et al demonstrated the clinical utility of rifampicin in chronic biofilm infections (Widmer, et al. 1990). Further studies also identified that quinolones retained activity in the presence of biofilms (Schwank, et al. 1998, Widmer, et al. 1991).

The addition of rifampicin to antimicrobial regimens has led to a significant improvement in success rates reported in the treatment of gram-positive prosthetic joint infection; in many instances comparable to that reported for two-stage exchange. In our experience combination treatment including rifampicin has resulted in successful treatment in up to 90% of patients (Aboltins, et al. 2007); however successful outcomes are associated with several factors. Higher success rates are reported where the causative organism is a staphylococcus species and when antibiotic therapy is continued for a protracted period; 12 months or greater, (Choong, et al. 2007, Widmer, et al. 1992). In contrast the rate of success is significantly diminished when a fistula is present, particularly in knee arthroplasty where successful outcomes have been reported in only 45-69% of patients. (Drancourt, et al. 1993).

The only randomised double-blinded control trial examining the role of rifampicin in the treatment of prosthetic device staphylococcal infections was conducted from 1992 through 1997. The study involved 33 patients with orthopaedic device infections and duration of symptoms less than one year. Patients were randomised to receive rifampicin 450mg and ciprofloxacin 750mg (twice daily) or ciprofloxacin and placebo. Rifampicin/ciprofloxacin combination was successful in all patients compared to 58% of patients who received ciprofloxacin alone (Zimmerli, et al. 1998). Subsequent studies corroborated these results with success rates of greater than 85% of patients treated with debridement and retention and rifampicin containing antibiotic treatment (Berdal, et al. 2005, Byren, et al. 2009, Rao, et al. 2003). The main limitations with the use of rifampicin are the high likelihood of generation of resistance when used without a second antibiotic and the hepatic and gastrointestinal toxicities (John, et al. 2009, Widmer, et al. 1990). Therefore careful, regular follow up of patients is necessary and the management these antibiotics should involve collaboration between Infectious Diseases Physicians and Orthopaedic Surgeons.

The investigation of newer agents for the treatment of prosthetic joint infection is ongoing. In guinea pig foreign-body infection model, John et al assessed the activity of newer agents including linezolid and daptomycin, alone and in combination with rifampicin. In this study

neither daptomycin nor linezolid had activity against adherent MRSA when used as monotherapy. When used in combination with rifampicin, daptomycin at a dose of 30mg/kg (corresponding to a dose of 6mg/kg in humans) cured 67% of cage infections. At this dose, no cases of rifampicin resistance emerged. Results were less encouraging for linezolid; even in combination with rifampicin, linezolid failed to cure any cage infection. Resistance to rifampicin emerged in 8% of cage infections treated with rifampicin-linezolid combinations (John, et al. 2009).
For gram-negative infections, ciprofloxacin has been shown to be effective in guinea pig tissue cage models(Widmer, et al. 1991). In a study of 28 patients with bone and joint infections secondary to gram-negative bacilli combination therapy with cefepime and fluoroquinolone obtained a cure in 79% of patients. However only 5 patients in this cohort had a prosthetic joint infection, two were treated with debridement and retention and only one of which was cured (the second patient died from a cause unrelated to the infection)(Legout, et al. 2006). In prosthetic joint infection secondary to gram negative bacilli, debridement and retention has yielded a success rate as low as 27% (Hsieh, et al. 2009b). This contrasts with our results where by infection free survival at 2 years was 94% in gram-negative infections when fluoroquinolone was used in conjunction with debridement and retention (Aboltins, et al. 2011). Again this is in the setting of short duration of symptoms (median 7 days) and prolonged oral antibiotic treatment (median 12 months).
The duration of antibiotic after debridement and retention varies in reported clinical studies ranging from six months to greater than 4 years. In a study by Laffer et al there was no difference in outcome in patients receiving three to six months of antibiotics compared with greater than six months (91% v 87% success). In this study patients were followed up for a median duration of 28 (range, 2–193) months and 55% of infections were caused by Staphylococcus species(Laffer, et al. 2006). In accordance with consensus guidelines, debridement and retention of the prosthetic joint should be considered in patients with a short duration of symptoms in the absence of implant loosening and soft tissue damage where antibiotics with biofilm activity are available (Laffer, et al. 2006, Matthews, et al. 2009, Trampuz & Zimmerli 2008, Zimmerli, et al. 2004).

6. Conclusion

Prosthetic joint infections involve a complex interplay between the biofilm forming microorganisms, host responses and the implant. These infections are an uncommon but devastating complication of arthroplasty. However with given the ageing population the number of patients requiring arthroplasty is set to increase exponentially. Clinical investigation is imperative to increase understanding, improve diagnosis, optimise treatment and ultimately prevent prosthetic joint infections. While 2-stage exchanges remains the most reliable and consistent treatment option in terms of successful outcomes, the advent of more accurate diagnostic tools and combining the use of newer antibiotic agents with debridement and retention of the prosthetic joint should be considered a viable treatment option rather than an alternative. However this works best where a clear treatment protocol has been established, that targets patients at the earliest onset of symptoms, where debridement is aggressive and treatment involves is a combined approach between infectious Diseases Physicians and Orthopaedic Surgeons. Results at our institution attest to the success of such a protocol.

7. References

Aalto, K., Osterman, K., Peltola, H. & Rasanen, J. Change in Erythrocyte sedimentation rate and c-reactive protein after total hip arthorplasty. *Clinical Orthopaedics and Related Research* 184, 118-120 (1984).

Aboltins, C.A., Dowsey, M.M., Buising, K.L., Peel, T.N., Daffy, J.R., Choong, P.F. & Stanley, P.A. Gram-negative prosthetic joint infection treated with debridement, prosthesis retention and antibiotic regimens including a fluoroquinolone. *Clin Microbiol Infect* 17, 862-867 (2011).

Aboltins, C.A., Page, M.A., Buising, K.L., Jenney, A.W.J., Daffy, J.R. & Choong, P.F.M. Treatment of staphylococcal prosthetic joint infections with debridement , prosthesis retention and oral rifampicin and fusidic acid. *Clinical Microbiology and Infection* 13, 586-591 (2007).

Ahnfelt, L., Herberts, P., Malchau, H. & Andersson, G.B.J. Prognosis of total hip replacement. *Acta Orthopaedica Scandinavica* 61, 2 26 (1990).

Amann, R. & Fuchs, B.M. Single-cell identification in microbial communities by improved fluorescence in situ hybridization techniques. *Nature Reviews Microbiology* 6, 339-348 (2008).

Amorena, B., Gracia, E., Monzon, M., Leiva, J., Oteiza, C., Perez, M., Alabart, J.L. & Hernandez-Yago, J. Antibiotic susceptibility assay for Staphylococcus aureus in biofilms developed in vitro. *Journal of Antimicrobial Chemotherapy* 44, 43-55 (1999).

Atkins, B.L., Athanasou, N., Deeks, J.J., Crook, D.W.M., Simpson, H., Peto, T.E.A., Lardy-smith, P.M.C. & Berendt, A.R. Prospective Evaluation of Criteria for Microbiological Diagnosis of Prosthetic-Joint Infection at Revision Arthroplasty. *Journal of Clinical Microbiology* 36, 2932-2939 (1998).

Bauer, T.W., Parvizi, J., Kobayashi, N. & Krebs, V. Diagnosis of periprosthetic infection. *J Bone Joint Surg Am* 88-A, 869-882 (2006).

Bengtson, S. & Knutson, K. The infected knee arthroplasty. *Acta Orthopaedica Scandinavica* 62, 301-311 (1991).

Bengtson, S., Knutson, K. & Lidgren, L. Treatment of Infected Knee Arthroplasty. *Clinical Orthopaedics and Related Research* 245, 173-178 (1989).

Berbari, E.F., Hanssen, A.D., Duffy, M.C., Steckelberg, J.M., Ilstrup, D.M., Harmsen, W.S. & Osmon, D.R. Risk factors for prosthetic joint infection: case-control study. *Clin Infect Dis* 27, 1247-1254 (1998).

Berbari, E.F., Marculescu, C., Sia, I., Lahr, B.D., Hanssen, A.D., Steckelberg, J.M., Gullerud, R. & Osmon, D.R. Culture-negative prosthetic joint infection. *Clinical Infectious Diseases* 45, 1113-1119 (2007).

Berbari, E.F., Osmon, D.R., Duffy, M.C., Harmssen, R.N., Mandrekar, J.N., Hanssen, A.D. & Steckelberg, J.M. Outcome of prosthetic joint infection in patients with rheumatoid arthritis: the impact of medical and surgical therapy in 200 episodes. *Clinical Infectious Diseases* 42, 216-223 (2006a).

Berbari, E.F., Osmon, D.R., Duffy, M.C.T., Harmssen, R.N.W., Mandrekar, J.N., Hanssen, A.D. & Steckelberg, J.M. Outcome of prosthetic joint infection in patients with rheumatoid arthritis: the impact of medical and surgical therapy in 200 episodes. *Clinical Infectious Diseases* 42, 216-223 (2006b).

Berdal, J.E., Skramm, I., Mowinckel, P., Gulbrandsen, P. & Bjornholt, J.V. Use of rifampicin and ciprofloxacin combination therapy after surgical debridement in the treatment of early manifestation prosthetic joint infections. *Clinical Microbiology and Infection* 11, 843-845 (2005).

Bori, G., Soriano, A., GarcÃ-a, S.n., Gallart, X., Casanova, L., Mallofre, C., Almela, M., MartÃ-nez, J.a., Riba, J. & Mensa, J. Low sensitivity of histology to predict the presence of microorganisms in suspected aseptic loosening of a joint prosthesis. *Modern Pathology* 19, 874-877 (2006).

Bottner, F., Wegner, a., Winkelmann, W., Becker, K., Erren, M. & Gotze, C. Interleukin-6, procalcitonin and TNF-alpha: markers of peri-prosthetic infection following total joint replacement. *J Bone Joint Surg Am* 89-Br, 94-99 (2007).

Bozic, K.J. & Ries, M.D. The impact of infection after total hip arthroplasty on hospital and surgeon resource utilization. *J Bone Joint Surg Am* 87-A, 1746-1751 (2005).

Brandt, C.M., Sistrunk, W.W., Duffy, M.C., Hanssen, a.D., Steckelberg, J.M., Ilstrup, D.M. & Osmon, D.R. Staphylococcus aureus prosthetic joint infection treated with debridement and prosthesis retention. *Clinical Infectious Diseases* 24, 914-919 (1997).

Byren, I., Bejon, P., Atkins, B.L., Angus, B., Masters, S., McLardy-Smith, P., Gundle, R. & Berendt, a. One hundred and twelve infected arthroplasties treated with 'DAIR' (debridement, antibiotics and implant retention): antibiotic duration and outcome. *Journal of Antimicrobial Chemotherapy* 63, 1264-1271 (2009).

Callaghan, J.J., Katz, R.P. & Johnston, R.C. One-Stage Revision Surgery of the Infected Hip. *Clinical Orthopaedics and Related Research* 369, 139-143 (1999).

Canner, G.C., Steinberg, M.E., Heppenstall, R.B. & Balderston, R. The infected hip after total hip arthroplasty. *J Bone Joint Surg Am* 66-A, 1393-1399 (1984).

Ceri, H., Olson, M.E., Stremick, C., Read, R.R. & Morck, D. The Calgary Biofilm Device : New Technology for Rapid Determination of Antibiotic Susceptibilities of Bacterial Biofilms. *Journal of Clinical Microbiology* 37, 1771-1776 (1999).

Choong, P.F., Dowsey, M.M., Carr, D., Daffy, J. & Stanley, P. Risk factors associated with acute hip prosthetic joint infections and outcome of treatment with a rifampinbased regimen. *Acta Orthop* 78, 755-765 (2007).

Clarke, M.T., Roberts, C.P., Lee, P.T.H., Gray, J., Keene, G.S. & Rushton, N. Polymerase Chain Reaction Can Detect Bacterial DNA in Aseptically Loose Total Hip Arthroplasties. *Clinical Orthopaedics and Related Research* 427, 132-137 (2004).

Colyer, R.a. & Capello, W.N. Surgical Treatment of the Infected Hip Implant. *Clinical Orthopaedics and Related Research* 298, 75-79 (1994).

Costerton, J.W. Bacterial Biofilms: A Common Cause of Persistent Infections. *Science* 284, 1318-1322 (1999).

Costerton, J.W., Lewandowski, Z., Caldwell, D.E., Korber, D.R. & Lappin-scott, H.M. Microbial biofilms. *Annual Reviews of Microbiology* 49, 711-745 (1995).

Crockarell, J.R., Hanssen, A.D., Osmon, D.R. & Morrey, B.F. Treatment of Infection with Debridement and Retention of the Components following Hip Arthroplasty

Treatment of Infection with Debridement and Retention of the Components following Hip Arthroplasty. *J Bone Joint Surg Am* 80-A, 1306-1313 (1998).

Cyteval, C., Hamm, V., Sarrabere, M.P., Lopez, F.M., Maury, P. & Taourel, P. Painful infection at the site of hip prosthesis: CT imaging. *Radiology* 224, 477-483 (2002).

De Man, F.H.R., Graber, P., Luem, M., Zimmerli, W., Ochsner, P.E. & Sendi, P. Broad-range PCR in selected episodes of prosthetic joint infection. *Infection* 37, 292-294 (2009).

Deacon, J.M., Pagliaro, A.J., Zelicof, S.B. & Horowitz, H.W. Current concepts review. Prophylactic use of antibiotics for procedures after total joint replacement. *J Bone Joint Surg Am* 78-A, 1755-1770 (1996).

Deirmengian, C., Greenbaum, J., Lotke, P.A., Booth, R.E. & Lonner, J.H. Limited Success with Open Debridement and Retention of Components in the Treatment of Acute Staphylococcus Aureus Infections After Total Knee Arthroplasty. *Journal of Arthroplasty* 18, 22-26 (2003).

Del Pozo, J.L. & Patel, R. Infection Associated with Prosthetic Joints. *New England Journal of Medicine* 361, 787-794 (2009).

Delank, K.S., Schmidt, M., Michael, J.W.P., Dietlein, M., Schicha, H. & Eysel, P. The implications of 18F-FDG PET for the diagnosis of endoprosthetic loosening and infection in hip and knee arthroplasty: results from a prospective, blinded study. *BMC Musculoskeletal Disorders* 7, 20-20 (2006).

Donlan, R.M. & Costerton, J.W. Biofilms : Survival Mechanisms of Clinically Relevant Microorganisms. *Clinical Microbiology and Infection* 15, 167-193 (2002).

Dowsey, M.M. & Choong, P.F. Obesity is a major risk factor for prosthetic infection after primary hip arthroplasty. *Clin Orthop Relat Res* 466, 153-158 (2008).

Dowsey, M.M. & Choong, P.F. Obese diabetic patients are at substantial risk for deep infection after primary TKA. *Clin Orthop Relat Res* 467, 1577-1581 (2009).

Drancourt, M., Stein, A., Argenson, J.N., Zannier, A., Curvale, G. & Raoult, D. Oral rifampin plus ofloxacin for treatment of Staphylococcus-infected orthopedic implants. *Antimicrobial Agents and Chemotherapy* 37, 1214-1218 (1993).

Fernandez Lopez, A., Luaces Cubells, C., García Garcia, J.J. & Fernandez Pou, J. Procalcitonin in pediatric emergency departments for the early diagnosis of invasive bacterial infections in febrile infants: results of a multicenter study and utility of a rapid qualitative test for this marker. *The Pediatric Infectious Disease Journal* 22, 895-903 (2003).

Fitzgerald, R.H., Nolan, D.R., Ilstrup, D.M., E., R., Washington, J.A. & Coventry, M.B. Deep wound sepsis following total hip arthroplasty. *J Bone Joint Surg Am* 59-A, 847-847 (1977).

Frances Borrego, A., Martinez, F.M., Cebrian Parra, J.L., Graneda, D.S., Crespo, R.G. & Lopez-Duran Stern, L. Diagnosis of infection in hip and knee revision surgery: intraoperative frozen section analysis. *International Orthopaedics* 31, 33-37 (2007).

Ghanem, E., Antoci, V., Jr., Pulido, L., Joshi, A., Hozack, W. & Parvizi, J. The use of receiver operating characteristics analysis in determining erythrocyte sedimentation rate and C-reactive protein levels in diagnosing periprosthetic infection prior to revision total hip arthroplasty. *Int J Infect Dis* 13, e444-449 (2009).

Giulieri, S.G., Graber, P., Ochsner, P.E. & Zimmerli, W. Management of infection associated with total hip arthroplasty according to a treatment algorithm. *Infection* 32, 222-228 (2004).

Graves, S., Davidson D, de Steiger R & A., T. Australian Orthopaedic Association National Joint Replacement Registry. Annual Report 2009. Adelaide: Australian Orthopaedic Association. (Adelaide, 2010).

Gristina, A.G. & Costerton, J.W. Bacterial adherence to biomaterials and tissue . The significance of its role in clinical sepsis to Biomaterials. *J Bone Joint Surg Am* 67-A, 264-273 (2009).

Grogan, T.J., Dorey, F., Rollins, J. & Amstutz, H.C. Deep sepsis following total knee arthroplasty. Ten-year experience at the University of California at Los Angeles Medical Center. *J Bone Joint Surg Am* 68-A, 226-234 (1986).

Haleem, A.A., Berry, D.J. & Hanssen, A.D. Mid-Term to Long-Term Followup of Two-stage Reimplantation for Infected Total Knee Arthroplasty. *Clinical Orthopaedics and Related Research* 428, 35-39 (2004).

Hanssen, A.D., Rand, J.A. & Osmon, D.R. Treatment of the infected total knee arthroplasty with insertion of another prosthesis: the effect of antibiotic-impregnated bone cement. *Clinical Orthopaedics and Related Research*, 44-55 (1994).

Hirakawa, K., Stulberg, B.N., Wilde, A.H., Bauer, T.W. & Secic, M. Results of 2-stage reimplantation for infected total knee arthroplasty. *Journal of Arthoplasty* 13, 22-28 (1998).

Hoeffel, D.P., Hinrichs, S.H. & Garvin, K.L. Molecular diagnostics for the detection of musculoskeletal infection. *Clinical Orthopaedics and Related Research*, 37-46 (1999).

Horan, T.C., Gaynes, R.P., Martone, W.J., Jarvis, W.R. & Emori, G.T. CDC Definitions of Nosocomial Surgical Site Infections, 1992: A Modification of CDC Definitions of Surgical Wound Infections. *Infection Control and Hospital Epidemiology* 13, 606-608 (1992).

Hsieh, P.-H., Lee, M.S., Hsu, K.-Y., Chang, Y.-H., Shih, H.-N. & Ueng, S.W. Gram-negative prosthetic joint infections: risk factors and outcome of treatment. *Clinical Infectious Diseases* 49, 1036-1043 (2009a).

Hsieh, P.H., Lee, M.S., Hsu, K.Y., Chang, Y.H., Shih, H.N. & Ueng, S.W. Gram-negative prosthetic joint infections: risk factors and outcome of treatment. *Clin Infect Dis* 49, 1036-1043 (2009b).

Inman, R.D., Gallegos, K.V., Brause, B.D., Redecha, P.B. & Christian, C.L. Clinical and microbial features of prosthetic joint infection. *American Journal of Medicine* 77, 47-53 (1984).

Insall, J.N., Thompson, F.M. & Brause, B.D. Two-stage reimplantation for the salvage of infected total knee arthroplasty. *J Bone Joint Surg Am* 65-A, 1087-1087 (1983).

Jackson, W.O. & Schmalzried, T.P. Limited role of direct exchange arthroplasty in the treatment of infected total hip replacements. *Clinical Orthopaedics and Related Research* 381, 101-105 (2000).

Jamsen, E., Stogiannidis, I., Malmivaara, A., Pajamaki, J., Puolakka, T. & Konttinen, Y. Outcome of prosthesis exchange for infected knee arthroplasty: the effect of treatment approach. *Acta Orthopaedica* 80, 67-77 (2009).

John, A.-K., Baldoni, D., Haschke, M., Rentsch, K., Schaerli, P., Zimmerli, W. & Trampuz, A. Efficacy of daptomycin in implant-associated infection due to methicillin-resistant Staphylococcus aureus: importance of combination with rifampin. *Antimicrobial Agents and Chemotherapy* 53, 2719-2724 (2009).

Jones, S.M., Morgan, M., Humphrey, T.J. & Lappin-Scott, H. Effect of vancomycin and rifampicin on methicillin-resistant Staphylococcus aureus biofilms. *Lancet* 357, 40-41 (2001).

Ko, P., Ip, D., Chow, K., Cheung, F., Lee, O. & Lam, J. The Role of Intraoperative Frozen Section in Decision Making in Revision Hip and Knee Arthroplasties in a Local Community Hospital. *Journal of Arthoplasty* 20, 189-195 (2005).

Krimmer, V., Merkert, H., von Eiff, C., Frosch, M., Eulert, J., Lohr, J.F., Hacker, J. & Ziebuhr, W. Detection of Staphylococcus aureus and Staphylococcus epidermidis in clinical Samples by 16S rRNA-Directed In Site Hybridization. *Journal of Clinical Microbiology* 37, 2667-2673 (1999).

Kurtz, S., Ong, K., Lau, E., Mowat, F. & Halpern, M. Projections of primary and revision hip and knee arthroplasty in the United States from 2005 to 2030. *J Bone Joint Surg Am* 89-A, 780-785 (2007).

Kurtz, S.M., Lau, E., Schmier, J., Ong, K.L., Zhao, K. & Parvizi, J. Infection burden for hip and knee arthroplasty in the United States. *Journal of Arthoplasty* 23, 984-991 (2008).

Kurtz, S.M., Ong, K.L., Lau, E., Bozic, K.J., Berry, D. & Parvizi, J. Prosthetic joint infection risk after TKA in the Medicare population. *Clinical Orthopaedics and Related Research* 468, 52-56 (2010).

Kwee, T.C., Kwee, R.M. & Alavi, A. FDG-PET for diagnosing prosthetic joint infection: systematic review and metaanalysis. *European Journal of Nuclear Medicine and Molecular Imaging* 35, 2122-2132 (2008).

Laffer, R.R., Graber, P., Ochsner, P.E. & Zimmerli, W. Outcome of prosthetic knee-associated infection: evaluation of 40 consecutive episodes at a single centre. *Clin Microbiol Infect* 12, 433-439 (2006).

Langlais, F. Can we improve the results of revision arthroplasty for infected total hip replacement? *J Bone Joint Surg Am* 85-Br, 637-640 (2003).

Langlais, F., Belot, N., Ropars, M., Thomazeau, H., Lambotte, J.C. & Cathelineau, G. Antibiotic cements in articular prostheses: current orthopaedic concepts. *International Journal of Antimicrobial Agents* 28, 84-89 (2006).

Larsson, S., Thelander, U.L.F. & Friberg, S. C-reactive protein (CRP) levels after elective orthopedic surgery. *Clinical Orthopaedics and Related Research* 275, 237-242 (1992).

Legout, L., Senneville, E., Stern, R., Yazdanpanah, Y., Savage, C., Roussel-Delvalez, M., Rosele, B., Migaud, H. & Mouton, Y. Treatment of Bone and Joint Infections Caused by Gram-Nagative Bacilli with a Cefepime-Fluoroquinolone Combination. *Clinical Microbiology and Infection* 12, 1030-1033 (2006).

Leunig, M., Chosa, E., Speck, M. & Ganz, R. A cement spacer for two-stage revision of infected implants of the hip joint. *International Orthopaedics* 22, 209-214 (1998).

Lim, S.-j., Park, J.-c., Moon, Y.-w. & Park, Y.-s. Treatment of Periprosthetic Hip Infection Caused by Resistant Microorganisms Using 2-Stage Reimplantation Protocol. *Journal of Arthroplasty* 24, 1264-1269 (2009).

Marculescu, C.E., Berbari, E.F., Hanssen, A.D., Steckelberg, J.M., Harmsen, S.W., Mandrekar, J.N. & Osmon, D.R. Outcome of prosthetic joint infections treated with debridement and retention of components. *Clinical Infectious Diseases* 42, 471-478 (2006a).

Marculescu, C.E., Berbari, E.F., Hanssen, A.D., Steckelberg, J.M., Harmsen, S.W., Mandrekar, J.N. & Osmon, D.R. Outcome of prosthetic joint infections treated with debridement and retention of components. *Clinical Infectious Diseases* 42, 471-478 (2006b).

Marculescu, C.E. & Cantey, J.R. Polymicrobial Prosthetic Joint Infections. *Clinical Orthopaedics and Related Research* 466, 1397-1404 (2008).

Mariani, B.D., Martin, D.S., Levine, M.J., Booth, R.E. & Tuan, R.S. The Coventry Award. Polymerase chain reaction detection of bacterial infection in total knee arthroplasty. *Clinical Orthopaedics and Related Research*, 11-22 (1996).

Matthews, P.C., Berendt, a.R., McNally, M.a. & Byren, I. Diagnosis and management of prosthetic joint infection. *British Medical Journal* 338, b1773-b1773 (2009).

McDonald, D.J., Fitzgerald, R.H. & Ilstrup, D.M. Two-stage reconstruction of a total hip arthroplasty because of infection. *J Bone Joint Surg Am* 71-A, 828-834 (1989).

McDowell, A. & Patrick, S. Evaluation of Nonculture Methods for the Detection of Prosthetic Hip Biofilms. *Clinical Orthopaedics and Related Research* 437, 74-82 (2005).

Miley, G.B., Scheller, A.D. & Turner, R.H. Medical and surgical treatment of the septic hip with one-stage revision arthroplasty. *Clinical Orthopaedics and Related Research* 170, 76-76 (1982).

Miller, T.T. Imaging of knee arthroplasty. *European Journal of Radiology* 54, 164-177 (2005).

Mirra, J.M., Amstutz, H.C., Matos, M. & Gold, R. The pathology of the joint tissues and its clinical relevance in prosthesis failure. *Clinical Orthopaedics and Related Research* 117, 221-240 (1976).

Mittal, Y., Fehring, T.K., Hanssen, A., Marculescu, C., Odum, S.M. & Osmon, D. Two-stage reimplantation for periprosthetic knee infection involving resistant organisms. *J Bone Joint Surg Am* 89-A, 1227-1231 (2007).

Monzon, M., Oteiza, C., Leiva, J., Lamata, M. & Amorena, B. Biofilm testing of Staphylococcus epidermidis clinical isolates: low performance of vancomycin in relation to other antibiotics. *Diagnostic Microbiology and Infectious Disease* 44, 319-324 (2002).

Moojen, D.J.F., Spijkers, S.N.M., Schot, C.S., Nijhof, M.W., Vogely, H.C., Fleer, A., Verbout, A.J., Castelein, R.M., Dhert, W.J.a. & Schouls, L.M. Identification of orthopaedic infections using broad-range polymerase chain reaction and reverse line blot hybridization. *J Bone Joint Surg Am* 89-A, 1298-1305 (2007).

Moran, E., Masters, S., Berendt, A.R., McLardy-Smith, P., Byren, I. & Atkins, B.L. Guiding empirical antibiotic therapy in orthopaedics: The microbiology of prosthetic joint infection managed by debridement, irrigation and prosthesis retention. *Journal of Infection* 55, 1-7 (2007).

Morrey, B.F., Westholm, F., Schoifet, S., Rand, J.A. & Bryan, R.S. Long-Term Results of Various Treatment Options for Infected Total Knee Arthroplasty. *Clinical Orthopaedics and Related Research* 248 120-128 (1989).

Moter, A. & Gobel, U.B. Fluorescence in situ hybridization (FISH) for direct visualization of microorganisms. *Journal of Microbiological Methods* 41, 85-112 (2000).

Murdoch, D.R., Roberts, S.a., G., V., Shah, M.a., Taylor, S.L., Morris, a.J. & Corey, G.R. Infection of orthopedic prostheses after Staphylococcus aureus bacteremia. *Clinical Infectious Diseases* 32, 647-649 (2001).

Nunez, L.V., Buttaro, M.a., Morandi, A., Pusso, R. & Piccaluga, F. Frozen sections of samples taken intraoperatively for diagnosis of infection in revision hip surgery. *Acta Orthopaedica* 78, 226-230 (2007).

Ong, K.L., Kurtz, S.M., Lau, E., Bozic, K.J., Berry, D.J. & Parvizi, J. Prosthetic joint infection risk after total hip arthroplasty in the Medicare population. *Journal of Arthoplasty* 24, 105-109 (2009).

Pandey, R., Berendt, A.R. & Athanasou, N.A. Histological and microbiological findings in non-infected and infected revision arthroplasty tissues. *Archives of Orthopaedic and Trauma Surgery* 120, 570-574 (2000).

Panush, R.S. & Petty, R.W. Inhibition of human lymphocyte responses by methylmethacrylate. *Clinical Orthopaedics and Related Research* 134, 356-356 (1978).

Petty, W. The effect of methylmethacrylate on the bacterial inhibiting properties of normal human serum. *Clinical Orthopaedics and Related Research*, 266-278 (1978).

Poss, R., Thornhill, T.S., Ewald, F.C., Thomas, W.H., Batte, N.J. & Sledge, C.B. Factors influencing the incidence and outcome of infection following total joint arthroplasty. *Clinical Orthopaedics and Related Research* 182, 117-126 (1984).

Poulsen, L.K., Ballard, G. & Stahl, D.a. Use of rRNA fluorescence in situ hybridization for measuring the activity of single cells in young and established biofilms. *Applied and Environmental Microbiology* 59, 1354-1360 (1993).

Pulido, L., Ghanem, E., Joshi, A., Purtill, J.J. & Parvizi, J. Periprosthetic joint infection: the incidence, timing, and predisposing factors. *Clinical Orthopaedics and Related Research* 466, 1710-1715 (2008).

Rand, J.A., Bryan, R., Morrey, B. & Westholm, F. Management of Infected Total Knee Arthroplasty. *Clinical Orthopaedics and Related Research* 205, 75-85 (1986).

Rao, N., Crossett, L.S., Sinha, R.K. & L., J. Long-term suppression of infection in total joint arthroplasty. *Clinical Orthopaedics and Related Research* 414, 55-60 (2003).

Rose, W.E. & Poppens, P.T. Impact of biofilm on the in vitro activity of vancomycin alone and in combination with tigecycline and rifampicin against Staphylococcus aureus. *Journal of Antimicrobial Chemotherapy* 63, 485-488 (2009).

Schafer, P., Fink, B., Sandow, D., Margull, A., Berger, I. & Frommelt, L. Prolonged bacterial culture to identify late periprosthetic joint infection: a promising strategy. *Clinical Infectious Diseases* 47, 1403-1409 (2008).

Schwank, S., Rajacic, Z., Zimmerli, W. & Blaser, J. Impact of bacterial biofilm formation on in vitro and in vivo activities of antibiotics. *Antimicrobial Agents and Chemotherapyy* 42, 895-898 (1998).

Shah, K., Mohammed, A., Patil, S., McFadyen, A. & Meek, R.M.D. Circulating cytokines after hip and knee arthroplasty: a preliminary study. *Clinical Orthopaedics and Related Research* 467, 946-951 (2009).

Sharma, D., Douglas, J., Coulter, C., Weinrauch, P. & Crawford, R. Microbiology of infected arthroplasty: implications for empiric peri-operative antibiotics. *Journal of Orthopaedic Surgery (Hong Kong)* 16, 339-342 (2008).

Shiau, a.L. & Wu, C.L. The inhibitory effect of Staphylococcus epidermidis slime on the phagocytosis of murine peritoneal macrophages is interferon-independent. *Microbiology and Immunology* 42, 33-40 (1998).

Shih, L.-Y., Wu, J.-J. & Yanc, D.-J. Erythrocyte Sedimentation Rate and C-reactive Protein Values in Patients with Total Hip Arthroplasty. *Clinical Orthopaedics and Related Research* 225, 238-246 (1987).

Smith, S.L., Wastie, M.L. & Forster, I. Radionuclide bone scintigraphy in the detection of significant complications after total knee joint replacement. *Clinical radiology* 56, 221-224 (2001).

Souli, M. & Giamarellou, H. Effects of Slime Produced by Clinical Isolates of Coagulase-Negative Staphylococci on Activities of Various Antimicrobial Agents. *Antimicrobial Agents and Chemotherapy* 42, 939-941 (1998).

Southwood, R.T., Rice, J.L., McDonald, P.J., Hakendorf, P.H. & Rozenbilds, M.A. Infection in experimental hip arthroplasties. *J Bone Joint Surg Am* 67-Br, 229-231 (1985).

Spangehl, M.J., Masri, B.A., Connell, J.X.O. & Duncan, C.P. Prospective Analysis of Preoperative and Intraoperative Investigations for the Diagnosis of Infection at the Sites of Two Hundred and Two Revision Total Hip Arthroplasties. *J Bone Joint Surg Am* 81-A, 672-683 (1999).

Steckelberg, J.M. & Osman, D.R. Prosthetic Joint Infections. in *Infections Associated with Indwelling Medical Devices, 3rd ed.* (eds. Waldvogel, F.A. & Bisno, A.L.) 173-209 ASM Press, 1-55581-177-9, Washington D.C, 2000.

Steckelberg, J.M. & Osmon, D.R. Prosthetic Joint Infections. in *Infections Associated with Indwelling Medical Devices* (eds. Waldvogel, F.A. & Bisno, A.L.) 173-209 ASM Press, Washington DC, 2000.

Stewart, P.S. & Costerton, J.W. Antibiotic resistance of bacteria in biofilms. *Lancet* 358, 135-138 (2001).

Surin, V.V., Sundholm, K. & Backman, L. Infection After Total Hip Replacement. *Journal of Bone and Joint Surgery: British Volume* 65, 412-418 (1983).

Swan, J., Dowsey, M., Babazadeh, S., Mandaleson, A. & Choong, P.F. Significance of sentinel infective events in haematogenous prosthetic knee infections. *ANZ J Surg* 81, 40-45 (2011).

Trampuz, A., Hanssen, A.D., Osmon, D.R., Mandrekar, J., Steckelberg, J.M. & Patel, R. Synovial fluid leukocyte count and differential for the diagnosis of prosthetic knee infection. *American Journal of Medicine* 117, 556-562 (2004).

Trampuz, A., Osmon, D.R., Hanssen, A.D., Steckelberg, J.M. & Patel, R. Molecular and antibiofilm approaches to prosthetic joint infection. *Clinical Orthopaedics and Related Research*, 69-88 (2003).

Trampuz, A., Piper, K.E., Jacobson, M.J., Hanssen, A.D., Unni, K.K., Osmon, D.R., Mandrekar, J.N., Cockerill, F.R., Steckelberg, J.M., Greenleaf, J.F. & Patel, R. Sonication of removed hip and knee prostheses for diagnosis of infection. *New England Journal of Medicine* 357, 654-663 (2007).

Trampuz, A. & Zimmerli, W. Diagnosis and treatment of implant-associated septic arthritis and osteomyelitis. *Current Infectious Disease Reports* 10, 394-403 (2008).
Trebse, R., Pisot, V. & Trampuz, A. Treatment of infected retained implants. *J Bone Joint Surg Am* 87-Br, 249-256 (2005).
Tsukayama, D.T., Estrada, R. & Gustilo, R.B. Infection after total hip arthroplasty. A study of the treatment of one hundred and six infections. *J Bone Joint Surg Am* 78-A, 512-523 (1996).
Tunney, M.M., Patrick, S., Curran, M.D., Ramage, G., Hanna, D., Nixon, J.R., Gorman, S.P., Davis, R.I. & And, N. Detection of prosthetic hip infection at revision arthroplasty by immunofluorescence microscopy and PCR amplification of the bacterial 16S rRNA gene. *Journal of Clinical Microbiology* 37, 3281-3290 (1999).
Vandercam, B., Jeumont, S., Cornu, O., Yombi, J.-C., Lecouvet, F.d.r., LefÃ¨vre, P., Irenge, L.o.M. & Gala, J.-L. Amplification-based DNA analysis in the diagnosis of prosthetic joint infection. *Journal of Molecular Diagnostics* 10, 537-543 (2008).
Wang, J.W. & Chen, C.E. Reimplantation of infected hip arthroplasties using bone allografts. *Clinical Orthopaedics and Related Research* 335, 202-202 (1997).
Wasielewski, R.C., Barden, R.M. & Rosenberg, A.G. Results of different surgical procedures on total knee arthroplasty infections. *Journal of Arthoplasty* 11, 931-938 (1996).
Widmer, A.F., Frei, R., Rajacic, Z. & Zimmerli, W. Correlation between In Vivo and In Vitro Efficacy of Antimicrobial Agents against Foreign Body Infections. *Journal of Infectious Diseases* 162, 96-102 (1990).
Widmer, A.F., Gaechter, A., Ochsner, P.E. & Zimmerli, W. Antimicrobial treatment of orthopedic implant-related infections with rifampin combinations. *Clinical Infectious Diseases* 14, 1251-1253 (1992).
Widmer, A.F., Wiestner, A., Frei, R. & Zimmerli, W. Killing of Nongrowing and Adherent Escherichia coli Determines Drug Efficacy in Device-Related Infections. *Antimicrobial Agents and Chemotherapy* 35, 741-746 (1991).
Wilson, M.G., Kelley, K. & Thornhill, T.S. Infection as a complication of total knee-replacement arthroplasty. Risk factors and treatment in sixty-seven cases. *J Bone Joint Surg Am* 72-A, 878-883 (1990).
Windsor, R.E., Insall, J.N., Urs, W.K., Miller, D.V. & Brause, B.D. Two-stage reimplantation for the salvage of total knee arthroplasty complicated by infection. Further follow-up and refinement of indications. *J Bone Joint Surg Am* 72-A, 272-278 (1990).
Woods, G.W., Lionberger, D.R. & Tullos, H.S. Failed total knee arthroplasty: Revision and arthrodesis for infection and noninfectious complications. *Clinical Orthopaedics and Related Research* 173, 184-184 (1983).
Wymenga, A.B., van Horn, J.R., Theeuwes, A., Muytjens, H.L. & Slooff, T.J. Perioperative factors associated with septic arthritis after arthroplasty. Prospective multicenter study of 362 knee and 2,651 hip operations. *Acta Orthopaedica Scandinavica* 63, 665-671 (1992).
Yang, K., Yeo, S.J., Lee, B.P. & Lo, N.N. Total knee arthroplasty in diabetic patients: a study of 109 consecutive cases. *Journal of Arthoplasty* 16, 102-106 (2001).
Zimmerli, W. Prosthetic-joint-associated infections. *Best Practice and Research Clinical Rheumatology* 20, 1045-1063 (2006).

Zimmerli, W., Trampuz, A. & Ochsner, P.E. Prosthetic-joint infections. *New England Journal of Medicine* 351, 1645-1654 (2004).

Zimmerli, W., Widmer, A.F., Blatter, M., Frei, R. & Ochsner, P.E. Role of rifampin for treatment of orthopedic implant-related staphylococcal infections: a randomized controlled trial. *Journal of the American Medical Association* 279, 1537-1541 (1998).

Zoccali, C., Teori, G. & Salducca, N. The role of FDG-PET in distinguishing between septic and aseptic loosening in hip prosthesis: a review of literature. *International Orthopaedics* 33, 1-5 (2009).

20

Infections in Hip and Knee Arthroplasty: Challenges to and Chances for the Microbiological Laboratory

Peter Schäfer[1], Bernd Fink[2], Dieter Sandow[1] and Lars Frommelt[3]
[1]MVZ Labor Ludwigsburg, Wernerstrasse 33, Ludwigsburg,
[2]Department of Joint Replacement, General and Rheumatic Orthopaedics, Orthopaedic Clinic Markgröningen, Kurt-Lindemann-Weg 10, Markgröningen,
[3]Institute for Infectiology, ENDO-Clinic Hamburg, Holstenstrasse 2, Hamburg
Germany

1. Introduction

Comprehensive algorithms have been devised to improve the management of periprosthetic joint infections of the hip and the knee (Gomez & Patel, 2011a, 2011b; Peel et al., 2011). There is still no single best method for diagnosis, as stressed for instance in a guideline published recently by the American Association of Orthopedic Surgeons (AAOS) (Della Valle et al., 2010). An important reason for this is lacking consensus on how to define arthroplasty infection accurately. Nevertheless, it is beyond dispute that microbiologic techniques play a key role in assessment for these infections.

The chapter consists of three sections. Firstly, a general introduction to the special nature of arthroplasty infection is given, which highlights the necessity of reliable microbiological diagnostics. Secondly, a critical appraisal of the various technical and interpretive aspects of microbiologic procedures is featured. Thirdly, our own diagnostic approaches are presented, and a prospect on probable useful developments in the future is offered.

2. Identification of infected implants: The need for microbiological testing

2.1 Epidemiology

Periprosthetic joint infections are a feared complication of hip and knee arthroplasty. Infection is supposed to be the underlying cause in about 15% of hip revision arthroplasties and 25% of knee revision arthroplasties (Bozic et al., 2009, 2010). Depending on the onset of infection after the primary implantation, periprosthetic infections have been defined as "early" (up to 3 months), "delayed" (3-24 months), and "late" (more than 24 months) after surgery (Zimmerli et al., 2004). However, a different classification makes more sense from the therapeutic point of view. According to this, infections which occur within 4 weeks after arthroplasty implantation are recognized as "early". These are most often caused by highly virulent organisms (e. g. *Staphylococcus aureus*) acquired during or shortly after implantation and can be treated with the prospect of survival of the implant. In contrast, infections which become manifest after more than 4 weeks ("late" infections) require removal of the prosthesis. Late infections are low-grade infections due to less virulent agents belonging to the normal skin flora (e. g. coagulase-negative staphylococci, *Propionibacterium* species, coryneform bacteria), which are mostly also attained during the operation procedure or are infections which result from hematogenous spreading from remote sites (Cui et al., 2007; Hanssen & Osmon, 2002; Virolainen et al., 2002).

2.2 Pathogenetic aspects

The characteristics of arthroplasty infection reflect a unique pathogenesis which is ultimately marked by two features: biofilm development and manifestation of a periprosthetic membrane.

2.2.1 Biofilms

Biofilm-forming bacteria share the ability to colonize foreign implant materials by initial attachment to the surface, followed by agglomeration in multi-cellular layers. During the accumulation process the bacteria excrete matrix substances into which the infectious agents themselves become embedded. Due to alterations in cellular metabolism, regulated by complex signal pathways within the biofilm, the bacteria switch from the planktonic state to a sessile condition in which proliferation rates are extremely low (Costerton et al., 1999; Donlan & Costerton, 2002; Donlan, 2005; Gristina & Costerton, 1985).

Infections involving biofilm formation are both difficult to identify and to treat. On one hand, the biofilm matrix provides a substantial barrier to host defense mechanisms and to diffusion of antibiotics. On the other hand, the low proliferation levels of the sessile organisms may dramatically impair their antibiotic susceptibility, especially to bactericidal agents (Jones et al., 2001; Monzon et al., 2002; Stewart & Costerton, 2001), and their cultivation for diagnostic purposes in vitro.

As biofilm formation is a gradual process, this mechanism is the characteristic feature of late, low-grade infections. Implants with an established biofilm are definitely subject to removal although the causative agents are less virulent by themselves than the bacteria which cause early arthroplasty infections.

2.2.2 Periprosthetic membrane

The periprosthetic membrane is the histomorphologic hallmark of joint implant failure. It is a seam of connective tissue which develops at the interface between the bone and the implant in the course of the inflammatory process that leads to septic or aseptic prosthetic loosening. Interestingly, there are four morphologic types which can be linked to different etiologies of inflammation. Of these, the infectious type (type II) is particularly often associated with periprosthetic infection. It is characterized by predominant infiltration with neutrophilic polymorphonuclear leukocytes (Krenn et al., 2011; Morawietz et al., 2006).

As the periprosthetic membrane must be removed if the surgical revision procedure is to be successful, it is ideal sample material for characterizing the type of inflammation by histology, thus providing valuable evidence for the underlying cause of implant loosening.

2.3 Inflammation parameters: Utility to detect infections

Early periprosthetic infections are mostly associated with typical clinical signs of infectious disease. However, in low-grade (late) infections the clinical symptoms and radiologic signs are often unspecific and therefore not suitable for ruling out aseptic implant failure

(Virolainen et al., 2002). Nuclear imaging techniques used to detect periprosthetic inflammation are generally regarded as optional tests which may be of use if the diagnosis cannot be established otherwise, but they are not recommended for routine application (Della Valle et al., 2010). In contrast, the following procedures do play important roles in patient assessment for arthroplasty infection.

2.3.1 Blood laboratory markers

Erythrocyte sedimentation rate (ESR) and C-reactive protein (CRP) level are the parameters most widely used for preoperative evaluation of patients with suspected arthroplasty infection. While sensitivity is mostly high, specificity is limited, especially in patients with systemic inflammatory diseases (e. g., rheumatoid arthritis) (Bottner et al., 2007; Della Valle et al., 2007; Fink et al., 2008; Greidanus et al., 2007; Kamme & Lindberg, 1981). Nevertheless, from the studies with reliable data the AAOS strongly recommends testing of both ESR and CRP in all patients assessed for arthroplasty infection (Della Valle et al., 2010).
Other inflammation markers (interleukin 6, procalcitonin, tumor necrosis factor α) are evaluated increasingly for periprosthetic infections, but at present there seems to be no advantage over CRP testing (Berbari et al., 2010; Bottner et al., 2007; Di Cesare et al., 2005).

2.3.2 Microscopic detection of inflammatory cells

Joint aspiration fluid. Total and differential white blood cell counts in synovial fluid are routinely determined in many settings. Some studies of knee patients have reported that total leukocyte counts or neutrophils percentages which exceed a certain cutoff level are highly indicative of arthroplasty infection. However, the thresholds differ considerably between studies (Della Valle et al., 2007; Ghanem et al., 2008; Trampuz et al., 2004).
In contrast, there are less data available for hip patients because aspiration of this joint is more prone to complications and is therefore only recommended if there is substantial clinical or laboratory evidence for infection (Della Valle et al., 2010; Schinsky et al., 2008).
Frozen tissue sections. Neutrophils are the predominant histomorphologic factor in periprosthetic infection (Krenn et al., 2011; Morawietz et al., 2006). As a consequence, the histologic diagnosis of probable infections is based on the tissue neutrophil concentration, as defined by i) the number of neutrophils in a high-power (400x) microscopic field, and ii) the minimum number of fields (usually 10) containing that concentration of neutrophils. The available studies report 5 or 10 neutrophils per high-power field as suitable thresholds for diagnosis of arthroplasty infection (Banit et al., 2002; Della Valle et al., 2007; Fehring & McAlister, 1994; Fink et al., 2008; Frances Borrego et al., 2007; Ko et al., 2005; Lonner et al., 1996; Nunez et al., 2007; Schinsky et al., 2008). Patients with inflammatory arthropathy, which often display tissue infiltration by neutrophils in the absence of infection, were excluded in some of these investigations (Fehring & McAlister, 1994; Ko et al., 2005; Pandey et al., 1999; Schinsky et al., 2008). However, all in all there is not enough information to enable a clear-cut preference of the lower or the higher threshold.
Despite the considerable advances in recent years with respect to the histomorphologic characterization of periprosthetic infections, it is not possible to treat affected patients sufficiently unless the causative microorganisms are identified precisely. Thus, customized local and systemic antibiotic therapy of a known infectious agent is inherently superior to calculated therapy because treatment failure arising from antibiotic resistance can be avoided (Bejon et al., 2010).

3. Microbiological diagnosis: Pros and cons of different approaches

Adequate microbiological procedures must reflect the special character of periprosthetic infections in order to identify the causative agents accurately. Although largely interdependent, eight issues which may influence the significance of microbiologic testing are addressed separately in the following: i) patient-specific factors, ii) the sample character, iii) the logistic interface between the clinic and the laboratory, iv) the method of sample processing, v) the means of identification, vi) the culture conditions, vii) the means of discriminating between infection and contamination, and viii) the stage at which sample materials are drawn (pre-operatively versus intra-operatively).

3.1 Patient-specific factors

3.1.1 Sample origin (hip versus knee)

Joint aspiration prior to revision arthroplasty is widely utilized. For knee patients the procedure is comparatively straightforward, whereas hip aspiration may impose a higher risk of iatrogenic infection. Thus, it is often argued that invasive diagnostic samples from hip patients should be obtained only if a there is a high probability of infection (Bozic et al., 2009, 2010).

Regarding periprosthetic tissue biopsies, the diagnostic sensitivity of pre-operative sampling may be lower in hip infections compared with knee infections (Fink et al., 2008; Meermans & Haddad, 2010; Williams et al., 2004), possibly because infected tissue is more difficult to assess without dislocating the joint.

3.1.2 Underlying systemic diseases

The definitive identification of microorganisms is especially important in patients with systemic inflammatory diseases because, as mentioned before, inflammation markers can be elevated in aseptic implant failure. At the same time, the differentiation between an infecting and a contaminating agent is challenging in these patients (see 3.7).

3.1.3 Previous antibiotic therapy

False-negative results of microbiological cultures and even PCR tests have been reported in patients who received antibiotic therapy within 2 weeks prior to obtaining intra-articular sample material (Achermann et al., 2010). Furthermore, it is also suggested that peri-operative antibiotic prophylaxis should be withheld if possible until samples for microbiological analysis have been obtained, but that the risk of false-negative sample results also should be weighed against the protective effect of pre-operative administration of antibiotic prophylaxis (Achermann et al., 2010; Engesaeter et al., 2003; Jämsen et al., 2009; Trampuz et al., 2007).

3.2 Sample character

3.2.1 Tissue swabs

In a report on hip and knee patients organisms cultured from swabs of sinus tracts showed no concordance with the culture results from specimens obtained intra-operatively (Sadiq et al., 2005). There are limited data which suggest that the results of superficial swabs show a reasonable correlation with culture yield from intra-operative tissue biopsy material (Cune et al., 2009). However, other studies have rated results from swab material as both insensitive and unspecific (Font-Vizcarra et al., 2010; Levine & Evans, 2001). Swabs cannot absorb nearly as much material as can be harvested from tissue biopsies or joint fluid, which alone would account for inferior sensitivity. Furthermore, as most etiologic agents of arthroplasty infections belong to the normal skin flora, it is hardly possible to discern between infectious strains and contaminants using swab material. In summary, tissue swabs cannot be recommended to assess prosthetic infections reliably.

3.2.2 Joint aspiration fluid

The overall significance of culture from pre-operative synovial fluid to detect periprosthetic infection is valued as high. However, sensitivity may be reduced if the infection does not involve the synovia or if the concentration of planktonic bacteria in the fluid is limited due to a mature biofilm. Furthermore, false positive results from skin flora occur (Barrack & Harris, 1993; Della Valle et al., 2007; Eisler et al., 2001; Fink et al., 2008; Lachiewicz et al., 1996; Malhotra & Morgan, 2004; Williams et al., 2004).

3.2.3 Periprosthetic tissue biopsies

Analysis of tissue biopsies offers the advantage that multiple samples can be obtained from different locations within the suspicious area. Repeated isolation of bacteria (e. g., isolation of the same organism in at least 2 tissue samples) increases the probability of infection. Thus, there are several reports in which higher sensitivity of tissue culture compared with synovial fluid culture is observed (Fink et al., 2008; Meermans & Haddad, 2010; Roberts et al., 1992; Sadiq et al., 2005; Williams et al., 2004).

3.3 Logistics between clinic and laboratory

Pre-analytical sampling errors have been claimed to contribute significantly to false-negative culture results, with highly sensitive PCR techniques being a means to overcome these drawbacks (Achermann et al., 2010). Guidelines devised by the German Society of Hygiene and Microbiology have proposed that periprosthetic sample material intended for microbiological cultivation should be processed within one hour post-drawing. Although such stringent demands are not realistic for the routine setting, it is indeed crucial to establish a standardized work flow between the clinic and the laboratory regarding the procedures of sample drawing, transportation to the laboratory, and specimen processing. The organizational structure in our laboratory comprises a courier service as well as evening and weekend laboratory duty, which ensures that over 95% of culture samples are processed within 6 hours post-operatively (see 4.1.1).

3.4 Sample processing

The efforts made to obtain significant sample material are futile if the laboratory process is not optimized. However, costs and benefits should be well-balanced.

3.4.1 Native material

The simplest way of tissue sample processing is mincing by a scalpel. This allows efficient investigation of multiple samples from each patient (see 3.2.3). If carried out under a laminar air flow workbench it is not highly prone to contamination (Atkins et al., 1998; Schäfer et al., 2008; Trampuz et al., 2006, 2007).
Some authors favor scraping the surface of the explanted material. This has been reported to be more sensitive than tissue culture but also liable to contamination (Bjerkan et al., 2009; Neut et al., 2003).

3.4.2 Blood culture vials

Automated incubation and fluorometric detection of bacterial growth improves sensitivity compared with conventional liquid culture broths (Font-Vizcarra et al., 2010; Levine & Evans, 2001). However, there are potential drawbacks. Firstly, the possibility to determine leukocyte counts is lost if no native material is saved. Secondly, if the sample volume falls short of three milliliters, standard aerobic and anaerobic blood culture bottles may lack sensitivity. Pediatric vials are optimized for culture of lower sample volumes, but it is possible that some anaerobic bacteria are missed due to the composition of the medium (Morello et al., 1991).

3.4.3 Sonication of explants

Sonication of explanted prosthesis components to disrupt bacterial biofilms has been assessed by several authors (Achermann et al., 2010; Kobayashi et al., 2006; Trampuz et al., 2003, 2007; Tunney et al., 1998). Culture of the sonication fluid appears to be more sensitive than native sample processing. However, it is cumbersome and not suitable for high-throughput analysis. The possible destruction of planktonic bacteria is an issue that has not been raised systematically to date, but may be of importance in cases of prosthetic infection caused by bacteria which do not establish classical biofilms (Sampedro et al., 2010). There also may be an increased risk of contamination (Holinka et al., 2011; Trampuz et al., 2006).

3.4.4 Bead mill processing of tissue biopsies

The bacterial yield using a bead mill is probably enhanced due to facilitated tissue disruption (Roux et al., 2011). However, careful evaluation of conditions for different bacterial species is necessary in order to avoid overheating of samples and mechanical disruption of planktonic bacteria. At present it cannot be decided whether bead mill processing offers significant advantages.

3.5 Identification of infectious agents

3.5.1 Conventional microbiological detection

Direct gram staining of periprosthetic samples is insensitive and therefore not recommended as a routine test (Banit et al., 2002; Parvizi et al., 2006; Spangehl et al., 1999). However, it can be useful in certain cases of early infection, where prompt treatment of agents which show characteristic morphology (e. g. *Clostridium perfringens*) is enabled.
Classic microbiologic culture confirms the presence of viable bacteria and permits testing for antibiotic susceptibility.

3.5.2 PCR strategies

Universal bacterial detection by PCR-based amplification of the 16S rRNA gene allows the identification of bacteria or fungi which are not viable by conventional culture methods. The overall sensitivity may be higher compared with culture (Bergin et al., 2010; Dempsey et al., 2007; Ince et al., 2004; Levine et al., 1995; Panousis et al., 2005; Tunney et al., 1999). On the other hand, singular specific PCR assays (Kobayashi et al., 2009; Piper et al., 2009; Tarkin et al., 2003) or multiplex assays (Achermann et al., 2010) are sensitive but limited to the organisms included in the test panel.

Although important antibiotic resistance mechanisms like methicillin resistance can be identified genotypically with PCR (Kobayashi et al., 2009; Tarkin et al., 2003), for most substance classes phenotypic susceptibility testing will be necessary in the foreseeable future.

There is no straightforward method to determine whether microbial DNA as detected by PCR reflects living organisms. On the other hand, it cannot be ruled out that previous therapy with antibiotics hampers the sensitivity not only of culture, but also of PCR (Achermann et al., 2010).

3.6 Culture conditions

3.6.1 Culture media

A combination of solid (usually blood agar, chocolate agar, and Schaedler agar) and liquid media (e. g. brain-heart infusion broth and Schaedler broth) is used by standard for aerobic and anaerobic cultivation. Solid media alone lack sensitivity to detect low-grade infections because because the medium eventually dries out. On the other hand, infections involving more than one agent can be overlooked if only broth media are utilized because slower-growing organisms may be inhibited in the presence of fast-growing bacteria.

3.6.2 Culture duration

"Standard" cultivation periods (mostly ≤ 7 days in the literature) are generally questionable in infections where biofilms are involved, due to low cell counts of planktonic bacteria and impaired growth rates of sessile organisms in the biofilm. However, the issue was not addressed for a long time. Prolonged cultivation for 14 days was described sporadically (Ince et al., 2004) and even included as a standard recommendation into German practice guidelines, but not assessed under controlled conditions. Thus, our group systematically evaluated a 14-day culture period with periprosthetic tissue samples from hip and knee patients (Schäfer et al., 2008).

Using the algorithm described under 3.1.1 to distinguish infecting agents from contaminating strains, only 74% of the infections (caused by "early" agents) were found within the first week of cultivation (Schäfer et al., 2008). In the second week we not only identified a significant amount of additional infections, but also a completely different spectrum of causative ("late") species (Table 1).

	isolated organisms	frequency (%)	median time to detection (days)
early species	*Staphylococcus aureus*	8.9	2
	coagulase-negative staphylococci	55.4	4
	Enterococcus species	3.8	2
	Streptococcus species	3.8	1.5
	Enterobacteriaceae	1.9	5
late species	coryneform bacteria	7.6	10
	Propionibacterium species	13.4	11
	Finegoldia species	3.2	8
	others	1.9	9.5

Table 1. Spectrum of bacteria detected over a 14-day cultivation period.

Regarding the late species, the sensitivity would have been merely 27% if cultures had been monitored for only 7 days (Fig. 1).

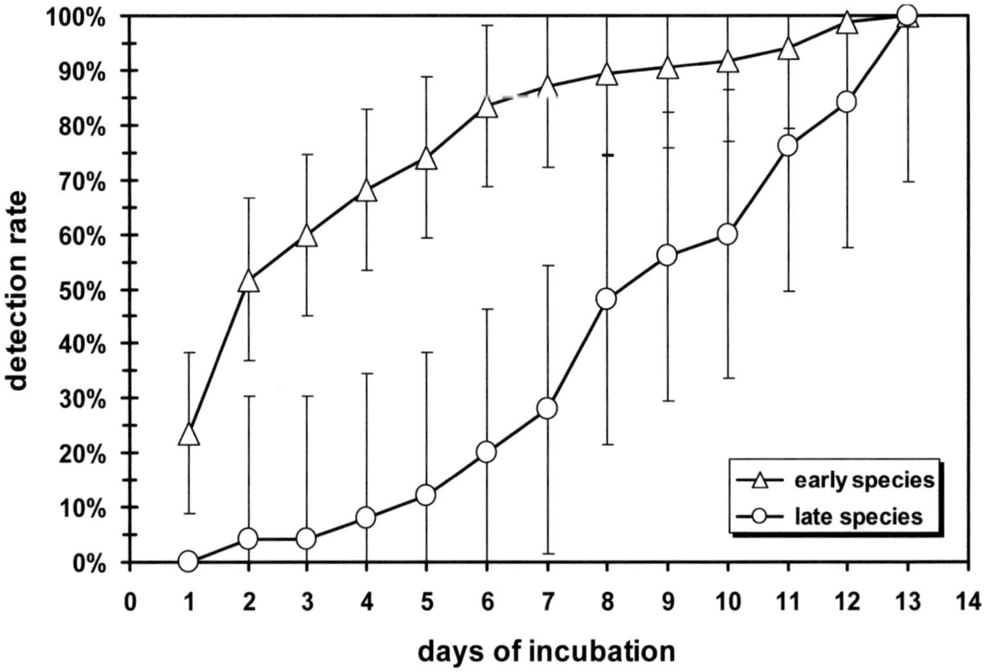

Fig. 1. Detection rates of early and late species depending on the cultivation period. Whisker bars span the Hall-Wellner 95% confidence intervals.

3.7 Discrimination between infection and contamination

There is no standardized procedure which would define infection over contamination accurately. Regarding tissue samples, usually a combined algorithm of neutrophil infiltration scores (2.3.2) and culture detection of identical organisms from multiple tissue samples is used. However, due to the missing consensus criteria the approaches vary considerably between studies (Atkins et al., 1998; Bori et al., 2007; Fink et al., 2008; Ko et al., 2005; Mirra et al., 1976; Pandey et al., 1999).

A problem we encountered was that the algorithms we have adopted to define infections (Atkins et al., 1998; Pandey et al., 1999; Virolainen et al., 2002) were evaluated in the context of "standard" microbiological cultivation periods. Thus, with prolonged culture duration (3.6.2) a larger amount of contaminants might have impaired the significance of this algorithm. However, our findings allowed us to refute the concern that prolonged culture of tissue biopsies could lead to over-proportional contamination rates (Schäfer et al., 2008). It became clear that among both the "early" and the "late" agents (Table 1) a highly significant correlation existed between positive histology and the number of culture-positive tissues (Fig. 2).

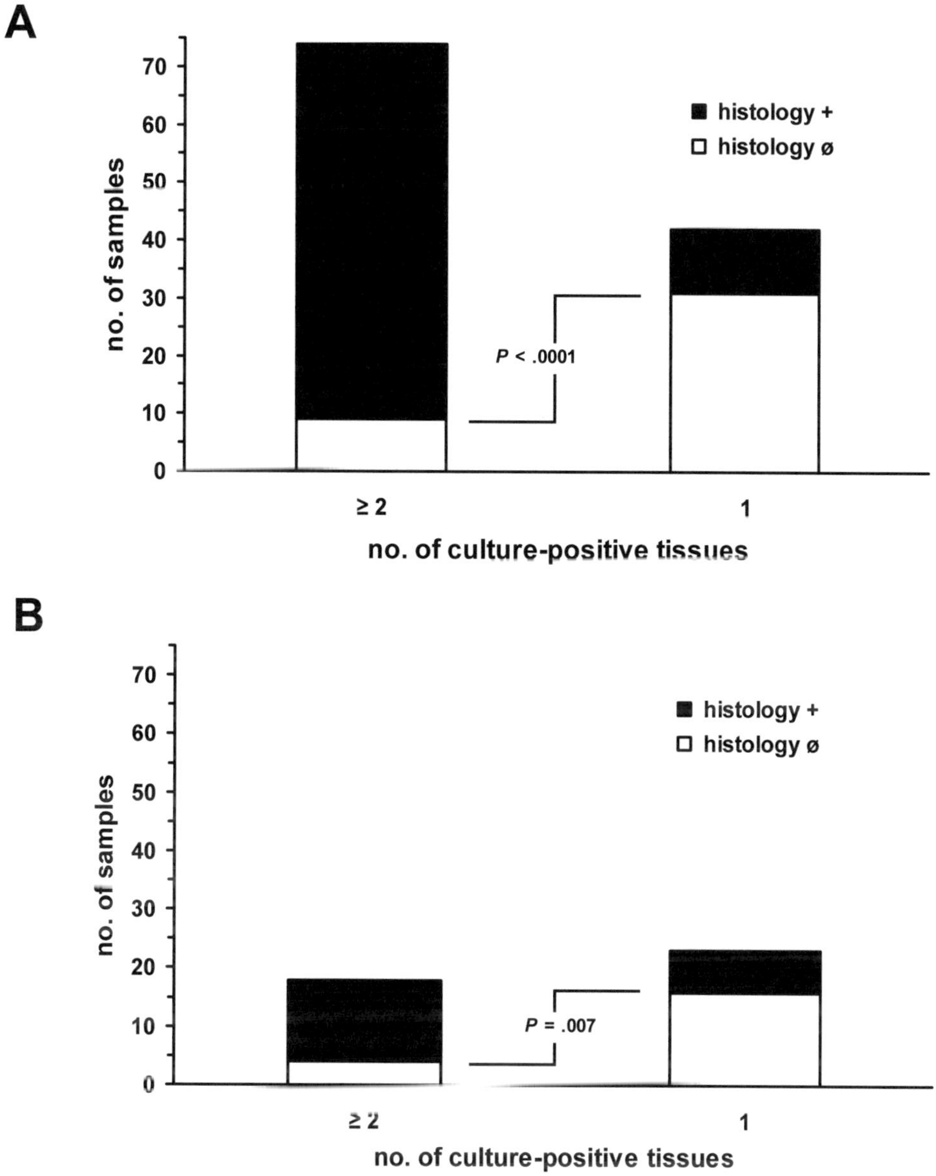

Fig. 2. Correlation between positive histology and the number of culture-positive tissue biopsies. (A) early species. (B) late species. Statistical significance was demonstrated by the χ^2 test.

3.8 Stage at which samples are attained

Although an additional risk and cost factor at first glance, preoperative evaluation of tissue samples in addition to joint aspiration can be helpful to identify the causative agent of arthroplasty infection accurately before the revision is carried out (Fink et al., 2008). This enables a one-stage replacement procedure, if clinically viable. Moreover, it allows to design an individual regimen of systemic and localized antibiotic treatment for two-stage approaches using cement spacers supplemented with antibiotics (Fink et al., 2011). However, the utility of pre-operative biopsies is controversial between studies, mainly due to differences regarding the number of biopsies obtained and the definitions of infection (Fink et al., 2008, 2009; Meermans & Haddad, 2010).

4. Our own approach and future prospects

4.1 The value of both pre-operative and intra-operative sampling

We are convinced that pre-operative identification of the causative agent is a key factor for successful eradication of arthroplasty infections. It enables the design of individualized systemic and localized antibiotic therapy, while intra-operative tissue samples confirm the diagnosis and allow modification of the systemic antibiotic regimen if necessary. The diagnostic workflows we have established to identify hip and knee infections are outlined below.

To minimize the effect of false-negative results, we call for an antibiotic-free interval of 4 weeks before sampling for microbiological diagnosis. At our clinic we withhold peri-operative antibiotic prophylaxis until samples have been drawn, and we have not experienced adverse outcomes.

4.1.1 Samples and diagnosis

An overview of the laboratory procedures is given in Table 2.

sample material	storage	detection method	processing method	no. of samples	definition of infection
synovial aspiration fluid	room temp.	14-day automated culture	pediatric blood culture vial		
tissue biopsies	4°C	14-day aerobic and anaerobic culture sheep blood agar chocolate agar Schaedler agar brain-heart infusion broth Schaedler broth	native	5	identical organisms in ≥ 2 samples
	-20°C	histological staining	frozen sections	5	≥ 5 neutrophils per 400 x field in 10 fields

Table 2. Overview over the laboratory methods used to detect arthroplasty infection.

The definitive diagnosis of arthroplasty infection is established with multiple tissue biopsies taken from the periprosthetic membrane and other macroscopically conspicuous sites during revision surgery. We have experienced that the inflammation process can be assessed with high reliability if 5 samples each are obtained for culture and for histologic analysis. The definition that i) growth of indistinguishable bacteria in ≥ 2 specimens or ii) microbial growth in one specimen combined with a histology score of 3+ (≥ 5 neutrophils per high-power field in 10 fields) (Atkins et al., 1998; Pandey et al., 1999; Virolainen et al., 2002) has proven feasible with respect to the clinical outcomes (Fink et al., 2008, 2009).

Until now we use native tissue biopsies for culture. Tissue mincing is simple to perform and not too prone to contamination if carried out under a laminar air flow workbench. In our opinion, the prolonged incubation period of 14 days we carry out before cultures are cleared is a decisive measure. The persuasiveness of this approach has been shown in detail in 3.6.2. Although it would be interesting to compare the allegedly most sensitive sonication culture method directly with prolonged tissue cultivation, we doubt that the cumbersome and potentially contamination-prone sonication concept would prove significantly superior to our own approach.

As we are convinced that prolonged cultivation over 14 days is the key to detecting infecting organisms with optimal sensitivity, we also currently refrain from using PCR techniques on a routine basis.

If overnight storage of unprocessed samples is necessary, which occurs in less than 5% of cases in our setting, tissue specimens are kept at 4°C and processed at the laboratory the next morning with highly reproducible results. Synovial fluid, when inoculated into pediatric blood culture vials immediately post-drawing, is stable for at least 24 hours at room temperature. Subsequent supplementation with the appropriate enhancing medium, which is necessary to cultivate blood-free sample fluids, can then be done at the laboratory.

Taken together, our diagnostic measures have contributed significantly to the high eradication rates we observe with the treatment of both hip and knee arthroplasty infections (Fink et al., 2008, 2009).

4.1.2 Hip infections

By default, we carry out two-stage revisions of infected hips in our clinic (Fink et al., 2009). Localized antibiotics applied via cement spacer and systemic antibiotics are customized for administration at the time of revision surgery (Fink et al., 2011).

The general sampling algorithm is depicted schematically in Fig. 3. In addition, we obtain pre-operative tissue biopsies for culture and histology if the joint aspiration culture is negative but the risk assessment suggests indicates septic implant failure.

4.1.3 Knee infections

We perform pre-operative tissue biopsies rather than joint aspiration if it is clear that revision operation is necessary due to an unstable implant (Fig. 4). Five biopsies for culture are obtained in a blind fashion without instillating fluid in the intra-articular space (to avoid possible losses in sensitivity due to sample dilution). Afterwards standard arthroscopy is performed to rule out possible joint damage, and during this process 5 additional tissue samples are obtained for histological analysis.

We define infection using the same combined culture and histology algorithm as in biopsy samples taken during revision surgery. Our experience is that pre-operative biopsies are more sensitive than culture from aspirated synovial fluid (Fink et al., 2008).

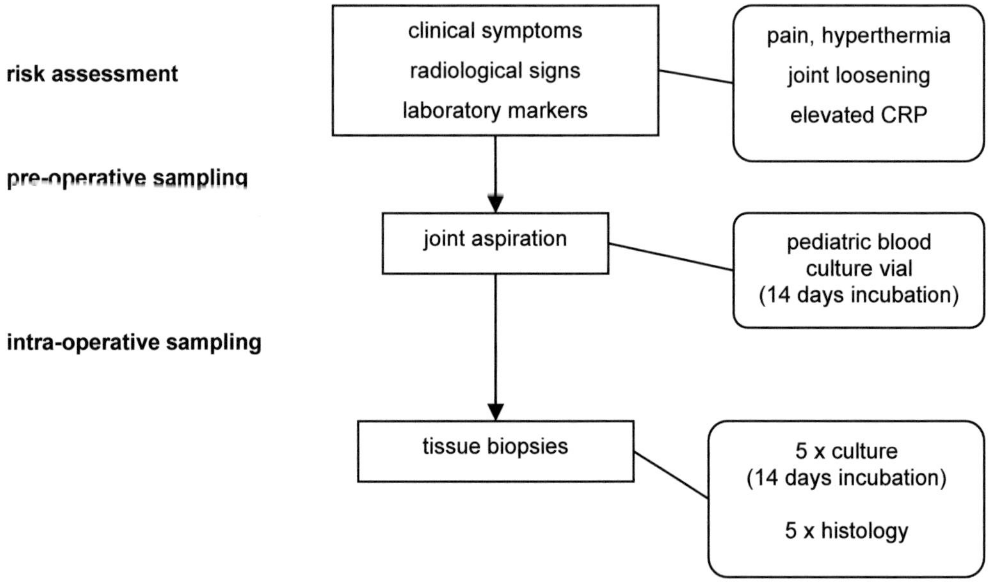

Fig. 3. Sampling algorithm for suspected periprosthetic hip infection. If joint aspiration cultures are negative but the risk assessment suggests indicates septic implant failure, pre-operative tissue biopsies are drawn additionally for culture and histology.

In stable implants, we do not undertake the risk of causing joint damage by blinded tissue biopsy. Instead, joint aspiration culture is performed, which has shown accuracy of 89% (Fink et al., 2008).

The pre-operative diagnostic approach of combined tissue culture histology has shown an accuracy of 98.6% compared to the definitive results obtained during revision surgery (Fink et al., 2008).

4.2 Future prospects

The detection of bacterial RNA rather than DNA by reverse transcription PCR is a potentially useful new approach to arthroplasty infection (Bergin et al., 2010). On one hand, RNA should be present only in viable bacteria and therefore indicate infections more accurately than DNA. On the other hand, the much shorter half-life of RNA should make its presence as a contaminant less likely. It remains to be seen whether this concept will prevail.

Rapid identification of bacteria and fungi to the species level by matrix-assisted laser desorption/ionization time-of-flight (MALDI-TOF) mass spectrometry is utilized increasingly. There are already promising data on the detection of *Staphylococcus epidermidis* in tissue samples of patients with periprosthetic joint infections (Harris et al., 2010). It appears that it should even be possible in the near future to prove clonal identity of strains from the same species isolated from different tissue samples with this technique. This should facilitate the decision whether bacteria isolated from multiple tissue biopsies are likely to be involved in infection or rather reflect contaminating strains.

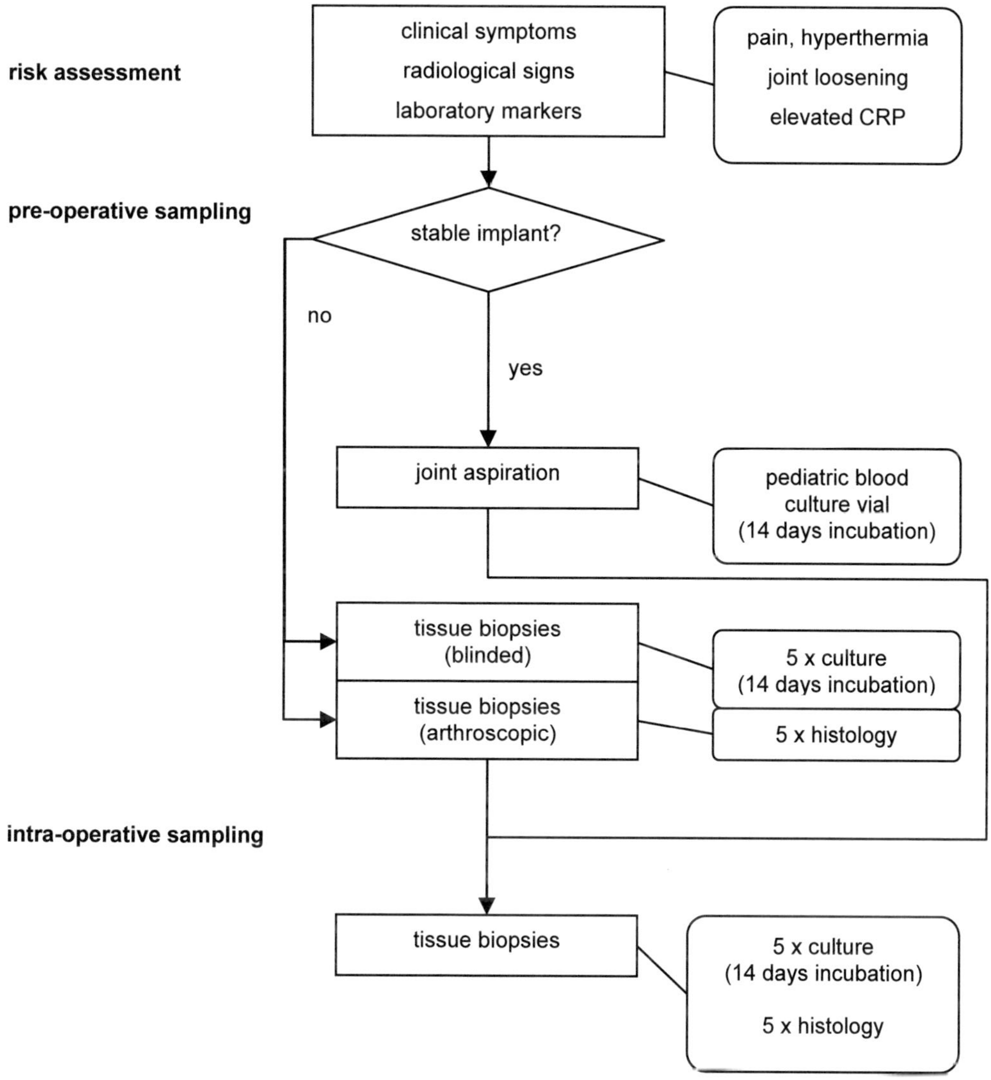

Fig. 4. Sampling algorithm for suspected periprosthetic knee infection.

5. References

Achermann, Y.; Vogt, M.; Leunig, M.; Wust, J. & Trampuz, A. (2010). Improved diagnosis of periprosthetic joint infection by multiplex PCR of sonication fluid from removed implants. *Journal of Clinical Microbiology,* Vol. 48, No. 4, (April 2010), pp. 1208-1214, ISSN 1098-660X

Atkins, B.L.; Athanasou, N.; Deeks, J.J.; Crook, D.W.; Simpson, H.; Peto, T.E.; McLardy-Smith, P. & Berendt, A.R. (1998). Prospective evaluation of criteria for microbiological diagnosis of prosthetic-joint infection at revision arthroplasty. The

OSIRIS Collaborative Study Group. *Journal of Clinical Microbiology,* Vol. 36, No. 10, (October 1998), pp. 2932-2939, ISSN 0095-1137

Banit, D.M.; Kaufer, H. & Hartford, J.M. (2002). Intraoperative frozen section analysis in revision total joint arthroplasty. *Clinical Orthopaedics and Related Research,* Vol. 401, (August 2002), pp. 230-238, ISSN 0009-921X

Barrack, R.L. & Harris, W.H. (1993). The value of aspiration of the hip joint before revision total hip arthroplasty. *Journal of Bone and Joint Surgery,* Vol. 75, No. 1, (January 1993), pp. 66-76, ISSN 0021-9355

Bejon, P.; Berendt, A.; Atkins, B.L.; Green, N.; Parry, H.; Masters, S.; McLardy-Smith, P.; Gundle, R. & Byren, I. (2010). Two-stage revision for prosthetic joint infection: predictors of outcome and the role of reimplantation microbiology. *Journal of Antimicrobial Chemotherapy,* Vol. 65, No. 3, (Mar 2010), pp. 569-575, ISSN 1460-2091

Berbari, E.; Mabry, T.; Tsaras, G.; Spangehl, M.; Erwin, P.J.; Murad, M.H.; Steckelberg, J. & Osmon, D. (2010). Inflammatory blood laboratory levels as markers of prosthetic joint infection: a systematic review and meta-analysis. *Journal of Bone and Joint Surgery,* Vol. 92, No. 11, (September 2010), pp. 2102-2109, ISSN 1535-1386

Bergin, P.F.; Doppelt, J.D.; Hamilton, W.G.; Mirick, G.E.; Jones, A.E.; Sritulanondha, S.; Helm, J.M. & Tuan, R.S. (2010). Detection of periprosthetic infections with use of ribosomal RNA-based polymerase chain reaction. *Journal of Bone and Joint Surgery,* Vol. 92, No. 3, (March 2010), pp. 654-663, ISSN 1535-1386

Bjerkan, G.; Witso, E. & Bergh, K. (2009). Sonication is superior to scraping for retrieval of bacteria in biofilm on titanium and steel surfaces in vitro. *Acta Orthopaedica,* Vol. 80, No. 2, (April 2009), pp. 245-250, ISSN 1745-3682

Bori, G.; Soriano, A.; Garcia, S.; Mallofre, C.; Riba, J. & Mensa, J. (2007). Usefulness of histological analysis for predicting the presence of microorganisms at the time of reimplantation after hip resection arthroplasty for the treatment of infection. *Journal of Bone and Joint Surgery,* Vol. 89, No. 6, (June 2007), pp. 1232-1237, ISSN 0021-9355

Bottner, F.; Wegner, A.; Winkelmann, W.; Becker, K.; Erren, M. & Götze, C. (2007). Interleukin-6, procalcitonin and TNF-alpha: markers of periprosthetic infection following total joint replacement. *Journal of Bone and Joint Surgery. British Volume,* Vol. 89, No. 1, (January 2007), pp. 94-99, ISSN 0301-620X

Bozic, K.J.; Kurtz, S.M.; Lau, E.; Ong, K.; Vail, T.P. & Berry, D.J. (2009). The epidemiology of revision total hip arthroplasty in the United States. *Journal of Bone and Joint Surgery,* Vol. 91, No. 1, (January 2009), pp. 128-133, ISSN 1535-1386

Bozic, K.J.; Kurtz, S.M.; Lau, E.; Ong, K.; Chiu, V.; Vail, T.P.; Rubash, H.E. & Berry, D.J. (2010). The epidemiology of revision total knee arthroplasty in the United States. *Clinical Orthopaedics and Related Research,* Vol. 468, No. 1, (January 2010), pp. 45-51, ISSN 0009-921X

Costerton, J.W.; Stewart, P.S. & Greenberg, E.P. (1999). Bacterial biofilms: a common cause of persistent infections. *Science,* Vol. 284, No. 5418, (May 1999), pp. 1318-1322, ISSN 0036-8075

Cui, Q.; Mihalko, W.M.; Shields, J.S.; Ries, M. & Saleh, K.J. (2007). Antibiotic-impregnated cement spacers for the treatment of infection associated with total hip or knee arthroplasty. *Journal of Bone and Joint Surgery,* Vol. 89, No. 4, (April 2007), pp. 871-882, ISSN 0021-9355

Cune, J.; Soriano, A.; Martinez, J.C.; Garcia, S. & Mensa, J. (2009). A superficial swab culture is useful for microbiologic diagnosis in acute prosthetic joint infections. *Clinical Orthopaedics and Related Research,* Vol. 467, No. 2, (February 2009), pp. 531-535, ISSN 0009-921X

Della Valle, C.; Parvizi, J.; Bauer, T.W.; Dicesare, P.E.; Evans, R.P.; Segreti, J.; Spangehl, M.; Watters, W.C., 3rd; Keith, M.; Turkelson, C.M.; Wies, J.L.; Sluka, P. & Hitchcock, K. (2010). Diagnosis of periprosthetic joint infections of the hip and knee. *Journal of the American Academy of Orthopaedic Surgeons,* Vol. 18, No. 12, (December 2010), pp. 760-770, ISSN 1067-151X

Della Valle, C.J.; Sporer, S.M.; Jacobs, J.J.; Berger, R.A.; Rosenberg, A.G. & Paprosky, W.G. (2007). Preoperative testing for sepsis before revision total knee arthroplasty. *Journal of Arthroplasty,* Vol. 22, No. 6 Suppl 2, (September 2007), pp. 90-93, ISSN 0883-5403

Dempsey, K.E.; Riggio, M.P.; Lennon, A.; Hannah, V.E.; Ramage, G.; Allan, D. & Bagg, J. (2007). Identification of bacteria on the surface of clinically infected and non-infected prosthetic hip joints removed during revision arthroplasties by 16S rRNA gene sequencing and by microbiological culture. *Arthritis Res Ther,* Vol. 9, No. 3, (May 2007), pp. R46, ISSN 1478-6362

Di Cesare, P.E.; Chang, E.; Preston, C.F. & Liu, C.J. (2005). Serum interleukin-6 as a marker of periprosthetic infection following total hip and knee arthroplasty. *Journal of Bone and Joint Surgery,* Vol. 87, No. 9, (Sep 2005), pp. 1921-1927, ISSN 0021-9355

Donlan, R.M. & Costerton, J.W. (2002). Biofilms: survival mechanisms of clinically relevant microorganisms. *Clinical Microbiology Reviews,* Vol. 15, No. 2, (April 2002), pp. 167-193, ISSN 0893-8512

Donlan, R.M. (2005). New approaches for the characterization of prosthetic joint biofilms. *Clinical Orthopaedics and Related Research,* Vol. 437, (August 2005), pp. 12-19, ISSN 0009-921X

Eisler, T.; Svensson, O.; Engström, C.F.; Reinholt, F.P.; Lundberg, C.; Wejkner, B.; Schmalholz, A. & Elmstedt, E. (2001). Ultrasound for diagnosis of infection in revision total hip arthroplasty. *Journal of Arthroplasty,* Vol. 16, No. 8, (December 2001), pp. 1010-1017, ISSN 0883-5403

Engesaeter, L.B.; Lie, S.A.; Espehaug, B.; Furnes, O.; Vollset, S.E. & Havelin, L.I. (2003). Antibiotic prophylaxis in total hip arthroplasty: effects of antibiotic prophylaxis systemically and in bone cement on the revision rate of 22,170 primary hip replacements followed 0-14 years in the Norwegian Arthroplasty Register. *Acta Orthopaedica Scandinavica,* Vol. 74, No. 6, (December 2003), pp. 644-651, ISSN 0001-6470

Fehring, T.K. & McAlister, J.A., Jr. (1994) Frozen histologic section as a guide to sepsis in revision joint arthroplasty. *Clinical Orthopaedics and Related Research,* Vol. 304, (July 1994), pp. 229-237, ISSN 0009-921X

Fink, B.; Makowiak, C.; Fuerst, M.; Berger, I.; Schäfer, P. & Frommelt, L. (2008). The value of synovial biopsy, joint aspiration and C-reactive protein in the diagnosis of late periprosthetic infection of total knee replacements. *Journal of Bone and Joint Surgery. British Volume,* Vol. 90, No. 7, (July 2008), pp. 874-878, ISSN 0301-620X

Fink, B.; Grossmann, A.; Fuerst, M.; Schäfer, P. & Frommelt, L. (2009). Two-stage cementless revision of infected hip endoprostheses. *Clinical Orthopaedics and Related Research,* Vol. 467, No. 7, (July 2009), pp. 1848-1858, ISSN 0009-921X

Fink, B.; Vogt, S.; Reinsch, M. & Buchner, H. (2011). Sufficient Release of Antibiotic by a Spacer 6 Weeks after Implantation in Two-stage Revision of Infected Hip Prostheses. *Clinical Orthopaedics and Related Research,* in press

Font-Vizcarra, L.; Garcia, S.; Martinez-Pastor, J.C.; Sierra, J.M. & Soriano, A. (2010). Blood culture flasks for culturing synovial fluid in prosthetic joint infections. *Clinical Orthopaedics and Related Research,* Vol. 468, No. 8, (August 2010), pp. 2238-2243, ISSN 0009-921X

Frances Borrego, A.; Martinez, F.M.; Cebrian Parra, J.L.; Graneda, D.S.; Crespo, R.G. & Lopez-Duran Stern, L. (2007). Diagnosis of infection in hip and knee revision surgery: intraoperative frozen section analysis. *International Orthopaedics,* Vol. 31, No. 1, (February 2007), pp. 33-37, ISSN 0341-2695

Ghanem, E.; Parvizi, J.; Burnett, R.S.; Sharkey, P.F.; Keshavarzi, N.; Aggarwal, A. & Barrack, R.L. (2008). Cell count and differential of aspirated fluid in the diagnosis of infection at the site of total knee arthroplasty. *Journal of Bone and Joint Surgery,* Vol. 90, No. 8, (August 2008), pp. 1637-1643, ISSN 1535-1386

Gomez, E. & Patel, R. (2011a). Laboratory diagnosis of prosthetic joint infection, Part I. *Clinical Microbiology Newsletter,* Vol. 33, No. 8, (April 2011), pp. 55-60, ISSN 0196-4399

Gomez, E. & Patel, R. (2011b). Laboratory diagnosis of prosthetic joint infection, Part II. *Clinical Microbiology Newsletter,* Vol. 33, No. 9, (May 2011), pp. 63-70, ISSN 0196-4399

Greidanus, N.V.; Masri, B.A.; Garbuz, D.S.; Wilson, S.D.; McAlinden, M.G.; Xu, M. & Duncan, C.P. (2007). Use of erythrocyte sedimentation rate and C-reactive protein level to diagnose infection before revision total knee arthroplasty. A prospective evaluation. *Journal of Bone and Joint Surgery,* Vol. 89, No. 7, (July 2007), pp. 1409-1416, ISSN 0021-9355

Gristina, A.G. & Costerton, J.W. (1985). Bacterial adherence to biomaterials and tissue. The significance of its role in clinical sepsis. *Journal of Bone and Joint Surgery,* Vol. 67, No. 2, (February 1985), pp. 264-273, ISSN 0021-9355

Hanssen, A.D. & Osmon, D.R. (2002). Evaluation of a staging system for infected hip arthroplasty. *Clinical Orthopaedics and Related Research,* Vol. 403, (October 2002), pp. 16-22, ISSN 0009-921X

Harris, L.G.; El-Bouri, K.; Johnston, S.; Rees, E.; Frommelt, L.; Siemssen, N.; Christner, M.; Davies, A.P.; Rohde, H. & Mack, D. (2010). Rapid identification of staphylococci from prosthetic joint infections using MALDI-TOF mass-spectrometry. *International Journal of Artificial Organs,* Vol. 33, No. 9, (September 2010), pp. 568-574, ISSN 1724-6040

Holinka, J.; Bauer, L.; Hirschl, A.M.; Graninger, W.; Windhager, R. & Presterl, E. (2011). Sonication cultures of explanted components as an add-on test to routinely conducted microbiological diagnostics improve pathogen detection. *Journal of Orthopaedic Research,* Vol. 29, No. 4, (April 2011), pp. 617-622, ISSN 1554-527X

Ince, A.; Rupp, J.; Frommelt, L.; Katzer, A.; Gille, J. & Löhr, J.F. (2004). Is "aseptic" loosening of the prosthetic cup after total hip replacement due to nonculturable bacterial pathogens in patients with low-grade infection? *Clinical Infectious Diseases*, Vol. 39, No. 11, (December 2004), pp. 1599-1603, ISSN 1537-6591

Jämsen, E.; Huhtala, H.; Puolakka, T. & Moilanen, T. (2009). Risk factors for infection after knee arthroplasty. A register-based analysis of 43,149 cases. *Journal of Bone and Joint Surgery*, Vol. 91, No. 1, (January 2009), pp. 38-47, ISSN 1535-1386

Jones, S.M.; Morgan, M.; Humphrey, T.J. & Lappin-Scott, H. (2001). Effect of vancomycin and rifampicin on meticillin-resistant Staphylococcus aureus biofilms. *Lancet*, Vol. 357, No. 9249, (January 2001), pp. 40-41, ISSN 0140-6736

Kamme, C. & Lindberg, L. (1981). Aerobic and anaerobic bacteria in deep infections after total hip arthroplasty: differential diagnosis between infectious and non-infectious loosening. *Clinical Orthopaedics and Related Research*, Vol. 154, (January-February 1981), pp. 201-207, ISSN 0009-921X

Ko, P.S.; Ip, D.; Chow, K.P.; Cheung, F.; Lee, O.B. & Lam, J.J. (2005). The role of intraoperative frozen section in decision making in revision hip and knee arthroplasties in a local community hospital. *Journal of Arthroplasty*, Vol. 20, No. 2, (February 2005), pp. 189-195, ISSN 0883-5403

Kobayashi, N.; Bauer, T.W.; Sakai, H.; Togawa, D.; Lieberman, I.H.; Fujishiro, T. & Procop, G.W. (2006). The use of newly developed real-time PCR for the rapid identification of bacteria in culture-negative osteomyelitis. *Joint Bone Spine*, Vol. 73, No. 6, (December 2006), pp. 745-747, ISSN 1778-7254

Kobayashi, N.; Inaba, Y.; Choe, H.; Iwamoto, N.; Ishida, T.; Yukizawa, Y.; Aoki, C.; Ike, H. & Saito, T. (2009). Rapid and sensitive detection of methicillin-resistant Staphylococcus periprosthetic infections using real-time polymerase chain reaction. *Diagnostic Microbiology and Infectious Disease*, Vol. 64, No. 2, (June 2009), pp. 172-176, ISSN 1879-0070

Krenn, V.; Morawietz, L.; Jakobs, M.; Kienapfel, H.; Ascherl, R.; Bause, L.; Kuhn, H.; Matziolis, G.; Skutek, M. & Gehrke, T. (2011). Joint endoprosthesis pathology: Histopathological diagnostics and classification. *Pathologe*, Vol. 32, No. 3, (May 2011), pp. 210-219, ISSN 0172-8113

Lachiewicz, P.F.; Rogers, G.D. & Thomason, H.C. (1996). Aspiration of the hip joint before revision total hip arthroplasty. Clinical and laboratory factors influencing attainment of a positive culture. *Journal of Bone and Joint Surgery*, Vol. 78, No. 5, (May 1996), pp. 749-754, ISSN 0021-9355

Levine, B.R. & Evans, B.G. (2001). Use of blood culture vial specimens in intraoperative detection of infection. *Clinical Orthopaedics and Related Research*, Vol. 382, (January 2001), pp. 222-231, ISSN 0009-921X

Levine, M.J.; Mariani, B.A.; Tuan, R.S. & Booth, R.E., Jr. (1995). Molecular genetic diagnosis of infected total joint arthroplasty. *Journal of Arthroplasty*, Vol. 10, No. 1, (February 1995), pp. 93-94, ISSN 0883-5403

Lonner, J.H.; Desai, P.; Dicesare, P.E.; Steiner, G. & Zuckerman, J.D. (1996). The reliability of analysis of intraoperative frozen sections for identifying active infection during revision hip or knee arthroplasty. *Journal of Bone and Joint Surgery*, Vol. 78, No. 10, (October 1996), pp. 1553-1558, ISSN 0021-9355

Malhotra, R. & Morgan, D.A. (2004). Role of core biopsy in diagnosing infection before revision hip arthroplasty. *Journal of Arthroplasty*, Vol. 19, No. 1, (January 2004), pp. 78-87, ISSN 0883-5403

Meermans, G. & Haddad, F.S. (2010). Is there a role for tissue biopsy in the diagnosis of periprosthetic infection? *Clinical Orthopaedics and Related Research,* Vol. 468, No. 5, (May 2010), pp. 1410-1417, ISSN 1528-1132

Mirra, J.M.; Amstutz, H.C.; Matos, M. & Gold, R. (1976). The pathology of the joint tissues and its clinical relevance in prosthesis failure. *Clinical Orthopaedics and Related Research,* Vol. No. 117, (June 1976), pp. 221-240, ISSN 0009-921X

Monzon, M.; Oteiza, C.; Leiva, J.; Lamata, M. & Amorena, B. (2002). Biofilm testing of Staphylococcus epidermidis clinical isolates: low performance of vancomycin in relation to other antibiotics. *Diagnostic Microbiology and Infectious Disease,* Vol. 44, No. 4, (December 2002), pp. 319-324, ISSN 0732-8893

Morawietz, L.; Classen, R.A.; Schröder, J.H.; Dynybil, C.; Perka, C.; Skwara, A.; Neidel, J.; Gehrke, T.; Frommelt, L.; Hansen, T.; Otto, M.; Barden, B.; Aigner, T.; Stiehl, P.; Schubert, T.; Meyer-Scholten, C.; König, A.; Ströbel, P.; Rader, C.P.; Kirschner, S.; Lintner, F.; Rüther, W.; Bos, I.; Hendrich, C.; Kriegsmann, J. & Krenn, V. (2006). Proposal for a histopathological consensus classification of the periprosthetic interface membrane. *Journal of Clinical Pathology,* Vol. 59, No. 6, (June 2006), pp. 591-597, ISSN 0021-9746

Morello, J.A.; Matushek, S.M.; Dunne, W.M. & Hinds, D.B. (1991). Performance of a BACTEC nonradiometric medium for pediatric blood cultures. *Journal of Clinical Microbiology,* Vol. 29, No. 2, (February 1991), pp. 359-362, ISSN 0095-1137

Neut, D.; Van Horn, J.R.; Van Kooten, T.G.; Van Der Mei, H.C. & Busscher, H.J. (2003). Detection of biomaterial-associated infections in orthopaedic joint implants. *Clinical Orthopaedics and Related Research,* Vol. No. 413, (August 2003), pp. 261-268, ISSN 0009-921X

Nunez, L.V.; Buttaro, M.A.; Morandi, A.; Pusso, R. & Piccaluga, F. (2007). Frozen sections of samples taken intraoperatively for diagnosis of infection in revision hip surgery. *Acta Orthopaedica,* Vol. 78, No. 2, (April 2007), pp. 226-230, ISSN 1745-3674

Pandey, R.; Drakoulakis, E. & Athanasou, N.A. (1999). An assessment of the histological criteria used to diagnose infection in hip revision arthroplasty tissues. *Journal of Clinical Pathology,* Vol. 52, No. 2, (February 1999), pp. 118-123, ISSN 0021-9746

Panousis, K.; Grigoris, P.; Butcher, I.; Rana, B.; Reilly, J.H. & Hamblen, D.L. (2005). Poor predictive value of broad-range PCR for the detection of arthroplasty infection in 92 cases. *Acta Orthopaedica,* Vol. 76, No. 3, (June 2005), pp. 341-346, ISSN 1745-3674

Parvizi, J.; Ghanem, E.; Menashe, S.; Barrack, R.L. & Bauer, T.W. (2006). Periprosthetic infection: what are the diagnostic challenges? *Journal of Bone and Joint Surgery,* Vol. 88 Suppl 4, (December 2006), pp. 138-147, ISSN 0021-9355

Peel, T.N.; Buising, K.L. & Choong, P.F. (2011). Prosthetic joint infection: challenges of diagnosis and treatment. *ANZ Journal of Surgery,* Vol. 81, No. 1-2, (January 2011), pp. 32-39, ISSN 1445-2197

Piper, K.E.; Jacobson, M.J.; Cofield, R.H.; Sperling, J.W.; Sanchez-Sotelo, J.; Osmon, D.R.; Mcdowell, A.; Patrick, S.; Steckelberg, J.M.; Mandrekar, J.N.; Fernandez Sampedro, M. & Patel, R. (2009). Microbiologic diagnosis of prosthetic shoulder infection by use of implant sonication. *Journal of Clinical Microbiology,* Vol. 47, No. 6, (June 2009), pp. 1878-1884, ISSN 1098-660X

Roberts, P.; Walters, A.J. & Mcminn, D.J. (1992). Diagnosing infection in hip replacements. The use of fine-needle aspiration and radiometric culture. *Journal of Bone and Joint Surgery. British Volume,* Vol. 74, No. 2, (March 1992), pp. 265-269, ISSN 0301-620X

Roux, A.L.; Sivadon-Tardy, V.; Bauer, T.; Lortat-Jacob, A.; Herrmann, J.L.; Gaillard, J.L. & Rottman, M. (2011). Diagnosis of prosthetic joint infection by beadmill processing of a periprosthetic specimen. *Clinical Microbiology and Infection,* Vol. 17, No. 3, (March 2011), pp. 447-450, ISSN 1469-0691

Sadiq, S.; Wootton, J.R.; Morris, C.A. & Northmore-Ball, M.D. (2005). Application of core biopsy in revision arthroplasty for deep infection. *Journal of Arthroplasty,* Vol. 20, No. 2, (February 2005), pp. 196-201, ISSN 0883-5403

Sampedro, M.F.; Huddleston, P.M.; Piper, K.E.; Karau, M.J.; Dekutoski, M.B.; Yaszemski, M.J.; Currier, B.L.; Mandrekar, J.N.; Osmon, D.R.; Mcdowell, A.; Patrick, S.; Steckelberg, J.M. & Patel, R. (2010). A biofilm approach to detect bacteria on removed spinal implants. *Spine,* Vol. 35, No. 12, (May 2010), pp. 1218-1224, ISSN 1528-1159

Schäfer, P.; Fink, B.; Sandow, D.; Margull, A.; Berger, I. & Frommelt, L. (2008). Prolonged bacterial culture to identify late periprosthetic joint infection: a promising strategy. *Clinical Infectious Diseases,* Vol. 47, No. 11, (December 2008), pp. 1403-1409, ISSN 1058-4838

Schinsky, M.F.; Della Valle, C.J.; Sporer, S.M. & Paprosky, W.G. (2008). Perioperative testing for joint infection in patients undergoing revision total hip arthroplasty. *Journal of Bone and Joint Surgery,* Vol. 90, No. 9, (September 2008), pp. 1869-1875, ISSN 1535-1386

Spangehl, M.J.; Masterson, E.; Masri, B.A.; O'connell, J.X. & Duncan, C.P. (1999). The role of intraoperative gram stain in the diagnosis of infection during revision total hip arthroplasty. *Journal of Arthroplasty,* Vol. 14, No. 8, (December 1999), pp. 952-956, ISSN 0883-5403

Stewart, P.S. & Costerton, J.W. (2001). Antibiotic resistance of bacteria in biofilms. *Lancet,* Vol. 358, No. 9276, (July 2001), pp. 135-138, ISSN 0140-6736

Tarkin, I.S.; Henry, T.J.; Fey, P.I.; Iwen, P.C.; Hinrichs, S.H. & Garvin, K.L. (2003). PCR rapidly detects methicillin-resistant staphylococci periprosthetic infection. *Clinical Orthopaedics and Related Research,* Vol. No. 414, (September 2003), pp. 89-94, ISSN 0009-921X

Trampuz, A.; Osmon, D.R.; Hanssen, A.D.; Steckelberg, J.M. & Patel, R. (2003). Molecular and antibiofilm approaches to prosthetic joint infection. *Clinical Orthopaedics and Related Research,* Vol. No. 414, (September 2003), pp. 69-88, ISSN 0009-921X

Trampuz, A.; Hanssen, A.D.; Osmon, D.R.; Mandrekar, J.; Steckelberg, J.M. & Patel, R. (2004) Synovial fluid leukocyte count and differential for the diagnosis of prosthetic knee infection. *American Journal of Medicine,* Vol. 117, No. 8, (October 2004), pp. 556-562, ISSN 0002-9343

Trampuz, A.; Piper, K.E.; Hanssen, A.D.; Osmon, D.R.; Cockerill, F.R.; Steckelberg, J.M. & Patel, R. (2006). Sonication of explanted prosthetic components in bags for diagnosis of prosthetic joint infection is associated with risk of contamination. *Journal of Clinical Microbiology,* Vol. 44, No. 2, (February 2006), pp. 628-631, ISSN 0095-1137

Trampuz, A.; Piper, K.E.; Jacobson, M.J.; Hanssen, A.D.; Unni, K.K.; Osmon, D.R.; Mandrekar, J.N.; Cockerill, F.R.; Steckelberg, J.M.; Greenleaf, J.F. & Patel, R. (2007). Sonication of removed hip and knee prostheses for diagnosis of infection. *New England Journal of Medicine,* Vol. 357, No. 7, (August 2007), pp. 654-663, ISSN 1533-4406

Tunney, M.M.; Patrick, S.; Gorman, S.P.; Nixon, J.R.; Anderson, N.; Davis, R.I.; Hanna, D. & Ramage, G. (1998). Improved detection of infection in hip replacements. A currently underestimated problem. *Journal of Bone and Joint Surgery. British Volume,* Vol. 80, No. 4, (July 1998), pp. 568-572, ISSN 0301-620X

Tunney, M.M.; Patrick, S.; Curran, M.D.; Ramage, G.; Hanna, D.; Nixon, J.R.; Gorman, S.P.; Davis, R.I. & Anderson, N. (1999). Detection of prosthetic hip infection at revision arthroplasty by immunofluorescence microscopy and PCR amplification of the bacterial 16S rRNA gene. *Journal of Clinical Microbiology,* Vol. 37, No. 10, (October 1999), pp. 3281-3290, ISSN 0095-1137

Virolainen, P.; Lähteenmäki, H.; Hiltunen, A.; Sipola, E.; Meurman, O. & Nelimarkka, O. (2002). The reliability of diagnosis of infection during revision arthroplasties. *Scandinavian Journal of Surgery,* Vol. 91, No. 2, (August 2002), pp. 178-181, ISSN 1457-4969

Williams, J.L.; Norman, P. & Stockley, I. (2004). The value of hip aspiration versus tissue biopsy in diagnosing infection before exchange hip arthroplasty surgery. *Journal of Arthroplasty,* Vol. 19, No. 5, (August 2004), pp. 582-586, ISSN 0883-5403

Zimmerli, W.; Trampuz, A. & Ochsner, P.E. (2004). Prosthetic-joint infections. *New England Journal of Medicine,* Vol. 351, No. 16, (October 2004), pp. 1645-1654, ISSN 1533-4406

21

Staphylococcus Infection Associated with Arthroplasty

Weisheng Ye, Wei Shang and Yaqiong Yang
Tianjin Orthopaedics Hospital
P. R. China

1. Introduction

Prosthetic joints improve the quality of life, but they may fail, necessitating revision or resection arthroplasty. The numbers of primary total hip and total knee arthroplastics have been increasing over the past decade, with nearly 800,000 such procedures performed in the United States in 2006 (Fig.1A)[1],with numbers projected to rise to 572,000 by 2030 and are expected to undergo a continuing rise, especially in light of an aging population[2]. Procedures to replace the shoulder, elbow, wrist, ankle, temporomandibular, metacarpophalangeal and interphalangeal joints are less commonly performed. The growth in the number of prosthetic joint replacement procedures provides new opportunities for infections to take hold.

The classification of the arthroplasty associated infection may distinguishes two major types—septic arthritis and osteomyelitis, which both involve the inflammatory destruction of joint and bone. The incidence of septic arthritis is between 2 and 10 in 100,000 in the general populace but may be as high as 30–70 per 100,000 in rheumatoid arthritis sufferers or recipients of prosthetic joints [3-5] and is more common in children than adults, and in males rather than females [6]. Haematogenous osteomyelitis most frequently effects children and the elderly [7]. In children, the incidence is typically between 1 in 5000 and 1 in 10,000 [8]. It has been argued that the incidence of haematogenous osteomyelitis is decreasing with an annual fall in childhood cases of 0.185 per 100,000 people recorded in Glasgow, Scotland between 1970 and 1997 [8-10]. Conversely, osteomyelitis resulting from direct infection is reportedly on the increase[10,11]. Local spread of infection from contiguous tissue to bone or direct infection can occur at any age, with foreign body implants a substantial risk factor [7].

Infection, although uncommon, is the most serious complication, occurring in 0.8 to 1.9% of knee arthroplasties[12-14] and 0.3 to 1.7% of hip arthroplasties[14-16]. The frequency of infection is increasing as the number of primary arthroplasties increases (Fig. 1B)[17]. These infections are increasingly difficult to treat with the rise in antibiotic-resistant forms.

2. Risk factors for infection

Patient-related risk factors for infection include previous revision arthroplasty or previous infection associated with a prosthetic joint at the same site, tobacco abuse, obesity, rheumatoid arthritis, a neoplasm, immunosuppression, and diabetes mellitus.

Surgical risk factors include simultaneous bilateral arthroplasty, a long operative time(>2.5 hours), and allogeneic blood transfusion.
Postoperative risk factors include woundhealing complications (e.g., superficial infection, hematoma, delayed healing, wound necrosis, and dehiscence), atrial fibrillation, myocardial infarction, urinary tract infection, prolonged hospital stay, and *S. aureus* bacteremia[12-15],[18-21].

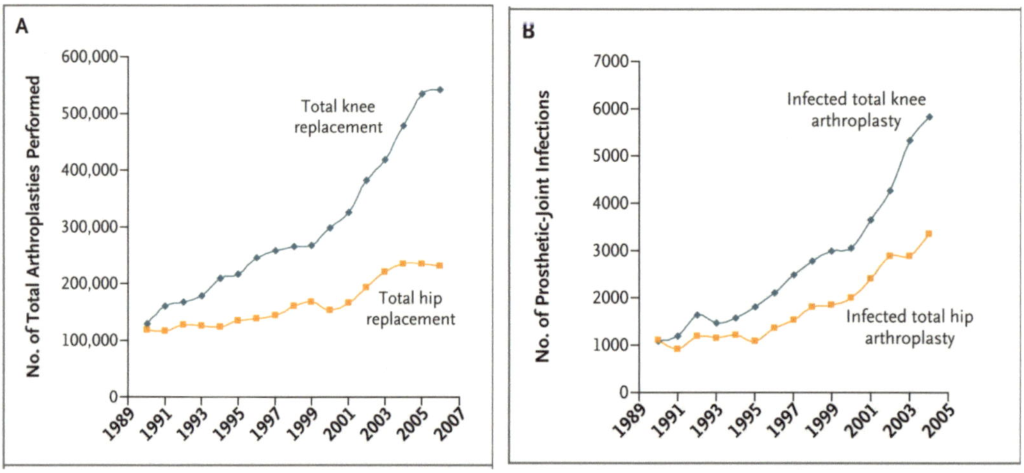

Fig. 1. Total Arthroplasties Performed and Prosthetic Infections, According to Procedure. Panel A shows the number of total arthroplasties performed from 1990 through 2006. Data are from the Centers for Disease Control and Prevention. Panel B shows the number of prosthetic joint infections from 1990 through 2004. Data are from Kurtz et al.

An increased rate of infection occurs in the pre-damaged joint and is also associated with particular predispositions of the patients (Table 1) [22-24]. In articular, a joint prosthesis is a high risk predisposition for an infection. Perioperatively the initial bacterial entry into the joints may occur. On the other hand the implanted foreign material causes in addition to the severe joint disease present an additional reduction in local resistance, which facilitates haematogenous infections. The prosthetic materials are also additional binding sites for various bacteria, and act as a starting point for prosthetic infections. Thus, in addition to the local conditions, the bacterial properties and their specific pathogenity have to be considered for understanding the whole mechanism of infection. Basically, a too late or not

Preexisting joint defects
Extraarticular infection
Diabetes mellitus
Immunosuppression
Higher age
Intraarticular injection or operation
HLA-B27, for reactive arthritis

Table 1. Predisposing factors

sufficiently cured joint infection can cause trophic and functional limitations or can even be the starting point of a progressive infection spreading in continuity, lymphogenic or haematogenic. In general, the detection and treatment of acute infectious arthritis is an acute emerging situation, in which a delay may progress to further septic inflammation[23].

3. Classification of the arthroplasty associated infection

The arthroplasty associated infection may distinguishes two major types—septic arthritis and osteomyelitis, which both cause serious morbidity and are often difficult to manage.

Septic arthritis is a joint disease typified by bacterial colonisation and rapid articular destruction[6]. Infiltration and growth of bacteria within the synovium results in inflammation with infiltration of leukocytes into the joint fluid [4]. The production of reactive oxygen species and host matrix metalloproteinases (MMPs), lysosomal enzymes and bacterial toxins contribute to the destruction of cartilage. This starts with degradation of host proteoglycans followed by collagen breakdown within hours of infection, and is mediated by polymorphonuclear leukocytes[3-5,24]. The containment of the inflammatory process within the joint results in increasing pressure, which impedes blood and nutrient supply to the joint exacerbating joint damage and facilitating destruction of cartilage and the synovium. Permanent destruction of articular cartilage and subchondral bone can occur rapidly, within just a few days[24].

Osteomyelitis describes a range of infections in which bone is colonized with microorganisms, with associated inflammation and bone destruction. Acute osteomyelitic foci are characterized by pus-forming inflammation at the site of microbial colonisation. Damage to bone matrix and compression and destruction of vasculature is also observed as the infection spreads to surrounding soft tissues, which can further exacerbate bone necrosis[7,10].Sections of dead bone, known as sequestra, can form which may then detach to form separate infectious foci which, due to the lack of vasculature, are protected from immune cells and antibiotics[7,10]. Such areas of dead, infected tissues that are inaccessible to antimicrobials or the immune response can lead to chronic persistence of the infection[10].

The principal routes of these infection involve: (I) haematogenous or lymphogenous seed of the pathogen, (II) contiguous, by contact with a neighboring infected site, (III) or direct, resulting from infiltration of bone, often following inj ury, surgery or implantation of a foreign body, such as joint repalcement[25]. The range of environments experienced by the bacterium differs for each route and hence the virulence factors that are involved in pathology may be different for each route of infection.

Another classification of arthroplasty associated infection distinguishes acute, chronic and reactive forms, which differ in their type of joint infection and their triggering bacteria.

Infection with virulent organisms (e.g., S. aureus and gram-negative bacilli) inoculated at implantation is typically manifested as acute infection in the first 3 months (or, with hematogenous seeding of the implant, at any time) after surgery, whereas infection with less virulent organisms (e.g., coagulase-negative staphylococci and P. acnes) is more often manifested as chronic infection several months (or years) postoperatively. The most common symptom of infection associated with a prosthetic joint is pain. In acute infection, local signs and symptoms (e.g., severe pain, swelling, erythema, and warmth at the infected joint) and fever are common. Chronic infection generally has a more subtle presentation, with pain alone, and it is often accompanied by loosening of the prosthesis at the bone–cement interface and sometimes by sinus tract formation with discharge.

Reactive arthritis is a postinfectious complication with no need of presence for viable pathogens in the joint. While reactive arthritis often simultaneously affect several joints, the presence of polyarthritic types of non reactive arthritis occur infrequently and then mostly as a result of several bacteriaemic phases.

Among joint infections, the knee is the most frequent localization than others. Infection occurs in 0.8 to 1.9% of knee arthroplasties[12-14]and 0.3 to 1.7% of hip arthroplasties[14-16]. However, hip joint infections are aggravated by the fact that they can exist over a long time with only poor symptoms. Basically, there are no differences in the bacterial spectrum among large joints.

4. Bacteria responsible for arthroplasty associated infection

A broad range of bacterial species have been isolated in cases of septic arthritis and osteomyelitis[26]. Pathogens cultured from septic joints include S. aureus, Streptococcus pyogenes, Streptococcus pneumoniae, Escherichia coli, Pseudomonas aeruginosa, Serratia marcescens, as well as Salmonella, Neisseria, Aerobacter, and Bacteroides species[4,24]. Staphylococcus and Streptococcus spp., Haemophilusinfluenzae, E. coli, P. aeruginosa, Salmonella and Mycobacterium spp. are all potential causes of osteomyelitis[7,10,27].

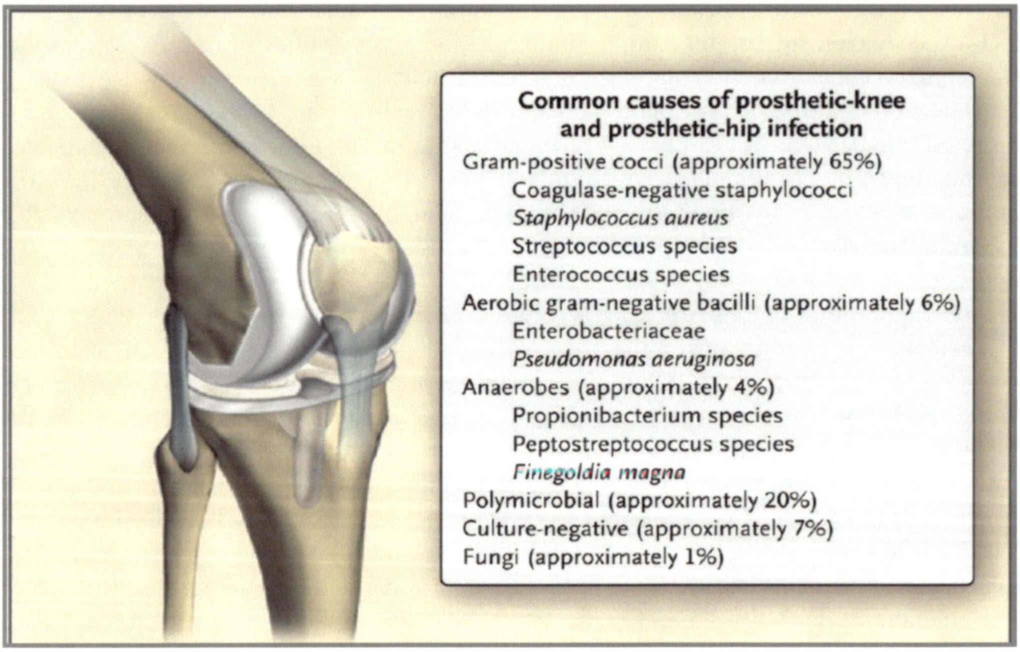

Fig. 2. Causes of Infection Associated with Prosthetic Joints

A small number of often otherwise nonvirulent bacteria contaminate the implant during surgery and persist as a biofilm despite a functional immune system and antimicrobial treatment. Commonly isolated microorganisms are shown. Unusual organisms that can also cause infection include (but are not limited to) Actinomyces israelii, Aspergillus fumigatus, Histoplasma capsulatum, Sporothrix schenckii, Mycoplasma hominis, Tropheryma whipplei, and mycobacterium (including tuberculosis), brucella, candida, corynebacterium, granulicatella, and abiotrophia species.

Some bacteria have preferences for certain infection routes and patterns. Infections not related to injuries or medical interventions (e.g. intraarticular puncture, joint replacement) are mostly resulting from often physiologic bacteriaemic periods.

S. aureus is the most commonly identified pathogen both in septic arthritis and osteomyelitis, by a substantial margin, regardless of type or route of infection [3,7,28]. Staphylococci (S. aureus and coagulase-negative staphylococcus species) account for more than half of cases of prosthetic-hip and prosthetic-knee infection[29](Fig. 2). Other bacteria

<table>
<tr><th>Bacteria</th><th>Typical mode of infection</th></tr>
<tr><td>Staphylococci</td><td></td></tr>
<tr><td>Staphylococcus aureus</td><td>NJI, PJI</td></tr>
<tr><td>Coagulase negative staphylococci</td><td>PJI</td></tr>
<tr><td>Streptococci</td><td></td></tr>
<tr><td>beta-hemolytic (e.g. Streptococcus pyogenes)</td><td>NJI, RA</td></tr>
<tr><td>Streptococcus pneumoniae</td><td>NJI</td></tr>
<tr><td>Enterobacteriaceae</td><td></td></tr>
<tr><td>Escherichia coli</td><td>NJI, PJI</td></tr>
<tr><td>Salmonella enterica</td><td rowspan="5">NJI, RAs</td></tr>
<tr><td>Shigella spec.</td></tr>
<tr><td>Yersinia spec.</td></tr>
<tr><td>Borrelia burgdorferi sensu lato</td></tr>
<tr><td>Neisseria gonorrhoeae</td></tr>
<tr><td>Pseudomonas aeruginosa</td><td>NJI, PJI</td></tr>
<tr><td>Bartonella henselae</td><td>NJI</td></tr>
<tr><td>Mycobacterium tuberculosis and other mycobacteria</td><td rowspan="3">NJI</td></tr>
<tr><td>Brucella spp.</td></tr>
<tr><td>Tropheryma whippelii</td></tr>
<tr><td>Campylobacter spp.</td><td rowspan="4">RAs</td></tr>
<tr><td>Chlamydia trachomatis</td></tr>
<tr><td>Mycoplasma pneumoniae</td></tr>
<tr><td>Ureaplasma urealyticum</td></tr>
</table>

Table 2. Bacteria responsible for (hip) joint infections

and fungi cause the remainder of cases[30,31]. Moreover, Staphylococcus aureus has the dominance in acute septic arthritis, and is particularly common in patients with rheumatoid arthritis[32]while coagulase -negative staphylococci can be found mainly in periprosthetic infections and after diagnostic arthroscopies.

Other gram-positive bacteria as causative agents for hip joint infections are streptococci, especially Streptococcus pyogenes, Enterococcus faecalis and Corynebacteria species. Propionibacterium acnes is a common cause of infection associated with shoulder arthroplasty[33].

A large number of different gram-negative rods act as infectious agents on joints. The group of enterobacteria contains a broad spectrum of pathogens. Salmonella enterica, Shigella species, and Yersinia species are classically described as pathogens for purulent and reactive forms of arthritis. Pseudomonas aeruginosa can be found more often in predisposed patients (e.g. diabetics). In otherwise healthy people it is associated with iatrogenic modes of infection during diagnostic procedures.

Campylobacter species, however, are classic agents of reactive arthritis, as well as the obligate intracellular bacteria Chlamydia trachomatis, Mycoplasma pneumoniae, and Ureaplasma urealyticum. From the spirochaetales only Borrelia burgdorferi sensu lato is relevant. Less commonly identified organisms for joint infections often accompanied with osteitis or osteomyelitis are Brucella species and Mycobacterium tuberculosis.

Up to 20% of cases are polymicrobial, most commonly involving methicillin -resistant S. aureus (MRSA) or anaerobes, such as Bacteroides fragilis[34]. Approximately 7% of cases are culture-negative, often in the context of previous antimicrobial therapy[35].

An overview is shown in Table 2[8].

Infection with virulent organisms (e.g., S. aureus and gram-negative bacilli) inoculated at implantation is typically manifested as acute infection in the first 3 months (or, with hematogenous seeding of the implant, at any time) after surgery, whereas infection with less virulent organisms (e.g., coagulase-negative staphylococci and P. acnes) is more often manifested as chronic infection several months (or years) postoperatively.

5. Interaction of staphylococci with bone

5.1 Genomic features of staphylococci associated with bone infections

A number of studies have attempted to identify an association between the possession of certain virulence genes by Staphylococci and invasive disease. Thus Peacock et al.[36]suggested that the possession of certain combinations of virulence factor genes is associated with invasive disease, and increased severity of infection following examination of a panel of 334 S. aureus isolates by PCR. The isolates comprised those from 179 healthy patients, 94 hospitalacquired isolates and 61 community-acquired isolates. Seven putative virulence genes, including the adhesin genes fnbA and cna, the toxin genes sej, eta and hlg, and icaA, which is involved in biofilm production, were found to be associated with invasive isolates. The association with specific types of invasive infection was not examined and indeed the small number of isolates examined in this study would have precluded such an analysis.

The genes for the fibronectin-binding proteins fnbA and fnbB have been reported to be present in 98% and 99% of clinical isolates, respectively, from a range of orthopaedic associated infections, whereas the cna gene, encoding the collagen -binding protein was identified in just 46% of isolates[37]. Another study by Peacock et al.[38]found the prevalence of both fnbA and fnbB genes, as opposed to just one of the two, to be significantly higher in invasive isolates than in 'carriage' strains in a panel of 163 strains, which included septic arthritis and osteomyelitis isolates. Genes encoding Panton-Valentine leukocidin were found to be present in 59 of 89 S. aureus isolates from cases of acute haematogenous osteomyelitis. The presence of pvl genes is associated with an increased risk of severe infection requiring intensive care, bacteremia and more severe systemic inflammation [39,40]. However, one of the problems with the above studies is that it is unclear how representative these strain collections are of those isolates carried in other establishments and regions across the world, since strain typing was not reported.

Strain typing studies of S. aureus, using multilocus sequence typing (MLST) and comparative genomic microarray hybridizations have so far failed to identify any specific clonal lineages associated with invasive disease. However, these studies did not use a collection of isolates from specific invasive diseases and therefore do not rule out the possibility that specific lineages or genes are associated with specific types of infection, such as osteomyelitis or septic arthritis.

To date, the only genome comparison study relevant to S. aureus bone infections has been done using comparative genome microarray hybridisations of the S. aureus UAMS-1 strain, isolated from an osteomyelitis patient, with a range of genome sequenced strains[41]. These authors found variations in the complement of adhesin, toxin, exoenzyme and regulatory genes. Although it is not possible to draw general conclusions about association with bone infection from characterisation of a single strain, the presence of fnbA, but not fnbB or the bone sialoprotein-binding gene bbp, in UAMS-1 suggest that fnbB and bbp are dispensable for bone infection, at least in certain genetic backgrounds. Thus at this juncture there is a lack of evidence to support or disprove an association between specific S. aureus lineages or specific genomic features and the pathogenesis of bone infections.

5.2 Bone as a target organ

In terrestrial vertebrates mature bone is made up of dense surface plates of bone, known as the cortices, and within these is a network of bone struts oriented to oppose loading forces, known as trabecular bone. Trabecular bone is typically replaced every 3–4 years, with the denser cortical bone taking over a decade to replace in adults. This process of continual remodelling is required to remove old bone and microfractures to ensure bone integrity and mineral homeostasis. The skeleton is a dynamic organ system, in a state of perpetual turnover which is continually remodelled by the actions of two cell types, osteoblasts and osteoclasts.

Osteoblasts are responsible for the deposition of bone matrix; they are found on bone surfaces and are derived from mesenchymal steoprogenitor cells. These cells secrete osteoid, a mixture of bone matrix proteins primarily made up of type I collagen (over 90%), proteoglycans such as decorin and biglycan, glycoproteins such as fibronectin, osteonectin and tenascin-C, osteopontin, osteocalcin and bone sialoprotein, oriented along stress lines. Osteoblasts are also thought to facilitate the mineralization of bone matrix, whereby hydroxyapatite, [Ca3(PO4)2]3·Ca[OH]2, crystals form, making up around 90% of bone matrix. It is thought that 'nucleators' are required to instigate mineralisation, and phosphate-containing matrix proteins like bone sialoprotein and osteopontin are likely to play such a role. Osteoblasts also produce tissue nonspecific alkaline phosphatase (TNAP) which cleaves phosphate esters to liberate free inorganic phosphate, which is key to the process of mineralisation[42].

Osteoblasts are not terminally differentiated, and some may form osteocytes and become implanted in the bone matrix, eventually ceasing the secretion of osteoid, whilst others undergo apoptosis. Osteocytes are also involved in bone maintenance, detecting stress within the bone through echanosensitive mechanisms located in extensive cellular projections, called canaliculi, that interconnect osteocytes[42]. Osteocytes are thought to respond to mechanical stress by undergoing apoptosis, leading to osteoclast recruitment and differentiation, possibly by alterations in the levels of soluble factors produced by the osteocyte. Candidates include transforming growth factor β (TGF-β), which may suppress osteoclastogenesis when produced by healthy osteocytes[43,44].

Osteoclasts, which are multinucleate cells derived from the acrophage-monocyte lineage, perform the opposing action of bone matrix removal. These cells express large quantities of a vacuolar-type H+-ATPase on their cell surface, along with chloride channel 7 (ClC 7)enabling localised hydrochloric acid secretion into a closed compartment, known as the resorption lacuna, and subsequent olubilisation of bone mineral. The cell is attached to the bone matrix by a sealing zone membrane to create this compartment, and fusion of acidified vesicles with the plasma membrane contributes further to acid release[45].Following mineral solubilisation, proteolysis of bone matrix proteins is then possible. Cathepsin K is centrally involved in degradation of bone matrix, it is highly expressed by osteoclasts and digests substrates such as collagen and osteonectin. Evidence from knock-out mouse and selective inhibitor experiments indicates that cathepsin L, and MMPs also play a role in degrading bone matrix[46]. Osteoclasts also secrete acid phosphatases, such as tartrate-resistant acid phosphatase(TRAcP), which is used as an osteoclast marker and is activated by cathepsin K cleavage. TRAcP is able to generate reactive oxygen species in addition to having phosphatase activity. The exact cellular function of TRAcP in bone resorption is not well understood, but serum TRAcP levels correlate with bone-resorptive activity, and TRAcP-deficient mice exhibit reduced osteoclastic bone resorption and increased bone mineralization.

The balance of activity between these two cell types is crucial to maintaining the proper homeostasis of bone turnover, and any shift in the relative levels of osteoblast and osteoclast activity can result in bone pathology. Infection with a pathogen such as S. aureus is capable of stimulating such a shift, mediated in part by induction of an inflammatory response. There is intimate interaction between the two cell types, with osteoblasts interpreting the majority of extracellular signals and subsequently modulating osteoclast differentiation and function[44].

Interaction between the RANK (receptor activator for nuclear factor κB) receptor, expressed by osteoclast precursors, and its cognate ligand, RANKL, expressed by osteoblasts is essential for osteoclastogenesis [44]. RANKL is a homotrimeric protein displayed on the membrane of osteoblasts, although it may be secreted following cleavage by MMPs 7 or 14, or ADAM (a disintegrin and metalloprotease domain). Suppression of MMP 14-mediated secretion enhances osteoclastogenesis[47,48]. The RANK receptor is a homotrimeric transmembrane protein belonging to the tumour necrosis factor (TNF) receptor superfamily. Following binding of RANKL to RANK, TRAF (TNF receptor-associated factor) adaptor proteins are recruited, with binding sites for TRAF2, TRAF5 and TRAF6 all present on RANK. TRAF6 seems to play a central role in RANK mediated osteoclast formation, and mice deficient in TRAF6 are osteopetrotic whereas TRAF2 and TRAF5 are relatively marginal players in osteoclastogenesis. Signalling via RANK, and these adaptor proteins, activates a number of transcription factors, including NFκB (nuclear factor κB), AP-

1(activator protein 1) and NFATc1 (nuclear factor of activated T-cells, cytoplasmic, calcineurin dependent 1) which drive osteoclast differentiation[44]. Osteoprotegrin (OPG) is an endogenous inhibitor of RANKL signalling, functioning as a decoy receptor that binds to RANKL and prevents its association with RANK.

5.3 Inflammation in bone infection

A number of host cytokines play a significant role in the pathogenesis of osteomyelitis, and there is strong evidence that production of these cytokines is induced by staphylococcal infection of bone, and that they directly contribute to bone destruction. In particular, the inflammatory cytokines tumour necrosis factor α (TNFα), interleukin 1 (IL-1) and IL-6 seem to be especially important in bone physiology and pathology. In patients with acute osteomyelitis, plasma levels of TNFα, IL-1β (the secreted form of IL-1) and IL-6 are all elevated. High levels of IL-1β, IL-6 and TNFα are also found in the synovial fluid of patients with septic arthritis. Interestingly, specific polymorphisms in the IL-1α and IL-6 genes have recently been found to be associated with an increased risk of osteomyelitis in the Greek population[49]. The most recently identified member of the IL-1 cytokine superfamily is IL-33, has been shown to expressed in differentiated osteoblasts and blocks osteoclast formation from bone marrow precursor cells[50].

A number of animal models of *S. aureus* osteomyelitis reveal that bone infection can lead to elevated levels of these cytokines both locally and systemically. Increased levels of IL-1β have been measured in the tibiae of 22-month-old rats experimentally implanted with *S. aureus* infected needles, and the same animals have increased circulating levels of IL-6[51]. In a murine osteomyelitis model, bone levels of IL-1β and IL-6 are significantly increased in the early post-infection period, with TNFα rising later during the infection. The local source of these cytokines is not fully clear. Production of IL-1β can be induced in human osteoblast-like cell lines by a variety of stimuli, including TNFα. However, infection of primary mouse osteoblasts with *S.aureus* results in increased transcription, but not increased protein synthesis or secretion of IL-1β. TNFα is detectable only at low levels in human osteoblasts derived from mesenchymal stem cells and the osteosarcoma cell line MG63.Infiltrating immune cells may therefore be a more likely source of IL-1β and TNFα in bone in response to infection. IL-6 however, is produced by osteoblasts in response to a variety of signals, including infection with *S. aureus* .

These cytokines have potent effects on the process of bone remodelling, and are strongly implicated in the pathology of osteomyelitis. Cell culture models support the view that IL-1 and TNFα stimulate the proliferation and differentiation of osteoclast progenitors into mature osteoclasts in the presence of osteoblasts. TNFα and IL-1β also stimulate osteoclast-mediated bone resorption, a process which may also require the presence of osteoblasts. Similarly, IL-6 increases bone resorption activity and osteoclast number in cultured mouse calvariae, and stimulates osteoclast differentiation in the presence of osteoblasts. In vivo, local administration of IL-1 and TNF antagonists in a non-human primate model of periodontitis results in significant reduction of osteoclast formation and bone destruction. Intravenous administration of TNFα and IL-1 in mice stimulates bone resorption in a dose-dependent fashion, and deletion of the murine IL-1R, TNF-R1 and TNF-R2 receptors and of caspase-1 significantly decreases osteoclast number and the area of bone resorption in calvariae following lipopolysaccharide (LPS) injection.

IL-1β and TNFα also inhibit the differentiation of mesenchymal stem cells into osteoblast-like cells, and suppress the accompanying mineralisation and increased expression of

alkaline phosphatase and procollagen I genes, although only TNFα inhibits osteonectin and osteopontin gene expression[52]. TNFα also decreases production of type I collagen and osteocalcin, and of alkaline phosphatase in a variety of osteoblast cell culture and bone tissue explant models, thereby reducing matrix deposition and mineralisation.
Surface-associated material (SAM) from *S. aureus* stimulates bone resorption and osteoclast formation, and blockade of IL-1 or TNFα signalling completely abolishes this bone resorption activity. Neutralisation of TNFα and IL-6 fully abolishes SAM-stimulated osteoclastogenesis, with antagonism of IL 1 having only a partial effect.
The effect of this SAM on osteoclast formation and stimulation of resorption does not require co-culture with osteoblasts, and does not require RANKL signaling[53]. *S.epidermidis* surface material can also induce bone resorption, by a mechanism that is strongly dependent on TNFα and, to a lesser extent, IL-1.Induction and release of these cytokines in response to pathogen-associated molecules involves two main classes of pattern recognition receptors (PRRs), the Toll-like receptors (TLRs) and NOD-like receptors (NLRs). The production of TNFα and IL-6 by murine macrophages in response to *S. aureus* cell wall preparations is dependent on TLR2, and TLR2-deficient mice exhibit reduced survival of intravenous *S. aureus* infections compared to wild-type counterparts. Signalling through TLRs, in response to microbial ligands such as LPS, 'primes' the cell for IL-1β production by inducing expression of the inactive, pro-form of the cytokine[54,55].IL-1β is synthesised as a 31-kDa precursor molecule, and is processed to produce a 17-kDa active molecule by caspase-1. Caspase-1 activation, and subsequent processing and release of active IL-1β involves assembly of a multiprotein complex known as the inflammasome. This complex consists of caspase-1, the adaptor protein ASC (apoptosis-associated speck-like protein containing a caspase recruitment domain (CARD)) and one of several NLR proteins, of which four are known to associate with inflammasomes[56].Each NLR responds to different activating signals, and although the exact recognition steps remain to be elucidated, reported stimuli include flagellin, anthrax lethal toxin, and muramyl dipeptide. A broad range of stimuli for NLRP3 (NLR family pyrin domain containing 3) have been reported, including *S. aureus*. Although NLRP3 and ASC are essential for IL-1β secretion by murine macrophages in response to *S. aureus,* the stimulating signal is as yet unknown, and deletionof the α-, β- and γ-toxins does not perturb production of the cytokine. The inflammasome is involved in cell death in response to bacterial invasion and although invasion of murine osteoblasts by *S. aureus* induces apoptosis, it is not established whether the inflammasome is involved.
Signalling in response to IL-1 and TNF binding of to their respective receptors leads to eventual activation of the NFκB transcription factor and JNK (c-Jun N-terminal kinase) and p38 MAPK(mitogen-activated protein kinase) signaling[57,58]. Studies with knockout mice have shown that at least one of the p50 or p52 NFκB subunits is required for IL-1-induced osteoclast formation and resorptive activity, indicating that much of the osteoclastogenic activity of IL-1 is dependent on NFκB. TNFα binds to two receptors, TNF type I (TNF-R1) and type II (TNF-R2) receptor which differ in their signaling mechanisms although there is substantial signalling crosstalk between the two receptors. Interestingly, the *S. aureus* virulence factor protein A, in addition to possession of immunoglobulin G-binding activity, is able to bind to the TNF-R1 receptor and stimulates downstream signalling and inflammation.
TNFα mediates the osteoclastogenic activity of RANKL. TNFα production by osteoclast progenitors is induced by RANKL and stimulates osteoclast differentiation in an autocrine manner. Signal transduction involves the activation of Janus family (JAK) tyrosine kinases

and subsequent phosphorylation and activation of STAT (signal transducers and activators of transcription) family transcription factors. IL-6 mediates bone resorption indirectly, and has no effect on isolated osteoclasts and IL-6 induction of osteoclastogenesis is dependent on the expression of the IL-6 receptor by osteoblasts, but not osteoclast progenitors.

It is clear that these cytokines have a prominent role in modulating bone turnover, and perturbation of their levels can have profound effects on this process. Although some mechanistic details are currently lacking, there is strong evidence that *S. aureus* infection of bone initiates local and systemic production of TNFα, IL-1 and IL-6 via host PRRs. Elevated levels of these cytokines then shift the homeostatic balance of bone turnover, increasing osteoclast differentiation and bone resorption and iminishing osteoblast-mediated bone matrix production and mineralisation, thereby driving bone destruction.

5.4 Staphylococcal invasion of bone cells

In addition to staphylococcal induction of inflammatory mediators that modulate the actions of osteoblasts and osteoclasts, bacteria of this genus are involved in more direct interactions with bone cells. Invasion and persistence of *S. aureus* in 'non-professional phagocytic' host cells in vitro has been described for many different cell types, including epithelial cells, endothelial cells and keratinocytes[59]. In cell culture systems, *S. aureus* is able to invade cultured osteoblasts from murine, human and embryonic chick sources, and *S. epidermidis* is also able to invade and grow within cultured osteoblasts. Electron microscopy has demonstrated the presence of bacteria within osteoblasts and osteocytes of embryonic chicks following injection with *S. aureus*, indicating that internalisation by bone cells also occurs in vivo. Intracellular bacteria inside osteoblasts and osteocytes in a patient with recurrent, long-term osteomyelitis of the fibula have been visualised by light and electron microscopy. More recently Stoodley et al. [60]have demonstrated *S. aureus* biofilms in an infected total joint arthroplasty. Although not reported in this paper the authors also identified *S. aureus* within host cells (personal communications, Stoodley). Thus the suggestion that internalisation of *S. aureus* by bone cells in vivo provides a protective niche for the bacterium, where it is shielded from immune effector mechanisms and antibiotics, may help to explain persistent cases of osteomyelitis. However, the true importance of intracellular staphylococci in clinical osteomyelitis has yet to be established.

S. aureus requires fibronectin-binding proteins (FnBPs) expressed on the surface of the bacterium to enable uptake by osteoblasts, and many other cell types. These proteins belong to a group of adhesions known as MSCRAMMs (microbial surface components recognising adhesive matrix molecules), which bind a range of extracellular matrix proteins including fibronectin, fibrinogen, collagen, elastin and bone sialoprotein. Mutants deficient in the two FnBPs, FnBPA and FnBPB invade host cells very poorly. Invasion is dependent on fibronectin binding by these proteins, and on the host cell integrin α5β1 receptor. *S. aureus* binds to fibronectin via FnBPs displayed on the bacterial surface, and fibronectin serves as a bridging molecule to the integrin α5β1 which acts as a "phagocytic"receptor. Alternative uptake mechanisms do exist in certain cell types, however, as *S. aureus* is still able to invade primary keratinocytes in the absence of FnBPs and uptake is not inhibited by blockade of integrin α5β1 binding to fibronectin. The mechanism of invasion also differs between *S. aureus* and *S. epidermidis* and the latter does not gain entry via the fibronectin-integrin α5β1 mechanism[61].

The level of expression of the alternative sigma factor, σ B, affects *fnbA* expression and the fibronectin binding ability of *S. aureus* strains and correlates with the level of internalization of bacteria by osteoblasts suggesting that σB-mediated up-regulation of FnBP expression may facilitate invasion[62].

Integrin $\alpha 5\beta 1$-mediated uptake of *S. aureus* requires remodelling of the actin cytoskeleton. The integrin-linked kinase, ILK, provides a link between $\alpha 5\beta 1$ and the cytoskeleton, and interacts with the cytoplasmic domains of β integrins and is subsequently activated. ILK activity is required for internalisation of *S. aureus* by epithelial cells. Recruitment of focal adhesion proteins, including the adaptor protein paxillin and the focal adhesion kinase, FAK, follows. Upon infection of HEK293T cells with *S. aureus* there is also recruitment of focal adhesion proteins, such as tensin, zyxin and vinculin to the site of bacterial attachment. FAK is recruited and tyrosine phosphorylated, and FAK-deficient cells are able to internalise *S. aureus* much less efficiently. Phosphorylation of downstream substrates of FAK, including cortactin, which is involved in actin cytoskeletal organisation, occurs during invasion, and interference with cortactin also reduces internalisation. So, signalling downstream of the integrin $\alpha 5\beta 1$ receptor, involving ILK and FAK, is important for *S. aureus* invasion, at least in certain cell types.

Physical contact between *S. aureus* and osteoblasts induces host cell expression of tumour necrosis factor apoptosis inducing ligand (TRAIL) . TRAIL is a member of the TNF cytokine family, and binds to two death domain -containing receptors, TRAIL receptors 1 and 2, which once activated recruit the FADD (Fas-associated protein with death domain) adaptor protein which in turn activates caspases 8 and −10 and commits the cell to an apoptotic pathway[63]. TRAIL produced by *S. aureus*-infected osteoblasts induces caspase-8 activation and apoptosis in cultured osteoblasts. Uninfected osteoblasts cultured alongside infected cells also express TRAIL[64]. TRAIL can induce apoptosis in human osteoclasts via TRAIL receptor 2, and also inhibits osteoclast differentiation. It is therefore possible that apoptosis of bone cells infected with *S. aureus*, and potentially of neighbouring uninfected cells may contribute to bone loss in osteomyelitis .

Growing experimental support indicates that staphylococcal invasion of osteoblasts, most likely via the FnBP-fibronectin-integrin α5β1 bridging mechanism in the case of *S. aureus*, may play a role in the pathogenesis of bone infections. This intracellular location may provide a protected environment for bacteria, aiding prolonged persistence by enabling evasion of antimicrobials and host immune mechanisms and possibly contributing to bone damage by inducing apoptosis of infected cells.

5.5 Staphylococcal virulence determinants

A number of animal models of bone implant infection, osteomyelitis and septic arthritis have been developed which have enabled the role of specific virulence factors in infections to be determined. As mentioned at the outset there are a number of routes of bone infection, i.e. haematogenous, contiguous and direct infection of bone, and models have been developed to mimic each of these routes of infection. This is important since the range of environments experienced by the bacterium differs for each route and hence the virulence factors that are involved in pathology may be different for each route of infection. The septic arthritis model developed by Tarkowski and colleagues in conjunction with defined isogenic mutants deficient in one or more virulence determinants, or with neutralising antibodies to virulence factors has proven to be particularly useful in elucidating the role of specific virulence determinants and host factors in bone infections. This model has shown that there is a plethora of virulence determinants involved in *S. aureus* septic arthritis. some of which are also involved in osteomyelitis. However, there is some controversy in this area

because whilst the murine septic arthritis model is well established and standardised a number of different models have been developed for osteomyelitis and the relevance of specific virulence factors to bone implant infections or osteomyelitis appears to be dependent on the particular model used. For example the collagen adhesin Cna has been shown to contribute to osteomyelitis by some workers but not by others and has been reported not to be important in orthopaedic device infections. The role of FnBPs has not been directly assessed in a model of osteomyelitis, but comparison of *S. aureus* strains with and without fibronectin-binding activity in a mouse osteomyelitis model suggests that fibronectin-binding strains may give rise to more severe bone infections. In the septic arthritis model, *S. aureus fnbA fnbB* mutants show no reduction in severity of arthritis, in contrast with *clfA clfB* mutants lacking the fibrinogen-binding clumping factors. However, the presence of the *fnb* genes results in greater weight loss and mortality, as well as higher serum levels of IL-6, indicating a role for FnBPs in the systemic inflammatory response.
One area of research that has received surprisingly little attention is that of the direct action of virulence factors on bone and bone cells. Work in our own laboratory has shown that *S.aureus* and *S. epidermidis* produce surface-associated proteins that can stimulate bone breakdown in an in vitro assay. These surface-associated proteins and capsular material appear to promote the formation and activation of the boneresorbing osteoclast. Interestingly, a proportion of the population have antibodies that can block the action of the *S. aureus* proteins and prevent bonebreakdown. The identity of the protein(s) in these mixtures which cause bone destruction has not been elucidated.

5.6 Small colony variants

Variant forms of *S. aureus*, known as small colony variants (SCVs), are associated with infections of bone and joint that may be particularly persistent, recurrent and refractory to antibiotic treatment[65]. These bacteria are mutant forms of *Staphylococcus* that may have an adaptive advantage enabling persistent bone colonisation.
SCV forms of coagulase-negative staphylococci, including *S. epidermidis*, *S. lugdunensis* and *S. capitis* have also been isolated from a range of infections. The SCV phenotype is characterised by slow growth, with colonies around 10-fold smaller than wild-type forms, often with decreased pigmentation, increased aminoglycoside resistance and some reports of reduced haemolytic activity[66]. The nature of these phenotypes can cause difficulty in detection and identification of the bacteria, and may contribute to an underestimation of the clinical prevalence of SCVs [67]. These phenotypes usually result from auxotrophy for hemin, menadione or thymidine and can be reversed by supplementation with these molecules. Mutations in the *hemB* and *menD* genes produce hemin and menadione auxotrophic strains with typical SCV phenotypes, and give rise to disruption of electron transport which is the basis of the growth deficiency, increased minoglycoside resistance and other phenotypes. SCVs can be selected for with gentamicin in vitro, and there is evidence that antibiotic therapy, in particular use of gentamicin beads, which are used in addition to debridement and systemic antibiotic therapy for osteomyelitis may select for SCVs in clinical situations. In a cohort of fourteen patients with confirmed *S. aureus* osteomyelitis, SCVs were isolated only from those four that had received gentamicin bead therapy, with the remaining ten patients harbouring normal *S. aureus* strains. Of the four SCVs, three were auxotrophic for hemin, and one for menadione. Only the patients harbouring SCVs had recurrent infections, although only patients whose gentamicin bead

therapy had failed were included in the study. SCVs have also been isolated from cases of infection of hip prostheses, and intracellular bacteria within host fibroblasts were identified in one of the five instances.
Clinically isolated SCVs with hemin auxotrophy, and defined *hemB* mutants, show enhanced intracellular persistence in a range of human cell types. The basis of this persistence is not established but may involve a number of possible mechanisms. *S. aureus hemB* mutants exhibit enhanced binding to fibrinogen and fibronectin, and transcribe and display more ClfA and FnBP on their surface, which may increase attachment and uptake by host cells. Transcriptional profiling of clinical and defined mutant SCVs reveals increased transcription of genes regulated by σ B, including adhesin genes, and down-regulation of exoprotein and toxin genes. The effect of increased σ B activity on MSCRAMM expression has been shown to correlate well with osteoblast invasion, adding weight to the argument that σ B-mediated upregulation of adhesins increases host cell invasion, at least in vitro, and that increased invasion by SCVs may be partially dependent on this mechanism. It has been argued that reduced production of toxins, particularly haemolysins, by SCVs also contributes to intracellular persistence by reducing the cytotoxic effect on host cells.
In a murine septic arthritis model, a defined stable *hemB* mutant, exhibiting the SCV phenotype, elicited more frequent and severe arthritis than the parental strain despite a reduced bacterial load in the kidney and joints. It has been argued that SCVs are therefore more virulent on a'per organism' basis and that enhanced protease production by *hemB* mutants may partially explain this. It may be that in clinical infections relatively small numbers of SCVs with enhanced virulence survive within tissues, possibly intracellularly, for extended periods and cause persistent infections. Clinically isolated SCVs are able to revert to the parent phenotype, although to what extent this may play a role in infections, and whether *S. aureus* may 'switch' between states in different in vivo situations is currently unclear.

6. Diagnostic approach

It is important to accurately diagnose prosthetic-joint–associated infection because its management differs from that of other causes of arthroplasty failure. Although there is no universally accepted definition of this type of infection, the criteria listed in Table 3 have been applied in a number of studies.

The presence of at least one of the following findings: • Acute inflammation detected on histopathological examination of periprosthetic tissue • Sinus tract communicating with the prosthesis • Gross purulence in the joint space • Isolation of the same microorganism from two or more cultures of joint aspirates or intraoperative periprosthetic-tissue specimens, isolation of the organism in substantial amounts (e.g., ≥20 CFU per 10 ml from the implant in a total volume of 400 ml of sonicate fluid), or both

Table 3. Criteria for the Diagnosis of a Prosthetic-Joint Infection.

Establishing the presence of acute infection or, in the presence of a draining sinus, chronic infection, is uncomplicated. In these situations, testing may be limited to that needed to establish the microbiologic diagnosis. Chronic infection manifested as localized joint pain alone poses more diagnostic difficulty, warranting additional testing. The criteria for interpreting laboratory and imaging findings in patients with a prosthetic joint are distinct from those applied in patients with a native joint. In addition to establishing the diagnosis, the identification of the involved organism or organisms and their antimicrobial susceptibility (i.e., on the basis of cultures of synovial fluid, periprosthetic tissue, the implant, or a combination of such cultures) is important in order to guide antimicrobial therapy.

C-Reactive Protein—In the absence of underlying inflammatory conditions, CRP measurement is the most useful preoperative blood test for detecting infection associated with a prosthetic joint. CRP testing has a sensitivity of 73 to 91% and a specificity of 81 to 86% for the diagnosis of prosthetic-knee infection with the use of a cutoff point of 13.5 mg per liter or more[68,69]. It has a sensitivity of 95% and a specificity of 62% for the diagnosis of prosthetichip infection with the use of a cutoff point of more than 5 mg per liter[70]. Although the CRP level and erythrocyte sedimentation rate are elevated after uncomplicated arthroplasty, the CRP level returns to the preoperative level within 2 months, whereas the erythrocyte edimentation rate may remain elevated for several months. A normal CRP level generally indicates an absence of infection, although false negative results may occur in patients who have been treated with antimicrobial agents or who have infection that is caused by low-virulenceorganisms such as *P. acnes*. Elevations in the peripheral -blood leukocyte count and levels of procalcitonin have low sensitivity for detecting infection.

Imaging—Plain radiography has low sensitivity and low specificity for detecting infection associated with a prosthetic joint[71]. Periprosthetic radiolucency, osteolysis, migration, or all of these features may be present on radiographs in patients with either infection or aseptic loosening of the prosthesis. Diagnostic studies with the use of computed tomography (CT) or magnetic resonance imaging (MRI) are hampered by artifacts produced by prostheses, although implants that are not ferromagnetic (i.e., titanium or tantalum) are associated with minimal MRI artifacts, and MRI scans of such implants provide good resolution for detecting soft-tissue abnormalities. Bone scans obtained after the administration of technetium-99m -labeled methylene diphosphonate are sensitive for detecting failed implants but nonspecific for detecting infection, and they may remain abnormal for more than a year after implantation.

Some studies suggest that combined bone and gallium-67 scans are more specific than bone scans alone. However, labeled-leukocyte imaging (e.g., leukocytes labeled with indium-111) combined with bone marrow imaging with the use of technetium -99m–labeled sulfur colloid is more accurate than bone imaging alone, combined bone and gallium-67 imaging, or labeledleukocyte and bone imaging when compared head to head, and it is considered the imaging test of choice when imaging is required[71]. 18F-fluorodeoxyglucose positron-emission tomography (PET) has a sensitivity of 82% and a specificity of 87% for the detection of prosthetic-knee or prosthetic-hip infection, on the basis of pooled data from several studies, but it is not widely available[72]. Newer imaging strategies such as scintigraphy with antigranulocyte monoclonal antibodies and hybrid imaging (e.g., combined PET and CT) (see Fig. 3)are under investigation.

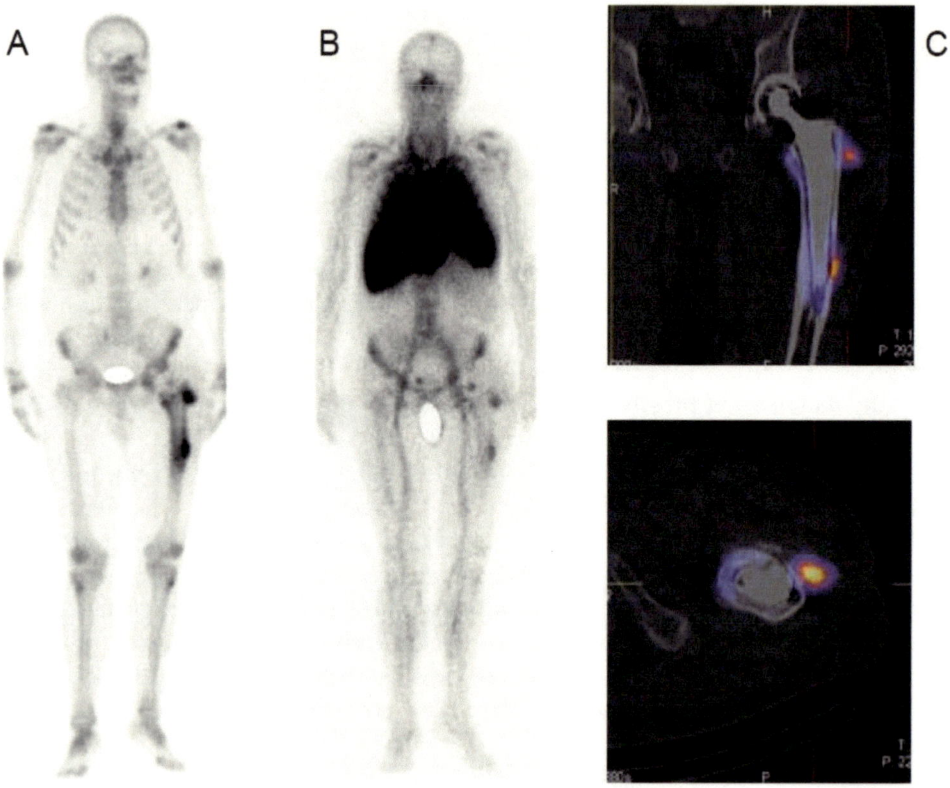

Fig. 3. Bone Scan, Labeled-Leukocyte Scan and Positron Emission Tomography/Computed Tomography Scan from a Patient with Prosthetic Joint Infection.
In Panel A, an anterior bone scan obtained after the administration of technetium-99m–labeled methylene diphosphonate shows diffusely increased activity around the femoral component of a left hip replacement, with foci of increased activity at the tip of the femoral component and around the tibia. In Panel B, a labeled leukocyte scan obtained after the administration of indium-111–labeled leukocytes shows accumulation of labeled leukocytes that is spatially congruent with the bone scan image shown in Panel A. In Panel C, 18F-fluoro-2-deoxyglucose positron emission tomography/computed tomography coronal and sagittal images show increased activity around the bone-prosthesis interface. Staphylococcus epidermidis and Finegoldia magna were isolated from the periprosthetic tissue. (Images courtesy of Carmen Vigil, M.D., and Jose Angel Richter, M.D., Department of Nuclear Medicine, University Hospital of Navarre, Pamplona, Spain.)

Synovial-Fluid Studies—If there is uncertainty about the diagnosis, the most useful preoperative diagnostic test is aspiration of joint synovial fluid for a total and differential cell count and culture. Aspiration should not be performed through overlying cellulitis. Hip aspiration may require imaging guidance. A synovial-fluid leukocyte count of more than 1.7×103 per cubic millimeter or a differential count with more than 65% neutrophils is consistent with prosthetic-knee infection. A synovial-fluid leukocyte count of more than 4.2×103 per cubic millimeter or more than 80% neutrophils is consistent with prosthetic-hip infection[73]. The leukocyte count cutoffs are dramatically lower than those used to diagnose native-joint infection. Synovial-fluid culture has a sensitivity of 56 to 75% and a specificity of 95 to 100%, and to achieve optimal sensitivity and specificity, it should be performed by means of inoculation into a blood-culture bottle. If an organism of questionable clinical significance is isolated, repeat synovial-fluid aspiration for culture should be considered. Previous antimicrobial treatment reduces the sensitivity.

Histopathological Examination of Periprosthetic Tissue—In patients in whom the diagnosis of prosthetic-joint–associated infection has not been established preoperatively, an intraoperative frozen section may be obtained to look for evidence of acute inflammation. In studies that used a polymorphonuclear-cell count ranging from more than 5 to 10 or more cells per high-power field as a positive test, sensitivity for infection ranged from 50 to 93% and specificity ranged from 77 to 100%; the rate of interobserver agreement was 86%.

Intraoperative Microbiologic Testing—Identification of the pathogen or pathogens is critical for choosing the antimicrobial regimen; if microbiologic testing has not been done preoperatively, specimens should be collected for microbiologic study at the time of surgery. Antimicrobial therapy should be discontinued at least 2 weeks before surgery, and perioperative antimicrobial coverage should be deferred until culture specimens have been collected. Cultures of sinus tract exudates should be avoided; these are often positive because of microbial skin colonization and correlate poorly with cultures of surgical specimens.

If periprosthetic tissue is obtained, collection of multiple periprosthetic-tissue specimens for aerobic and anaerobic bacterial culture is imperative because of the poor sensitivity of a single culture and to distinguish contaminants from pathogens. A study that used mathematical modeling to estimate yield based on the number of cultures concluded that to maximize accuracy, five or six specimens should be submitted for culture, and two or three culturepositive samples would be considered to be diagnostic.

Periprosthetic-tissue cultures may be falsely negative because of previous antimicrobial therapy, leaching of antimicrobial agents from antimicrobial -impregnated cement, biofilm growth on the surface of the prosthesis (but not in the surrounding tissue), a low number of organisms in tissue, an inappropriate culture medium, an inadequate culture incubation time, or a prolonged time to transport the specimen to the laboratory. Because of poor sensitivity, neither intraoperative swab cultures nor Gram's staining of the periprosthetic tissue is recommended. Fungal cultures, mycobacterial cultures, or both may be considered (e.g., if bacterial cultures are negative in a patient with apparent infection), but they are not routinely recommended.

Microorganisms form a biofilm on the prosthesis; therefore, if the prosthesis is removed, obtaining a sample from its surface is useful for microbiologic diagnosis. The implant is removed and transported to the laboratory in a sterile jar. After the addition of Ringer's solution, the container is vortexed and sonicated (frequency, 40 kHz; power density, 0.22 W per square centimeter) for 5 minutes in a bath sonicator, and the resultant fluid is cultured. This technique is more sensitive than and as specific as multiple periprosthetic-tissue cultures for diagnosing infection of a prosthetic hip, knee, or shoulder, provided that an appropriate cutoff for significant results is applied. This technique is particularly helpful in patients who have received previous antimicrobial therapy. In a study involving patients receiving antimicrobial agents within 2 weeks before surgery, the sensitivity of periprosthetic-tissue culture was 45%, whereas the sensitivity of sonicate-fluid culture was 75% ($P<0.001$). Sonication in bags is not recommended because of the potential for contamination.

6.1 Treatment

The goal of treatment is to cure the infection, prevent its recurrence, and ensure a pain-free, functional joint. This goal can best be achieved by a multidisciplinary team consisting of an orthopedic surgeon, an infectious-disease specialist, and a clinical microbiologist. On the basis of clinical experience, the use of antimicrobial agents alone, without surgical intervention, ultimately fails in most cases. Careful surgical débridement is critical. A general approach to surgical management is outlined in Figure 4; different centers and surgeons may use slightly different strategies. Chronic infections require resection arthroplasty either as a onstage exchange (i.e., removal of the infected prosthesis and reimplantation of a new prosthesis during the same surgical procedure) or a two-stage exchange (i.e., removal of the infected prosthesis and administration of systemic antimicrobial agents with subsequent implantation of a new prosthesis, usually between 6 weeks and 3 months after the first stage). Case series have suggested improved outcomes with a one-stage exchange when polymethylmethacrylate impregnated with one or more antimicrobial agents is used. A spacer impregnated with one or more antimicrobial agents may be used to maintain the leg at its correct length and to control infection during the prosthesis-free interval of a two-stage exchange. In a randomized trial involving patients with infection associated with hip arthroplasty, the use of a vancomycinloaded spacer (as compared with no spacer) resulted in a lower rate of recurrent infection (11% vs. 33%, P = 0.002)[74].

Patients who have had symptoms of infection for fewer than 3 weeks, who present with infection within 3 months after implantation or who have hematogenous infection, and who have a well-fixed, functioning prosthesis, without a sinus tract, and with an appropriate microbiologic diagnosis (Fig. 4) may be candidates for débridement and retention of the prosthesis. The addition of rifampin is recommended in cases of rifampin-susceptible staphylococcal infection. In a small, randomized trial comparing different antibiotic regimens in patients with staphylococcal infection of prosthetic knees or hips or osteosynthetic implants, salvage of the implant was successful in all 12 patients treated for 3 to 6 months with rifampin and ciprofloxacin, as compared with successful salvage in 7 of 12 patients treated with ciprofloxacin alone for 3 to 6 months (P = 0.02).

When unacceptable joint function is anticipated after surgery or the infection has been refractory to multiple surgical attempts at cure, resection arthroplasty with creation of a pseudarthrosis for hips (Girdlestone resection) or arthrodesis for knees may be considered. If the patient is not a candidate for surgery, antimicrobial suppression may be attempted; this approach is unlikely to cure infection, so the use of antimicrobial agents is often continued indefinitely.

In brief, information about antimicrobial susceptibility should be used to confirm the activity of any antimicrobial agent used for therapy. Data from randomized trials on the optimal duration of treatment are lacking. The therapeutic approach has to be selected in accordance with the mode of infection (NJI, PJI, RA), the expected or found pathogens, and their resistance. It should be remembered that the slowed growth of bacteria in a biofilm on surfaces of joint prosthesis may additionally reinforces antibiotic resistance. Responsible for such an increase against antibacterial substances are changes in cell wall synthesis, which limits the effect of beta-lactam antibiotics and glycopeptides, and the occurrence of bacterial variants with modifications of other metabolic activities, with implications for the action of quinolones, aminoglycosides, and tetracyclines. In principle, the spectrum of available antibiotics is limited by the specific pharmacokinetic requirements in the treatment of joint infections. This applies particularly to chronic infections and prosthesis infections.

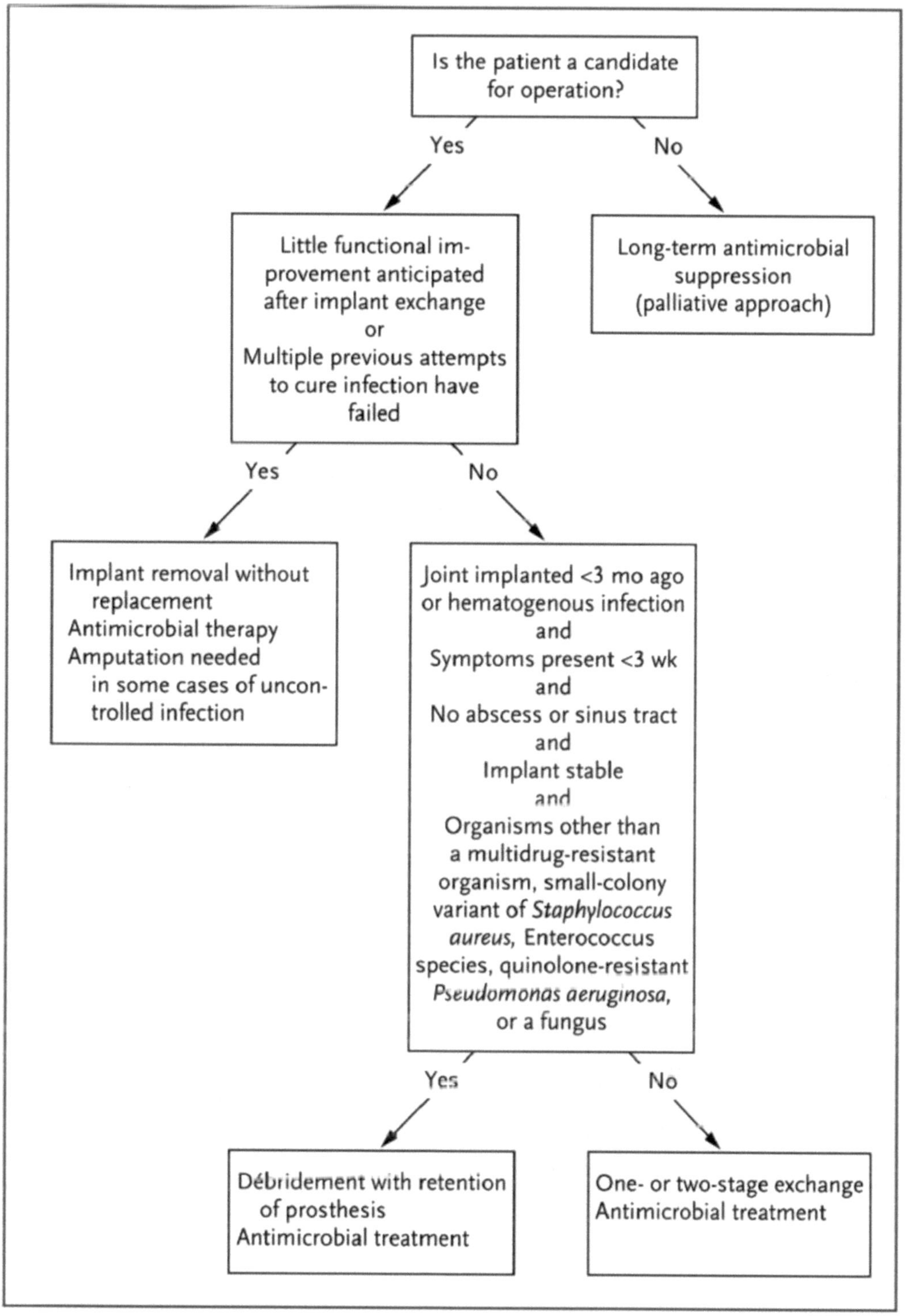

Fig. 4. Algorithm for the Treatment of Infection Associated with a Prosthetic joint

<table>
<tr><th rowspan="2">Organism</th><th colspan="2">Antibiotics</th></tr>
<tr><th>Native joint infection</th><th>Prosthetic joint infection</th></tr>
<tr><td>Methicillin resistant Staphylococcus aureus</td><td rowspan="2">(I) First choice:
Vancomycin 2× 1 g/d
Linezolid 2× 600 mg/d
(II) Alternatives:
Cotrimoxazol, Doxycyclin,
Clindamycin, Rifampicin (always in combination)</td><td rowspan="2">(I) First choice (in combination with Rifampicin 600–900 mg):
Vancomycin 2× 1 g/d
Teicoplanin 800 mg/d for the first 1–4 days, than 800 mg every 2 days
Fluoroquinolone (e.g. Ciprofloxacin 2× 500–750 mg/d)
Fusidinsäure 3× 500 mg/d
(II) Alternatives:
Linezolid, Quinupristin/Dalfopristin</td></tr>
<tr><td>Methicillin resistant coagulase negative staphylococci</td></tr>
<tr><td>Methicillin sensitive Staphylococcus aureus</td><td rowspan="2">(I) First choice:
beta-lactamase stable penicillin (e.g. Flucloxacillin 4× 2–3 g/d, Nafcillin 4× 2 g/d)
Clindamycin 3× 600–900 mg/d
(II) Alternatives:
Cefazolin, Vancomycin</td><td rowspan="2">(I) First choice (in combination with Rifampicin 600–900 mg):
Flucloxacillin 4× 2–3 g/d
Fluoroquinolone (e.g. Ciprofloxacin 2× 500–750 mg/d)
(II) Alternatives (in combination with Rifampicin):
Cefazolin, Vancomycin</td></tr>
<tr><td>Methicillin sensitive coagulase negative staphylococci</td></tr>
<tr><td>beta-hemolytic Streptococci</td><td>(I) First choice:
Penicillin G 6× 2 million units/d
Ampicillin 3× 2 g/d
(II) Alternatives:
Clindamycin, Cefazolin</td><td>(I) First choice
Penicillin G 6× 4–5 million units/d
Ampicillin 3× 4 g/d
(II) Alternatives:
Vancomycin, Ceftriaxon</td></tr>
<tr><td>Enterococcus spec.</td><td>(I) First choice:
Ampicillin 3× 2 g/d
Vancomycin 2× 1 g /d
(II) Alternatives:
Linezolid</td><td>(I) First choice
Ampicillin 3× 4 g/d
Vancomycin 2× 1 g /d
Teicoplanin 800 mg/d for the first 1–4 days, than 800 mg every 2 days
(II) Alternatives:
Linezolid</td></tr>
<tr><td>Escherichia coli</td><td>(I) First choice:
Ampicillin/Sulbactam 4× 3 g/d
(II) Alternatives:
Cefazolin, Fluoroquinolone (e.g. Ciprofloxacin), Gentamicin, Cotrimoxazole</td><td rowspan="3">(I) First choice:
Ciprofloxacin 2× 500–750 mg/d
Cefotaxime 3–4× 2 g/d
Piperacillin/Tazobactam 3× 4 g/0,5g/d
(II) Alternatives:
Imipenem, Meropenem</td></tr>
<tr><td>Proteus mirabilis</td><td>(I) First choice:
Ampicillin 3× 2 g/d
Fluoroquinolone (e.g. Ciprofloxacin 2× 500–750 mg/d)
(II) Alternatives:
Cefazolin, Cotrimoxazole, Gentamicin</td></tr>
<tr><td>Proteus vulgaris
Proteus rettgeri
Morganella morganii</td><td>(I) First choice:
Cefotaxime 3–4× 2 g/d
Imipenem 4× 500 mg/d
Fluoroquinolone (e.g. Ciprofloxacin 2× 500–750 mg/d)
(II) Alternatives:
Ampicillin, Gentamicin, free or fixed combination of beta-lactam/beta-lactamase inhibitor (e.g. combinations with Combactam or as Ampicillin/Sulbactam, Piperacillin/Tazobactam, Ticarcillin/Clavulanate)</td></tr>
<tr><td>Serratia marcescens</td><td>(I) First choice:
Cefotaxime 3–4× 2 g/d
(II) Alternatives:
Fluoroquinolone (e.g. Ciprofloxacin)
Gentamicin, Imipenem</td><td rowspan="2">I) First choice:
Ceftazidim 3× 2 g/d
+ Fluoroquinolone (e.g. Ciprofloxacin 2× 500–750 mg/d)
(II) Alternatives:
Imipenem, Meropenem</td></tr>
<tr><td>Pseudomonas aeruginosa</td><td>(I) First choice:
Piperacillin 4× 3 g/d
Imipenem 4× 500 mg/d
(II) Alternatives:
Fluoroquinolone (e.g. Ciprofloxacin)
Tobramycin, Amikacin</td></tr>
<tr><td>Anaerobe infection</td><td>(I) First choice:
Clindamycin 3× 600–900 mg/d
Imipenem 4× 500 mg/d
Metronidazole 3× 500 mg/d
(II) Alternatives:
free or fixed combination of beta-lactam/beta-lactamase inhibitor (e.g. combinations with Combactam or as Ampicillin/Sulbactam, Piperacillin/Tazobactam, Ticarcillin/Clavulanate)</td><td>First choice:
Clindamycin 3× 600–900 mg/d
Piperacillin/Tazobactam 3× 4 g/0,5g/d
Imipenem 4× 500 mg/d</td></tr>
</table>

(all given dosages are for healthy adults of 70 kg with normal liver and kidney function)

Table 4. Antibiotics for therapy of infectious arthritis

Lysostaphin is a 27 kDa endopeptidase that was first isolated from a culture of Staphylococcus simulans by Schindler & Schuhardt. The enzyme kills the organism by hydrolysing a pentaglycine cross-bridge structure unique to the staphylococcal cell wall. As the cell wall cross-bridges of S. aureus are composed of a high proportion of pentaglycine, both proliferating and quiescent S. aureus cells are highly sensitive to lysostaphin. Lysostaphin kills meticillin-susceptible S. aureus (MSSA) and MRSA equally well and has been demonstrated to be a potent therapeutic agent for S. aureus infections in various animal studies. In the USA, two therapeutic products formulated with recombinant lysostaphin for topical use have entered clinical studies. And recombinant lysostaphin is expected to be a potential alternative therapy for S. aureus infection[78].

For an overview of common substances and therapeutic regimes, see Table 4.

In patients undergoing débridement with retention of the prosthesis, 3-month courses of treatment for infection associated with hip prostheses and 6-month courses for infection associated with knee prostheses are often used. Oral therapy can be used if the agent has good oral bioavailability (e.g., quinolones, rimethoprim- sulfamethoxazole, and tetracyclines). In patients undergoing a two-stage exchange, systemic antimicrobial therapy is often administered for 4 to 6 weeks. Commercially available, preblended, polymethylmethacrylate impregnated with an antimicrobial agent is indicated for use in the second stage of a two-stage revision after elimination of active infection. Although it is not standard clinical practice, two studies involving a long period between the initial and second stages suggest that when a polymethylmethacrylate spacer impregnated with one or more antimicrobial agents or impregnated beads are used, the administration of systemic antimicrobial therapy for 2 weeks may be sufficient or systemic therapy may even be unnecessary[75,76].

6.2 Prophylaxis

In addition to good aseptic technique and procedures in the operating room, the administration of intravenous antimicrobial agents immediately before surgery minimizes the risk of infection. Cefazolin at a dose of 1 g (2 g if the patient weighs ≥ 80 kg) every 8 hours or cefuroxime at a dose of 1.5 g, followed by 750 mg every 8 hours is recommended routinely; vancomycin at a dose of 15 mg per kilogram every 12 hours (assuming normal renal function) is used in patients with a β-lactam allergy or MRSA colonization. Prophylaxis should begin within 60 minutes before surgical incision (within 120 minutes if vancomycin is used) and should be completed within 24 hours after the end of surgery. The entire antimicrobial dose should be infused before inflation of a tourniquet[77].

7. References

[1] National Hospital Discharge Survey: survey results and products. Atlanta: Centers for Disease Control and Prevention; 2009 [Accessed July 24, 2009]. http://www.cdc.gov/nchs/nhds/nhds_products.htm

[2] Lee K. Goodman S.B. Current state and future of joint replacements in the hip and knee. Expert Rev. Med. Devices 2008;5:383–393. [PubMed: 18452388]

[3] Goldenberg D.L. Septic arthritis. Lancet 1998;351:197–202. [PubMed: 9449882]

[4] Nade S. Septic arthritis. Best. Pract. Res. Clin. Rheumatol. 2003;17:183–200. [PubMed: 12787520]

[5] Stott N.S. Paediatric bone and joint infection. J. Orthop. Surg. (Hong Kong) 2001;9:83–90. [PubMed: 12468850]

[6] Levine M. Siegel L.B. A swollen joint: why all the fuss? Am. J. Ther. 2003;10:219–224. [PubMed: 12756429]
[7] Lew D.P. Waldvogel F.A. Osteomyelitis. Lancet 2004;364:369–379. [PubMed: 15276398]
[8] Weichert S. Sharland M. Clarke N.M. Faust S.N. Acute haematogenous osteomyelitis in children: is there any evidence for how long we should treat? Curr. Opin. Infect. Dis. 2008;21:258–262. [PubMed: 18448970]
[9] Blyth M.J. Kincaid R. Craigen M.A. Bennet G.C. The changing epidemiology of acute and subacute haematogenous osteomyelitis in children. J. Bone Joint Surg. Br. 2001;83:99–102. [PubMed: 11245548]
[10] Lazzarini L. Mader J.T. Calhoun J.H. Osteomyelitis in long bones. J. Bone Joint Surg. Am. 2004;86-A: 2305–2318. [PubMed: 15466746]
[11] Gillespie W.J. Epidemiology in bone and joint infection. Infect. Dis. Clin. North Am. 1990;4:361–376. [PubMed: 2212594]
[12] Jämsen E, Huhtala H, Puolakka T, Moilanen T. Risk factors for infection after knee arthroplasty: a register-based analysis of 43,149 cases. J Bone Joint Surg Am 2009;91:38–47.
[13] Peersman G, Laskin R, Davis J, Peterson M. Infection in total knee replacement: a retrospective review of 6489 total knee replacements. Clin Orthop Relat Res 2001;392:15–23. [PubMed: 11716377]
[14] Pulido L, Ghanem E, Joshi A, Purtill JJ, Parvizi J. Periprosthetic joint infection: the incidence, timing, and predisposing factors. Clin Orthop Relat Res 2008;466:1710–5. [PubMed: 18421542]
[15] Choong PF, Dowsey MM, Carr D, Daffy J, Stanley P. Risk factors associated with acute hip prosthetic joint infections and outcome of treatment with a rifampin-based regimen. Acta Orthop 2007;78:755- 65. [PubMed: 18236181]
[16] Phillips JE, Crane TP, Noy M, Elliott TS, Grimer RJ. The incidence of deep prosthetic infections in a specialist orthopaedic hospital: a 15-year prospective survey. J Bone Joint Surg Br 2006;88:943–8. [PubMed: 16799001]
[17] Kurtz SM, Lau E, Schmier J, Ong KL, Zhao K, Parvizi J. Infection burden for hip and knee arthroplasty in the United States. J Arthroplasty 2008;23:984–91. [PubMed: 18534466]
[18] Murdoch DR, Roberts SA, Fowler VG Jr, et al. Infection of orthopedic prostheses after *Staphylococcus aureus bacteremia*. Clin Infect Dis 2001;32:647–9. [PubMed: 11181131]
[19] Berbari EF, Hanssen AD, Duffy MC, et al. Risk factors for prosthetic joint infection: case-control study. Clin Infect Dis 1998;27:1247–54. [PubMed: 9827278]
[20] Bongartz T, Halligan CS, Osmon DR, et al. Incidence and risk factors of prosthetic joint infection after total hip or knee replacement in patients with rheumatoid arthritis. Arthritis Rheum 2008;59:1713–20. [PubMed: 19035425]
[21] Dowsey MM, Choong PF. Obesity is a major risk factor for prosthetic infection after primary hip arthroplasty. Clin Orthop Relat Res 2008;466:153–8. [PubMed: 18196388]
[22] Kaandorp CJ, Krijnen P, Moens HJ, Habbema JD, van Schaardenburg D. The outcome of bacterial arthritis: a prospective community-based study. Arthritis Rheum. 1997; 40:884–92.

[23] Kaandorp CJ, van Schaardenburg D, Krijnen P, Habbema JD, van de Laar MA. Risk factors for septic arthritis in patients with joint disease. A prospective study. Arthritis Rheum. 1995; 38:1819–25.
[24] Shirtliff ME, Mader JT. Acute septic arthritis. Clin Microbiol Rev. 2002; 15: 527–44.
[25] Udo Geipel. Pathogenic organisms in hip joint infections. International Journal of Medical Sciences 2009; 6(5):234-240.
[26] Jose L. Del Pozo, M.D., Ph.D. and Robin Patel, M.D. Infection Associated with Prosthetic Joints. N Engl J Med. 2009 August 20; 361(8): 787–794.
[27] Bennet G.C. Bennet S.J. Infection of bone and joint. Surgery (Oxford) 2006;24:211–214.
[28] Ciampolini J. Harding K.G. Pathophysiology of chronic bacterial osteomyelitis. Why do antibiotics fail so often? Postgrad. Med. J. 2000;76:479–483. [PubMed: 10908375]
[29] Trampuz A, Piper KE, Jacobson MJ, et al. Sonication of removed hip and knee prostheses for diagnosis of infection. N Engl J Med 2007;357:654–63. [PubMed: 17699815]
[30] Marculescu CE, Berbari EF, Cockerill FR III, Osmon DR. Fungi, mycobacteria, zoonotic and other organisms in prosthetic joint infection. Clin Orthop Relat Res 2006;451:64–72. [PubMed: 16906078]
[31] Unusual aerobic and anaerobic bacteria associated with prosthetic joint infections. Clin Orthop Relat Res 2006;451:55–63. Idem. [PubMed: 16906072]
[32] Berbari EF, Osmon DR, Duffy MC, et al. Outcome of prosthetic joint infection in patients with rheumatoid arthritis: the impact of medical and surgical therapy in 200 episodes. Clin Infect Dis 2006;42:216–23. [PubMed: 16355332]
[33] Piper KE, Jacobson MJ, Cofield RH, et al. Microbiologic diagnosis of prosthetic shoulder infection by use of implant sonication. J Clin Microbiol 2009;47:1878–84. [PubMed: 19261785]
[34] Marculescu CE, Cantey JR. Polymicrobial prosthetic joint infections: risk factors and outcome. Clin Orthop Relat Res 2008;466:1397–404. [PubMed: 18421538]
[35] Berbari EF, Marculescu C, Sia I, et al. Culture-negative prosthetic joint infection. Clin Infect Dis 2007;45:1113–9. [PubMed: 17918072]
[36] Peacock S.J. Moore C.E. Justice A. Kantzanou M. Story L. Mackie K. O'Neill G. Day N.P. Virulent combinations of adhesin and toxin genes in natural populations of Staphylococcus aureus. Infect. Immun. 2002;70:4987–4996. [PubMed: 12183545]
[37] Arciola C.R. Campoccia D. Gamberini S. Baldassarri L. Montanaro L. Prevalence of cna, fnbA and fnbB adhesin genes among Staphylococcus aureus isolates from orthopedic infections associated to different types of implant. FEMS Microbiol. Lett. 2005;246:81–86. [PubMed: 15869965]
[38] Peacock S.J. Day N.P. Thomas M.G. Berendt A.R. Foster T.J. Clinical isolates of Staphylococcus aureus exhibit diversity in fnb genes and adhesion to human fibronectin. J. Infect. 2000;41:23–31. [PubMed: 10942636]
[39] Bocchini C.E. Hulten K.G. Mason E.O. Gonzalez B.E. Hammerman W.A. Kaplan S.L. Panton-Valentine leukocidin genes are associated with enhanced inflammatory response and local disease in acute hematogenous Staphylococcus aureus osteomyelitis in children. Pediatrics 2006;117:433–440. [PubMed: 16452363]
[40] Sdougkos G. Chini V. Papanastasiou D.A. Christodoulou G. Tagaris G. Dimitracopoulos G. Spiliopoulou I. Methicillin-resistant Staphylococcus aureus

producing Panton–Valentine leukocidin as a cause of acute osteomyelitis in children. Clin. Microbiol. Infect. 2007;13:651–654. [PubMed: 17371535]

[41] Cassat J.E. Dunman P.M. McAleese F. Murphy E. Projan S.J. Smeltzer M.S. Comparative genomics of Staphylococcus aureus musculoskeletal isolates. J. Bacteriol. 2005;187:576–592. [PubMed: 15629929]

[42] van de Lest C.H. Vaandrager A.B. Mechanism of cell-mediated mineralization. Curr. Opin. Orthop. 2007;18:434–443.

[43] Henriksen K. Neutzsky Wulff A.V. Bonewald L.F. Karsdal M.A. Local communication on and within bone controls bone remodeling. Bone 2009;44:1026–1033. [PubMed: 19345750]

[44] Matsuo K. Irie N. Osteoclast–osteoblast communication. Arch. Biochem. Biophys. 2008;473:201–209. [PubMed: 18406338]

[45] Vaananen H.K. Laitala-Leinonen T. Osteoclast lineage and function. Arch. Biochem. Biophys. 2008;473:132–138. [PubMed: 18424258]

[46] Everts V. Korper W. Hoeben K.A. Jansen I.D. Bromme D. Cleutjens K.B. Heeneman S. Peters C. Reinheckel T. Saftig P. Beertsen W. Osteoclastic bone degradation and the role of different cysteine proteinases and matrix metalloproteinases: differences between calvaria and long bone. J. Bone Miner. Res. 2006;21:1399–1408. [PubMed: 16939398]

[47] Boyce B.F. Xing L. Functions of RANKL/RANK/OPG in bone modeling and remodeling. Arch. Biochem. Biophys. 2008;473:139–146. [PubMed: 18395508]

[48] Hikita A. Yana I. Wakeyama H. Nakamura M. Kadono Y. Oshima Y. Nakamura K. Seiki M. Tanaka S. Negative regulation of osteoclastogenesis by ectodomain shedding of receptor activator of NfkappaB ligand. J. Biol. Chem. 2006;281:36846–36855. [PubMed: 17018528]

[49] Tsezou A. Poultsides L. Kostopoulou F. Zintzaras E. Satra M. Kitsiou-Tzeli S. Malizos K.N. Influence of interleukin 1alpha (IL-1alpha), IL-4, and IL-6 polymorphisms on genetic susceptibility to chronic osteomyelitis. Clin. Vaccine Immunol. 2008;15:1888–1890. [PubMed: 18971305]

[50] Jochen Schulze.Thomas Bickert.F. Timo Beil.et al. Interleukin-33 is Expressed in Differentiated Osteoblasts and Blocks Osteoclast Formation from Bone Marrow Precursor Cells. Journal of Bone and Mineral Research.

[51] Garcia-Alvarez F. Navarro-Zorraquino M. Castro A. Grasa J.M. Pastor C. Monzon M. Martinez A. Garcia-Alvarez I. Castillo J. Lozano R. Effect of age on cytokine response in an experimental model of osteomyelitis. Biogerontology 2009;10:649–658. [PubMed: 19123052]

[52] Lacey D.C. Simmons P.J. Graves S.E. Hamilton J.A. Proinflammatory cytokines inhibit osteogenic differentiation from stem cells: implications for bone repair during inflammation. Osteoarthritis Cartilage 2008;17:735–742. [PubMed: 19136283]

[53] Lau Y.S. Wang W. Sabokbar A. Simpson H. Nair S. Henderson B. Berendt A. Athanasou N.A. Staphylococcus aureus capsular material promotes osteoclast formation. Injury 2006;37(Suppl. 2):S41–S48. [PubMed: 16651071]

[54] Creagh E.M. O'Neill L.A. TLRs, NLRs and RLRs: a trinity of pathogen sensors that co-operate in innate immunity. Trends Immunol. 2006;27:352–357. [PubMed: 16807108]

[55] Kahlenberg J.M. Lundberg K.C. Kertesy S.B. Qu Y. Dubyak G.R. Potentiation of caspase-1 activation by the P2×7 receptor is dependent on TLR signals and requires NF-kappaB-driven protein synthesis. J. Immunol. 2005;175:7611–7622. [PubMed: 16301671]
[56] Ting J.P.Y. Willingham S.B. Bergstralh D.T. NLRs at the intersection of cell death and immunity. Nat. Rev. Immunol. 2008;8:372–379. [PubMed: 18362948]
[57] Arend W.P. Palmer G. Gabay C. IL-1, IL-18, and IL-33 families of cytokines. Immunol. Rev. 2008;223:20–38. [PubMed: 18613828]
[58] Dinarello C.A. Immunological and inflammatory functions of the interleukin-1 family. Annu. Rev. Immunol. 2009;27:519–550. [PubMed: 19302047]
[59] Garzoni C. Kelley W.L. Staphylococcus aureus: new evidence for intracellular persistence. Trends Microbiol. 2009;17:59–65. [PubMed: 19208480]
[60] Stoodley P. Nistico L. Johnson S. Lasko L.A. Baratz M. Gahlot V. Ehrlich G.D. Kathju S. Direct demonstration of viable Staphylococcus aureus biofilms in an infected total joint arthroplasty. A case report. J. Bone Joint Surg. Am. 2008;90:1751–1758. [PubMed: 18676908]
[61] Khalil H. Williams R.J. Stenbeck G. Henderson B. Meghji S. Nair S.P. Invasion of bone cells by Staphylococcus epidermidis. Microbes Infect. 2007;9:460–465. [PubMed: 17331787]
[62] Mitchell G. Lamontagne C.A. Brouillette E. Grondin G. Talbot B.G. Grandbois M. Malouin F. Staphylococcus aureus SigB activity promotes a strong fibronectin-bacterium interaction which may sustain host tissue colonization by small-colony variants isolated from cystic fibrosis patients. Mol. Microbiol. 2008;70:1540–1555. [PubMed: 19007412]
[63] Mahalingam D. Szegezdi E. Keane M. Jong S. Samali A. TRAIL receptor signalling and modulation: Are we on the right TRAIL? Cancer Treat. Rev. 2009;35:280–288. [PubMed: 19117685]
[64] Reott M.A. Ritchie-Miller S.L. Anguita J. Hudson M.C. TRAIL expression is induced in both osteoblasts containing intracellular Staphylococcus aureus and uninfected osteoblasts in infected cultures. FEMS Microbiol. Lett. 2008;278:185–192. [PubMed: 18070069]
[65] von Eiff C. Peters G. Becker K. The small colony variant (SCV) concept – the role of staphylococcal SCVs in persistent infections. Injury 2006;37(Suppl. 2):S26–S33. [PubMed: 16651068]
[66] Sendi P. Proctor R.A. Staphylococcus aureus as an intracellular pathogen: the role of small colony variants. Trends Microbiol. 2009;17:54–58. [PubMed: 19162480]
[67] von Eiff C. Staphylococcus aureus small colony variants: a challenge to microbiologists and clinicians. Int. J. Antimicrob. Agents 2008;31:507 510. [PubMed: 18180148]
[68] Fink B, Makowiak C, Fuerst M, Berger I, Schäfer P, Frommelt L. The value of synovial biopsy, joint aspiration and C-reactive protein in the diagnosis of late periprosthetic infection of total knee replacements. J Bone Joint Surg Br 2008,90:874–8. [PubMed: 18591595]
[69] Greidanus NV, Masri BA, Garbuz DS, et al. Use of erythrocyte sedimentation rate and C-reactive protein level to diagnose infection before revision total knee arthroplasty: a prospective evaluation.J Bone Joint Surg Am 2007;89:1409–16. [PubMed: 17606776]

[70] Müller M, Morawietz L, Hasart O, Strube P, Perka C, Tohtz S. Diagnosis of periprosthetic infection following total hip arthroplasty – evaluation of the diagnostic values of pre- and intraoperative parameters and the associated strategy to preoperatively select patients with a high probability of joint infection. J Orthop Surg 2008;3:31.

[71] Love C, Marwin SE, Palestro CJ. Nuclear medicine and the infected joint replacement. Semin Nucl Med 2009;39:66–78. [PubMed: 19038601]

[72] Kwee TC, Kwee RM, Alavi A. FDG-PET for diagnosing prosthetic joint infection: systematic review and metaanalysis. Eur J Nucl Med Mol Imaging 2008;35:2122–32. [PubMed: 18704405]

[73] Schinsky MF, Della Valle CJ, Sporer SM, Paprosky WG. Perioperative testing for joint infection in patients undergoing revision total hip arthroplasty. J Bone Joint Surg Am 2008;90:1869–75. [PubMed: 18762646]

[74] Cabrita H, Croci A, De Camargo O, De Lima A. Prospective study of the treatment of infected hip arthroplasties with or without the use of an antibiotic-loaded spacer. Clinics (Sao Paulo) 2007;62:99– 108. [PubMed: 17505692]

[75] Whittaker JP, Warren RE, Jones RS, Gregson PA. Is prolonged systemic antibiotic treatment essential in two-stage revision hip replacement for chronic Gram-positive infection? J Bone Joint Surg Br 2009;91:44–51. [Erratum, J Bone Joint Surg Br 2009;91:700.]. [PubMed: 19092003]

[76] Stockley I, Mockford BJ, Hoad-Red-dick A, Norman P. The use of two-stage exchange arthroplasty with depot antibiotics in the absence of long-term antibiotic therapy in infected total hip replacement. J Bone Joint Surg Br 2008;90:145–8. [PubMed: 18256078]

[77] Bratzler DW, Houck PM. Antimicrobial prophylaxis for surgery: an advisory statement from the National Surgical Infection Prevention Project. Am J Surg 2005;189:395–404. [PubMed: 15820449]

[78] Xin-Yi Yang. Cong-Ran Li. Ren-Hui Lou. et al. In vitro activity of recombinant lysostaphin against Staphylococcus aureus isolates from hospitals in Beijing, China. Journal of Medical Microbiology (2007), 56, 71–76.

22

Arthroplasty in HIV/SCD Carriers

J. Bahebeck, D. Handy Eone, B. Ngo Nonga and T. Kingue Njie
University Hospitals of Yaoundé
Cameroun

1. Introduction

Due to the growing of HIV pandemic in the world and especially in Africa during the last two decades, it has become more and more frequent to find HIV infected patients with an absolute indication of arthroplasty. In fact, the indication of arthroplasty in these patients may be a very challenging issue. Even though all of these patients are not immune depressed, due to the known natural history of HIV carriage, the risk of future immune depression remain and logically the risk of immediate, early, or late infection of arthroplastic implants and subsequent loosening or worse, generalized infection. The literature on this question remains very scarce ; the first section of this chapter will present a classification of HIV carriers elected to Arthroplasty, describe protective measures for each class of patients, and present immediate , short and mid term expected results, based an a systematic analysis, and Authors own experience. The second section will be focused on arthroplasty in sickle cell disease (SCD) carriers, as these types of patients usually demand arthroplasty at the end stage of secondary vascular necrosis, the most frequent adult joint complication of their genetic condition. Lastly, as Very few, if any, is known in case where both conditions (HIV & SCD) are combined in the same patient demanding arthroplasty, a short section will be proposed.

Section A: Arthroplasty in HIV carriers

- Introduction
- Pathogenesis of HIV infection
- Work up and classification of HIV carriers elected for arthroplasty
- General principles & practices of antiretroviral therapy
- Antiretroviral therapy in HIV carriers demanding arthroplasty
- Prophylactic antibiotic therapy in HIV carriers undergoing arthroplasty
- Section A Summary

Due to the spreading of HIV worldwide during the latest decades, it had become more and more frequent in the orthopaedic practice, to indicate an arthroplasty, especially of the hip, in patients living with HIV. This virus has been incriminated by many authors as a possible causal agent in the case of bone's aseptic necrosis. The profiles of the HIV infected patients are variable: some are previous known carriers, other are discovered at the time of the preoperative workup. The duration of the preoperative antiretroviral treatment vary also from one patient to another. Anyhow, the main question for the orthopedic surgeon is to find out what is the level of the immune system of a person living with HIV and who is a candidate for an arthroplasty? In another words, what is the infection risk of the implant, whether immediately, in the short, the mid and even the long term? These questions may be better understood through a review of the pathogenesis of HIV infection.

1.1 Pathogenesis of HIV Infection

HIV infection is due to the introduction of the related virus in the body mainly through unprotected sexual intercourses, secondly through blood transfusion, and more rarely through other ways. Sometimes the patient may present a minor inflammatory syndrome lasting for few days with a complete recovery and no detectable virus for a long period. In some people, the virus will spread into the body fluids and organs and will slowly, but surely, destroy a specific type of lymphocytes, named CD4; the problem is that, CD4 are the hard ware of the body immune system and thus, the protector against numerous common infectious agents. With time, and after many years, no matter the apparent normal clinical state, the CD4 lymphocytes count which is normally above 500 Cells/Ml, will decrease progressively with a proportional depression of the HIV carrier immunity. If nothing is done, the general status of the patient will decompensate with severe weight loss, anemia and fatigue. He will develop opportunistic infections or tumors which are exceptional in an immune competent person. The most common opportunistic diseases are from the skull to the foot: brain toxoplasmosis, mouth and esophageal candidiasis, lung tuberculosis and pneumocystoses, intestinal cryptosporidiosis, leg and generalized Kaposi angiosarcomas, and various lymphomas. At this stage, the majority of patients are killed by a combination of these diseases and their complications. It is obvious that clinical pictures of HIV carriers are numerous, depending on the level of the immune depression; a classification is therefore necessary. The WHO-AIDS has proposed such a classification based both on the clinical picture and biological markers. However, as far as arthroplasty is concerned, the extreme majority of demanders of this surgery look clinically well; therefore, except in case where they declare themselves, if a systematic sample of HIV serologogy is not done, the surgeon may be taking the risk of a major surgical procedure in an advanced immune depressed patient. In our practice where the HIV carriage is up to 10% into the general population, HIV screening is mandatory before any elective arthroplasty. No matter the result, the benefice is defendable. In fact, in one hand, negative patients may at least undergo an auto transfusion program while, in the other hand, virus carriers will be classified and appropriately managed before or during arthroplasty. Such classification is mainly based on immunological work up, since, as it had been said above, quite all patients look healthy.

1.2 Work up and classification of HIV carriers elected for arthroplasty

After the diagnosis is done and an indication of arthroplasty is made, especially into the areas of high HIV carriage in the general population, the Orthopedic Surgeon should obtain an inform consent from his patient about this uncomfortable matter. In twelve years practice in our community, we have not had any of our patients for hip arthrosplasty resisting to the above arguments, but as with all medical information, discretion is the rule. If the patient is a known HIV carrier already on antiretroviral treatment, we will look up for his latest CD4 count and viral load. In the other cases, the screening is mandatory; if the patient is seronegative, he is managed conventionally with the advantage of auto transfusion program, provided hepatitis B and C serology are negative. In HIV positive screened patients, the next step is the confirmation western-Blot test; if the latest is negative; the patient is qualified as non HIV carrier and managed as usual. In case of confirmed HIV carriage by western-Blot test, the next step is the CD4 lymphocytes count and the viral load measurement by up to date procedures. The CD4 lymphocyte count is the key point for HIV carriers classification. Patients with less than 500 CD4 lymphocytes / ML are considered immune depressed and named **class A arthroplasty demanders.** Depending on whether this count is above 300, les than 300 with no opportunistic disease, or less than 300 with an opportunistic disease, Class A patients are further sub divided **A1, A2 or A3**. Non immune depressed HIV seropositive Patients with low infection risk are classified **B**; if they were known before and under treatment, they are sub-divided **B1**, if they have more than 500 CD4/ML with no treatment, they are sub-divided **B2**. This makes a total of 5 classes of arthroplasty demanders living with the virus (**B1, B2, A1, A2, A3**) and thus, who need specific protective measures and especially, antiretroviral therapy (ARVT).

1.3 General principles of antiretroviral therapy

Antiretroviral therapy (ARVT) was introduced in the early nineties with the aim to act against the multiplication of the HIV and therefore, to stop the destruction of the CD4 lymphocytes and subsequent immune depression. The drugs are numerous, but have been considered based on their action into 3 main classes which are: antiproteasis, nucleoside inhibitor of reverse transcriptases and non nucleoside inhibitor of reverse transcriptase. Into the middle of the decade, it clearly appeared that none of these classes could solely stop the viral replication and that, in the contrary, the triple combination was efficient. Shortly after, the common presentation became a triple antiretroviral fixed combination drugs commonly named TRITHERAPY.

There are two most common combinations that are: Efavirenz, Zidovudine and Lamivudine into one hand, and on the other hand, Niverapine, Stadivudine and Lamivudine. In case of drug resistance, a second line combination of Indinavir, Zidovudine and Lamivudine is proposed. The first line treatment, which is commonly used, has shown that besides few sides effects seen at the beginning of the treatment, that combination is usually well tolerated thereafter and it is efficient. In a large majority of patients the CD4 level will rise above 500/ML after weeks to months and the virus will be undetectable in the peripheral blood, making them significantly less contagious to their sexual partners. Many institutions in our country give drugs only to severely immune depressed carriers defined as AIDS patients. Moderately immune depressed and non immune depressed carriers are not treated. Therefore, it remained a question weather this policy does not favor the spreading of the disease through the world? Anyway, whenever an arhtroplasty is demanded by a HIV carrier, a different protocol of ARVT should be associated.

1.4 Antiretroviral therapy in HIV carriers demanding arthroplasty

Finally, 5 types of HIV carriers have been considered among arthroplasty demanders; they may need a similar number of protocols regarding ARVT.

1. **B1** Arthroplasty demanders are already known as HIV carriers and under ARVT; they should never stop their treatment even the day before and after surgery. There is nothing to do more, compare to non carriers patients. Exceptionally, if their CD4 count is low, they are referred to their physician to find out if this low count is due to drug resistance or to a non compliant attitude. The surgery should be delayed, and the issue corrected by a second line protocol ARVT.
2. Type **B2** arthroplasty demanders (HIV carriers with >500 CD4 lymphocytes/ML): they are not immune depressed no matter their viral load; they should be managed

according to the protocol of their physicians. Into our own practice, they will be operated with no ARVT and will be placed on treatment only if the CD4 count fall below 500/ML during the follow-up. After they have started with ARVT, they will continue it forever.

3. Type **A1** patients, (HIV carriers with 300 to 499 CD4 lymphocytes/ML), as they are moderately immune depressed, should be placed on ARVT shortly after the CD4 count results and they should undergo surgery without delay. Although it is not recommend by the official policy, we believe that they do need treatment before they undergo major surgery to give them a protection which may be needed anyway in the future.
4. Type **A2** arthroplasty demanders (HIV carriers with less than 300 CD4 lymphocytes/ML , but with no opportunistic disease), who are by definition asymptomatic, but severely immune depressed, are placed on ARVT and their surgery postponed for a few weeks till the CD4 lymphocytes/ML above 300 is obtained. Exceptionally in the emergency setting, the arthroplasty should not be postponed but the patient must be protected by a prolonged antibioprophylaxis which is actually an antibiotherapy.
5. Type **A3** arthroplasty demanders (HIV carriers with less than 300 CD4 lymphocytes/ML, but with an opportunistic disease) are first treated for their opportunistic disease, various prophylaxes, ARVT and the surgery postponed as above.

In all the cases, prophylactic antibiotic therapy should also be considered.

1.5 Prophylactic antibiotic therapy in HIV carriers undergoing arthroplasty

The aim of classical **prophylactic antibiotic therapy (PATB)** is to keep the surgical site under antibiotic protection during the short period of decrease immune response around the perioperative period. This period, which is less than 72 hours in a normal individual, may be prolonged in cases of immune depressed HIV carriers. Our previous study has shown that there is no significant difference in rates of post-operative infections between immune depressed and non immune depressed patients when we extend **PATB** to 10 ten days ,what we call **prolonged prophylactic antibiotherapy**, **(PPATB)** as one would expect. Although there were only few cases of arthroplasty in this serie. Finally, as far as arthroplasty demanders are concerned, two different regiments of prophylactic antibiotic therapy are to be considered, that is:

1. The classical regiment of PATB with intravenous cefuroxime (or any other second generation cephalosporin); 1.5g at the anesthesia induction, followed by 750 mg every 12h within not more than 72 hours. This is indicated for class B arthroplasty demanders.
2. The extended regiment of **PPATB** into which the above regiment is maintained during 10 days. This is indicated for all class A arthroplasty demanders.

1.6 Section A summary

Finally, combined protective measures of HIV carriers demanding atrhroplasty may be summarized as follow (table I), depending of their classification:

1. B2 patients should continue their previous ARVT and, get normal PABT during the arthroplasty which should not be delayed.
2. B1 may wait to start ARVT when the CD4 count will cross the 500 line; they should undergo normal PABT and their arthroplasty with no delay.
3. A1 patients should start an ARVT and get their arthroplasty not delayed but under protective PPABT.

4. A2 patients should start the ARVT and the arthroplasty delayed when they cross the 300 line in their CD4 count; the surgery should be protected by a PPABT.
5. A3 patient should first be treated for their opportunist disease and later on managed as A2.

With these measures, we think that the results of arthroplasty in HIV carriers should be comparable to HIV seronegative counterparts.

	Definition	ARVT?	PABT?	PPABT?
B1	HIV +, under ARVT	YES	YES	NO
B2	HIV+, CD4>500	NO	YES	NO
A1	HIV+, 300<CD4<500	YES	NO	YES
A2	HIV+, CD4<300 no opportunist infection-	YES	NO	YES
A3	HIV+,CD4<300 & some opportunist infection	YES	NO	YES

Table 1. Summarizing the use of ARVT, PABT, & PPABT in the five type HIV carriers demanders of arthroplasty

2. Section B: Arthroplasty in SCD carriers

- Definition & history of SCD
- Physiopathology of SCD & related secondary avascular necrosis
- Diagnosis and classification of SCD
- Work-up and management of SCD systemic acute complications
- Section B summary

2.1 Definition & history of SCD

SCD is a chronic hemolytic hemoglobinopathy that is genetically transmitted. During a crisis, red blood cells become sickle-shaped increasing blood viscosity, slowing blood flow, and consequently plugging small blood vessels creating widespread thromboembolic tissue infarction.

This genetic disease which is the most frequent genetic disease in black people, is also the most common cause of femoral head necrosis in them. In fact, SCD touches up to 0.74% of the births in sub-Saharan Africa, while this number is 10-20 times less in Europe and North America. In Nigeria, an estimated 45,000 to 90,000 babies are born each year with SCD. The African blacks are the main victims but the disease is also distributed in the south of Italy, Greece, Turkey, the Arabian Gulf, especially Saudi Arabia, and the Indian subcontinent. In the United States SCD occurs in approximately 1 out of every 500 African American births. People in the USA with sickle-cell disease number 90,000 of which 80,000 are black and 10,000 are Hispanic. The state with the highest sickle-cell population was New York with 8000, followed by Florida with 7500, and Texas with 6700 people with SCD. FLOUZAT-LACHANIETTE et al. report a series of SCD patients developing secondary avascular necrosis that originated from Africa, the United States of America, the Indian subcontinent, the Persian Gulf and from Mediterranean countries. Multifocal secondary vascular necrosis was found to occur in at least 64 percent of patients.

2.2 Physiopathology of SCD & related secondary avascular necrosis

Herrick first described the characteristic sickle-shaped erythrocytes in 1910 and Pauling and colleagues identified the abnormal hemoglobin (HbS) and coined the term "molecular disease" in 1949 . Hemoglobin A is normally found in the adult and is composed of four globular protein subunits the α and β globins. A fetal form or hemoglobin F is also found, normally, in small proportion in the adult. In SCD, an inappropriate substitution of valine for glutamine at the sixth position of the β globin chain produces hemoglobin S that polymerizes at low oxygen tensions. This causes the red cell to sickle which increases viscosity in the microvasculature and leads recurrent episodes of vaso-occlusion. These recurring episodes of widespread infarcts in patients homozygous for the sickle cell gene (HbSS) cause life-threatening conditions such as renal failure, acute chest syndrome, autosplenectomy, immune deficiency and infection all leading to an early death. As far as heavy surgery and especially arthroplasty is concerned in SCD patients; the key points and the difference with non SCD patients will therefore be focused into the prevention, the monitoring, and if needed, the management of the above cited acute systemic complications.

But SCD complications are not just acute; these repeated cycles of hypoxia and inflammation due to sickling cause chronic musculo-skeletal pain and finally secondary avascular necrosis of bone ends, especially, femoral and humeral heads, and less frequently, femoral condyles. This secondary avascular necrosis, at the end stages, causes severe chronic joints pain and functional impairment, for which very few solutions except of arthroplasties are currently available. In deed, secondary avascular necrosis is the leading indication of arthroplasty in SCD carriers. Secondary avascular necrosis doesn't occur only in homozygous HbSS patients; it is also common in heterozygous SCD clinically asymptomatic carriers with AS hemoglobin. In to the other hand, other types of abnormal hemoglobin such as HbC (Substitution of a lysine for glutamine at the 6th position of the β-globin chain) are also found in some patients with similar effects. Finally, secondary avasular necrosis due to SCD is therefore not exclusively observed in homozygous SS patients (HbSS); it should also be suspected in various other heterozygous forms; especially, HbAS and HbSC carriers.

2.3 Diagnosis and classification of SCD and related secondary avascular necrosis

To specifically diagnose SCD, cheap and widely available techniques such as hemoglobin electrophoresis or chromatography accurately determine the levels of HbA, HbF, HbS and HbC.

For secondary avascular necrosis and bony lesions due to SCD, standard X-ray, C-T Scan, Isotope Scan, and MRI are indicated in various stages for diagnosis and staging. However, the FICAT- ARLET classification is the must commonly used world wide. It is divided in four stages as below.

FICAT-ARLET classification of AVN (17):

Stage I: MRI changes

Stage II: Sclerotic and cystic changes
Stage III : Collapse
Stage IV: Osteoarthritis on both sides

2.4 Work-up and management of SCD systemic acute complications

2.4.1 General

Preoperatively the HbS level should be of less than 30% of the circulating hemoglobin before major surgery such as Arthroplasty; however, VICHINSKY et al., have shown in a randomized controlled trial that, exchange transfusion may not be necessary to avoid complications. In all cases, it is prudent to take the preoperative hemoglobin concentration to 100 g/L and to keep it at this level in the early postoperative phase; this objective may be obtained by ordinary transfusion of normal red blood cells as it may be confirmed by post transfusion electrophoresis or chromatography. This will also reduce the risk of peri-operative thromboembolic complications. The above target hemoglobin level may be rich by preoperative oral folic acid of few weeks, in those SCD patients with less than 30% of HbSS during the initial work-up; however, at least postoperatively, blood transfusion will be needed. It should be clear that, to the best of current literature, there is no place for autologous blood transfusion in SCD patients; these patients should always be managed with homologous bank blood products. In the other hand, Reduction of HbS concentrations may be obtained by the chronically use of hydroxycarbamide because this increases the concentration of fetal hemoglobin (HbF) which reduces hemolysis and prevents vaso-occlusion. It is also well known that that hypothermia, acidosis, hypoxemia and dehydration should be avoided pre and postoperatively.

2.4.2 Acute chest syndrome

Acute chest syndrome is a specificity of SCD and affects around 20% of the patients. A combination of thoracic pain, fever and infiltrates on thoracic x ray characterizes this syndrome. The etiology is multifactorial including pulmonary embolism, microvascular occlusion and infection Severity varies, but 13% of patients require mechanical ventilation and 3% may die. In a post operative period of any arthroplasty procedure in SCD patient, this syndrome should be seriously considered in establishing etiologies of acute chest pain. In fact, it prevention and management include respiratory support, antibiotics, blood transfusions and deep venous thromboses prophylaxis/therapy. At times corticosteroids may be indicated.

2.4.3 Infection

Susceptibility to infection is an issue in SCD. Many of these patients are immunocompromised because of autosplenectomy and osteonecrotic tissues tend to be colonized by Gram negative organisms. Several organisms have been identified as important causes of infection including S pneumoniae, H influenza, and non-typhi Salmonella species and appropriate antibiotic prophylaxis and immunization must be instituted in these patients. Therefore, a systematic preoperative investigation should be undertaken prior to any Arthroplasty procedure in a SCD patient to rule out occult infection; this should a least include urine culture, ENT consultation and dental examination and corrections. If there is a suspicion of infectious foyers a full antibiotic treatment should be undertaken with normalization of biological markers prior to the joint procedure. After arthroplasty, bone fragments from joint resection and reaming should also be send for bacterial analysis; if positive, a specific antibiotic testing should be undertaken. Subsequently, a long term antibiotic therapy should be undertaken in collaboration with the infectious diseases team, and till the normalization of biological infectious markers.

2.5 Section B summary

Finally, arthroplasties of the Hip, the knee, the shoulder or any other joint may commonly be demanded by SCD patients, mainly due the high frequency secondary avascular necrosis as a chronic complication of their genetic condition. The procedure may be performed with at least acceptable results, provided the following precautions are properly taken:

- Conventional biological work-up and especially, the hemoglobin types/ratios, and comprehensive research of occult infections.
- Preoperative treatment of any occult or evident infection
- Enhancement of the fetal hemoglobin ratio by chronic preoperative administration of hydroxycarbamide.
- Enhancement of the total Hemoglobin level to 100G/ml preoperatively, by chronic oral folic acid, and maintaining it so per and post operatively by homologous red blood cells
- Optimal oxygenation during the early post operative period
- Optimal fluid infusion during the early post-operative period
- Adequate warming during the early post-operative period
- Avoiding any acidosis state by blood gas control and correction during the early post operative period
- Culture of bone resection/reaming products and subsequent long standing and targeted post arthroplasty antibiotic therapy
- Avoiding autologous blood transfusion

3. Section C: Arthroplasty in HIV & SCD carriers

- Introduction
- HIV carriage in SCD patients
- Antiretroviral therapy in SCD patients
- Summary of section C

3.1 Introduction

After sexual intercourse, blood transfusion had been considered as one the possible pathway HIV contamination. Into the other hand, due acute episodes and chronic anemia, SCD patient had been to be more frequently transfused than normal hemoglobin carriers; it therefore appear rational to hypothesize that SCD patients present a higher risk of HIV infection. The literature on this matter is very scars; and the clinical experience does not confirm this theorical thinking.This may be due to at least a reduction on the transfusion rate in sickles and a better safety of blood banking systems. In the other hand, both HIV &

SCD have been incriminated as high risk factor or secondary aseptic necrosis, mainly of the hip. Provided the standard treatment of aseptic necrosis of the Hip is total hip arthroplasty, it become evident although rare and not reported currently, combination of both condition (SCD& HIV) in patients demanding arthroplasty, may in the next future, become a challenging issue. There is no evidence base on this precise issue; however, since the above both section A and B have been focused respectively on arthroplasty in HIV carriers in one hand, and in another one, Arthroplasty in SCD, knowing about HIV carriage in SCD patients may help to set up our thinking regarding arthroplasty in patients with both conditions.

3.2 HIV carriage in SCD patients

As it has been said above, the literature on HIV carriage in SCD patients is very scars, due to the paucity of patients themselves. In fact, the clinical experience in Central Africa where HIV carriage is higher than 10% in general population, shows that this rate is not significantly higher in homozygous HbSS patients. Further more, as the large majority of HbSS homozygous patients are also sexually active, it make sense to believe that the HIV infection in these specific set, is got through the same pathways with the general population. One of the rare related paper we could found regarding this matter is the one of Bagasra O et al; it suggests that, in patients with both SS and HIV-1 infection, the retroviral disease may be ameliorated by host factors of which absence of splenic function prior to HIV-1 contamination may be one. In another term, this author assume that HbSS carriage makes the body more resistant to HIV process as into his experimental case-control study of ten years follow-up, both the CD4 count and the Viral load were better in HbSS patients with HIV infection compare to HbAA counter part with the same viral infection. This may be explained by the fact that, as the spleen and lymph nodes are major sites of human immunodeficiency virus type 1 replication, mutation, and genetic variation in vivo; and as a major portion of this lymphatic tissue, such as the spleen, is removed or otherwise is unavailable for invasion by the HIV-1 virus, the course of this infection is altered. The clinical consequence is a prolonged symptom-free interval or even increased survival that we experience in daily clinical follow up of homozygous HbSS patients. Into the contrary, as it was reported by Sellier P et al, no significant difference in HIV infection progression is observed between heterozygous SCD carriers with HIV and their normal Hemoglobin counter part with the same virus.

Therefore, as far as HIV carriage is concerned in SCD patients, we should always distinguish homozygous patients in which, the expected course of retroviral process is slow than usual in one side, and in the other side, heterozygous patient in which it does not differ from that of the non SCD-non HIV patients. The same differentiation may be necessary regarding the management of antiretroviral therapy (ARVT) in this field.

3.3 Antiretroviral therapy in SCD patients

If we agree to distinguish Homozygous patients from their heterozygous counterpart regarding the HIV carriage, it makes sense to do the same in the matter of ARVT.

Regarding first homozygous HbSS patients, to the best of our knowledge, no evidence exist on the use of ARVT on them. However, on observing a short cohort of 5 patients in our practice at the Central Hospital of Yaoundé in Cameroun in to the last 5 years, our standard

protocol of ARVT has been well tolerated by homozygous HbSS patients, provided all the other measures of SCD control are well conducted.
In the contrary, we have more heterozygous SCD patients with HIV carriage under ARVT; as said above; the tolerance and efficiency of ARVT on them does not differ from the general non SCD population.

3.4 Summary of section C

There is very little evidences and experience on how to manage patients demanding arthroplasty, in cases where they are simultaneously HIV and SCD carriers. This little experience shows that those who are heterozygous should be managed as non SCD patients. In those who are homozygous, a simultaneous protocol of SCD care protocol as presented in section B, should be added.

4. References

[1] Bagasra O, Steiner RM, Ballas SK, Castro O, Dornadula G, Embury S, Jungkind D, Bobroski L, Kutlar A, Burchott S. Viral burden and disease progression in HIV-1-infected patients with sickle cell anemia. Am J Hematol. 1998 Nov;59(3):199-207

[2] J. Bahebeck a,*, D. Handy Eone b, B. Ngo Nonga c, T. Ndjie Kingue d, M. Sosso: Implant orthopaedic surgery in HIV asymptomatic carriers: Management and early outcome. Injury, Int. J. Care Injured 40 (2009) 1147–1150.

[3] Bahebeck J,. Atangana R, Techa A, Monny-Lobe M, Sosso M, Hoffmeyer P. Relative rates and features of musculoskeletal complications in adult sicklers. Acta Orthop Belg 2004, 70(2): 107-111.

[4] Brousseau DC, Panepinto JA, Nimmer M, Hoffmann RG. The number of people with sickle-cell disease in the United States: national and state estimates. Am J Hematol. 2010 Jan;85(1):77-8.

[5] Ficat RP, Arlet J. Functional investigation of bone under normal conditions. In: Ficat RP, Arlet J, Hungerford DS (eds): Ischemia and necroses of bone. Baltimore, MD, Williams and Wilkins. 1980. 29-52.

[6] Flouzat-Lachaniette CH, Roussignol X, Poignard A, Mukasa MM, Manicom O, Hernigou P. Multifocal joint osteonecrosis in sickle cell disease. Open Orthop J. 2009,15;3:32-5.

[7] Gutierrez F, Padilla S, Masia M, et al. Osteonecrosis in patients infected with HIV: clinical epidemiology and natural history in a large case series from Spain. J Acquir Immune Defic Syndr. 2006;42(3):286–292. [PubMed]

[8] Harrison WJ, Lewis CP, Lavy CB. Wound healing after implant surgery in HIV-positive patients. J Bone Joint Surg Br. 2002;84(6):802–806. [PubMed]

[9] Hernigou P, Zilber S, Filippini P, Mathieu G, Poignard A, Galacteros F. Total THA in adult osteonecrosis related to sickle cell disease. Clin Orthop Relat Res 2008, 466(2): 300-308.

[10] Hoekman P, van de Perre P, Nelissen J, Kwisanga B, Bogaerts J, Kanyangabo F. Increased frequency of infection after open reduction of fractures in patients who

are seropositive for human immunodeficiency virus. J Bone Joint Surg Am. 1991;73(5):675–679. [PubMed]

[11] Jeong Joon Yoo, Sae Hyung Chun,Young Sam Kwon, Kyung-Hoi Koo, Kang Sup Yoon, Hee Joong Kim. Operations about Hip in Human Immunodeficiency Virus-Positive Patients. Clin Orthop Surg. 2010 March; 2(1): 22–27.

[12] Keruly JC, Chaisson RE, Moore RD. Increasing inicidence of avascular necrosis of the hip in HIV-infected patients. J Acquir Immune Defic Syndr. 2001;28(1):101–102. [PubMed]

[13] Lehman CR, Ries MD, Paiement GD, Davidson AB. Infection after total joint arthroplasty in patients with human immunodeficiency virus or intravenous drug use. J Arthroplasty. 2001;16(3):330–335. [PubMed]

[14] Mahoney CR, Glesby MJ, DiCarlo EF, Peterson MG, Bostrom MP. Total hip arthroplasty in patients with human immunodeficiency virus infection: pathologic findings and surgical outcomes. Acta Orthop. 2005;76(2):198–203. [PubMed]

[15] Miller KD, Masur H, Jones EC, et al. High prevalence of osteonecrosis of the femoral head in HIV-infected adults. Ann Intern Med. 2002;137(1):17–25. [PubMed]

[16] Morse CG, Mican JM, Jones EC, et al. The incidence and natural history of osteonecrosis in HIV-infected adults. Clin Infect Dis. 2007;44(5):739–748. [PubMed]

[17] Paiement GD, Hymes RA, LaDouceur MS, Gosselin RA, Green HD. Postoperative infections in asymptomatic HIV-seropositive orthopedic trauma patients. J Trauma. 1994;37(4):545–550. [PubMed]

[18] Parvizi J, Sullivan TA, Pagnano MW, Trousdale RT, Bolander ME. Total joint arthroplasty in human immunodeficiency virus-positive patients: an alarming rate of early failure. J Arthroplasty. 2003;18(3):259–264. [PubMed]

[19] Platt OS, Brambilla DJ, Rosse WF et al. Mortality in sickle cell disease : life expectancy and risk factors for early death. N Engl J Med. 1994;330:1639-44

[20] Rees DC, Williams TN ,Gladwin MT. Sickle-cell disease. Lancet 2010, 376: 2018–31.

[21] Ries MD, Barcohana B, Davidson A, Jergesen HE, Paiement GD. Association between human immunodeficiency virus and osteonecrosis of the femoral head. J Arthroplasty. 2002;17(2):135–139. [PubMed]

[22] Scribner AN, Troia-Cancio PV, Cox BA, et al. Osteonecrosis in HIV: a case-control study. J Acquir Immune Defic Syndr. 2000;25(1):19–25. [PubMed]

[23] Sellier P, Masson E, Zini JM, Simoneau G, Magnier JD, Evans J, Bergmann JF : Disease progression in HIV-1 infected patients heterozygous for the sickle hemoglobin gene. AIDS. 2009 Nov 13;23(17):2362-4.

[24] Taylor LE, Stotts NA, Humphreys J, Treadwell MJ, Miaskowski C. A review of the literature on the multiple dimensions of chronic pain in adults with sickle cell disease. J Pain Symptom Manage. 2010;40(3):416-35.

[25] Vichinsky EP, Haberkern CM, Neumayr L, Earles AN, Black D, Koshy M, Pegelow C, Abboud M, Ohene-Frempong K, Iyer RV. A comparison of conservative and aggressive transfusion regimens in the perioperative management of sickle cell disease. The Preoperative Transfusion in Sickle Cell Disease Study Group. N Engl J Med. 1995;333:206–213.

[26] Vichinsky EP, Neumayr LD, Earles AN, Williams R, Lennette ET, Dean D, Nickerson B, Orringer E, McKie V, Bellevue R, Daeschner C, Manci EA. Causes and outcomes of the acute chest syndrome in sickle cell disease. National Acute Chest Syndrome Study Group. N Engl J Med, 2000;342:1855-1865.

Part 5

Arthroplasty of Spine and Upper Extremity

23

Cervical Disc Arthroplasty

Bruce V. Darden
OrthoCarolina Spine Center, Charlotte
USA

1. Introduction

For more than 50 years, anterior cervical discectomy and fusion (ACDF) has been the workhorse procedure for cervical degenerative pathology. (Bailey & Badgely, 1960; Cloward, 1961; Robinson & Smith, 1955) The procedure has yielded successful results clinically in multiple large series. (Bohlman et al, 1993; Gore & Sepic, 1984) Advances in allograft and cage techniques as well as the use of anterior plating systems have diminished complications in ACDF. However, concerns about adjacent segment degeneration (ASD) have tempered some enthusiasm for the procedure. Gore et al (Gore & Sepic, 1998) reviewed a series of 50 ACDF patients followed long term. Almost universally, the patients developed ASD. One-third of the cohort developed recurrent pain with half of the symptomatic group requiring additional surgery. Hilibrand et al (Hilibrand et al, 1999) evaluated a group of 374 patients undergoing ACDF. They showed a 2.9% per year risk of development of symptomatic ASD, with two thirds of the symptomatic patients requiring additional surgery. Goffin et al (Goffin et al, 1995) prospectively followed a series of ACDF patients who underwent the procedure for either a degenerative or traumatic condition. Follow up was for five to nine years. Sixty percent of the patients developed ASD, equally distributed between the older degenerative population and the younger traumatic population, providing evidence that fusion may accelerate degenerative changes. Goffin et al (Goffin et al, 2004) reviewed a larger series of ACDF patients followed for an average of 8.3 years. In this group, 92% of the patients developed ASD, though they had a much lower rate of additional surgical procedures, 6.1% for the entire length of follow-up, distinctly lower than Hilibrand et al. Numerous cadaveric biomechanical studies (Eck et al, 2002; Pospiech et al, 1999) evaluating adjacent level intradiscal pressures and range of motion in simulated fusion models have shown that both increase after fusion. These altered biomechanics may thus accelerate ASD.

Against this background, centers began experimenting with cervical disc arthroplasty in the 1980s. Cummins and collaborators at the Frenchay Hospital, Bristol, England developed a metal-on-metal ball and socket arthroplasty and implanted it on a small series of patients in the 1990s. (Cummins et al, 1998) The arthroplasty underwent a number of design changes and is now known as Prestige. Bryan, in the US, developed a one piece metal-on-polymer device called the Bryan Cervical Disc Replacement, initially evaluated clinically in Europe. (Goffin et al, 2002) ProDisc-C arthroplasty is a metal-on-polyethylene implant adopted from the ProDisc-L lumbar disc arthroplasty developed by Thierry Marnay. (Delamarter & Pradhan, 2004) Since these first three devices have been developed, the number of cervical disc arthroplasties has proliferated. The literature in this nascent field is limited, but growing each year.

2. Types of cervical disc arthroplasty

It is beyond the scope of this chapter to catalogue all of the cervical disc arthroplasties available; the devices with the most clinical experience will be discussed.

2.1 Prestige

The technology from the early designs of Cummins et al was acquired by Medtronic Sofamor Danek (Memphis, Tennessee) and rebadged Prestige. With Prestige I, the initial ball and socket design which was entirely fabricated from stainless steel, was converted to a ball and trough design, allowing limited translation. The anterior flanges were diminished in size and a locking screw added to prevent bone screw backout. Prestige II was further modified by again reducing the anterior flange and modifying the endplates to allow bone ingrowth. Prestige ST was the design evaluated in the United States as part of the Food and Drug Administration (FDA) investigational device evaluational (IDE) study. This arthroplasty incorporates the features of Prestige II with further shortened anterior flanges. The final design is Prestige LP, a major change from its predecessors. Instead of stainless steel, the Prestige LP is made from a titanium ceramic composite, preserving the ball and trough bearing design. It has a titanium plasma spray on the endplates for bone ingrowth, as well as two pairs of rails allowing immediate fixation. The flange and locking bone screws have been removed. The Prestige LP, being made of titanium, has a better compatibility than stainless steel in MRI imaging. (Figure 1)

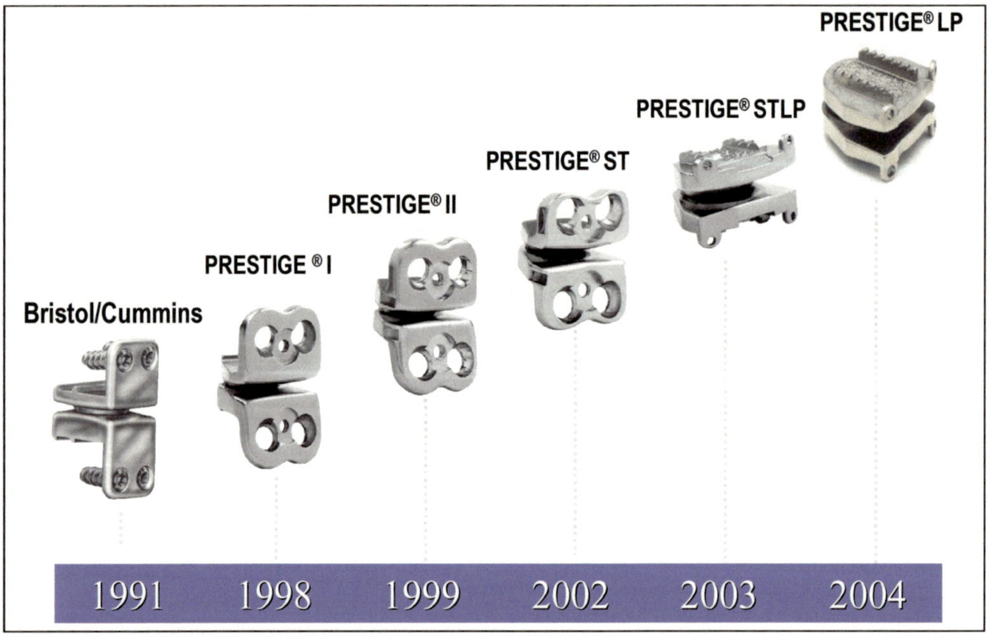

(Courtesy of Medtronic Sofamor Danek, Memphis, Tennessee)

Fig. 1. Prestige Cervical Disc evolution

2.2 Bryan Cervical Disc Prosthesis

Bryan Cervical Disc Prosthesis (Medtronic Sofamor Danek, Memphis, Tennessee) consists of a nucleus made of polyurethane between two titanium alloy endplates in a clamshell configuration. (Figure 2) There are two bearing surfaces in the arthroplasty at the interfaces between the nucleus and the endplates. A polyurethane sheath attaches to the endplates and surrounds the nucleus. Sterile saline is injected between the outer sheath and the nucleus as lubricant. The endplates have a titanium porous coating for bone ingrowth and a small flange anteriorly to prevent posterior migration.

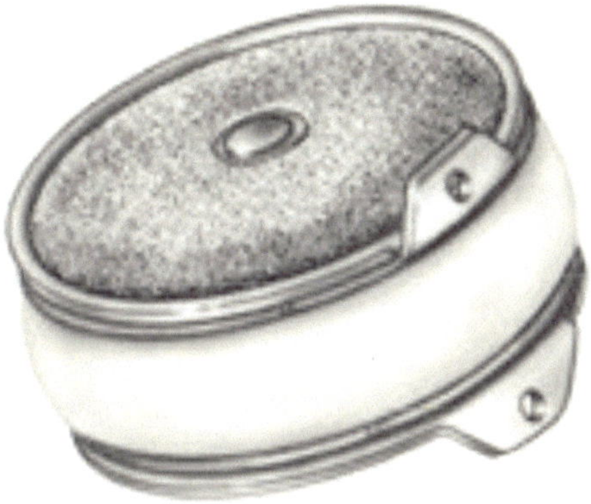

(Courtesy of Medtronic Sofamor Danek, Memphis, Tennessee)

Fig. 2. Bryan Cervical Disc Prosthesis

2.3 ProDisc-C

ProDisc-C Cervical Disc Prosthesis (Synthes, West Chester, Pennsylvania) has a ball and socket design, with endplates made of a cobalt-chrome alloy. The endplates have keels for immediate fixation and titanium plasma spray backing for bone ingrowth. The bearing surface has an articulating dome of ultra high molecular weight polyethylene (UHMWPE) attached to the inferior endplate and a concave polished socket integral to the superior endplate. (Figure 3)

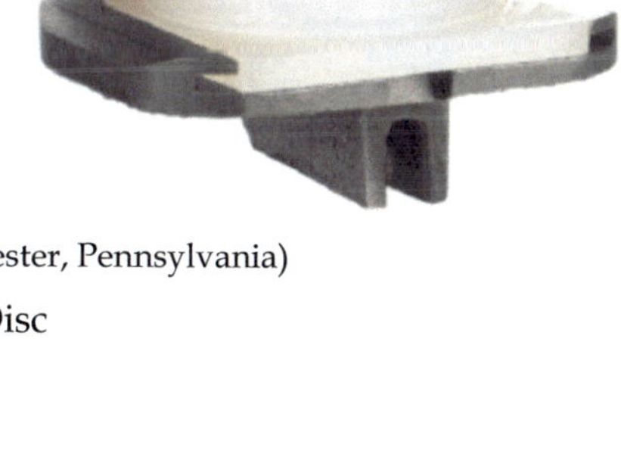

(Courtesy of Synthes, West Chester, Pennsylvania)

Fig. 3. ProDisc-C Cervical Disc

2.4 Porous-Coated Motion (PCM) Cervical Arthroplasty

The Porous-Coated Motion (PCM) Cervical Arthroplasty (Cervitech, Rockaway, New Jersey) consists of two cobalt-chrome-molybdenum (CoCrMo) endplates that have a titanium calcium phosphate porous coated backing for bone ingrowth. The device is inserted by a "press-fit" method, but the endplates have transverse serrated rows of teeth that resist migration. The bearing surface is an ultra high molecular weight polyethylene (UHMWPE) convex insert of large radius of curvature attached to the inferior endplate which articulates with the polished CoCrMo concave surface of the superior endplate. (Figure 4)

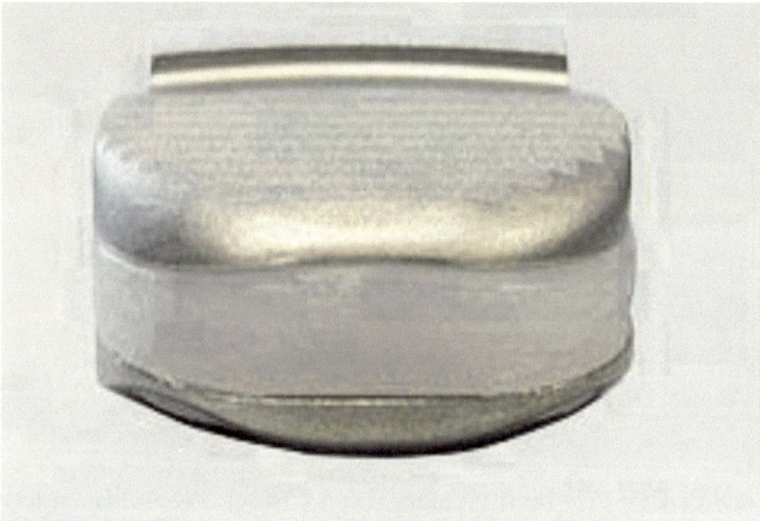

(Courtesy of Paul McAfee, MD)

Fig. 4. Porous Coated Motion (PCM) Cervical Arthroplasty

3. Biomechanics

Cervical disc arthroplasty attempts to replicate the normal kinematics of the subaxial cervical spine, defined as the segments from C3 to C7. The subaxial cervical spine contributes 60% of the flexion/extension motion of the cervical spine with each segment accounting for between 14 to 22 degrees of motion (Dvorak et al, 1993; Dvorak et al, 1991; Penning, 1978). The flexion/extension arc, together with translational movements due to slight relative facet motion, results in coupled motions. Coupled motions also occur with lateral bending and thus axial rotation. These coupled motions result in differences in the center of rotation of each motion segment. Since the center of rotation is not fixed, there are instantaneous centers of rotation. (ICR) Penning (Penning, 1978) established normalized ICR for each segment, which were further defined by Amevo et al (Amevo et al, 1991) The normalized ICR for each segment are shown in figure 5 (Bogduk & Mercer, 2000) and are grossly posterior and inferior to the center of the caudal vertebral endplate. Arthroplasty designs with a ball and socket articulation have a predetermined center of rotation (ie: ProDisc-C). These more constrained designs have to be implanted more precisely to match the physiologic center of rotation to avoid increased strain on the facet joints. (Darden & Raposo, pending)

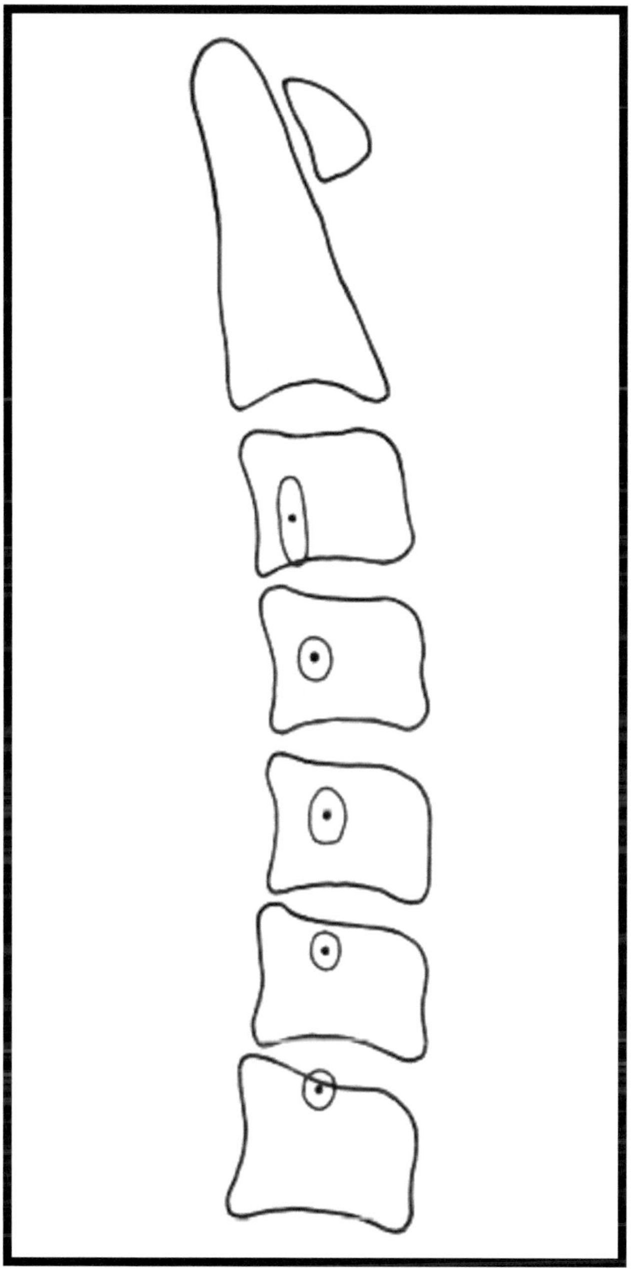

(Reprinted from: Bogduk N, Mercer S. Clin Biomechanics, 2000)

Fig. 5. Mean instantaneous axes of rotation for each motion segment of the cervical spine depicted with a dot. Two standard deviation range of distribution is located within the enclosed circles shown.

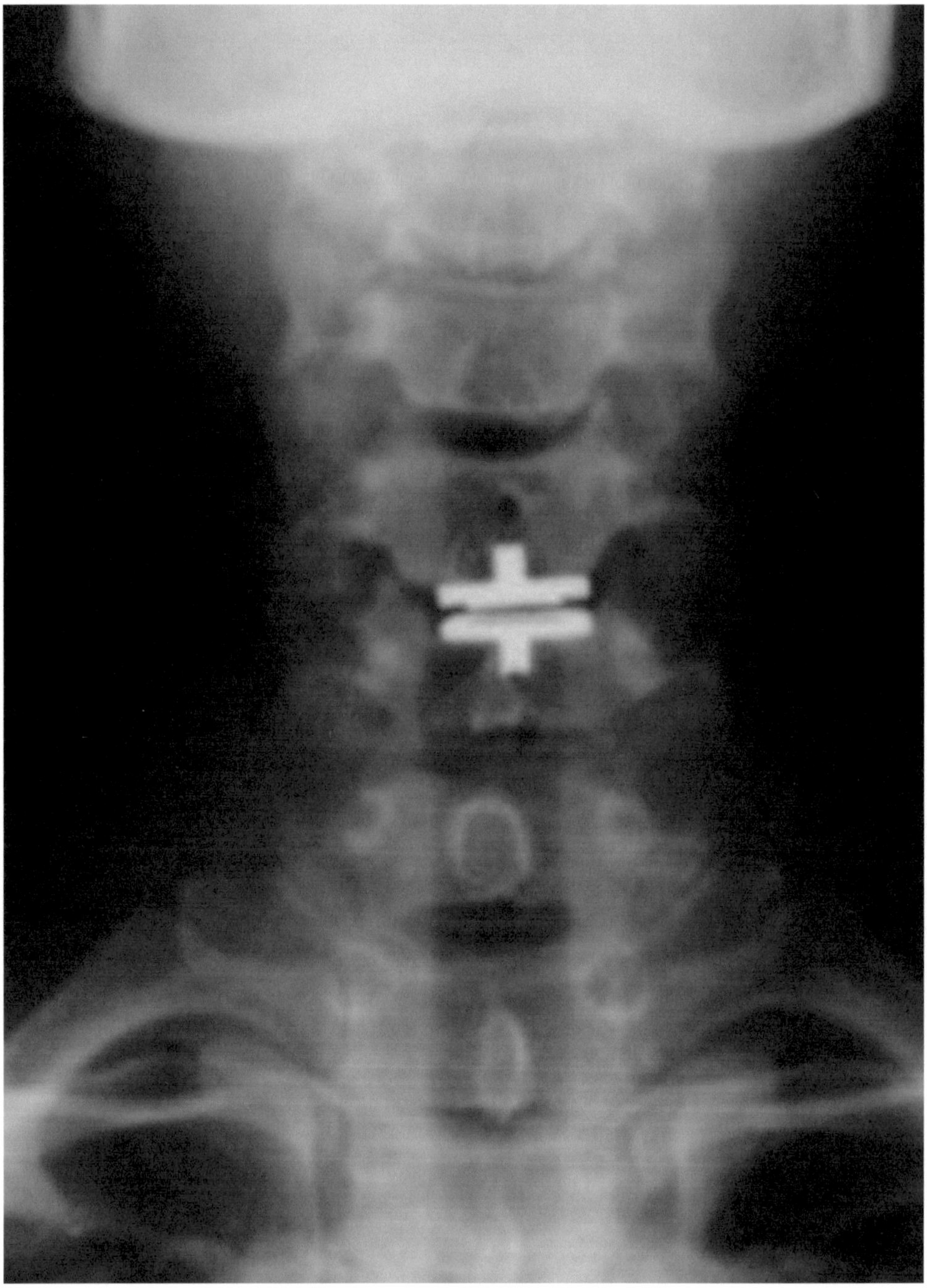

Fig. 6-A.

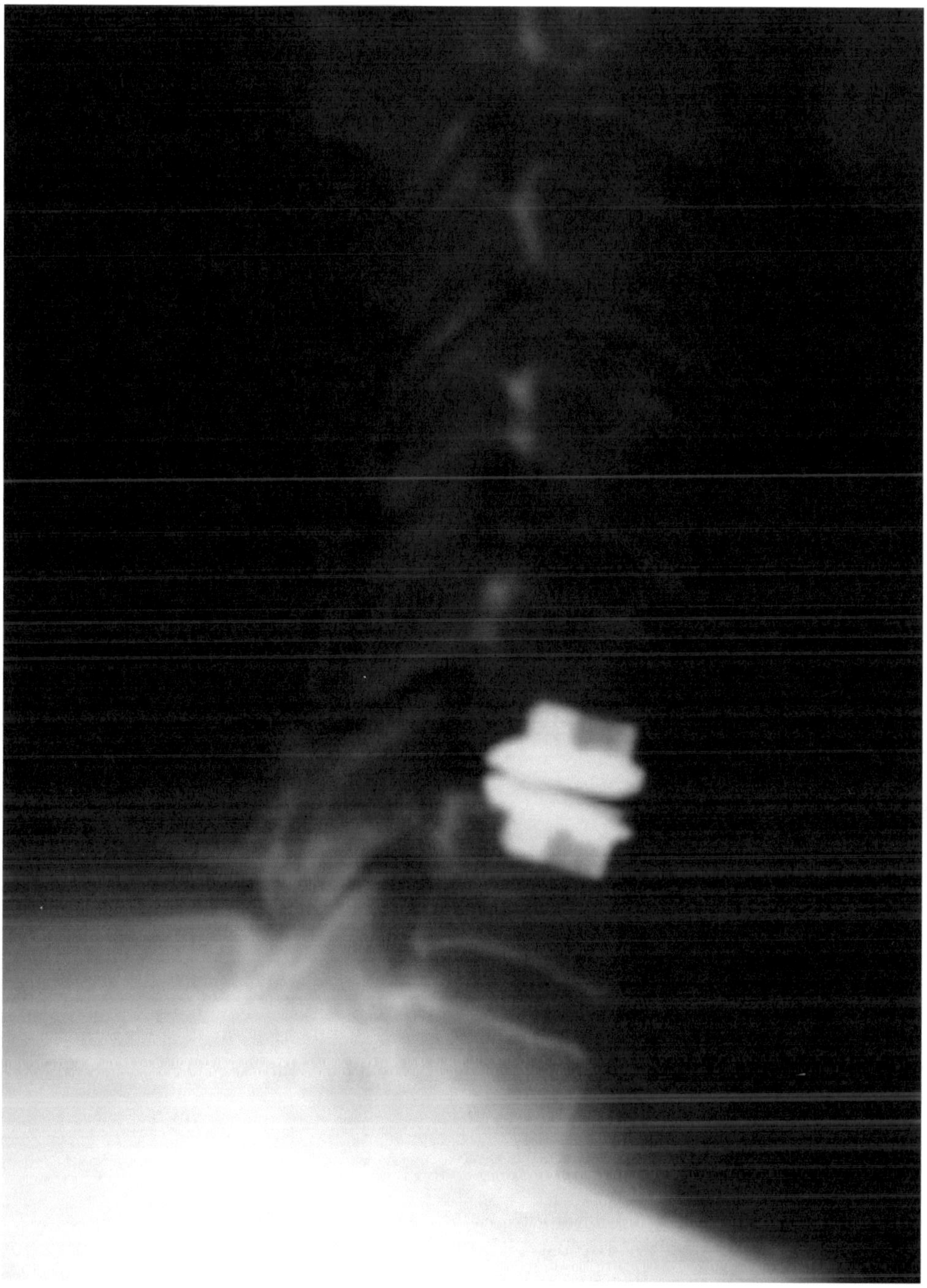

Fig. 6-B.

Fig. 6-A, B. AP and lateral radiographs of ProDisc-C

In the cervical spine, the dominant plane of motion is sagittal. Constraint is therefore defined as limitation of anterior-posterior translational motion. (Huang et al, 2003) An unconstrained arthroplasty would allow unrestricted motion while a fully constrained arthroplasty would allow only flexion/extension without any anterior-posterior translation. However, compared to large joints, the differences in constraint in cervical disc arthroplasties are limited. (Darden & Raposo, pending) (Table 1)

	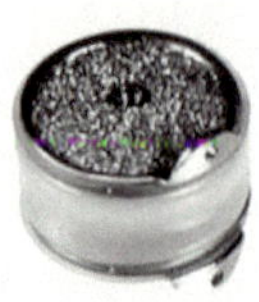	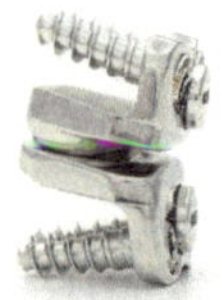	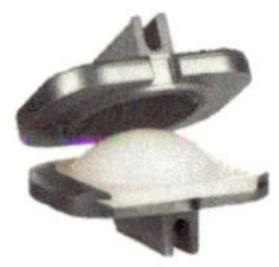	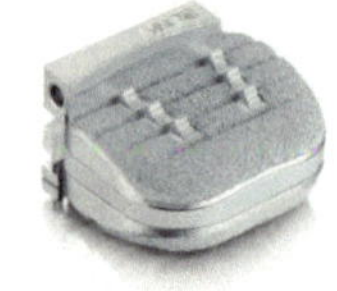
Implant	**Bryan®**	**Prestige ST®**	**Prodisc-C®**	**PCM-V®**
Manufacturer	Medtronic Sofamor Danek,	Medtronic Sofamor Danek	Synthes	Cervitech
Bearing surface materials	Metal-on-poly; Titanium end plates, polycarbonate urethane nucleus	Metal-on-metal; Stainless steel	Metal-on-poly; Chrome cobalt, UHMWPE	Metal-on-poly; chrome cobalt, UHMWPE
Bearing surface geometry	Biconvex nucleus articulating with upper and lower endplates	Ball and trough design	Ball and socket design	Ball and socket design (shallow sphere)
Primary (immediate) fixation	Milling technique creates concave endplate surfaces to fit convex endplates of the device.	Anterior flanges with screws	Keels	LP: Press-fit, ridges
Degree of constraint	Unconstrained	Semi-constrained	Semi-constrained	Semi-constrained
Relative constraint	Least	Less	Most	Less
Implant center or rotation	Variable; lies at center of the mobile nucleus	Variable; superior to disc space	Fixed; inferior to disc space	Variable; inferior to disc space

Table 1. Summary of implant features and design characteristics.

A number of arthroplasties have been evaluated biomechanically versus simulated fusion in human cadaveric models. These routinely show increased adjacent segment motion and increased adjacent segment disc pressures in the fusion simulations compared to cervical disc arthroplasty. (DiAngelo et al, 2003; Dmitriev et al, 2005)

4. Clinical results

As a result of the US FDA IDE studies, there have been a number of thorough clinical evaluations of cervical disc arthroplasty. These trials have been designed as non-inferiority studies, comparing cervical disc arthroplasty to ACDF. The Prestige ST results at two years follow-up were reported by Mummaneni et al. (Mummaneni et al, 2007) The study, similar to all of the FDA IDE studies, was a prospective, randomized, multicenter trial comparing Prestige ST cervical disc arthroplasty to ACDF for one level pathology. Five hundred forty-one patients were enrolled with 1:1 randomization; over 75% of patients were available for two-year follow-up. There were no statistically significant differences in the revision surgeries at the index level (3.4% ACDF, 1.9% Prestige ST). However, the rate of surgery at adjacent levels was statistically higher for ACDF (3.4% versus 1.1%, p=0.0492). Neurological success, defined as maintenance or improvement in the neurological exam, was better with Prestige ST (92.8%) than ACDF (84.3%). Clinically, the patients were evaluated by Short-form 36 (SF-36), Visual Analogue Scale (VAS) and the Neck Disability Index (NDI). While both groups improved significantly from the preoperative state, there was no statistically significant difference between the groups at final follow-up. Overall success was defined as an NDI improvement ≥ 15 points, maintenance of the neurological status and the absence of implant-related adverse events. The arthroplasty group showed overall success in 79.3% of the patients compared to 67.8% in the ACDF group. As a sidebar, the Prestige ST patients were able to return to work on average at 45 days postoperatively, compared to 61 days for the ACDF patients.

A small prospective study compared results for Prestige LP and ACDF at a minimum of two years follow-up. Single and multilevel procedures were evaluated by VAS, NDI, SF-36 and Japanese Orthopedic Association scores. Clinically, while both groups improved significantly, there was no statistical difference between them. Motion was preserved in the Prestige LP group at a mean of 13.9° on flexion/extension lateral radiographs of two years. (Peng et al, 2011)

For the Bryan Cervical Disc Replacement, Goffin et al reported on the European experience, a multicenter, prospective, nonrandomized study, including both single-level and multi-level implants. Ninety-eight patients were evaluated at the 4 to 6 year follow-up point, 89 single-level patients and 9 two-level patients. The patients maintained improvement clinically at all evaluation periods. Approximately 90% of the patients had good or excellent results by Odum's criteria. The success rate for the arthroplasties, estimated by Kaplan-Meier analysis was 94% at 7 years postoperatively. One patient had removal of the arthroplasty for progressive spinal cord compression due to posterior osteophytes. (Goffin et al, 2010)

The Bryan FDA IDE study results at two years were published by Heller et al (Heller et al, 2009). Four hundred sixty-three patients enrolled, with 242 having a single-level Bryan Cervical Disc Replacement and 221 having single-level ACDF. The Bryan patients had statistically significantly improved NDI and VAS scores compared to the ACDF group at two years follow-up. Other clinical parameters improved equally between the two groups. Overall success at final follow-up was better in the Bryan patients (82.6%) versus the ACDF controls (72.7%), (p=0.010). As with the Prestige IDE patients, the Bryan patients returned to work sooner than did the ACDF patients.

Riew et al (Riew et al, 2008) evaluated a subset of patients enrolled in the Prestige ST or Bryan IDE studies that were determined to have a cervical myelopathy, defined as being hyperreflexic, having clonus or having a Nurick grade ≥ 1. In most of the patients, the cause of the myelopathy was a disc herniation. Because of enrollment criteria, multilevel cervical disease or patients with ossification of the posterior longitudinal ligament (OPLL) were excluded. A total of 107 patients in both studies were deemed myelopathic and underwent cervical disc arthroplasty. Compared to the ACDF patients, arthroplasty patients with myelopathy showed similar clinical improvement. There were no arthroplasty patients who deteriorated neurologically, suggesting that myelopathy confined to a single disc level without OPLL or retrovertebral osteophytes can be treated successfully with cervical disc arthroplasty.

Murrey et al (Murrey et al, 2009) published the two year ProDisc-C IDE study. The study was structured similarly to the Prestige ST and Bryan studies, with 209 patients enrolled, 103 who underwent ProDisc-C arthroplasty and 106 who had an ACDF. Both groups showed improvement by all clinical after parameters; NDI, SF-36, VAS arm and neck pain scores and neurological success. A significant difference was in the rate of re-operation: 8.5% in the ACDF group versus 1.8% in the ProDisc-C group (p= 0.033).

Delamarter et al further evaluated the ProDisc-C IDE patients as well as 136 patients who received ProDisc-C in the continued access phase of the study, with a minimum of four years follow-up. (Delamarter et al, 2010) Demographic data remained similar between the arthroplasty and ACDF groups. All clinical parameters improved equally in both groups at all follow-up periods (p<.0001). A significant difference in the study was the rate of secondary surgical procedures. At the four year follow-up point, 12 (11.3%) of the ACDF patients had additional surgery, while only three (2.9%) of the ProDisc-C patients required further procedures (p=.0292). The ACDF patients primarily required additional surgery for pseudoarthrosis at the index level; however, six (5.6%) ACDF patients had surgery at an adjacent level. Three ProDisc-C patients were converted to fusion for axial pain. No ProDisc-C patients had to have surgery at adjacent levels. In the continued access arm of the study, one ProDisc-C patient required additional surgery to reposition the implant and two were converted to fusion for axial neck pain.

Pimenta et al (Pimenta et al, 2007) prospectively evaluated patients undergoing the PCM cervical disc replacement. Seventy-one single-level and 69 multi-level arthroplasties were performed. While both groups improved, the multi-level patients showed improved scores compared to the single-level patients. The mean NDI improvement was better in the multi-level PCM group (p=0.021). While the overall IDE results have yet to be reported, Philips et al (Phillips et al, 2009) showed in a small set of the IDE patients that arthroplasty was viable at levels adjacent to a prior fusion.

5. Radiographic results

Heterotopic ossification (HO) has initially been reported in the Bryan Cervical Disc Replacement (Bartels & Donk, 2005; Leung et al 2005; Solas et al, 2005) but as the literature expands, no disc arthroplasty has proven immune to this problem. (Figure 7) McAfee et al characterized the severity of HO with a simple scale, modified from lumbar disc arthroplasty findings. The scale ranged from grade 0 (no HO) to grade IV -(complete ankylosis). (McAfee et al, 2003) (Table 2) Delamarter et al described three patients that developed grade IV HO in the ProDisc-C IDE study by 24 months, with two additional patients developing grade IV HO by 48 months. Non-steroidal anti-inflammatory drugs (NSAIDs) were not part of the study protocol. Interestingly in the continued access arm of the study, in which NSAIDs were more commonly used, no patients developed ankylosis at the index level. (Delamarter et al, 2010) Mehren et al (Mehren et al, 2006) evaluated the rate of HO at two centers performing cervical disc arthroplasty. Approximately one third of patients postoperatively showed no sign of HO, while almost 20% of patients had HO that lead to restrictions in motion. Nine percent of the patients had grade IV HO, with most of the patients having had multilevel procedures. There was a difference in the overall rate of grade IV HO between the two centers, 12.8% versus 5.2%. The center with the lower HO

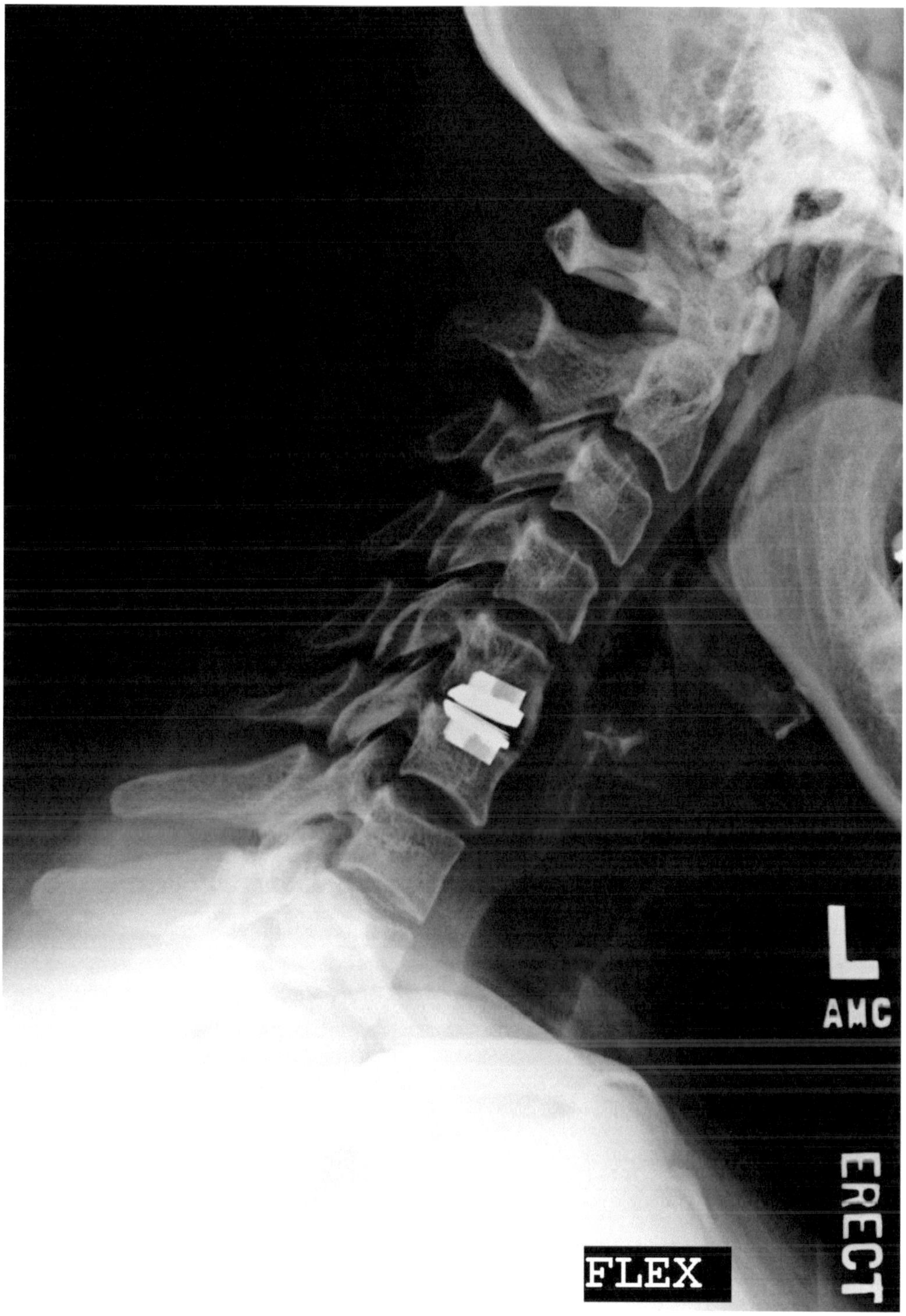

Fig. 7. Lateral flexion radiography- implanted ProDisc-C with heterotopic ossification, preserved motion.

rate routinely prescribed NSAID use postoperatively. Yi et al (Yi et al, 2010) studied the rate of HO according to the arthroplasty type. They found the following HO rates: Bryan 21.0%, Mobi-C (LDR Medical, Troyes, France) 52.5% and ProDisc-C 71.4%. The only two patients that developed grade IV HO were in the Bryan group. All patients routinely received postoperative NSAIDs.

Grade 0	No HO present
Grade I	HO is detectable in front of the vertebral body but not in the anatomic interdiscal space
Grade II	HO is growing in to the disc space. Possible affection of the function of the prosthesis
Grade III	Bridging ossifications which still allow movement of the prosthesis
Grade IV	Complete fusion of the treated segment without movement in flexion/extension

HO indicates Heterotopic ossification

(modified from McAfee et al, 2003)

Table 2. Characterisation of the Different Grades of Heterotopic Ossification (HO) in Total Cervical Disc Replacement

In all the clinical studies evaluating cervical disc arthroplasty and HO, there has been no correlation between the development of HO and the clinical results. Barbargallo et al (Barbargallo et al, 2010) specifically looked at this aspect of cervical disc arthroplasty. They found an overall rate of HO development of 42% and no difference in the functional scores in patients with or without HO. Segmental range of motion of ≥ 3° was preserved in 93.8% of patients with HO.

6. Complications

All of the large clinical series published on cervical disc arthroplasty have not reported any severe neurological injuries, such as quadriplegia. The rate of revision surgery at the index level has been acceptably low. None of the cervical disc arthroplasty series have had implants removed for infection.

Concerns of wear debris and local and remote inflammatory changes in cervical disc arthroplasty have been expressed. *In vitro* wear tests have been submitted to the United States FDA as part of the clinical approval process. Generally, wear debris volume has been in the range of 10% of that produced by large joint arthroplasties. Anderson et al (Anderson et al 2004) published *in vitro* wear testing on the Bryan Cervical Disc Replacement using a custom cervical spine simulator on six disc assemblies. At 10 million cycles, the mean mass loss was 1.76% and a mean height loss of 0.75%. At 40 million cycles there was an 18% mass loss. Wear particles were elliptical in shape and larger than typical particles in large joint arthroplasties. Anderson studied local and remote wear debris and the subsequent inflammatory response using an *in vivo* caprine model with implanted Bryan arthroplasties. Sacrificed animals at up to twelve months showed an increase in extracellular wear debris. No apparent inflammatory response was seen locally or distally in these animals.

Clinically, there have been scattered case reports of osteolysis after cervical disc arthroplasty implantation. Tumialan and Gluf reported on a 30-year-old man who underwent a ProDisc-C arthroplasty at C5-6. (Tumialan & Gluf, 2011) He had an uneventful postoperative course until he developed worsening neck pain at nine months. Repeat imaging studies by 15 months showed a progressive osteolysis process in the vicinity of the superior endplate and keel. Work-up for infection was negative. The patient underwent explantation of the arthroplasty and conversion to a fusion. The implant was studied after removal and no defects or unusual wear was noted. The authors hypothesized that the most likely cause of the osteolysis was an immune mediated process. Longer study periods are needed to determine the significance of wear changes and the rate of osteolysis of cervical disc arthroplasty.

7. Conclusions

Cervical disc arthroplasty has been one of the most closely scrutinized surgical procedures in the last decade. Short-term prospective clinical studies show cervical disc arthroplasty to be at least the equivalent of ACDF for degenerative pathology. There is some evidence that cervical disc arthroplasty may play a role in diminishing adjacent segment disease. However, the long-term efficacy and safety of cervical disc arthroplasty await further clinical studies.

8. References

[1] Amevo B, Worth D, Bogduk N. (1991) Instantaneous axis of rotation of the typical cervical motion segments: a study in normal volunteers. *Clinical Biomechanics* Vol. 6: pp. 111-117

[2] Anderson PA, Sasso RC, Rouleau JP et al. (2004) The Bryan Cervical Disc: wear properties and early clinical results. *Spine Journal,* 4(6): 5303-5309

[3] Bailey R, Badgely C. (1960) Stabilization of the cervical spine by anterior fusion. *Journal of Bone and Joint Surgery Am,* 42(4): 565-594

[4] Barbargallo GM, Corbino LA, Olindo G, et al. (2010) Heterotopic ossification in cervical disc arthroplasty: Is it clinically relevant? *Evidence-Based Spine Care Journal,* 1(1):15-20

[5] Bartels RH, Donk R. (2005) Fusion around cervical disc prosthesis: Case report. *Neurosurgery,* 57:E194

[6] Bogduk N, Mercer S. (2000) *Clinical Biomechanics,* 15(9): 633-648

[7] Bohlman HH, Emery SE, Goodfellow DB, et al. (1993) Robinson anterior cervical discectomy and arthrodesis for cervical radiculopathy: long term follow-up of one hundred and twenty-two patients. *Journal of Bone and Joint Surgery Am,* 75: 1298-1307

[8] Cloward RD. (1961) Treatment of acute fractures and fracture dislocations of cervical spine by vertebral body fusion: a report of cases. *Journal of Neurosurgery*, 118: 205-209

[9] Cummins BH, Robertson JT, Gill SS. (1998) Surgical experience with an implanted artificial cervical joint. *Journal of Neurosurgery*, 88: 943-948

[10] Delamarter RB, Pradhan BB. (2004) Indications for cervical spine prostheses, early experiences with ProDisc-C in the USA. *Spine Art*, 1:7-9

[11] Delamarter RB, Murrey D, Janssen MI et al. (2010) Results of 24 months from the prospective, randomized, multicenter investigation device exemption trial of ProDisc-C versus anterior cervical discectomy and fusion with 4-year follow-up and continued access patients. *SAS Journal*, 4: 122-128

[12] DiAngelo DJ, Robertson JT, Metcalf NH et al. (2003) Biomechanical testing of an artificial cervical joint and an anterior cervical plate. *Journal of Spinal Disorders and Tech*, 16(4): 314-323

[13] Dmitriev AE, Cunningham BW, Hu N et al. (2005) Adjacent level intradiscal pressure and segmental kinematics following a cervical total disc arthroplasty: An in vitro human cadaveric model. *Spine*, 30: 1165-1172

[14] Dvorak J, Panjabi MM, Grob D et al. (1993) Clinical validation of functional flexion/extension radiographs of the cervical spine. *Spine*, 18:120-127

[15] Dvorak J, Panjabi MM, Novotny JE et al. (1991) In vivo flexion/extension of the normal cervical spine. *Journal of Orthop Res*, 9: 828-834

[16] Eck JC, Humphreys SC, Lim T, et al. (2002) Biomechanical study on the effect of cervical spine fusion on adjacent level intradiscal pressure and segment motion. *Spine*, 27: 2431-2434

[17] Goffin J, VanLoo J, VanCalenbergh F et al. (2010) A clinical analysis of 4-6 year follow-up results after cervical disc replacement using the Bryan Cervical Disc Prosthesis. J *Neurosurgery Spine*, 12 (3) 261-9

[18] Goffin J, Geusens E, Vantomme N, et al. (2004) Long-term follow-up after interbody fusion of the cervical spine. *Journal of Spinal Disorders and Techniques*, 17(2) 79-85

[19] Goffin J, Casey A, Kehr P, et al. (2002) Preliminary clinical experience with the Bryan cervical disc prosthesis. *Neurosurgery*, 51(3) 840-845.

[20] Goffin J, Van Loon J, VanCalenbergh F, et al. (1995) Long-term results after anterior cervical fusion and osteosynthetic stabilization for fractures and/or dislocation of the cervical spine. *Journal of Spinal Disorders and Techniques*, 8: 500-508

[21] Gore DR, Sepic SB. (1998) Anterior discectomy and fusion for painful cervical disc disease: a report of 50 patients with an average follow-up of 21 years. *Spine*, 23: 2047-2051

[22] Gore DR, Sepic SB. (1984) Anterior cervical fusion for degenerated or protruded discs: A review of one hundred forty-six patients. *Spine*, 9:667-71

[23] Heller JG, Sasso RC, Papadopoulos SM, Anderson PA, Fessler RG et al. (2009) Comparison of Bryan Cervical Disc Arthroplasty with anterior cervical decompression and fusion. *Spine*, 34(2) 101- 107

[24] Huang RC, Girardi FP, Cammisa FP et al. (2003) The implications of constraint in lumbar total disc replacement. *Journal of Spinal Disorders and Techniques,* 16(4): 412-417

[25] Hilibrand AS, Carlson GD, Palumbo MA, et al. (1999) Radiculopathy and myelopathy at segments adjacent to the site of a previous anterior cervical arthrodesis. *Journal of Bone and Joint Surgery Am,* 81: 519-528

[26] Mehren, Suchomel et al. (2006) Heterotopic ossification in total cervical artificial disc replacement. *Spine,* 31(24) 2802-2806

[27] Leung C, Casey et al. (2005) Clinical significance of Heterotopic ossification in cervical disc replacement: a prospective multi-center clinical trial. *Neurosurgery,* 57:759-631 discussion 763

[28] McAfee, Cunningham et al. (2003) Classification of Heterotopic ossification (HO) in artificial disk replacement. *Journal of Spinal Disorders and Techniques* 16: 384-9

[29] Mummaneni et al. Clinical and radiographic analysis of cervical disc arthroplasty compared with allograft fusion: A randomized controlled trial. *Journal of Neurosurgery –Spine,* Vol. 6, pp 198-209

[30] Murrey et al. (2009) Results of the prospective, randomized, controlled Food and Drug Administration Investigational Device Exemption Study of the ProDisc-C total disc replacement versus anterior discectomy and fusion for the treatment of one level symptomatic cervical disc disease. *Spine Journal,* Vol. 9, pp 275-286

[31] Peng CW, Yue WM, Abdul B et al. (2011) Intermediate results of the Prestige LP cervical disc replacement: clinical and radiological analysis with minimum two-year follow-up. *Spine,* 36 (2): E 105-111

[32] Pospiech J, Stolke D, Wilke HJ et al. (1999) Intradiscal pressure recordings in the cervical spine. *Neurosurgery,* 44: 379-384.

[33] Phillips FM, Allen TR, Regen JJ, et al. (2009) Cervical disc replacement in patients with and without previous adjacent level fusion surgery: A prospective study. *Spine,* 34 (6) 556-565

[34] Pimenta L, McAfee PC, Cappuccino A, et al. (2007) Superiority of multilevel cervical arthroplasty outcomes versus single level outcomes: 229 consecutive PCM prostheses. *Spine,* 32 (12) 1337-1344

[35] Penning L. (1978) Normal movements of the cervical spine. *Am J Roentgenol,* 130: 317-326

[36] Raposo J, Darden BV. (publication pending) Biomechanics of cervical disc arthroplasty. *The Cervical Spine, 5th Edition.* Editor Edward Benzel, Lippincott, Williams and Wilkins

[37] Riew KD, Buchowski JM, Sasso R, Zdeblick T, Metcalf NH, Anderson PA. (2008) Cervical disc arthroplasty compared with arthrodesis for the treatment of myelopathy. *Journal of Bone and Joint-A,* Vol. 90: pp 2351-2361

[38] Robinson R, Smith G. (1955): Anterolateral cervical disc removal and interbody fusion for cervical disc syndrome. *Bull. John Hopkins Hospital,* 96:223-224

[39] Sola S, Hebecker R, Knoop M et al. (2005 suppl) Bryan cervical disc prosthesis- three years follow-up. *European Spine Journal,* 14:38

[40] Tumialan LM and Gluf, Wm. (2011) Progressive vertebral body osteolysis after cervical arthroplasty. *Spine,* 36(14):973-8

[41] Yi S, Kim KN, Yang MS, et al. (2010) Difference in occurrence of Heterotopic ossification according to prosthesis type in the cervical artificial disc replacement. *Spine,* 35(16):1556-1561

24

Lumbar Spinal Arthroplasty: Clinical Experience

Fred H. Geisler
Chicago Back Institute, Swedish Covenant Hospital, N. Francisco, Chicago, IL USA

1. Introduction

Lumbar spinal arthroplasty was first reported in clinical settings more than 10 years ago by Griffith et al [1]. This early experience was acquired with the first lumbar artificial disc, the CHARITÉ I, in patients with degenerative disc disease. Since that time, a randomized controlled trial comparing arthroplasty with the CHARITÉ Artificial Disc vs. anterior lumbar interbody fusion with the BAK Cage and iliac crest bone was completed. Multiple other lumbar arthroplasty devices have been developed subsequent to the CHARITÉ and are undergoing or completing clinical trials.

Unlike other spinal medical devices, lumbar discs are required by the Food and Drug Administration to complete randomized controlled trials (RCT) prior to market approval in the United States. As a result, lumbar arthroplasty devices have undergone more scrutiny and clinical evaluation than any other spinal medical devices. Specifically, a new device, the ProDisc-L, was granted FDA approval in 2006 and was described in a recent peer-review publication[2]. In addition, the Maverick Total Disc Arthroplasty System (Medtronic Sofamor Danek), Kineflex Lumbar Disc (SpinalMotion), and FlexiCore Intervertebral Disc (SpineCore/Stryker) lumbar discs have both completed their randomized enrollments and are currently in continued access (non-randomized) mode.

All these ongoing and completed randomized clinical trials have generated a large body of evidence on the safety and efficacy of arthroplasty for lumbar spine in clinical applications and, in many cases, in Level-1 publications.

The safety and efficacy of arthroplasty are not the only parameters discussed in the >60 clinical papers published over the last 6 years. In fact, significant insights were developed in the impact of arthroplasty on sagittal alignment and motion, possible adverse events and reoperation, as well as optimal patient selection and indication. Surgical technique and health economics papers have also been generated in an effort to fully understand the clinical and societal impact of this new technology. This review paper is aimed at providing an overview of all the existing clinical data related to spinal arthroplasty.

2. Materials and methods

A search was conducted on the OVID and COCHRANE Library database to collect all clinical data relevant to spinal arthroplasty. Specifically, the following keywords were used:

(CHARITÉ Artificial Disc or ProDisc-L or Maverick Total Disc Arthroplasty System or KineFlex or FlexiCore Intervertebral Disc) and (disc) and (lumbar). The search was limited to English-language papers. Preclinical, biomechanical, and review papers were excluded from the final paper selection. In addition, papers describing obsolete devices (CHARITÉ I and CHARITÉ II) were also excluded from the study. A total of 60 papers were analyzed herein and subdivided by key topic, as following: 1) General clinical outcomes; 2) Radiographic Analysis: Range of motion, heterotopic ossification and sagittal balance analyses; 3) facet and adjacent-level degeneration; 4) Revisions and revision strategies; 5) Surgical technique; 6) Complications; 7) Special patient population analyses; and 8) Health economics evaluations.

3. Results

3.1 General clinical outcome results

General clinical outcome results were available for the CHARITÉ Artificial Disc, the ProDisc-L, the Maverick Total Disc Arthroplasty System, and the FlexiCore Intervertebral Disc. However, level-1 data was only available for the CHARITÉ Artificial disc and the ProDisc-L, as the final study FDA IDE results for the Maverick Total Disc Arthroplasty System and the FlexiCore Intervertebral Disc have yet to be published.

The CHARITÉ Artificial Disc manuscripts described clinical outcomes as early as 1 year [3] and up to 13 years post-operative[4]. The short/medium term papers included herein typically disclosed early analyses from single sites involved in the CHARITÉ Artificial Disc IDE study comparing arthroplasty with CHARITÉ Artificial Disc vs. anterior interbody fusion with BAK cage and autograft [3, 5, 6]. The complete RCT at 2-year follow-up included 205 arthroplasty and 99 fusion patients, and was thoroughly described in two manuscripts, one focused on clinical outcomes[7], the other on radiographic outcomes[8]. Three additional medium- and long-term studies were also found: 2 papers with 10-year follow-up [4, 9] and one with an average of 6.6 year follow-up [10].

Safety and efficacy of arthroplasty was demonstrated in all short- and medium-term studies. Specifically, at 2-years post-operative, Blumenthal and McAfee reported no device-related complications and a reoperation rate of 5.4% (vs. 9.1% in the control arm). Efficacy was also demonstrated using validated disability (ODI) and pain (VAS) clinical outcomes tools. At 2 years, the reduction in ODI reached 48.5% (vs. 42.4% in the control group) and the absolute reduction in VAS reached 40.6 points (vs. 34.1 points in the control group) [7, 8].

Two of the three long-term studies confirmed these findings. Lemaire et al reported 10-year follow-up results in 100 patients. [4] This study included 54 patients operated at one level, 45 patients operated at two levels and one patient operated at 3 levels. Overall, authors reported excellent or good clinical outcomes in 90% cases. In a second long-term study, David et al presented 10-year data on 106 patients[9]. Only one-level surgeries were performed in this study. Excellent or good clinical outcome was obtained in 82.1% patients. Both papers thus concluded that arthroplasty was a viable option for disc degeneration.

Recently, a third, medium-term paper was published by Ross et al, describing the long-term effect of arthroplasty in 160 patients (226 CHARITÉ Artificial Discs). This paper reported a cumulative survival rate at 156 months of 35% and a mean ODI score improvement of 14%. Implant removal was also described in 12 patients[10]. These relatively poor findings were further discussed in two Letters to the Editors, which pointed out mathematical inconsistencies and overall clinical flaws in the manuscript, and further highlighted the need of proper surgical technique and patient selection for optimal clinical outcome [11, 12].

The ProDisc-L manuscripts described clinical outcomes as early as 3 months[13] and up to 8.7 years post-operative [14]. As described above for CHARITÉ Artificial Disc, The short-term papers typically disclosed early findings from one or two of the sites that participated in the randomized controlled trial comparing ProDisc-L against a 360 degree fusion[13, 15-21]. The complete RCT at 2-year follow-up included 161 arthroplasty and 75 fusion patients [2]. The long-term data included 64 patients operated at one site, of which 55 were available between 7 and 11 years post-operative, for clinical and radiographic follow-up[14]. All these studies concluded similarly that disc arthroplasty, at all evaluated time points, was safe and resulted in complication and/or re-operation rates comparable to those generally accepted for spinal surgery (complication rate of 9% at 8.7 years[14]; there were no major complications, but a reoperation rate of 3.7% at 2 years was reported[2]). In addition to safety, efficacy of spinal arthroplasty was also shown herein as all cases presented significant improvements in pain and disability. The final RCT data reported improvements in the arthroplasty group in Visual Analogue Scores (VAS) for pain by an average 39-mm, and in disability, as determined by the Oswestry Disability Index (ODI), by 28 points. It is worth noting, however, that the ODI tool utilized in this RCT was not the validated and widely accepted ODI methodology Version 1.0 as defined by Fairbanks et al[22]. In a Letter to the Editor, Fairbanks denounced the use of the so-called Oswestry Disability Index in the ProDisc-L study and thus cast doubt on the validity of the disability improvement outcomes observed herein[23].

The 2 clinical data publications on the MAVERICK device were both based on the same data set of 64 patients, collected at one site[24, 25]. The clinical outcomes were described using the ODI Version 1.0 and VAS scores. The efficacy of arthroplasty was once again demonstrated using these tools, as ODI scores decreased by an average of 20.7 points and VAS scores by 4.4 points. As for the FlexiCore Intervertebral Disc, only one paper was recently published[26]. This manuscript describes the clinical outcomes of 44 patients, of which only 6 were available for 2-year follow-up. While the clinical relevance of this data may therefore be questionable, authors still concluded that the device may be safe and efficacious but that the data was not representative of the entire patient cohort.

3.2 Radiographic analyses: Range of motion, heterotopic ossification and sagittal balance analyses

Radiographic evaluations such as ROM, heterotopic ossification, and sagittal balance have been broadly analyzed for the CHARITÉ Artificial Disc, the ProDisc-L, as well as the Maverick Total Disc Arthroplasty System.

Unlike other clinical and radiographic outcomes, accurate measurement of ROM was shown to be challenging and, to some extent, subjective, as patient positioning, imaging staff training, and other factors unrelated to the actual motion potential of the spine were shown to impact final readings [27]. Using ProDisc-L cases, Lim et al evaluated different methodologies and associated error margins for the measurement of ROM from radiographic images. Specifically, Lim et al concluded that a ROM of at least 4.6 degs must be observed in order to be 95% certain that a given device had any sagittal motion at all. Similarly, changes needed to be at least 9.6 degs in ROM in order to confirm at 95% that change in motion really happened[28, 29]. These technical limitations might explain the inconsistent ROM data, particularly for ProDisc-L cases, found in the published literature. The flexion-extension ROM results from the 2-year RCT were determined at 7.7 degrees and 4.67 degrees and characterized as a normal ROM [2]. However, at 8.7 years post-operative, Huang et al reported a ROM less than that reported in asymptomatic normal individuals, with an average motion of 3.8 degs [30]. In a 2006 prospective study on 41 patients with 2 year follow-up, Leivseth et al also reported that the device fails to restore normal segmental motion, while another retrospective study on 26 patients concluded that sagittal balance and ROM significantly improved after lumbar arthroplasty[31].

Less controversy was observed when reviewing ROM data for the CHARITÉ Artificial Disc. A complete manuscript was dedicated to the radiographic data of the 2-year RCT of the CHARITÉ Artificial Disc [8]. In this study, arthroplasty patients had a 13.6% increase in motion from preoperative to the 2-year post-operative time point. The ROM also correlated to device placement, as poor device placement resulted in a statistically significant reduction in motion. At 10-year follow-up, David reported an average 10.1 degs ROM, a value very similar to the 10.3 degs reported by Lemaire et al in their 10-year follow-up study[4, 9].

Le Huec et al published the only data available on radiographic findings after arthroplasty with the Maverick Total Disc Arthroplasty System. In their study, Le Huec et al broadened their analysis to include sagittal alignment and pelvic tilt[24, 32]. Using data related to 35 patients at an average 14 months post-operative, authors showed maintenance of overall lordosis and unchanged sacral and pelvic tilts, following arthroplasty.

More recently, a study by Tournier comparing all three - CHARITÉ Artificial Disc, ProDisc-L and Maverick Total Disc Arthroplasty System - further refined the analyses from LeHuec on pelvic and sagittal tilt. In this study, authors found no difference in ROM between prostheses and observed maintenance of sagittal balance before and after surgery with all devices. However, modifications of the lumbar curvature were observed[33].

The issue of heterotopic ossification in clinical cases of lumbar arthroplasty has been presented by McAfee et al and, more recently, by Tortolani et al[34, 35]. In his 2003 paper, McAfee introduced a novel method to characterize spinal heterotopic ossification. This methodology was applied by Tortolani et al in reviewing the 276 arthroplasty patients from the CHARITÉ Artificial Disc RCT (randomized and non-randomized cases). From this analysis, 4.3% cases of heterotopic ossification were noted. However, heterotopic ossification was not related to range of motion, as the authors concluded that no difference in the range of motionat 24-months post-operatively was found between the patients who had and those who did not have heterotopic ossification.

3.3 Facets and adjacent-level degeneration

Facet degeneration is currently a contraindication for arthroplasty. However, a few publications have investigated the impact of arthroplasty on index-level facet joints, as

well as adjacent-level discs, in order to determine whether the added motion at the index level could slow down the natural progression of the disease at the facets and the adjacent-level joints.
Three long-term analyses evaluated adjacent-level degeneration, one with ProDisc-L at 8.7 years, and the other two with the CHARITÉ Artificial Disc at 10 years follow-up. In the ProDisc-L study, 24% cases developed adjacent level degeneration by the latest follow-up time point. A correlation was also found between a low range of motion and the prevalence of adjacent level degeneration: all patients with adjacent-level degeneration had a ROM l ess than 5 degrees, while only 59% of patients without adjacent-level degeneration had a ROM less than 5 degrees [36]. Lemaire et al and David reported 2 (2%) and 3 (2.8%) cases of adjacent-level degeneration at the latest time point, respectively[4, 9]. Lemaire et al and David also disclosed 11 cases (11%) and 5 cases (4.7%) with facet arthrosis at the latest time point, respectively.
The issue of facet degeneration was also recently discussed in a short-term study. From a 13-patient case series with 12 months follow-up, Trouillier et al alluded to possible maintenance of facet joint integrity following arthroplasty with CHARITÉ Artificial Disc based on the favorable results from their series[37]. At the other end of the spectrum, Shim et al, at the 3-year time point, observed 36.4% and 32.0% increase in index level facet degeneration and 19.4% and 28.6% adjacent level disc degeneration with the CHARITÉ Artificial Disc and the ProDisc-L, respectively.

3.4 Revision and revision strategies

The issue of possible revisability of arthroplasty devices represented a key concern when the first artificial disc, the CHARITÉ Artificial Disc, was introduced to the market. As such, multiple papers have focused on this issue and provided surgical and clinical insights to ensure appropriate approaches to revision surgery.
The first description of appropriate revision for a CHARITÉ Artificial Disc was presented by David[38]. In this single-case example, a CHARITÉ Artificial Disc was replaced at 9.5 years post-operative with another CHARITÉ Artificial Disc. The author concluded that revision of the disc with another disc could be safely and adequately performed and was thus an alternative to a revision fusion procedure. David also noted that, due to the inherent difficulty of an anterior approach, only experienced surgeons should undertake this operation. Further revision and explantation of the disc were also described by McAfee et al and Leary et al [39, 40]. McAfee et al confirmed Davids experience and concluded that arthroplasty with the CHARITÉ Artificial Disc did not preclude any further procedures at the index level during primary insertion, with nearly one third being revisable to a new motion-preserving prosthesis and just over two thirds being successfully converted to ALIF and/or posterior pedicle screw arthrodesis, the original alternative procedure. Leary further implied that technical errors in position and sizing of the implant were largely to blame for further revision surgery. Finally, Punt et al reviewed 75 revision cases from the Dutch experience (estimated by the authors at approximately more than 1000 Dutch patients). In this series, patients were fused posteriorly either with removal of the disc or without removal of the disc. No statistically significant difference was observed between these 2 groups[41]. This paper included patients previously described by Van Ooij et al[42].

3.5 Surgical technique

The appropriate surgical technique with the CHARITÉ Artificial Disc as well as the ProDisc-L was presented in 2 separate publications. Geisler et al provided a detailed account of the surgical technique for the CHARITÉ Artificial Disc, and dedicated an entire section of the paper to patient selection and preoperative planning, two critical aspects of successful spinal arthroplasty[43]. Authors also strongly recommended the availability of a spinal access surgeon to perform the approach, especially in revision cases. Finally, appropriate midline identification and positioning of the device also represented a critical discussion point in this paper. For the ProDisc-L, Gumbs et al retrospectively reviewed 64 cases of open retroperitoneal exposures and concluded that the approach was safe and, as discussed by Geisler et al, required a multidisciplinary team, such as an orthopedic and an access or general surgeon, to minimize complication rates[44].

3.6 Complications

Complications from spinal arthroplasty have also been reported for all three devices. Most complications requiring revision surgery were resolved by either fusion and/or disc replacement surgery. Interestingly, the causes of these complications seemed to be device-specific (i.e.; due to the design and/or make of the device).

For the ProDisc-L, the major complication described in the literature referred to the vertical split fracture of the vertebral body following total disc replacement. This occurrence was described by Shim et al in 2 separate cases that were not revised or treated surgically, but experienced prolonged back pain as a result[45]. An additional complication in the form of acquired spondylolysis was described by Schulte et al[46]. Authors attributed this complication to inaccurate implant size and positioning.

For the CHARITÉ Artificial Disc, the key complications were observed on the earlier devices, which were gamma sterilized in air and thus had a potential for oxidation of the core polyethylene nucleus [38]. Complications due to this oxidation process were described by Van Ooij et al (and Punt et al, as this paper reiterate data from the Van Ooij patient population)[41, 42]. This issue was resolved with a process change in 1998 to gamma sterilization in nitrogen. In a review of the RCT patient population, Geisler et al also evaluated the rate of neurological complications in the arthroplasty group vs. fusion group. The rate of neurological complication was described as exceedingly low in both groups with no statistically significant differences between groups.

While little has been published so far on the Maverick Total Disc Arthroplasty System, one article described an early removal of the Maverick Total Disc Arthroplasty System [47]. This removal was performed one year after implantation due to severe persistent back pain. Intraoperatively, gross metallosis around the articulation of the device was observed. The revision was successful and included a 360 degs fusion. Metallosis was thus cited as a potential complication for devices consisting of a metal-on-metal design. Zeh et al presented an additional potential complication: due to this metal-on-metal structure of the Maverick Total Disc Arthroplasty System, cobalt and chromium ions from the device were being released into the bloodstream [48]. In this study, cobalt and chromium ions from subjects implanted with the Maverick Total Disc Arthroplasty System were evaluated and compared to ion levels in total hip arthroplasty (THA) patients. Zeh et al found that concentrations of Cr/Co measured in the serum were similar in terms of their level to the values measured in THA metal-on-metal combinations or exceed those values reported in the literature. As a result, while Zeh et al did not recommend holding back with the implantation of the device, they did suggest long-term clinical evaluations to determine the clinical impact of high ion levels in serum and also recommended discussions with patients on the potential health effects of the prosthesis.

3.7 Special patient population analyses

The clinical outcomes for selective patient populations (e.g.; smokers, >60yr old) were discussed in multiple papers, more specifically for the ProDisc-L device. Bertagnoli et al lead these efforts with 4 publications presenting clinical data on arthroplasty with ProDisc-L in patients with: 1) single-level arthroplasty[15]; 2) multi-level arthroplasty[16]; 3) patients 60-years or older[49]; 4) smokers [50]; and 5) arthroplasty cases adjacent to a fused level [51]. While Bertagnoli et al repeatedly stated the importance of proper patient selection in each and every paper, all the results presented in these studies concluded that spinal arthroplasty with ProDisc-L successfully addressed low-back pain in these specific patient populations. Hannibal et al recently compared one- vs. two-level arthroplasty cases at the 2-year follow-up to try and establish whether one-level cases were experiencing greater clinical improvements as compared to the two-level cases. This hypothesis was not verified as differences in clinical improvements between one- and two-level cases were marginal [52]. Yaszay et al approached the problem from a different angle and evaluated patients outcomes based on a radiographic observation, i.e.; preoperative disc height [53]. Yaszay et al observed that patients with greater disc collapse experienced a greater benefit from total disc replacement, as compared to patients with less collapsed intervertebral discs. On average, patients in all of Bertagnoli et al and Yaszay et al series showed significant clinical improvement following arthroplasty.

Using the CHARITÉ Artificial Disc IDE RCT patient population, sub-analyses by patient types were also published by Guyer et al and Geisler et al. Specifically, patients were stratified by age at surgery (18-45 vs. 46-60) or whether they had had prior surgery or not[54, 55]. In both cases, there was no difference in clinical outcome between groups, whether patients were 18-45 or 46-60, or whether patient did or did not have prior surgery. Along the same trend, Geisler et al also evaluated the clinical outcomes of those patients from the CHARITÉ Artificial Disc RCT that did not improve with arthroplasty and needed revision surgery to a fusion. These patients (7.1% of all arthroplasty cases) did not improve, despite the revision surgery, further highlighting the importance of proper patient selection, and possibly, the fact that patient selection still remains a somewhat approximate science(59)[56].

3.8 Health economics evaluations

The impact of spinal arthroplasty on health care economics were reviewed for both the CHARITÉ Artificial Disc and the ProDisc-L. Guyer et al analyzed the costs related to a CHARITÉ Artificial Disc arthroplasty compared to: 1) an anterior fusion with autograft: 2) anterior fusion with rhBMP-2 (Infuse Bone Graft and LT-Cages) as well as 3) instrumented posterior lumbar interbody fusion. This analysis included the cost of revision surgery at the rate estimated in the published literature. Guyer et al concluded that all fusion procedures were more costly than the arthroscopy approach by 12.0% (ALIF with autograft) to 36.5% (ALIF with rhBMP-2 and posterior fusion)[57].

A similar analysis by Levin et al evaluated the costs of 1- and 2-level arthroplasty vs. 360 degs fusion. This study did not include possible needs for revisions. Nevertheless, one-level arthroplasty cases were found to be less costly than one-level fusions ($35,592 for arthroplasty vs. $46,280 for 360 deg fusion) while two-level cases were similar for both groups ($55,524 for arthroplasty vs. $56,823 for fusion)[58].

4. Discussion

From 2002 to 2008, a significant volume of data was made available on the clinical impact of arthroplasty. Sixty studies related to the clinical use of arthroplasty were published in peer-reviewed papers, of which 35 described data collected prospectively and 18 represented data from multi-center studies. The total number of patients described in the literature for spinal arthroplasty is difficult to evaluate, since many studies are early data releases or sub-analyses of the main randomized controlled trials performed for each new device. Thus, a given patient population might have been discussed in multiple papers. Overall, however, it was estimated that approximately 1,600 patients were included in the current literature.

The RCTs for the ProDisc-L and the CHARITÉ Artificial Disc both demonstrated the non-inferiority of the arthroplasty procedure, compared to their respective controls (ALIF for CHARITÉ Artificial Disc, 360 degs fusion for ProDisc-L. The complete RCT data for Maverick Total Disc Arthroplasty System and FlexiCore Intervertebral Disc are not yet published.) For some specific clinical outcomes such as pain, disability, and hospital stay, arthroplasty patients experienced greater clinical outcomes at some of the follow-up time points. For the CHARITÉ Artificial Disc RCT, arthroplasty patients fared statistically better than fusion on pain and disability for all but the 24-month follow-up time point. Hospital stay was also significantly shorter in the CHARITÉ Artificial Disc group as compared to the fusion group. As for ProDisc-L, pain scores were statistically better in the investigational cohort as compared to control. In addition, most other case series, for any of the given arthroplasty products, including those with short- and long-term follow-up data, presented favorable overall outcomes for spinal lumbar arthroplasty.

The issues of range of motion, heterotopic ossification, and sagittal balance have also drawn significant attention. While accurate and reproducible measurement of the lumbar ROM may be a significant limitation to collect meaningful data, average ROM at the 2-year time point throughout the studies evaluated herein were at ~ 7-10 degs. In addition, restoration of sagittal balance was observed for each device, the CHARITÉ Artificial Disc, the ProDisc-L as well as the Maverick Total Disc Arthroplasty System.

This review contained however somewhat contradictory data on the issue of facet and adjacent-level degeneration. While two of the 10year studies showed very small instances of facet and/or adjacent-level degeneration, others reported nearly a 1/3 of all cases with either CHARITÉ Artificial Disc or ProDisc-L developing changes in facet morphology. The inconsistency in these results points at potential surgeon-specific techniques and approaches that may impact the long-term benefits of both procedures.

Surgeon-specific variability in technique and proficiency was also cited in cases of revision. In fact, a study by Regan et al evaluating the occurrence of revision in low-volume vs. high-volume center, confirmed that surgeon in low-volume centers may incur greater peri-operative complications, however none that affected long-term outcomes[59]. Nevertheless, revisions were often found to be associated with technical errors, such as errors in positioning or sizing of the implant.

This critical importance of proper technique was in fact described in the 2 technique papers discussed herein. Both these publications stressed the importance of proper patient selection, a recurrent theme in almost all arthroplasty discussions.

Three types of major complications were described or foreseen in the current literature: 1) vertebral body split due to the ProDisc-L keel design; 2) oxidation of the core polymer nucleus, a problem specific to first generation CHARITÉ I prosthesis; and 3) metallosis and long-term impact of metal ions in the body. While the issue of metallosis and metal ions still needs to be thoroughly investigated, the problems related to vertebral body split only occurred once in the published literature, and as such, may represent a rare occurrence, and that of core oxidation, has been since resolved with new sterilization techniques following which core oxidation of the polymer nucleus is not observed. Thus, possible complications related to devices with metal-on-poly designs seem to be fairly limited.

Finally, low rates of complication and adverse event were observed for most of all analyzed patients. For the ProDisc-L, smokers as well as patients 60 years of age seemed to experience similar benefit from the procedure. In all these studies, however, authors reiterated the importance of proper patient selection, thus concluding that, while all analyzed patient types experienced clinical benefit from the procedure, specific care must be given to only operate on appropriate patients.

Finally, no technology is sustainable in today's market place if its cost is prohibitive. Thus, the impact of arthroplasty on health economics was also investigated. Both, the CHARITÉ Artificial Disc and the ProDisc-L study came up at a lower cost than their fusion controls, whether potential revision costs were included or not. No data on cost exists yet for the Maverick Total Disc Arthroplasty System and the FlexiCore Intervertebral Disc.

5. TDR surgery

The typical diseased lumbar segment considered for artificial disc technologies at L4-L5 or L5-S1 has advanced degenerative disc disease with loss of vertical height and lordosis, dehydration changes, adjacent Modic endplate changes, and little motion on dynamic studies (see Figure 1). The natural progression of degenerative disease disc limits the joint mobility and this biomechanical fact places more forces on the adjacent levels then in the normal situation. The artificial lumbar disc, by restoring normal motion, height, and lordosis, will decrease the forces on the adjacent levels. Thus, theoretically, levels adjacent to a dynamically stabilized level may have beneficial effects compared to the natural history of the unoperated degenerative state. Clearly some patients will benefit from the decreased force on the adjacent vertebral level(s) following a dynamic stabilization (arthroplasty) compared to a static stabilization (fusion). Estimates of the rate and groups of patients at maximum benefit will need to await long-term clinical follow up studies with lumbar arthroplasty devices similar to the hip and knee arthroplasty registries. Also, although a dynamically stabilized level can be converted to a fusion, a fused level cannot be converted to a dynamic joint. Thus, artificial technology can be thought of as a definitive procedure for the vast majority of patients that can be converted to a fusion if the pain and functional goals are not met or degenerative changes occur in the posterior elements and the arthrodesis level is believed to be the pain generator.

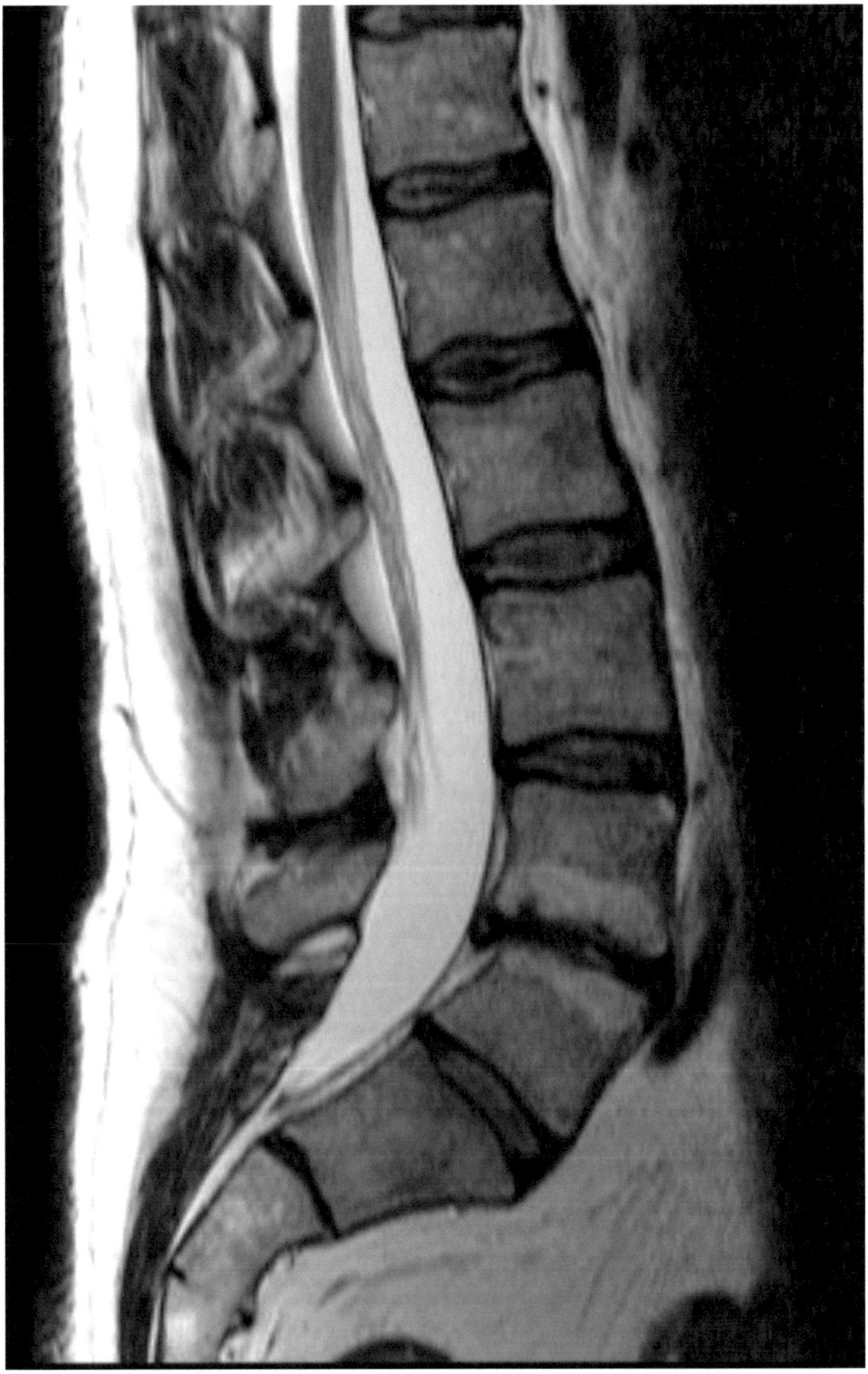

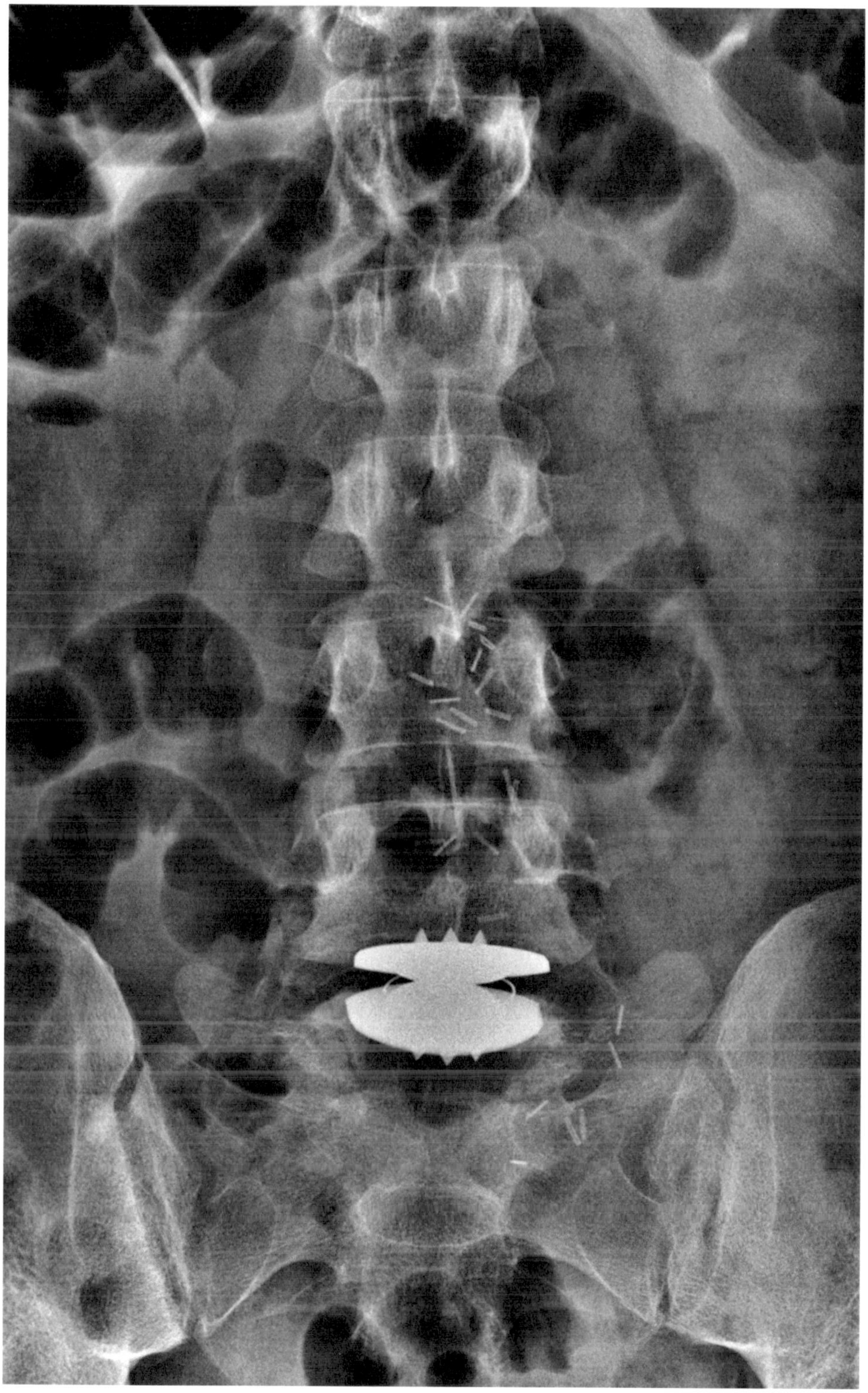

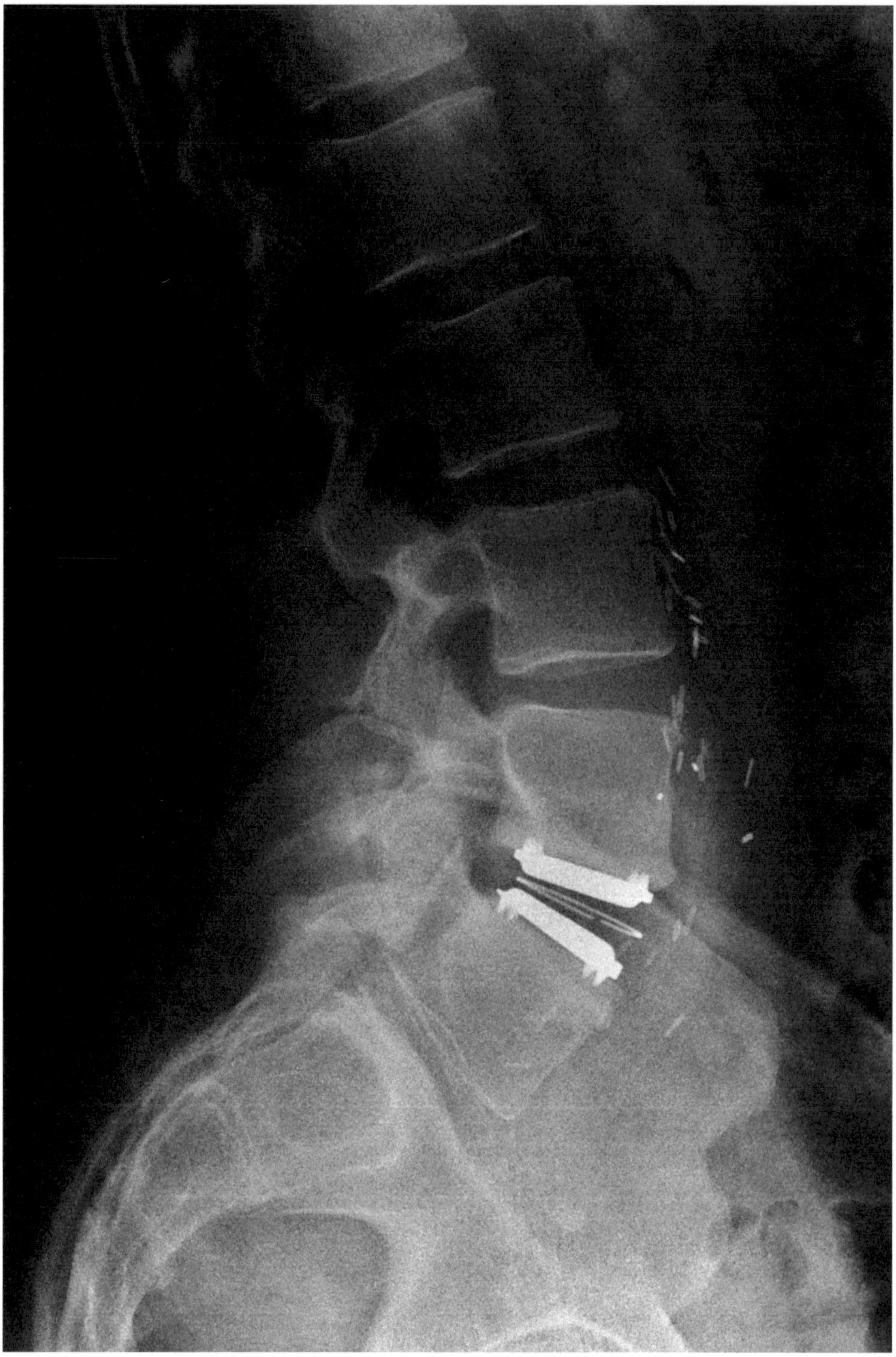

Fig. 1. Typical radiographies for a TDR patient. 1a. Pre-operative MRI. 1b. Post-operative A-P radiography. 1c. Post-operative lateral radiography.

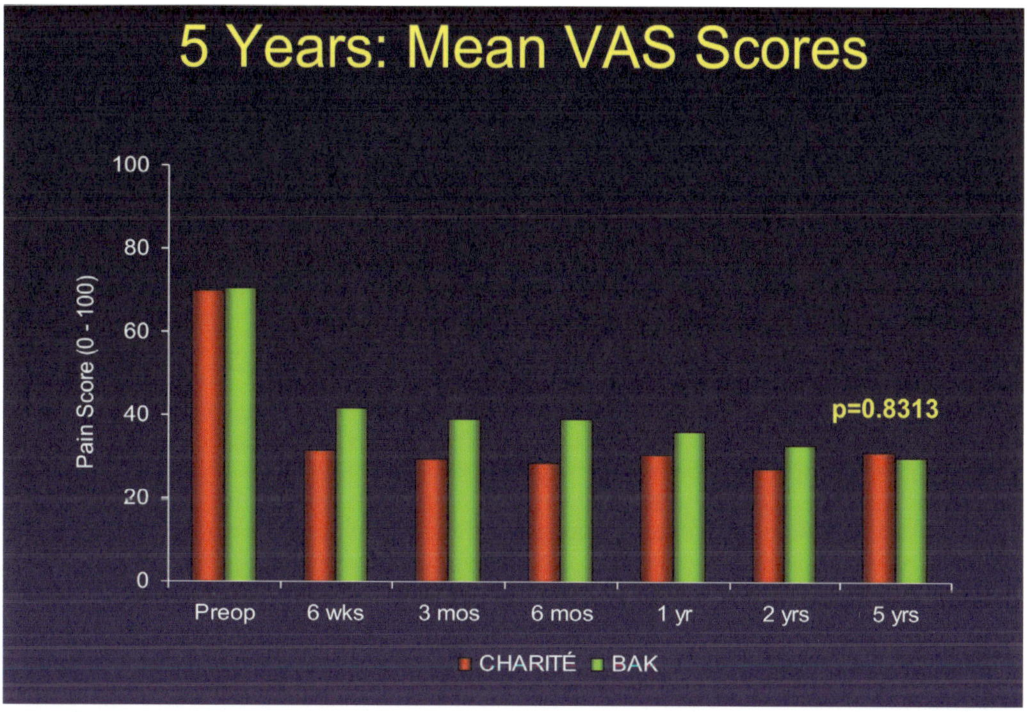

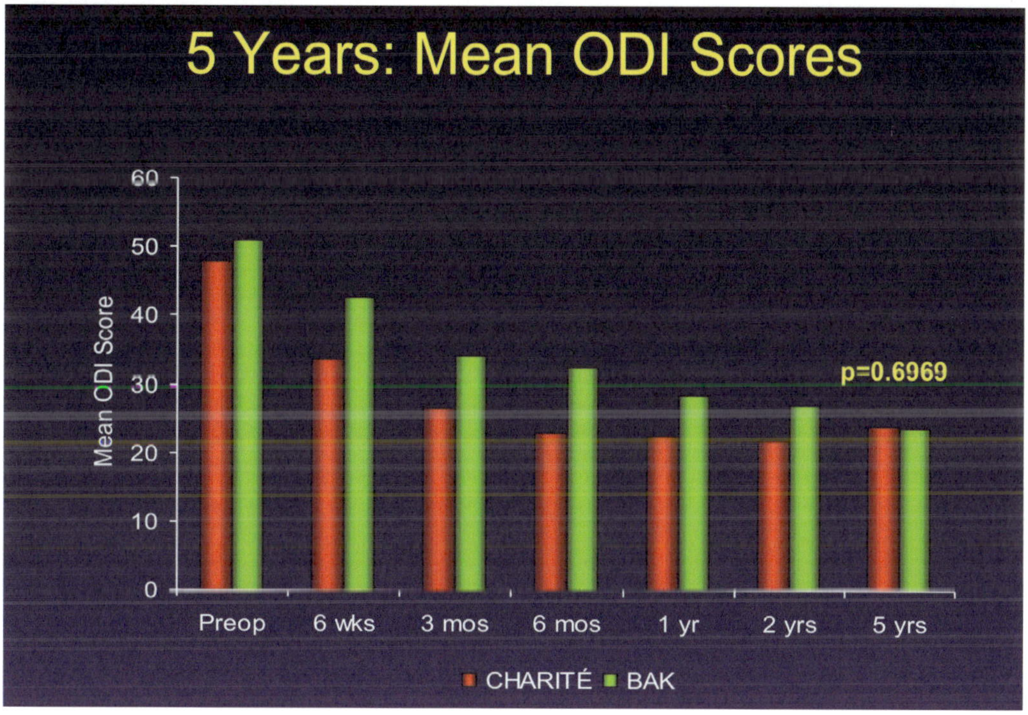

Fig. 2. Five years results from the Charité FDA IDE prospective randomized study. 2a. ODI. 2b. VAS.

6. Revision techniques

If a CHARITÉ artificial disc were required to be revised, there would be two options available. One approach would be anterior reoperation. This would involve dissecting the retroperitoneal area and dealing with the post-op scarring and hence increased risk of great vessel damage, ureteral damage, and damage to the sympathetic nerves compared to a case without prior dissection and scarring in the retroperitoneal space. A revision allows removal, position adjustment or size change of the CHARITÉ artificial disc. The plastic core would be removed first, and then the metal endplates are separated from the bony endplates by using a chisel between them and levering away from the bone into the disc space. This would allow the placement of another artificial disc in the disc space or the conversion to a fusion. Alternately, a posterior operation with rod-screw stabilization and posterior lateral fusion could be used to fuse the lumbar segment, which would use the CHARITÉ artificial disc as an anterior load share device. As with all surgical decision making, understanding the biomechanical reasoning and etiology of clinical failure is of the utmost importance. In patients with recurring or persistent pain the characterization of the pain generator is often more important than the exact surgical technique used. Radiologic studies such as dynamic A-P and Lat x-ray and multislice CT will aid in understanding failure of the device or progression of the degenerative anatomic changes. Radiologic and provocative studies, including discography, anesthetic or negative discography, nerve root blocks, epidural injections, and facet injections may all be utilized to identify the anatomic site of the pain generator.

7. Long-term follow-up of TDR patients

The initial CHARITÉ was planned with a 2-year follow-up period. At the request of the FDA the follow-up period was extended to 5-years and the sites requested to participate in the "new" 2 to 5 year follow-up period. Multiple sites did participate in this extended reporting period and formed the basis of the 5-year CHARITÉ results. The CHARITÉ 5-year ODI and VAS results (Figure 2a and 2b respectively) were substantially the same as the 2-years follow-up results[60]. Despite the prospective collection of the these results, critics formulated objections to these reported good results[61].

8. Conclusion

Overall, there were only minor differences between devices in terms of overall clinical and radiographic outcome. Significant improvements in clinical outcomes were seen with all evaluated devices, regardless of make or design. An average maintenance of motion post-operatively was described, along with relatively low rates of revision. Differences between devices were mostly apparent in complication types: one potential complication for devices with keels was vertebral body split, while devices with metal-on-metal designs could cause metallosis and ion release in the serum. As for metal-on-poly devices, degradation of the polymer core was also mentioned as a potential complication, albeit one that is not relevant for the current metal-on-poly devices. Specific emphasis was found in most of all publications on proper technique and patient selection, regardless of implant design. Finally, arthroplasty was found to be less costly than fusion.

9. References

[1] Griffith SL, Shelokov AP, Buttner-Janz K, LeMaire JP, Zeegers WS. A multicenter retrospective study of the clinical results of the LINK SB Charite intervertebral

prosthesis. The initial European experience. *Spine.* Aug 15 1994;19(16):1842-1849.
[2] Zigler J, Delamarter R, Spivak JM, et al. Results of the prospective, randomized, multicenter Food and Drug Administration investigational device exemption study of the ProDisc-L total disc replacement versus circumferential fusion for the treatment of 1-level degenerative disc disease. *Spine (Phila Pa 1976).* May 15 2007;32(11):1155-1162; discussion 1163.
[3] McAfee PC, Fedder IL, Saiedy S, Shucosky EM, Cunningham BW. SB Charite disc replacement: report of 60 prospective randomized cases in a US center. *J Spinal Disord Tech.* Aug 2003;16(4):424-433.
[4] Lemaire JP, Carrier H, Sari Ali E, Skalli W, Lavaste F. Clinical and Radiological Outcomes With the CHARITÉ™ Artificial Disc: A 10-Year Minimum Follow-Up. *J Spinal Disord.* 2005;18(4):353-359.
[5] Guyer RD, McAfee PC, Hochschuler SH, et al. Prospective randomized study of the Charite artificial disc: data from two investigational centers. *Spine J.* Nov-Dec 2004;4(6 Suppl):252S-259S.
[6] Geisler FH, Blumenthal SL, Guyer RD, et al. Neurological complications of lumbar artificial disc replacement and comparison of clinical results with those related to lumbar arthrodesis in the literature: results of a multicenter, prospective, randomized investigational device exemption study of Charite intervertebral disc. Invited submission from the Joint Section Meeting on Disorders of the Spine and Peripheral Nerves, March 2004. *J Neurosurg Spine.* Sep 2004;1(2):143-154.
[7] Blumenthal SL, McAfee PC, Guyer RD, et al. A Prospective, Randomized, Multicenter Food and Drug Administration Investigational Device Exemptions Study of Lumbar Total Disc Replacement with the CHARITÉ™ Artificial Disc Versus Lumbar Fusion Part I: Evaluation of Clinical Outcomes. *Spine.* 2005;30(14):1565-1575.
[8] McAfee PC, Cunningham B, Holsapple GA, et al. A Prospective, Randomized, Multicenter Food and Drug Administration Investigational Device Exemptions Study of Lumbar Total Disc Replacement with the CHARITÉ™ Artificial Disc Versus Lumbar Fusion Part II: Evaluation of Radiographic Outcomes and Correlation of Surgical Technique Accuracy with Clinical Outcomes. *Spine.* 2005;30(14):1576-1583.
[9] David T. Long-term results of one-level lumbar arthroplasty: minimum 10-year follow-up of the CHARITE artificial disc in 106 patients. *Spine (Phila Pa 1976).* Mar 15 2007;32(6):661-666.
[10] Ross R, Mirza AH, Norris HE, Khatri M. Survival and clinical outcome of SB Charite III disc replacement for back pain. *J Bone Joint Surg Br.* Jun 2007;89(6):785-789.
[11] Guyer RD, Blumenthal SL. Survival and clinical outcome of SB Charite III disc replacement for back pain. *J Bone Joint Surg Br.* Dec 2007;89(12):1673; author reply 1673-1674.
[12] Scott-Young MN. Survival and clinical outcome of SB Charite III disc replacement for back pain. *J Bone Joint Surg Br.* Dec 2007;89(12):1674; author reply 1674 1675.
[13] Bertagnoli R, Kumar S. Indications for full prosthetic disc arthroplasty: a correlation of clinical outcome against a variety of indications. *Eur Spine J.* Oct 2002;11 Suppl 2:S131-136.

[14] Tropiano P, Huang RC, Girardi FP, Cammisa FP, Jr., Marnay T. Lumbar total disc replacement. Seven to eleven-year follow-up. *J Bone Joint Surg Am.* Mar 2005;87(3):490-496.
[15] Bertagnoli R, Yue JJ, Shah RV, et al. The treatment of disabling single-level lumbar discogenic low back pain with total disc arthroplasty utilizing the Prodisc prosthesis: a prospective study with 2-year minimum follow-up. *Spine (Phila Pa 1976).* Oct 1 2005;30(19):2230-2236.
[16] Bertagnoli R, Yue JJ, Shah RV, et al. The treatment of disabling multilevel lumbar discogenic low back pain with total disc arthroplasty utilizing the ProDisc prosthesis: a prospective study with 2-year minimum follow-up. *Spine (Phila Pa 1976).* Oct 1 2005;30(19):2192-2199.
[17] Chung SS, Lee CS, Kang CS. Lumbar total disc replacement using ProDisc II: a prospective study with a 2-year minimum follow-up. *J Spinal Disord Tech.* Aug 2006;19(6):411-415.
[18] Delamarter RB, Fribourg DM, Kanim LE, Bae H. ProDisc artificial total lumbar disc replacement: introduction and early results from the United States clinical trial. *Spine (Phila Pa 1976).* Oct 15 2003;28(20):S167-175.
[19] Tropiano P, Huang RC, Girardi FP, Marnay T. Lumbar disc replacement: preliminary results with ProDisc II after a minimum follow-up period of 1 year. *J Spinal Disord Tech.* Aug 2003;16(4):362-368.
[20] Zigler JE, Burd TA, Vialle EN, Sachs BL, Rashbaum RF, Ohnmeiss DD. Lumbar spine arthroplasty: early results using the ProDisc II: a prospective randomized trial of arthroplasty versus fusion. *J Spinal Disord Tech.* Aug 2003;16(4):352-361.
[21] Zigler JE. Lumbar spine arthroplasty using the ProDisc II. *Spine J.* Nov-Dec 2004;4(6 Suppl):260S-267S.
[22] Fairbank JC, Pynsent PB. The Oswestry Disability Index. *Spine (Phila Pa 1976).* Nov 15 2000;25(22):2940-2952; discussion 2952.
[23] Fairbank JC. Use and abuse of Oswestry Disability Index. *Spine (Phila Pa 1976).* Dec 1 2007;32(25):2787-2789.
[24] Le Huec JC, Mathews H, Basso Y, et al. Clinical results of Maverick lumbar total disc replacement: two-year prospective follow-up. *Orthop Clin North Am.* Jul 2005;36(3):315-322.
[25] Le Huec JC, Basso Y, Aunoble S, Friesem T, Bruno MB. Influence of facet and posterior muscle degeneration on clinical results of lumbar total disc replacement: two-year follow-up. *J Spinal Disord Tech.* Jun 2005;18(3):219-223.
[26] Sasso RC, Foulk DM, Hahn M. Prospective, randomized trial of metal-on-metal artificial lumbar disc replacement: initial results for treatment of discogenic pain. *Spine (Phila Pa 1976).* Jan 15 2008;33(2):123-131.
[27] Cunningham BW, McAfee PC, Geisler FH, et al. Distribution of in vivo and in vitro range of motion following 1-level arthroplasty with the CHARITE artificial disc compared with fusion. *J Neurosurg Spine.* Jan 2008;8(1):7-12.
[28] Lim MR, Girardi FP, Zhang K, Huang RC, Peterson MG, Cammisa FP, Jr. Measurement of total disc replacement radiographic range of motion: a comparison of two techniques. *J Spinal Disord Tech.* Jun 2005;18(3):252-256.
[29] Lim MR, Loder RT, Huang RC, et al. Measurement error of lumbar total disc replacement range of motion. *Spine (Phila Pa 1976).* May 1 2006;31(10):E291-297.

[30] Huang RC, Girardi FP, Cammisa Jr FP, Tropiano P, Marnay T. Long-term flexion-extension range of motion of the prodisc total disc replacement. *J Spinal Disord Tech.* Oct 2003;16(5):435-440.
[31] Chung SS, Lee CS, Kang CS, Kim SH. The effect of lumbar total disc replacement on the spinopelvic alignment and range of motion of the lumbar spine. *J Spinal Disord Tech.* Jul 2006;19(5):307-311.
[32] Le Huec J, Basso Y, Mathews H, et al. The effect of single-level, total disc arthroplasty on sagittal balance parameters: a prospective study. *Eur Spine J.* Jun 2005;14(5):480-486.
[33] Tournier C, Aunoble S, Le Huec JC, et al. Total disc arthroplasty: consequences for sagittal balance and lumbar spine movement. *Eur Spine J.* Mar 2007;16(3):411-421.
[34] McAfee PC, Cunningham BW, Devine J, Williams E, Yu-Yahiro J. Classification of heterotopic ossification (HO) in artificial disk replacement. *J Spinal Disord Tech.* Aug 2003;16(4):384-389.
[35] Tortolani PJ, Cunningham BW, Eng M, McAfee PC, Holsapple GA, Adams KA. Prevalence of heterotopic ossification following total disc replacement. A prospective, randomized study of two hundred and seventy-six patients. *J Bone Joint Surg Am.* Jan 2007;89(1):82-88.
[36] Huang RC, Tropiano P, Marnay T, Girardi FP, Lim MR, Cammisa FP, Jr. Range of motion and adjacent level degeneration after lumbar total disc replacement. *Spine J.* May-Jun 2006;6(3):242-247.
[37] Trouillier H, Kern P, Refior HJ, Muller-Gerbl M. A prospective morphological study of facet joint integrity following intervertebral disc replacement with the CHARITE Artificial Disc. *Eur Spine J.* Feb 2006;15(2):174-182.
[38] David T. Revision of a Charite artificial disc 9.5 years in vivo to a new Charite artificial disc: case report and explant analysis. *Eur Spine J.* Jun 2005;14(5):507-511.
[39] Leary SP, Regan JJ, Lanman TH, Wagner WH. Revision and explantation strategies involving the CHARITE lumbar artificial disc replacement. *Spine (Phila Pa 1976).* Apr 20 2007;32(9):1001-1011.
[40] McAfee PC, Geisler FH, Saiedy S, et al. Revisability of the CHARITÉ Artificial Disc Replacement - Analysis of 688 Patients Enrolled in the U.S. IDE Study of the CHARITÉ Artificial Disc. *Spine.* 2006 2006;31(11):1217-1226.
[41] Punt IM, Visser VM, van Rhijn LW, et al. Complications and reoperations of the SB Charite lumbar disc prosthesis: experience in 75 patients. *Eur Spine J.* Jan 2008;17(1):36-43.
[42] van Ooij A, Oner FC, Verbout AJ. Complications of artificial disc replacement: a report of 27 patients with the SB Charite disc. *J Spinal Disord Tech.* Aug 2003;16(4):369-383.
[43] Geisler FH. Surgical Technique of Lumbar Artificial Disc Replacement with the CHARITE™ Artificial Disc. *Neurosurgery.* 2005;56:ONS46-57.
[44] Gumbs AA, Shah RV, Yue JJ, Sumpio B. The open anterior paramedian retroperitoneal approach for spine procedures. *Arch Surg.* Apr 2005;140(4):339-343.
[45] Shim CS, Lee S, Maeng DH, Lee SH. Vertical split fracture of the vertebral body following total disc replacement using ProDisc: report of two cases. *J Spinal Disord Tech.* Oct 2005;18(5):465-469.
[46] Schulte TL, Lerner T, Hackenberg L, Liljenqvist U, Bullmann V. Acquired spondylolysis after implantation of a lumbar ProDisc II prosthesis: case report and review of the literature. *Spine (Phila Pa 1976).* Oct 15 2007;32(22):E645-648.

[47] Francois J, Coessens R, Lauweryns P. Early removal of a Maverick disc prosthesis: surgical findings and morphological changes. *Acta Orthop Belg.* Feb 2007;73(1):122-127.

[48] Zeh A, Planert M, Siegert G, Lattke P, Held A, Hein W. Release of cobalt and chromium ions into the serum following implantation of the metal-on-metal Maverick-type artificial lumbar disc (Medtronic Sofamor Danek). *Spine (Phila Pa 1976).* Feb 1 2007;32(3):348-352.

[49] Bertagnoli R, Yue JJ, Nanieva R, et al. Lumbar total disc arthroplasty in patients older than 60 years of age: a prospective study of the ProDisc prosthesis with 2-year minimum follow-up period. *J Neurosurg Spine.* Feb 2006;4(2):85-90.

[50] Bertagnoli R, Yue JJ, Kershaw T, et al. Lumbar total disc arthroplasty utilizing the ProDisc prosthesis in smokers versus nonsmokers: a prospective study with 2-year minimum follow-up. *Spine (Phila Pa 1976).* Apr 20 2006;31(9):992-997.

[51] Bertagnoli R, Yue JJ, Fenk-Mayer A, Eerulkar J, Emerson JW. Treatment of symptomatic adjacent-segment degeneration after lumbar fusion with total disc arthroplasty by using the prodisc prosthesis: a prospective study with 2-year minimum follow up. *J Neurosurg Spine.* Feb 2006;4(2):91-97.

[52] Hannibal M, Thomas DJ, Low J, Hsu KY, Zucherman J. ProDisc-L total disc replacement: a comparison of 1-level versus 2-level arthroplasty patients with a minimum 2-year follow-up. *Spine (Phila Pa 1976).* Oct 1 2007;32(21):2322-2326.

[53]Yaszay B, Bendo JA, Goldstein JA, Quirno M, Spivak JM, Errico TJ. Effect of intervertebral disc height on postoperative motion and outcomes after ProDisc-L lumbar disc replacement. *Spine (Phila Pa 1976).* Mar 1 2008;33(5):508-512; discussion 513.

[54] Guyer RD, Geisler FH, Blumenthal SL, McAfee PC, Mullin BB. Effect of age on clinical and radiographic outcomes and adverse events following 1-level lumbar arthroplasty after a minimum 2-year follow-up. *J Neurosurg Spine.* Feb 2008;8(2):101-107.

[55] Geisler FH, Guyer RD, Blumenthal SL, et al. Effect of previous surgery on clinical outcome following 1-level lumbar arthroplasty. *J Neurosurg Spine.* Feb 2008;8(2):108-114.

[56] Geisler FH, Guyer RD, Blumenthal SL, et al. Patient selection for lumbar arthroplasty and arthrodesis: the effect of revision surgery in a controlled, multicenter, randomized study. *J Neurosurg Spine.* Jan 2008;8(1):13-16.

[57] Guyer RD, Tromanhauser SG, Regan JJ. An economic model of one-level lumbar arthroplasty versus fusion. *Spine J.* Sep-Oct 2007;7(5):558-562.

[58] Levin DA, Bendo JA, Quirno M, Errico T, Goldstein J, Spivak J. Comparative charge analysis of one- and two-level lumbar total disc arthroplasty versus circumferential lumbar fusion. *Spine (Phila Pa 1976).* Dec 1 2007;32(25):2905-2909.

[59] Regan JJ, McAfee PC, Blumenthal SL, et al. Evaluation of Surgical Volume and the Early Experience with Lumbar Total Disc Replacement as Part of the IDE Study of the CHARITÉ™ Artificial Disc. *Spine.* Sept 1, 2006 2006;31(19):2270-2276.

[60] Guyer RD, McAfee PC, Banco RJ, et al. Prospective, randomized, multicenter Food and Drug Administration investigational device exemption study of lumbar total disc replacement with the CHARITE artificial disc versus lumbar fusion: five-year follow-up. *Spine J.* May 2009;9(5):374-386.

[61] van den Eerenbeemt KD, Ostelo RW, van Royen BJ, Peul WC, van Tulder MW. Total disc replacement surgery for symptomatic degenerative lumbar disc disease: a systematic review of the literature. *Eur Spine J.* Aug 2010;19(8):1262-1280.

25

Shoulder Hemiarthroplasty in Proximal Humerus Fractures

José Hernández Enríquez, Xavier A. Duralde and Antonio J. Pérez Caballer
[1]*Orthopaedics Department, Hospital Infanta Elena, Valdemoro*
[2]*Orthopaedics Department, Peachtree Orthopaedic Clinic, Atlanta GA*
[3]*Orthopaedics Department, Hospital Infanta Elena, Valdemoro*
[1,3]*Spain*
[2]*USA*

1. Introduction

We present a review of the most recent published articles related to shoulder hemiarthroplasty in proximal humerus fractures. Four-part proximal humerus fractures represent between 2% and 10% of all proximal fractures where displacement occurs as a result of the muscular deforming force.

Hemiarthroplasty is indicated in patients with four-part fractures and in elderly patients with osteoporotic bone who have fracture-dislocations. In both groups of patients, obtaining a secure stable reduction using internal fixation techniques is difficult, and the rate of osteonecrosis can range from 13% to 35% in four-part fractures. Hemiarthroplasty can also be considered in patients with three-part fractures and fracture-dislocations when bone quality is poor and the degree of conminution precludes satisfactory reduction and internal fixation. Headsplitting proximal humerus fractures in elderly patients also should be treated with hemiarhroplasty. Primary replacement can be considered in younger patients with four-part proximal fractures if acceptable redution cannot be obtained.

The important surgical principles when performing a hemiartroplasty for four-part proximal humeral fractures include the following: the use of a deltopectoral approach, allowing preservation of the deltoid origin and insertion; restoration of humeral length and retroversion; and secure fixation of the tuberosities to the prosthesis, to the shaft and to one another.

Results of hemiarthroplasty for four-part proximal humerus fractures are somewhat difficult to interpret, specifically because other proximal humerus fracture patterns often are included in published series. Wide variation in outcomes measurements also makes comparisons between studies difficult. Despite these limitations, hemiarthroplasty offers reliable pain relief and reasonable levels of patient satisfaction, but only modest functional results. Limited use with activities of daily living below shoulder level may be reliably obtained but overhead use is not typical following this surgery.

Significant residual pain generally tends to be associated with moderate activity: minimal pain occurs at rest. Even when motion and functional results are limited, pain relief is reported to be consistent.

Reports of patient satisfaction vary widely, in part because of the numerous scales used to measure outcomes and satisfaction. High satisfaction rates seem to correlate more with pain relief than with range of motion of functional outcomes. Even studies with poor functional results report high patient satisfaction if pain relief is acceptable.

The prognostic factors have been shown to be the age, the delay between injury and surgery, preoperative neurologic deficit, history of cigarette smoking, excessive alcohol consumption and female sex. Tuberosity position and healing may be the most important factors in determining outcome.

Recently the use of the Reverse Total Shoulder Replacement has been recommended in selected cases of proximal humeral fracture. Although the indications and results of this technique are not well known yet, this may offer an advantage in selected cases over traditional Humeral Head Replacement. Any possible advantages of this technique must be weighed against increased risks and the known results of humeral head replacement.

Humeral head replacement is indicated for a select group of proximal humeral fractures depending on the severity and pattern of the fracture as well as bone quality and cuff integrity (Compito et al 1994). The results of this surgery are dependent on patient factors, timing of surgery, and technical factors associated with the performance of the operation. The majority of fractures of the proximal humerus can be treated nonoperatively but a full 15% of cases will require some type of operative interventio (Young et al 1985, Zuckerman et al 2007). Neer's fracture classification has generally served as a reliable guide to fracture managemen (Neer et al 1970, 1970). The more severe the injury, the higher the risk of avascular necrosis of the humeral head, malunion, or nonunion of the fracture. When indicated, early surgical intervention leads to superior results and avoids many complications associated with delayed management (Demirhan et al 2003, Duralde & Leddy 2010).

Operative treatment options for proximal humeral fractures include various forms of open or closed reduction and fixation versus prosthetic replacement. The introduction of the proximal humeral locking plate has expanded the indications for ORIF as patients with osteoporotic bone can now be better managed utilizing this plate for fixation (Duralde & Leedy 2010). Even cases of late avascular necrosis following ORIF can be managed effectively with hardware removal and prosthetic replacement as long as the tuberosities have healed in a relatively anatomic position (Boileau et al 2001). Similarly advances in the technique of closed reduction and percutaneous pinning have increased the indications for this modality (Jaberg et al 1992). ORIF remains a good option for displaced 2-part fractures, 3-part fractures (even in the face of osteoporosis), and impacted valgus 4-part fractures of the proximal humerus (Bastian & Hertel 2009, Duralde & Leedy 2010). Four-part fractures in young patients are preferably treated with a locking plate but if stable fixation cannot be attained, humeral head replacement is indicated. A group of fractures remain, however, that are not amenable to this modality and require prosthetic replacement for adequate management.

Prosthetic replacement for proximal humeral fractures remains the treatment of choice for 4-part fracture dislocations, head-split fractures, and head impaction fractures of ›40%. These fractures represent between 2 and 10% of proximal humeral fractures (Zuckerman & Sajadi 2007). It remains a good option in comminuted 3-part fractures especially in elderly patients with poor bone quality or a high degree of comminution (Bigliani 1990). Humeral head replacement is contraindicated in cases of active infection, severe nerve palsy to the deltoid and rotator cuff, and in patients unable to comply with the postoperative rehabilitation

program. In patients with known chronic large rotator cuff tears, the results of humeral head replacement for fracture are poor (Compito et al 1994) and this may be an indication for the use of a Reverse Total Shoulder Arthroplasty (RTSA). Indications and technical recommendations for the use of the RTSA in this setting are not clearly defined but this represents an area of exciting new research (Franke et al 2002, Wall & Walch 2007).
Prosthetic replacement for proximal humerus fractures is a challenging operation with variable results reported in the orthopaedic literature especially in terms of patient function (Robinson et al 2003). This procedure is performed uncommonly even by shoulder specialists. Anatomic landmarks are lost due to fracture of the tuberosities away from the humeral shaft making proper placement of prosthesis in terms of height and version a challenge. Tuberosities may be comminuted and the deforming pull of the rotator cuff tendons represents a challenge to fracture healing. Excellent results following humeral head replacement for fracture are associated with proper implant selection and insertion, anatomic tuberosity healing, and early rehabilitation to restore motion and strength[3]. Conversely, poor results are most commonly associated with tuberosity malunion or nonunion and improper humeral stem positioning (Boliieau et al 2002, Demirhan et al 2003, Esen et al 2009, Frankle et al 2001, Robinson et al 2003). Other important factors include the timing of surgery, patient age, tobacco and alcohol use, and female sex. Despite intensive study and improvements in patient selection, prosthetic design, and surgical technique, functional results remain variable. Wide variation in outcomes measurements also makes comparisons between studies difficult. Despite these limitations, hemiarthroplasty offers reliable pain relief and reasonable levels of patient satisfaction, but only modest functional results. Limited use with activities of daily living below shoulder level may be reliably obtained but overhead use is not typical following this surgery. Good to excellent results remain between 75-85% despite these challenges (Bigliani 1990, Goldman et al 1995, Green et al 1993, Kontakis et al 2008, Moeckel et al 1992, Robinson et al 2003, Tanner & Cofield 1983). High satisfaction rates seem to correlate more with pain relief than with range of motion or functional outcomes. Even studies with poor functional results report high patient satisfaction if pain relief is acceptable. Certainly, the more prepared the surgeon finds him or herself in the management of the patient with a severely displaced proximal humeral fracture, the better the chance of success. The purpose of this article is to review the preoperative evaluation, describe the surgical technique required for successful placement of the prosthesis and fixation of the tuberosities, and outline a safe postoperative rehabilitation program. We will review current results and complications associated with the technique of humeral head replacement and Reverse total shoulder arthroplasty for proximal humeral fractures.

2. Shoulder arthroplasty for proximal humerus fractures

2.1 Preoperative evaluation

Adequate preoperative evaluation is critical in the management of patients with displaced proximal humerus fractures. The surgeon must have a good working knowledge as to the mechanism of injury and level of energy associated as this will give an indication of possible neurovascular injuries. The surgeon should attempt to determine whether the injury represents a fracture or a fracture/dislocation and evaluation of all available radiographic studies is beneficial. Previous history of osteoporosis will give an indication as to the quality of bone available for fixation. Past history of rotator cuff disease is helpful as a large rotator cuff tear will be associated with poor results with a humeral head replacement and may be an indication for reverse ball and socket prosthesis.

Physical examination may be limited in the acute fracture setting because of pain and swelling. The area of bruising is most commonly seen in the chest as well as the arm distal to the deltoid muscle. Bruising in the area of the deltoid itself is indicative of either direct trauma to this area or perforation of the deltoid by one of the fracture fragments. Neurovascular examination is typically limited because of pain and the status of the axillary nerve often cannot be determined prior to surgery. Distal pulses should be evaluated and compared to the contralateral side. Differences in distal pulses may be an indication for arteriogram. Displacement of the shaft medially in the area of the brachial plexus is also in indication to obtain an arteriogram prior to open reduction internal fixation. Range of motion testing is of no benefit in the acute fracture setting.

Radiographic examination should be limited to a trauma series which does not require the patient to move the arm. Three orthogonal views as described by Neer can adequately evaluate the fracture in the majority of cases (Neer 1990). (Figure 1) These include an AP view in the scapular plane, a transthoracic lateral view, and a Valpeau axillary view. All of these X-rays can be taken without removal of the arm from the sling. CT scan has been shown to improve the accuracy of fracture classification and is very beneficial in preoperative planning (Shrader et al 2005). (Figure 2)

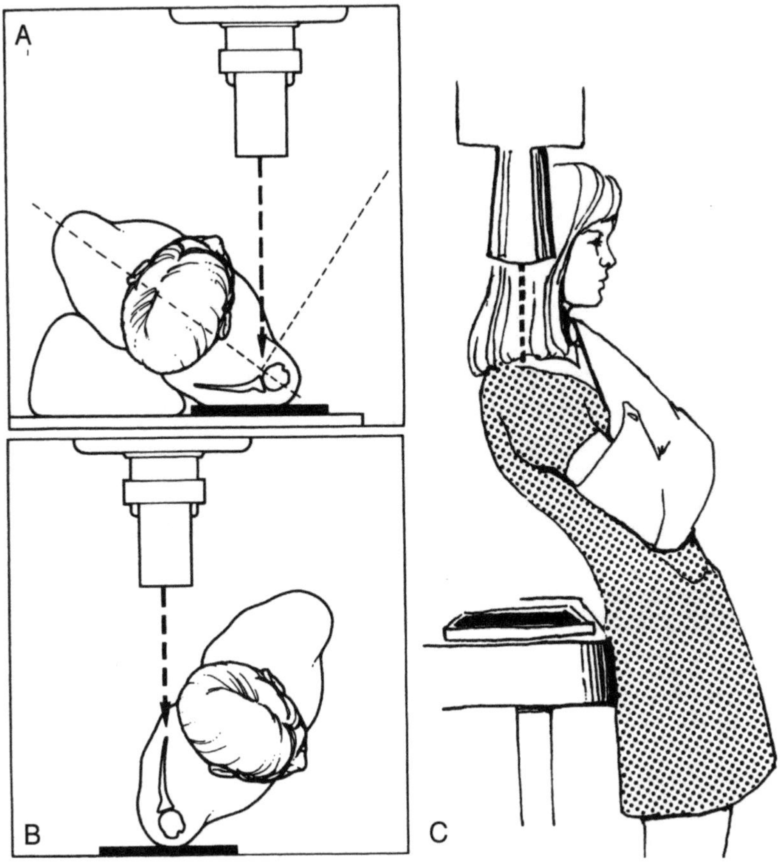

Fig. 1.

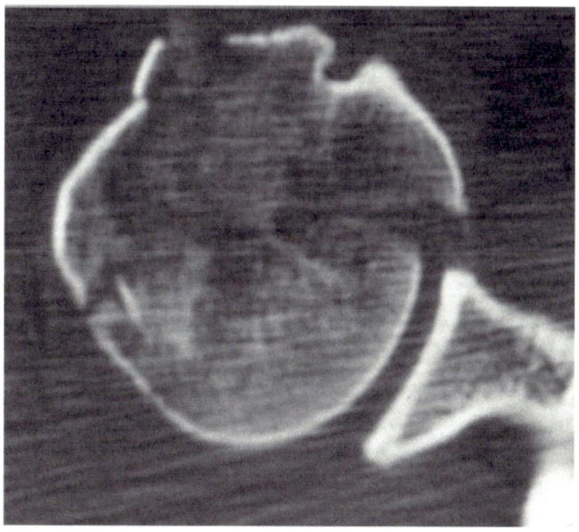

Fig. 2.

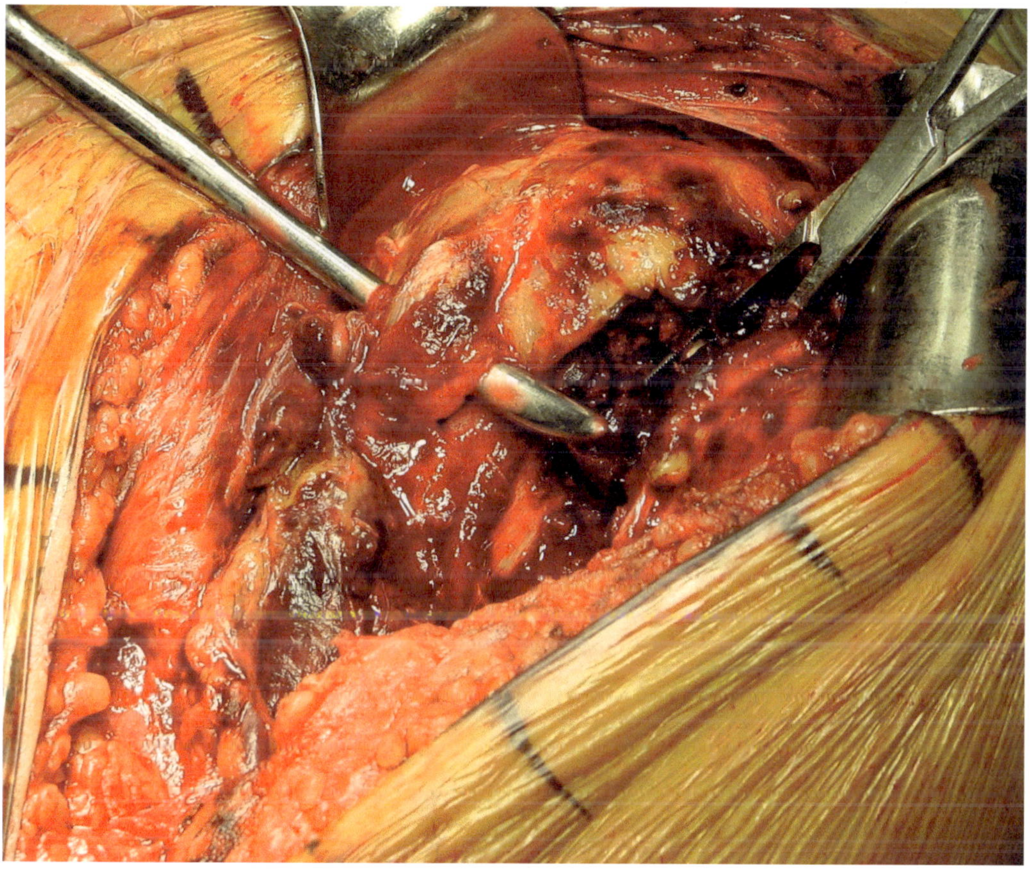

Fig. 3.

Arthroplasty for proximal humerus fractures is typically indicated for head split and head indentation fractures ›40% fractures, displaced 4-part fractures of the proximal humerus, and 4-part fracture/dislocations. In these cases, the proximal humerus does fracture in a very characteristic pattern. The fracture line between the greater and lesser tuberosity typically lies directly posterior to the bicipital groove so that the lesser tuberosity fracture typically also contains the bicipital groove and a small portion of the greater tuberosity. (Figure 3) The remainder of the greater tuberosity often fractures away from the shaft and lesser tuberosity with a characteristic "V" shaped pattern of bone leaving a distinctive defect in the proximal shaft which can be used in realigning the fracture fragments anatomically. (Figure 4) Variable amounts of head fragment may still be attached to a tuberosities. A small portion of the calcar typically stays attached to the humeral head fragment. (Figure 5)

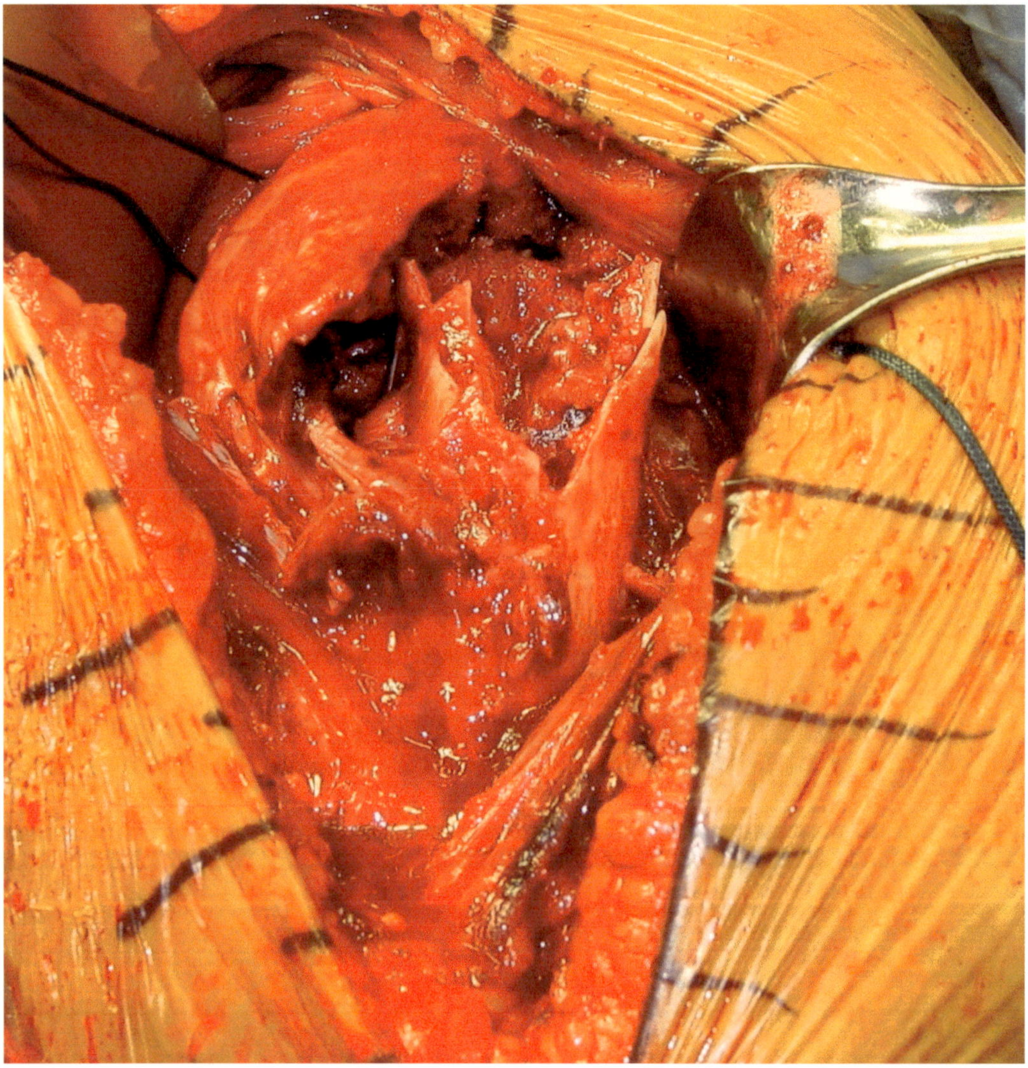

Fig. 4.

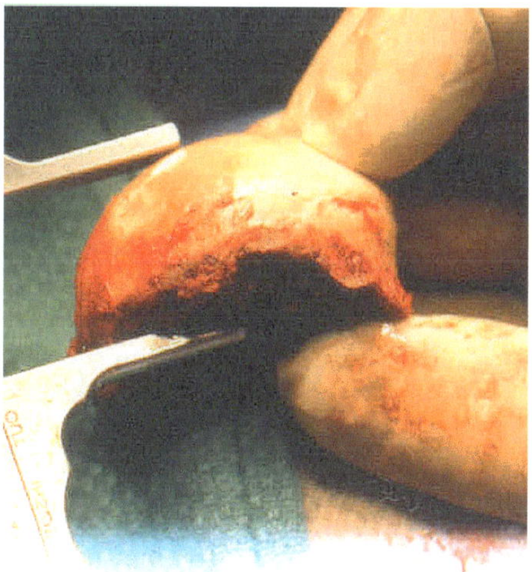

Fig. 5.

2.2 Operative technique

Key goals in prosthetic replacement for proximal humerus fractures include atraumatic exposure of the fracture site with protection of the deltoid origin and insertion while avoiding further devascularization of the fracture fragments, proper positioning of the prosthesis both in terms of height and version, and secure anatomic fixation of the tuberosities. The exact indications for the use of reverse prosthesis in the management of proximal humerus fractures is not well understood currently and is undergoing a period of development and research. Surgery is recommended within 7-10 days after the patient is cleared medically. Delay beyond this time makes dissection more challenging due to early fibrosis. Surgery must be followed by a safe physical therapy program which allows adequate healing of the tuberosities while avoiding excessive stiffness.

This surgery is typically performed under interscalene block anesthesia and general anesthesia. Relaxation during surgery decreases the pull of the pectoralis major and improves exposure. Interscalene block is contraindicated in the face of documented neurologic injury. This block results in excellent postoperative pain relief when indicated. The patient is placed in the beach chair position with the back of the table elevated approximately 30°. The patient is placed at the edge of the operating table with a bolster along the medial border of the scapula to stabilize this structure during surgery. Lateral placement of the arm allows extension off of the table for exposure and access to the humeral shaft. A well-padded neurosurgical head rest allows increased exposure and access to the superior shoulder and a short arm board supports the elbow without blocking access to the arm. All bony prominences are well-padded. A fluoroscan is utilized from above to allow evaluation of the fracture itself and tuberosity positioning. (Figure 6) Broad-spectrum antibiotics are routinely used. Surgical approach is planned to contribute minimal additional trauma to the soft tissues and vascular structures in the area of the proximal humerus. In situations in which the humeral head is displaced into the axilla in the area of the brachial plexus, caution must be exercised in its removal as this can result in hemorrhage. Assistance from a vascular surgeon may be required in such cases.

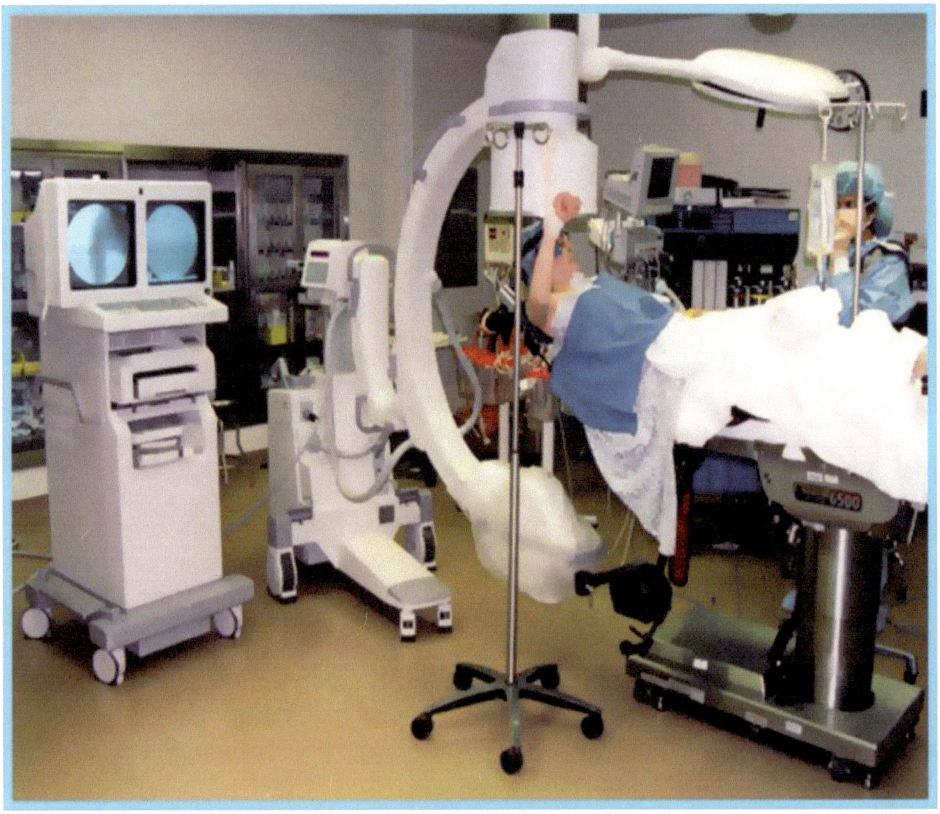

Fig. 6.

2.3 Surgical exposure

A deltopectoral incision is made beginning at the level superior to the coracoid and passing to a point directly anterior to the deltoid insertion. (Figure 7) The fat stripe over the cephalic vein is identified and carefully incised avoiding injury to the vein. With the edema encountered in acute fractures, blunt dissection can be carried through the deltopectoral interval dissecting the cephalic vein laterally with the deltoid down to the level of the fracture site itself. Fracture hematoma is evacuated and the anatomy of the fracture is now examined. The conjoined tendon is retracted medially and the deltoid is retracted laterally. The deltoid origin and insertion are preserved. Landmarks which assist in identification of critical structures include the coracoid which has been named "the lighthouse of the glenoid" and the biceps tendon which has been called "the highway to the glenoid". The coracoacromial ligament is identified at the lateral edge of the coracoid and can be followed to the subacromial space. The base of the coracoid can be palpated and helps guide the surgeon to the glenoid. The biceps tendon can be identified in the pectoralis insertion on the humeral shaft and followed into the fracture site. The fracture line between the lesser and greater tuberosities is typically immediately posterior to this tendon. The axillary nerve must be identified and protected throughout the procedure. The nerve is palpated anteriorly along the inferior border of the subscapularis and laterally along the undersurface of the deltoid muscle. Continuity of this nerve can be verified using the Tug Test (Flatow & Bigliani 1992) and is reassuring that the nerve has not been lacerated by fracture fragments.

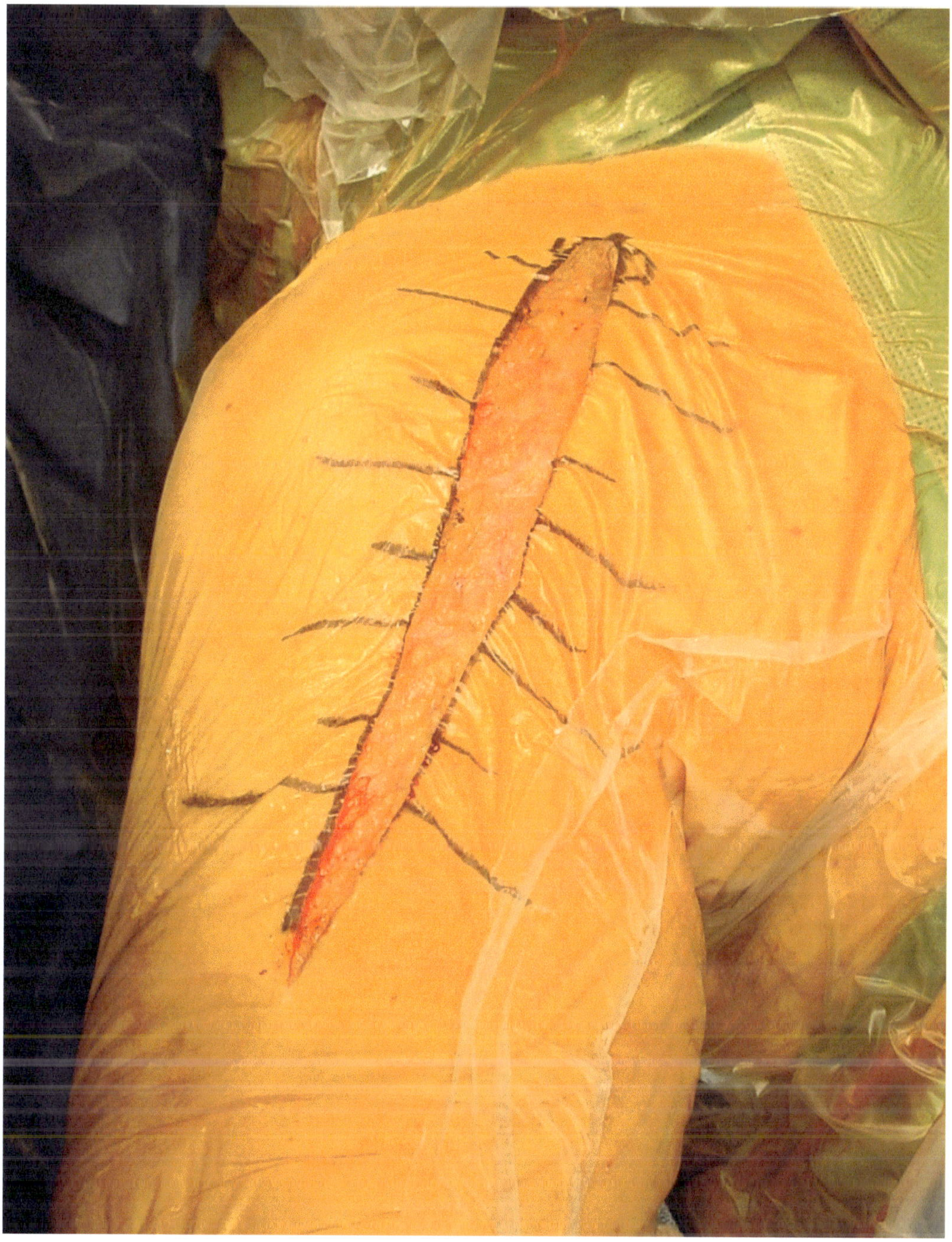

Fig. 7.

2.4 Control of fracture

The first step in controlling the 4-part proximal humerus fracture is to control the tuberosities. The lesser tuberosity is displaced medially by the pull of the subscapularis while the greater tuberosity is displaced posterosuperiorly by the pull of the infraspinatus and teres minor muscles. Heavy nonabsorbable sutures are passed through the subscapularis tendon to control the lesser tuberosity and through the infraspinatus tendon to control the greater tuberosity. (Figure 8) A bone hook or clamp may be necessary to reduce the greater tuberosity so that a suture can be passed through the cuff tendon. Abduction of the humerus relaxes the deltoid and assists with exposure of the greater tuberosity. Sutures are not placed through the greater tubersoity itself as bone quality may be poor and this will lead to further comminution. The rotator cuff tendon is often stronger than the bone itself and should be utilized for both mobilization and later fixation. The fracture line between the tuberosities is followed up to the rotator cuff. The rotator cuff can then be split in line with its fibers in continuity with this fracture line. This will leave a small strip of supraspinatus tendon attached to the anterior fragment. This fragment includes the lesser tuberosity, bicipital groove, and a small portion of the greater tuberosity. Attached to it are the subscapularis tendon, the rotator interval, and a small strip of the

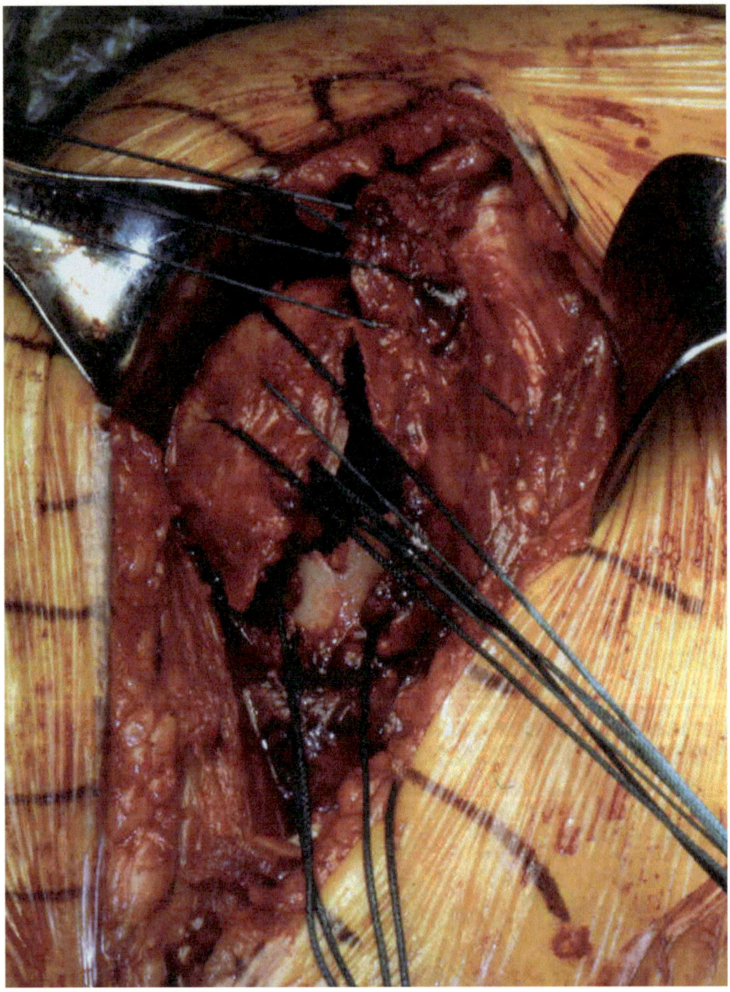

Fig. 8.

supraspinatus tendon. The remainder of the supraspinatus as well as the entire infraspinatus and teres minor tendons will be attached to the posterior fragment. Splitting the supraspinatus in line with its fibers to the level of the glenoid now allows exposure of the glenoid as well as the humeral head.
The humeral head is now removed and placed on the back table where it can be measured in terms of height and diameter. (Figure 9) Any missing fragments from the humeral head are typically still connected to the tuberosities and must be removed to allow adequate reduction of these tuberosities under the prosthetic humeral head. Removal of these portions of the humeral head is necessary but debulking of the tuberosity fragments is contraindicated as this may compromise tuberosity healing and positioning. The humeral head is also carefully inspected to determine the amount of calcar attached medially. The size of this fragment is indicative of the amount of missing shaft medially and will help determine the exact positioning of the prosthesis. The prosthetic humeral head should be positioned superior to the shaft a distance equal to the amount of the calcar bone left attached to the humeral head. Placement of the humeral head directly onto the humeral shaft ignoring the size of this calcar fragment will result in positioning of the head too low relative to the shaft. All cancellous bone in the humeral head can now be harvested and used for bone grafting of the tuberosities prior to fixation.

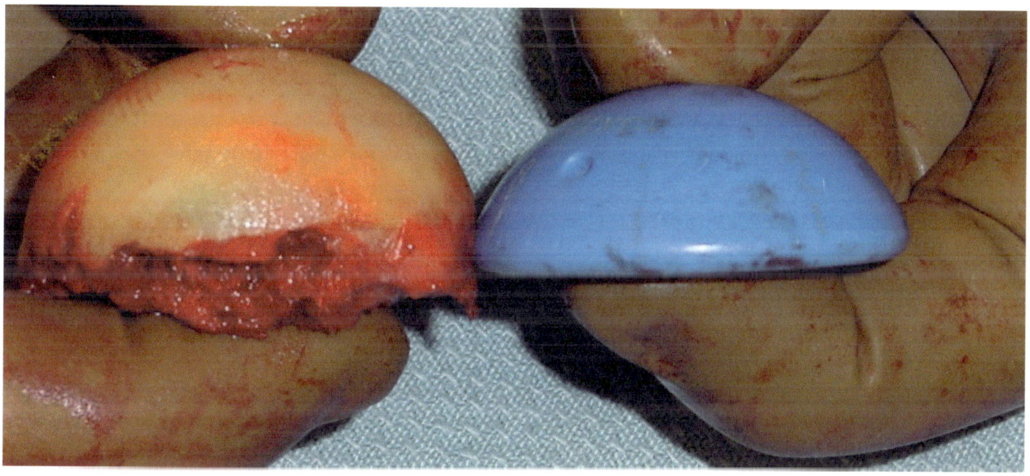

Fig. 9.

2.5 Prosthetic selection

Adequate prosthetic selection is determined by measuring the humeral head and canal. The proximal humeral shaft can be delivered into the operative site by extension, adduction and external rotation of the arm and placement of the elbow onto the short arm board. This allows access to the proximal humeral canal which can be measured with reamers. Minimal reaming is required. If there is no significant shaft comminution associated with the fracture, a standard length prosthetic stem on the order of 130 mm is adequate and a long stem prosthesis is not required. A prosthetic system which allows use of a narrow stem is preferred as this will allow room for bone grafting and tuberosity reduction and healing. Prostheses with a broad proximal collar often do not allow enough room for tuberosity reduction without debulking and compromises the healing ability of these tuberosities. Ingrowth material on the proximal stem may be beneficial to tuberosity healing. The prosthetic stem must be narrow enough to allow adequate insertion into the humerus and avoid proud placement of the prosthesis. Prosthetic humeral head size is determined by measuring the patient's humeral head at the time of surgery both in terms of height and diameter. In prosthetic systems with an offset humeral head, placement of the maximum offset is recommended posteriorly or posterosuperiorly to allow placement of the greater tuberosity under the humeral head in this location. Appropriate head sizing will help reestablish anatomic tension on the rotator cuff tendons after tuberosity repair.

2.6 Prosthetic positioning

Adequate positioning of the prosthesis both in terms of height and version is critical towards the success of this procedure and in reestablishing relatively normal anatomy for the patient postoperatively. Distortion of the normal proximal humeral anatomy by displacement of the tuberosities represents a challenge for determination of proper stem and head height. This positioning is important to reestablish the normal resting length of the deltoid muscle. There are multiple options for determining adequate height for the prosthesis. The superior margin of the pectoralis insertion typically is 56 mm from the superior aspect of the greater tuberosity and is a fairly standard measurement in patients of varying sizes (Murachovsky et al 2006). This measurement will allow the surgeon to determine whether he is in the generally correct range for prosthetic height. As mentioned previously, the size of the fragment of calcar on the humeral head will indicate the height of the prosthetic head relative to the shaft. In cases in which the greater tuberosity does not have significant comminution, the greater tuberosity fragment can be interdigitated back in the "V" shaped defect just posterior to the bicipital groove. The humeral head must be placed just superior to the greater tuberosity in this location and by reducing the greater tuberosity to the shaft, the surgeon can determine proper head height. (Figure 10[a] and 10[b]) Tension on the biceps tendon has been recommended as a guide for the prosthetic height but is less exact. The biceps can be tenodesed at this time and removed from the joint. Finally, some prosthetic systems do allow preoperative templating relative to the contralateral arm with jigs which can be utilized for determining height. These systems are often unwieldy and difficult to use. Placement of the prosthesis too low will result in inferior subluxation of the humeral head relative to the glenoid and cause weakness in elevation. Proud placement of the prosthesis will lead to overstuffing of the joint, superior subluxation, pain, and stiffness. Anatomic version of the humeral head has been generally reported between 20 and 40° of retroversion. Placing the prosthesis in less retroversion places less tension on the greater tuberosity fragment during internal rotation and may benefit healing. Version of approximately 20° is recommended for this reason and can be determined relative to the patients' forearm. In prosthetic systems with a posterior fin of the prosthesis positioned 180° from the medial calcar portion of the stem, this posterior fin should generally be located just posterior to the bicipital groove. The humeral stem is generally cemented in place to avoid subsidence and malrotation because the stabilizing effect typically afforded by the tuberosities has been lost due to the fracture.

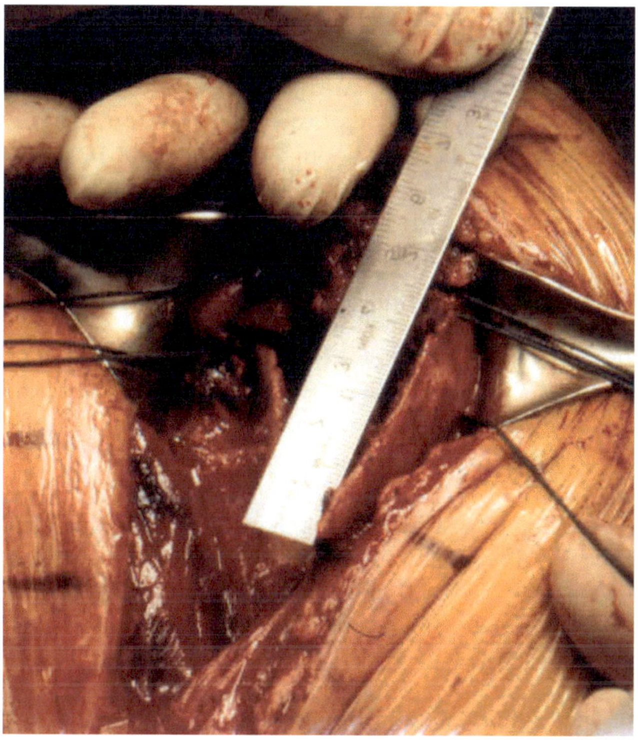

Fig. 10a.

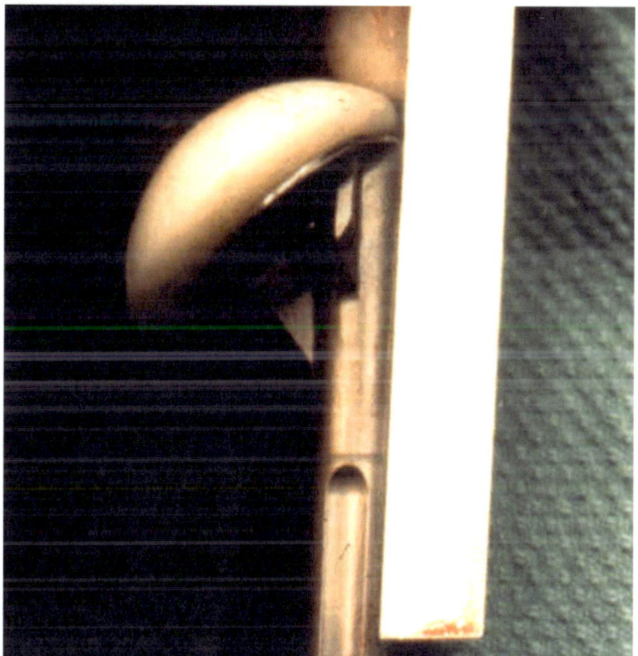

Fig. 10b.

2.7 Tuberosity fixation

Postoperative function is most closely tied to anatomic healing of the tuberosities. The success of tuberosity healing is directly related to the adequacy of reduction and fixation of the tuberosities at the time of surgery. Tuberosity healing is a major challenge and greater tuberosity pull off remains the most common complication of this surgery (Boileau et al 2002). The tuberosities must heal to each other and to the shaft as well as to the ingrowth material of the humeral prosthesis. A variety of fixation techniques have been reported but techniques recommended by both Frankle and Boileau have demonstrated superior biomechanical resistance to deforming forces (Boileau et al 2000, Frankle et al 2002). The tuberosities are repaired utilizing a suture technique which fixes these tuberosities to each other, to the prosthesis, and to the shaft of the humerus. The placement of these sutures and drill holes for their placement is necessary prior to cementing the humeral stem in place. Drill holes in the shaft include the one drill hole anterior to the bicipital groove, two drill holes straddling the bicipital groove, and one drill hole posterior to the bicipital groove. (Figure 11) In cases in which the "V" shaped fragment of the greater tuberosity is of adequate size, small drill holes between this fragment and the humeral shaft just posterior to the bicipital groove can be utilized for a figure of 8 reduction suture. (Figure 12) This suture does not resist deforming forces but is used for anatomic reduction of the tuberosity. #5 polyester nonabsorbable sutures are placed through the anterior drill hole and through the posterior drill hole respectively. One #5 polyester suture is passed through the holes straddling the bicipital groove in such a way that both ends of this suture pass out from the canal with a small loop of suture inside the canal. While the cement for stem fixation is curing, morcelized bone graft is packed into the proximal canal just above the cement. (Figure 13) These small fragments are fixed to the cement while the cement is setting. This creates a bony surface for healing to the tuberosities. The greater tuberosity is repaired first. One or two cerclage sutures of #5 polyester suture are placed through the rotator cuff at the bone tendon junction and around the anterior stem of the prosthesis. The #5 polyester suture from the anterior drill hole in the shaft is then passed diagonally across the prosthesis and through the rotator cuff tendon at the bone-tendon interface to fix the greater tuberosity to the shaft and to resist vertically directed deforming forces against the tuberosity. (Figure 14) The greater tuberosity is fixed to the posterior aspect of the fin on the stem just inferior to the humeral head utilizing the cerclage sutures passed around the prosthesis. The bone graft is inserted between the prosthesis and the greater tuberosity to restore bulk to the tuberosity and to assist with healing. The posterior shaft suture is then passed diagonally across the prosthesis and passed through the subscapularis tendon at the bone-tendon junction. One to two cerclage sutures between the greater tuberosity and lesser tuberosity are then used to reduce the lesser tuberosity to the stem just underneath the humeral head anterior to the prosthetic fin. Again bone graft is used as needed and the cerclage sutures are tied. The suture from the posterior shaft to the lesser tuberosity is then tied. The rotator cuff split made previously during exposure is closed using nonabsorbable figure of 8 sutures. By making that split through the supraspinatus tendon, good tissue is available for repair anteriorly and posteriorly to help resist greater tuberosity pull-off. Finally, the two suture limbs at the bicipital groove distally are passed in a figure of 8 fashion over the rotator interval and rotator cuff split to firmly repair these to each other and to the shaft. (Figure 15) The stability and strength of the repair is then tested by taking the arm through gentle range of motion. (Figure 16) Adequacy of reduction of the tuberosity fragments can be verified fluoroscopically. The continuity of the axillary nerve can be verified using the Tug test. Suction drains are placed deep to the deltoid and a layered closure is performed.

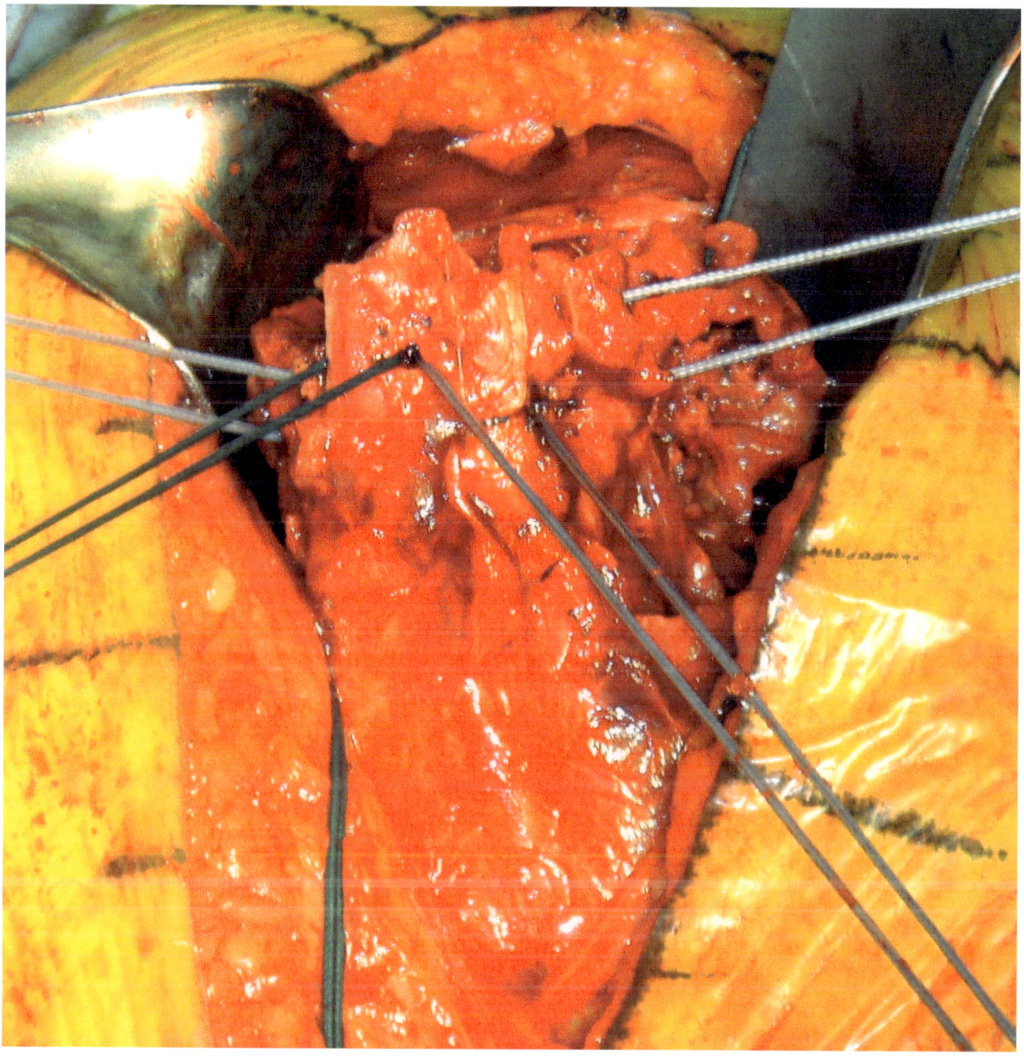

Fig. 11.

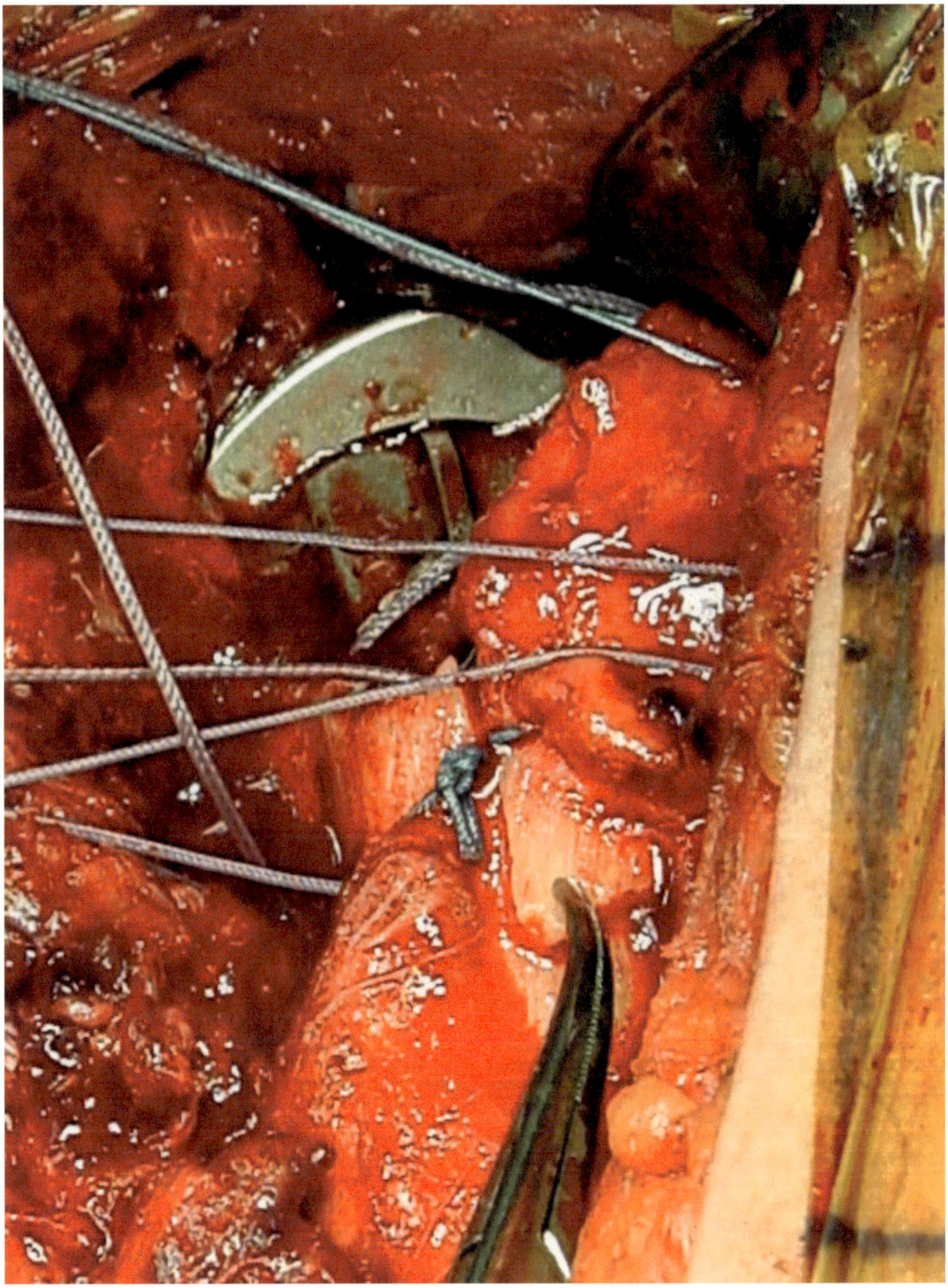

Fig. 12.

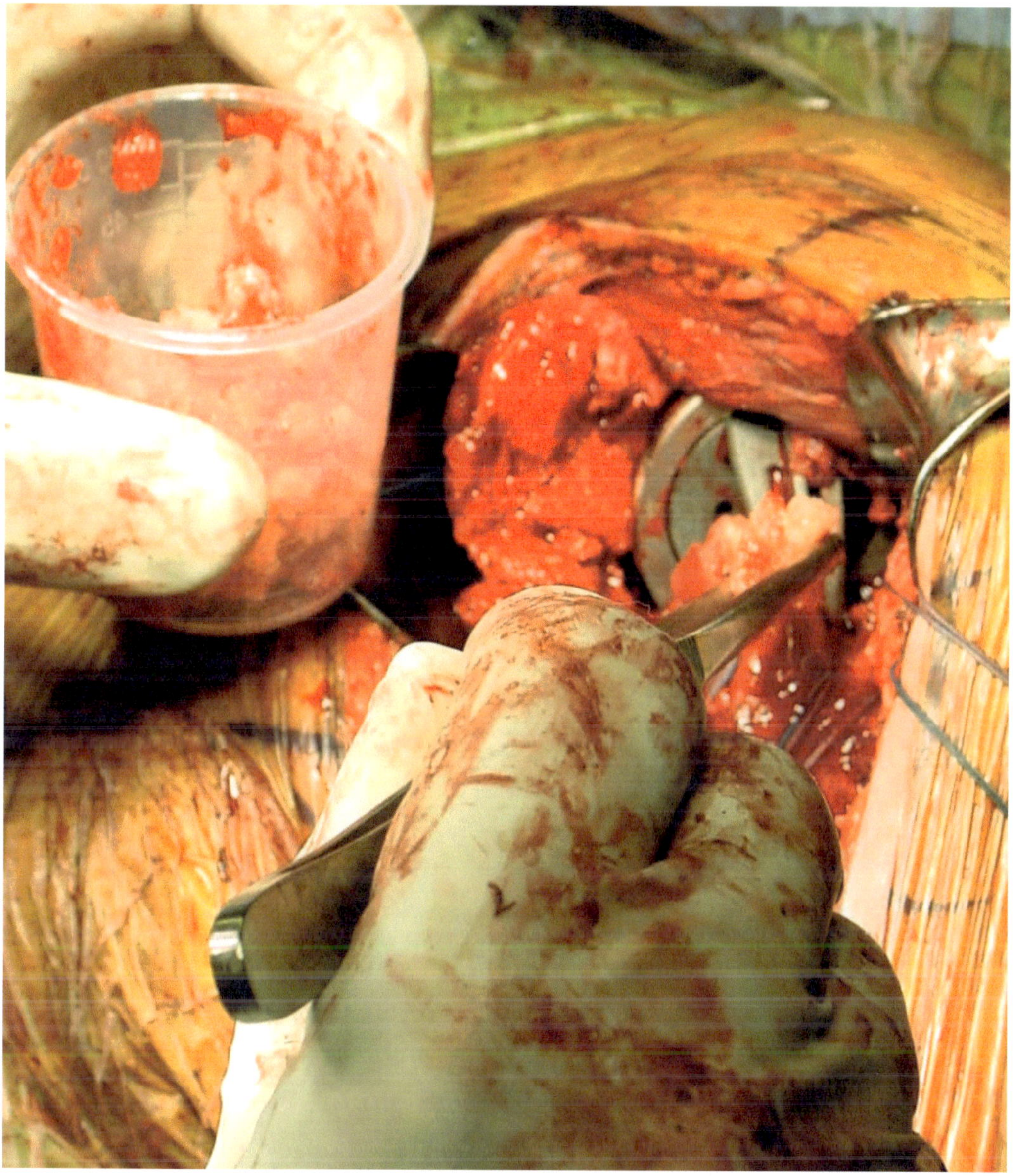

Fig. 13.

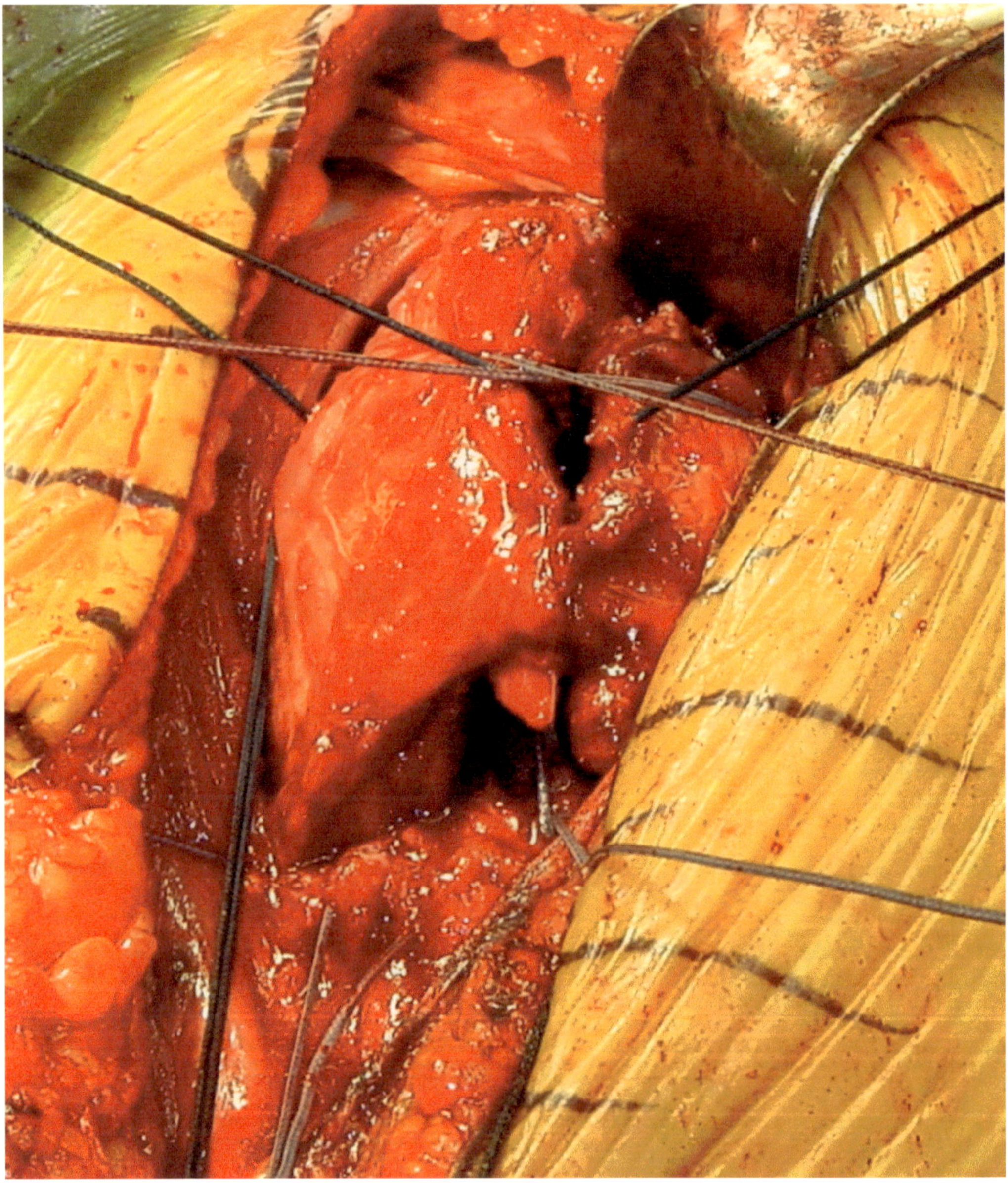

Fig. 14.

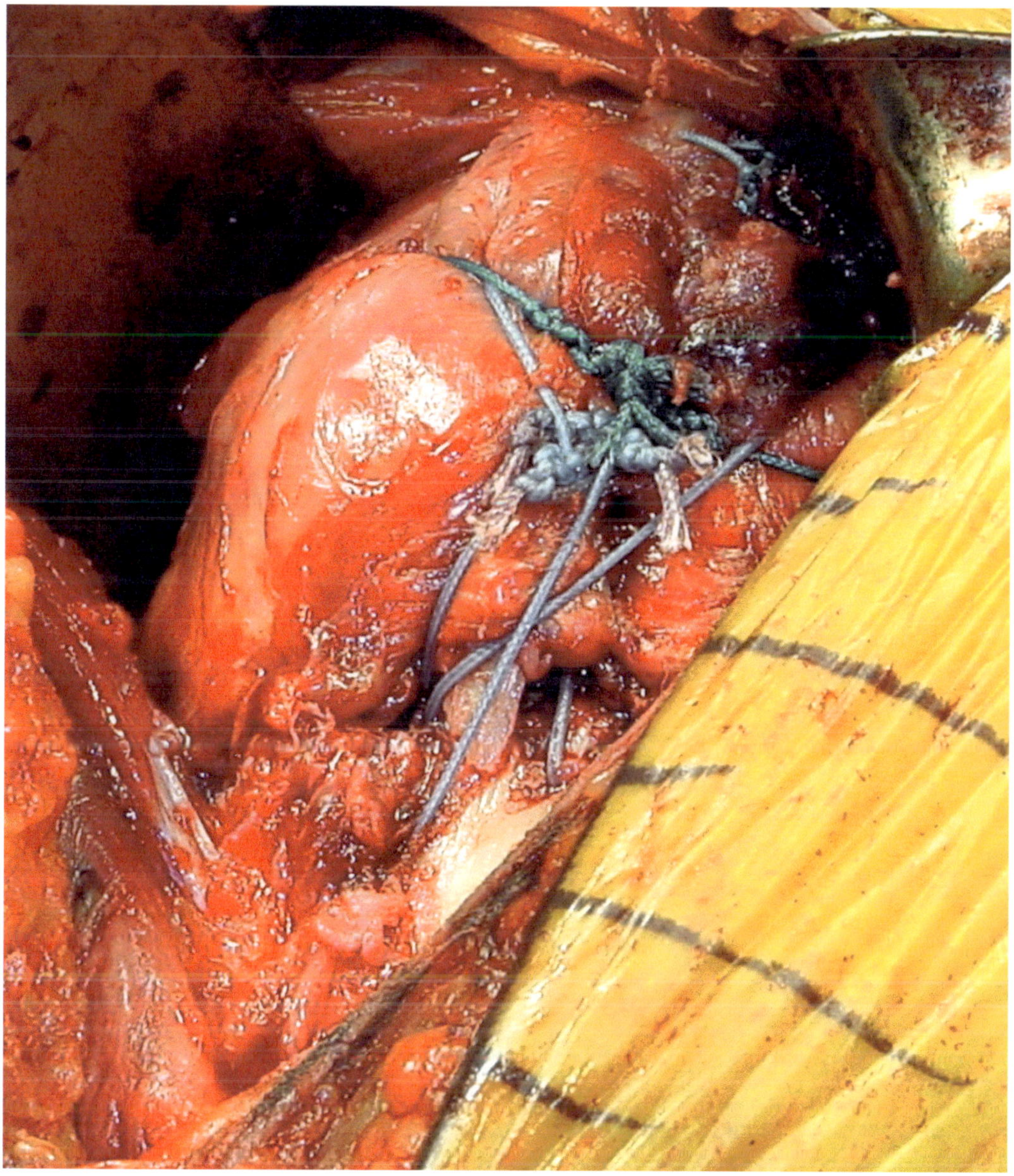

Fig. 15.

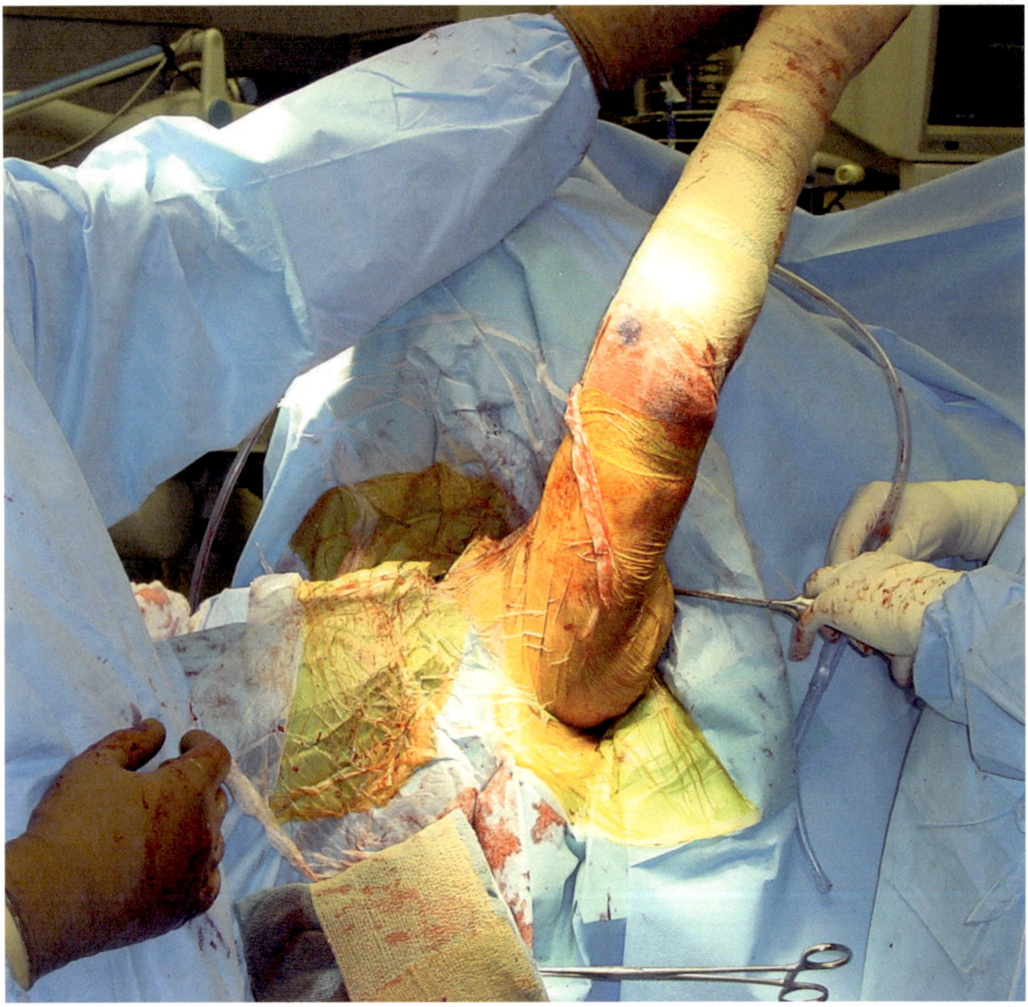

Fig. 16.

2.8 Reverse prosthesis for fracture

Indications for the use of the reverse total shoulder arthroplasty in the management of displaced proximal humerus fractures is in evolution. This prosthesis is generally not recommended in younger patients and it's use has most often been reported in patients around the age of 70. It should be considered in cases with a relatively poor prognosis with use of the humeral head replacement including elderly patients (›75), patients with pre-existing large rotator cuff tears, and patients whose fracture care has been delayed. These patients are at particular risk for poor tuberosity healing (Boileau et al 2002). Use has been spurred by variability in functional results of the humeral head replacement in the management of these complex fractures. The technique of reverse prosthesis in this situation is relatively straightforward (Wall & Walch 2007). The dissection up to removal of the humeral head is identical to that described previously for standard humeral head replacement. The deltopectoral approach is preferred over the superior approach for this indication as it permits easier rehabilitation and allows the surgeon to address any distal humeral shaft comminution that may be present. The exposure of the glenoid is easier than usual as the tuberosities are displaced away from the shaft and the glenoid can be clearly visualized at the time of surgery. The capsule and labrum are released from the glenoid to allow clear exposure of the glenoid rim. The glenoid is reamed according to the specifications of the particular prosthesis. The glenoid baseplate is placed slightly inferiorly and inclined caudally to help avoid notching of the lateral scapular border. Standard placement of the glenosphere is indicated. Humeral stem placement is dictated by soft tissue tension as in standard cases. Minimal or no pistoning of the stem relative to glenosphere should be present with adequate tension across the deltoid. Tension on the tuberosities will also influence the determination of stem height. Version is generally recommended at 0-20° of retroversion but can be altered to allow for optimal tuberosity reduction. In cases in which the supraspinatus is still attached to the greater tuberosity, the tendon insertion may require release in order to mobilize the tuberosity distally enough to reach the shaft and prosthesis. Similar suture fixation is recommended with cerclage sutures between the tuberosities and the prosthesis as well as the vertically aligned sutures diagonally between the shaft and the greater and lesser tuberosities. (Figure 17[a] and 17[b]) Prostheses with proximal ingrowth may help tuberosity union. Tuberosity repair should decrease incidence of prosthetic instability and allow improved external rotation postoperatively. Currently limited information as to the benefits of tuberosity healing is available in this setting (Bufquin et al 2007). Following tuberosity fixation with either the reverse prosthesis or standard humeral head replacement, suction drainage in indicated to avoid hematoma formation. The deltopectoral interval is closed and the skin is closed in a layered fashion.

Postoperative rehabilitation is geared toward allowing adequate tuberosity healing while helping the patient to regain flexibility in a reasonable and safe fashion. During the first six weeks following surgery the tuberosities are vulnerable to avulsion from active use or extreme range of motion with passive stretching. A protective ultrasling is indicated for the first six weeks following surgery holding the arm in neutral rotation to limit tension on the greater tuberosity fragment. The patient is allowed to perform gentle pendulum exercises with passive external rotation exercises utilizing a stick. Range of motion exercises of the elbow, wrist, and fingers are encouraged with gentle active use of these joints.

Once tuberosity healing can be verified radiographically, active use of the arm can be instituted. This typically occurs at approximately six weeks following surgery. Active-assisted exercises are begun in the supine position along with passive stretching under the supervision of a physical therapist. Light activities of daily living are allowed with the elbow at the side with progression of this as active function increases. Between weeks 6 and 12, exercises are characterized by gentle stretching with isometric strengthening for muscle reeducation. Beginning at 12 weeks, a resistive exercise program can be started below shoulder level with advancement to above shoulder exercises once the patient's strength increases.

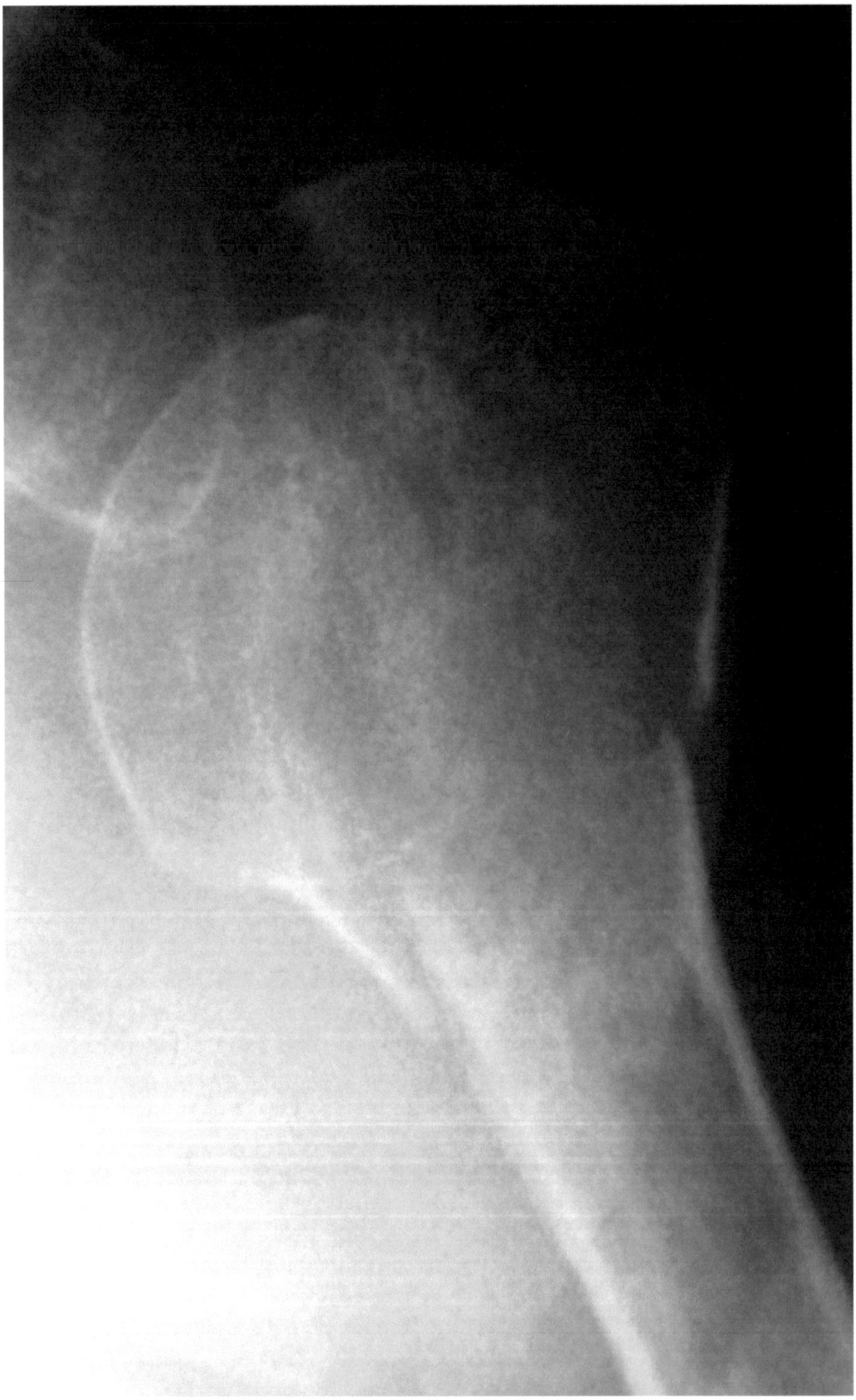

Fig. 17a.

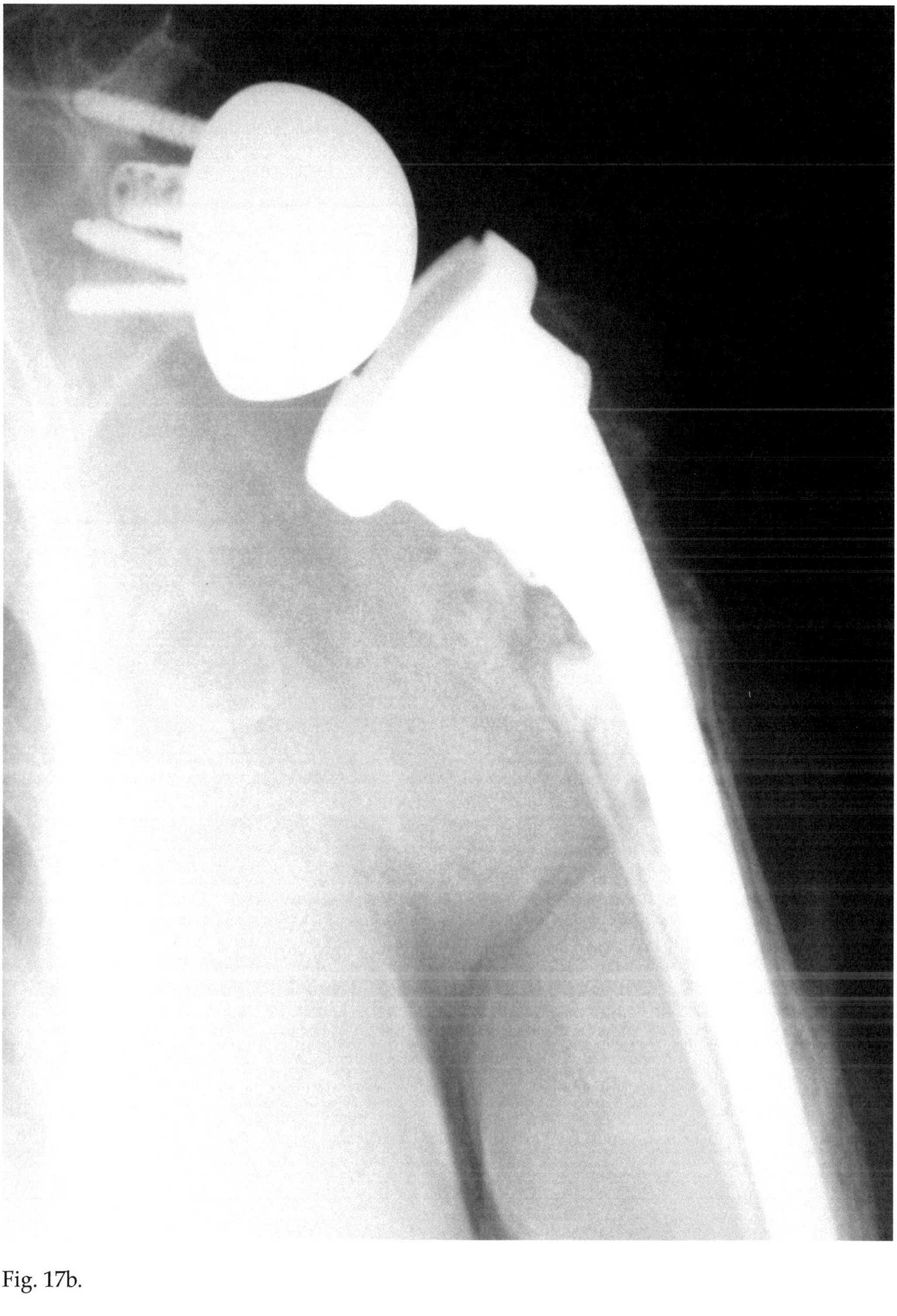

Fig. 17b.

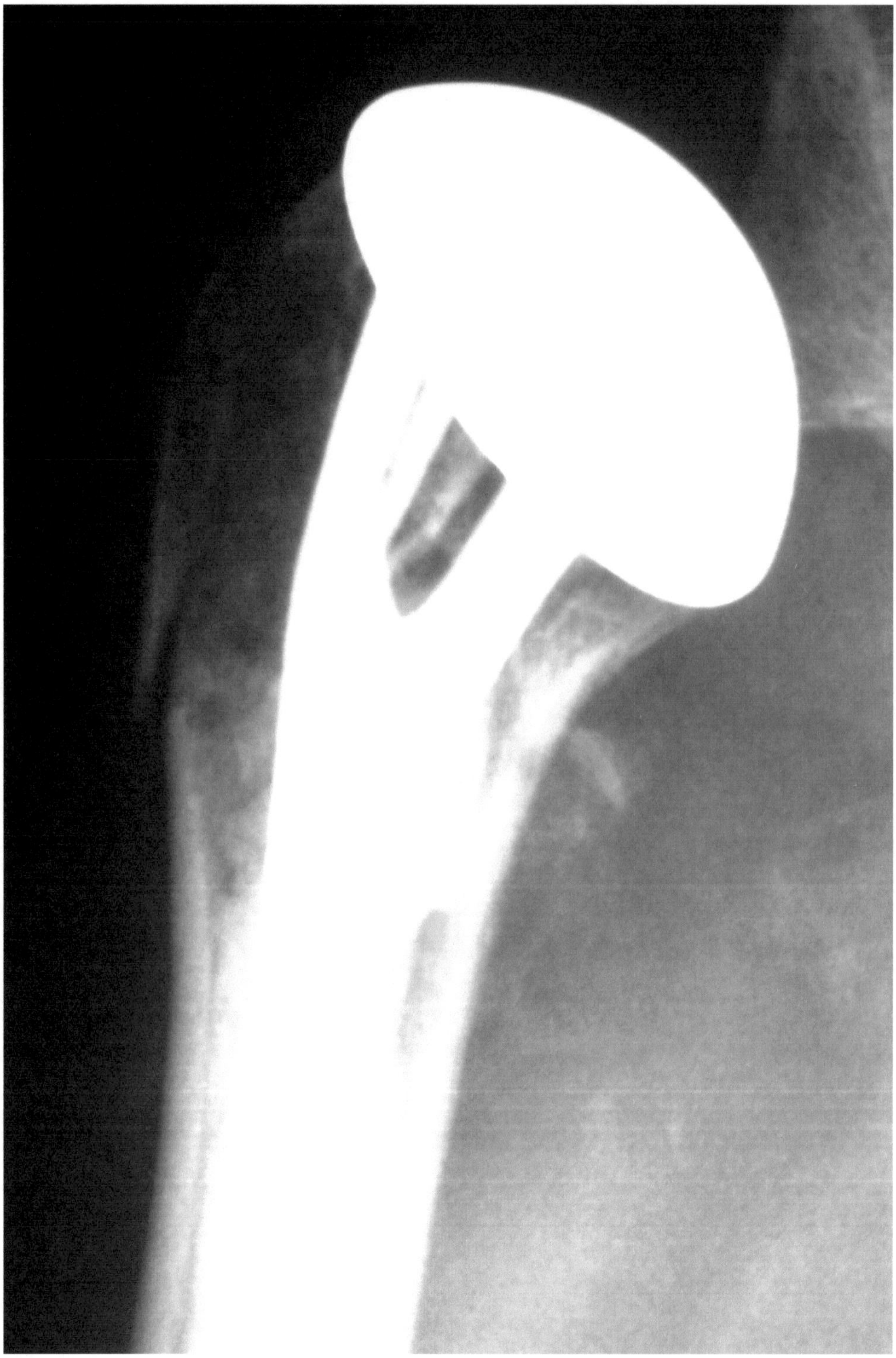

Fig. 18.

3. Results

Complex displaced three and four-part fractures, fracture-dislocations, and fractures with a humeral head split are at risk for the development of malunion and osteonecrosis, especially after internal fixation. Shoulder hemiarthroplasty or, recently, reverse total shoulder arthroplasty is indicated for the treatment of some of these complex fractures (Voos et al 2010).

In spite of advanced patient age, tuberosity healing can be achived by reattachment and bone grafting around specific Reverse Fracture prosthesis, according to Boileau et al. Successful peri-prosthetic tuberosity healing is associated with restoration of both active elevation and external rotation (Boileau et al 2010). (Figure 18)

3.1 Pain relief

Pain relief is the most predictable outcome following hemiarthroplasty for four-part proximal humerus fractures. Many authors have supported this finding, with 61% to 97% of patients reporting complete patiens reporting pain relief. Significant resifual pain generally tends to be associated with moderate activity; minimal pain occurs at rest. Even when motion and functional results are limited, pain relief is reported to be consistent (Young et al 2010).

3.2 Patient satisfaction

Reports of patient satisfaction vary widely, from 58% to 92,% , in part because of the numerous scales used to mesure outcome and satisfaction. High satisfaction rates seem to correlate more with pain relief than with range of motion or functional outcomes. Even studies with poor functional results report high patient satisfaction if pain relief is acceptable (Young et al 2010).

3.3 Prognostic factors

Patient age has been shown to be predictive of outcome. Younger patients have improved results, gaining more rang of motion and a higher level of functional return. These improved results are attributed, in part, to motivation and compliance with postoperative rehabilitation and a more structurally intact rotator cuff.

Another prognostic factor is the delay between injury and surgery. A long delay between the time of injury and surgery has been shown to result in poorer postoperative range of motion and decreased functional outcomes. Although the time frames vary across studies, surgery within 1 week of injury seems to be associated with improved outcomes.

Other preoperative factors that correlate with a poor result are preoperative neurologic deficit, a history of cigarette smoking, excesve alcohol consumption, and female sex. Poorer results associated with the latter are somewhat controversial because in the studies that identified ths finding, women were significantly older than men, which is a significant contounding variable.

Tuberosity position and healing may be the most important factors in determining outcome. Greater tuberosity malunion is the most common complication associated with hemiarthroplasty for four-part proximal humerus fractures. Final tuberosity position of more than 5 mm above or more than 10 mm below the prosthetic head is associated with poor results. A final position of more than 2 cm below the prosthetic humeral head also has been associated with a poor functional result. The best range of motion has been reported to occur if the tuberosity is between 10 and 16 mm below the humeral head. Although these results differ somewhat, a nonanatomic final positiion of the tuberosity generally is believed to interfere with rotator cuff function and compromise range of motion and function. Lesser tuberosity malunion has received much less attention as a factir affecting outcome and does not appear to be as significant as greater tuberosity position (Zuckerman & Sajadi 2007).

Studying the clinical and radiologic parameters that can explain unsatisfactory results, final tuberosity malposition correlates with unsatisfactory results as well as superior migration of the prosthesis, poor position of the greater tuberosity and women over age 75 years (likely with osteopenic bone) (Boileau et al 2002).

At least five compelling reasons exist to reattach the tuberosities and obtain bone healing when performing a reverse shoulder prosthesis: 1) humeral length is restored and thus the deltoid is tensioned optimally; 2) joint stability is improved as a function of the restored humeral length and reconstructed anterior and posterior soft tissue walls; 3) the risk of of infection is reduced as the subacromial dead-space is minimised and the surrounding soft-tissues are better vascularised. 4) better primary implant stability reduces the probability of humeral implant loosening and 5) active (specifically external) rotation is restored, crucial for activities of daily living in elderly patients (Boileau et al 2010).

3.4 Avoiding pitfalls and complications

Complications following hemiarthroplasty for acute proximal humerus fractures include infection, neurologic injury, preiprosthetic fracture, instability, tuberosity malunion and nonunion, rotator cuff tear, heterotopic ossification, glenoid erosion, and stiffness. Although the incidence of any specific complication is relatively low, the cumulative incidence represents at least 15%.

The incience of infection and wound healing problems is about 4% and includes acute postoperative infections and subacute delayed presentations within 6 months of the procedure. Factors that increase the risk of infection include the need for a second operation performed within a short period of time and a compromise immune system. Preventing infection requires meticulous attention to surgical preparation and drapping, particularly because of the potential contamination from the axilla. Perioperative antibiotics are indicated. Meticulous handling of soft tissues also is important. The fact that these injures occur more commonly in enderly patients whose tissues are more sensitive to injury and surgery further emphasizes its importance. If wound problems develop early in the postoperative course, treatment should be aggresive, including additional antibiotics and surgical debridement, if necessary (Young et al 2010).

Instability following hemiarthroplasty also can be a significant problem. The definition of instability varies widely, which affects the reported incidence of this problem. Several factors predispose patients to the development of instability, including component malposition, rotator cuff compromise, and tuberosity problems. Of these, component malposition is a critically important predisposing factor. Instability may result if the humeral component is placed too high or too low, resulting in secondary impingement or poor soft-tissue tension, respectively. Improper placement of the component in excessive anteversion or retroversion may lead to dislocation and tuberosity failure (Voos et al 2010).

If the component is placed in an incorrect amount of version or if humeral length is not properly restored, the risk of instability is greater. Careful attention to positioning the component intraoperatively and managining that position during cementing is essential. Inserting the component in proper version requires the use of consistent landmarks. Obtaining proper version and length during cementing can be difficult; therefore, we find the use of intraoperative fracture jigs to be beneficial. Component malposition can be prevented if a reliable method to obtain and mantain malposition during insertion is used. We believe that cemented fixation of these components is mandatory to mantain position, particularly in the absense of mataphyseal bony support (Young et al 2010).
The so-called "unhappy triad," involves prosthesis with excessive height and retroversion and the greater tuberosity is positioned too low. This combination was frequently associated with poor functional results and persistent pain and stiffness. Studies have also demonstrated that acute reconstruction (less than four weeks after the injury) results in better functional outcomes because of the ease of tuberosity reconstruction (Boileau et al 2000).
Rotator cuff compromise also causes instablity and usually develops as a result of tuberosity compromise. Preventing this problem requires secure fixation and proper positioning of the tuberosity. If the tuberosity becomes detached, particularly in the early postoperative period, instability often can result. Detachment of the lesser tuberosity compromises anterior support and can result in anterior instability (Young et al 2010).
Detachment of the greater tuberosity can result in significant superior and anterior instability. Although posterior instability can occur, it is less common. Factors that predispose patients to tuberosity detachment are inadequate tuberosity fixation and noncompliance with the postoperative rehabilitation. Secure tuberosity fixation and reattachment using the priciples (transverse, longitudinal, and cerclage fixation) will decrease the risk of fixation failure. A supervised, structured rehabilitaion program also can limit the potential for patient noncompliance. The treatment of instability following tuberosity failure can be difficult. If detachment is identified early, reattachment should be considered. Tuberositiy detachment identified more than 6 months after surgery is more probelmatic. Mobilization and attachment of tuberosities can be quite difficult at this time. If the patient reports significant pain and demonstrates instability, the revision surgery, possibly to a reverse shoulder arthroplasty, may be necessary.
Tuberosity nonunion is another significant complication following hemiarthroplasty. The factors that predispose patients to nonunion are related to the method of reattachment, particularly the ability to obtain proper reduction and secure fixation. The quality of bone and soft tissue also affect fixation. The significance of tuberosity nonunion can vary, but generally relates to the degree of migration and displacement. Limited amounts of migration and displacement frequently result in weakness and limited motion but not instability. With significant displacement, the patient will demonstrate weakness and limited motion, as well as instability and pain. The best approach to prevent tuberosity nonunion is use of an optimal method of reattachment.
Malunion of the greater or lesser tuberosity can occur, although probably with less frequency than nonunion. Malunion usually occurs as a result of either inadequate reduction at the time of surgery or inadequate fixation, which allows migration of the fragment with healing into a malunited position. Thus, proper positioning of the tuberosity

intraoperatively is mandatory to avoid these problems. If necessary, intraoperative radiographs should be obtained to confirm the position. Radiographs also should be obtained early in the postoperative period to ensure that migration has not occurred. Malunion of the greater tuberosity is a much more significant problem than that of the lesser tuberosity. Posterior or superior displacement of the greater tuberosity restricts motion and can be a source of pain. Treatment of tuberosity malunion depends on functional significance. If significant pain and limited motion can be attributed to tuberosity malunion, surgical management consisting of osteotomy, mobilization, and reattachment to a more anatomic position can be considered. If the component is not in an optimal position, the component revision may be necessary. These procedures tend to be difficult and, clearly, the most effective treatment of tuberosity malunion is prevention.

Heterotopic ossification following hemiarthroplasty for acute fractures is relatively common, although it generally is not clinically significant. Small areas of heterotopic ossification an reactive bone can develop, but these generally do not interfere with function or compromise outcomes. However, more extensive ossification, particularly in the subacromial space, or bone bridging from the acromion to the proximal humerus can be significant. The factors that predispose to clinically heterotopic ossification include high-energy injuries (fracture-dislocations) and delays in surgery longer than 10 to 14 days after the acute injury. Heterotopic ossification also can develop when the procedure is performed after an early failure of internal fixation. The second procedure, particularly when it is performed 2 to 4 weeks after the initial procedure, carries a signinficant increased risk of heterotopic ossification. Whenever possible, it is important to take measures to prevent the formation of heterotopic bone. At the time of the initial surgery, meticulous technique to minimize soft-tissue trauma is important. The timing of surgery also is important. Whenever possible, the "at risk" period should be avoided. For those patients who are felt to be at high risk for heterotopic bone development, prophylactic measures can be considered, including anti-inlammatory medications postoperatively and/or the use of single-dose radiation therapy. The use of preventive measures has to be balanced with the potential to interfer with tuberosity healing and should be individualized for each patient (Young et al 2010).

Plausinis et al reported the complicationes that took place after humeral head replacement and included infection, neurologic injury, intraoperative fracture, instability, tuberosity malunion and nonunion, rotator cuff tear, heterotopic ossification, glenoid erosion, and stiffness. When technical factors such as tuberosity malunion or component malpositioning are considered as postoperative complications, the incidence of complications is relatively high (Plausinis et al 2005).

Cazeneuve et al described the clinical and radiological outcome of 36 fractures at a mean of 6.6 years (1 to 16) in which the mean Constant score was 58.5 and was reduced to 53 points with the further follow-up. A total of 23 patients (63%) had radiological evidence of loosening of the glenoid component. Nevertheless, only one patient had aseptic loosening of the baseplate at 12 years' follow-up (Cazeneuve et al 2010).

Wall et al reported a series of 186 with 191 retained reverse total shoulder arthroplasty prostheses who were followed for an average of 39.9 months. Overall, the average Constant score improved from 23 points before surgery to 60 points at the time of follow-up and 173 of the 186 patients were satisfied or very satisfied with the result. Dislocation (fifteen cases) and infection (eight cases) were the most common complications among the 199 shoulders that were followed for two years or were revised prior to the minimum two-year follow-up. Patients who received the reverse prosthesis at the time of a revision arthroplasty had a higher complication rate than did those who received the reverse prosthesis at the time of a primary arthroplasty. The most common complications were dislocation (fifteen cases; prevalence, 7.5%) and infection (eight cases; prevalence, 4.0%). Glenoid fractures, postoperative humeral fractures, symptomatic hardware, musculocutaneous nerve palsy, radial nerve palsy, glenoid sphere loosening, and glenoid base loosening also occurred in five or fewer cases each (Wall & Walch 2007).

To evaluate functional outcome after hemiarthroplasty for displaced proximal humeral fractures and to review whether prosthesis type, intraoperative technique or previous ipsilateral shoulder surgery could affect the outcome, Fallatah et al reviewed the medical records and radiographs of patients who had undergone hemiarthroplasty for proximal humeral fractures between 1992 and 2000. They concluded that soft tissue status and operative technique played an important role in late postoperative pain and range of motion. Hemiarthroplasty after failed open reduction and internal fixation is associated with inferior results (Fallatah et al 2008).

In the retrospective study of Gallinet D et al, forty patients were treated by shoulder replacement for three- or four-part displaced fractures of the proximal humerus between 1996 and 2004. Twenty-one had a hemiarthroplasty and 19 were treated by reverse prosthesis. The reverse prosthesis group showed better results in terms of abduction, anterior elevation and Constant score. Rotation was better in the hemiarthroplasty group. They concluded that in three- or four-part displaced proximal humerus fracture, arthroplasty did not ensure recovery of pretrauma shoulder function. Management is therefore to be decided in terms of outcome predictability and rapid recovery of daily comfort for elderly patients (Gallinet et al 2009).

Hemiarthroplasty can provide good functional results, but depends on tuberosity union quality and this often necessitates a prolonged immobilization. Reverse prostheses provide reliable, rapid and predictable results in terms of abduction, anterior elevation and pain relief, but impaired rotation; this impacts quality of life and long-term implant durability (glenoid notching).

Reverse prostheses should thus prove advantageous in the treatment of complex fractures of the proximal humerus if these two drawbacks can be resolved and at present seem indicated on condition that the patient is no younger than 70 years of age (Gallinet et al 2009).

Compito et al reviewed the important factors for a successful outcome, including gentle soft tissue technique, secure placement of the prosthesis with proper version and height, secure tuberosity reconstruction, meticulous rotator cuff repair, and a motivated patient who is able to understand and perform the rigorous postoperative rehabilitation. Unsatisfactory results are associated with tuberosity detachment, prosthetic loosening, inadequate or noncompliant rehabilitation, preoperative nerve injury, humeral malposition, dislocation, deep infection, and ectopic hone formation (Compito et al 1994).

On the basis of the current literature, Voos et al list arthroplasties for the treatment of complex proximal humeral fractures in descending order with regard to their clinical success as follows: (1) hemiarthroplasty in a patient with reconstructible tuberosities, (2) reverse total shoulder arthroplasty in a patient with reconstructible tuberosities, (3) reverse

total shoulder arthroplasty in a patient without reconstructible tuberosities, and (4) hemiarthroplasty in a patient without reconstructible tuberosities (Voos et al 2010).
This review covers the indications, technique, results, and complications associated with the use of prostheses for proximal humeral fractures. Meticulous technique, especially in regards to tuberosity fixation, is necessary for successful reconstruction. The use of the Reverse Total Shoulder prosthesis is in evolution but does offer exciting options in the management of these difficult patients (Voos et al 2010).

4. References

[1] Antuña SA, Sperling JW, Cofield RH. Shoulder hemiarthroplasty for acute fractures of the proximal humerus: a minimum five-year follow-up. J Shoulder Elbow Surg. 2008;17(2):202-9.
[2] Bastian JD, Hertel R. Osteosynthesis and hemiarthroplasty of fractures of the proximal humerus: Outcomes in a consecutive case series. J Shoulder Elbow Surg 2009;19:216-219.
[3] Bigliani LU. Fractures of the proximal humerus. In: Rockwood CA, Green DP, eds. Fractures in Adults. 3rd ed. Philadelphia, Pa: JB Lippincott Completed/mh; 1990:871-927.
[4] Boileau P, Krishnan SG, Tinsi L, et al. Tuberosity malposition and migration: Reasons for poor outcomes after hemiarthroplasty fro displaced fractures of the proximal humerus. J Shoulder Elbow Surg 2002;11(5): 401-412.
[5] Boileau P, Trojani C, Walch G, Krishnan SG, Romeo A, Sinnerton R. Shoulder arthroplasty for the treatment of the sequelae of fractures of the proximal humerus. J Shoulder Elbow Surg 2001;10:299-308.
[6] Boileau P, Walch G, Krishnan SG. Tuberosity osteosynthesis and hemiarthoplasty for four-part fractures of the proximal humerus. Tech Shoulder Elbow Surg 2000;1:96-109.
[7] Boileau P, Moineau N, Brassart, Clavert, Favard L, Sirveaux F, O´Shea K. Reverse Shoulder Fracture-Prosthesis for the treatment of proximal humeral fractures in elderly patients. Shoulder Concepts 2010:231-43.
[8] Bufquin T, Hersan A, Hubert L, Massin P. Reverse shoulder arthroplasty for the treatment of three- and four-part fractures of the proximal humerus in the elderly: a prospective review of 43 cases with a short-term follow-up. J Bone Joint Surg. 2007 Apr;89(4):516-20.
[9] Cazeneuve JF, Cristofari DJ. The reverse shoulder prosthesis in the treatment of fractures of the proximal humerus in the elderly. J Bone Joint Surg. 2010;92(4):535-9.
[10] Compito CA, Self EB, Bigliani LU. Arthroplasty and acute shoulder trauma. Reasons for success and failure. Clin Orthop 1994;307:27-36.
[11] Demirhan M, Kilicoglu O, Altinel L, Eralp L, Akalin Y. Prognostic factors in prosthetic replacement for acute proximal humerus fractures. J Orthop Trauma 2003;17(3):181-189.
[12] Duralde XA, Leddy LR. The results of ORIF of displaced unstable proximal humeral fractures using a locking plate. J Shoulder Elbow Surg 2010;19:480-488.

[13] Esen E, Dogramaci Y, Gultekin S, Deveci MA, et al. Factors affecting results of patients with humeral proximal end fractures undergoing primary hemiarthroplasty: A restrospective study in 42 patients. Injury 2009;40:1336-1341.

[14] Fallatah S, Dervin GF, Brunet JA, Conway AF, Hrushowy H. Functional outcome after proximal humeral fractures treated with hemiarthroplasty. Can J Surg. 2008;51(5):361-5.

[15] Flatow EL, Bigliani LU. Locating and protecting the axillary nerve in the shoulder surgery; the Tug Test. Orthop Rev. 1992;21:503-505.

[16] Frankle M, Siegal S, Pupello D, et al. The reverse shoulder prosthesis for glenohumeral arthritis associated with severe rotator cuff deficiency. A minimum two-year follow-up study of sixty patients. J Bone Joint Surg Am 2005;87(8):1697-1705.

[17] Frankle MA, Ondrovic LE, Markee BA, Harris ML, Lee WE 3rd. Stability of tuberosity reattachment in proximal humeral hemiarthroplasty. J Shoulder Elbow Surg 2002;11(5):413-420.

[18] Frankle MA, Greenwald DP, Markee BA, Ondrovic LE, Lee WE 3rd. Biomechanical effects of malposition of tuberosity fragments on the humeral prosthetic reconstruction for four-part proximal humerus fractures. J Shoulder Elbow Surg 2001;10(4):321-326.

[19] Gallinet D, Clappaz P, Garbuio P, Tropet Y, Obert L. Three or four parts complex proximal humerus fractures: hemiarthroplasty versus reverse prosthesis: a comparative study of 40 cases. Orthop Traumatol Surg Res. 2009 Feb;95(1):48-55.

[20] Goldman RT, Koval KJ, Cuomo F, et al. Functional outcomes after humeral head replacement for acute three and four-part proximal humerus fractures. J Shoulder Elbow Surg 1995;4:81-86.

[21] Green A, Bamard L, Limbrid RS. Humeral head replacement for acute, four-part proximal humerus fractures. J Shoulder Elbow Surg 1993;2:249-254.

[22] Hawkins RJ, Switlyk P. Acute prosthetic replacement for severe fractures of the proximal humerus. Clin Orthop 1993;289:156-160.

[23] 23 Huffman GR, Itamura JM, McGarry MH, Duong L, et al. Neer Award 2006: Biomechanical assessment of inferior tuberosity placement during hemiarthroplasty for four-part proximal humeral fractures. J Shoulder Elbow Surg 2008;17(2):189-196.

[24] Jaberg H, Warner JJ, Jakob RP. Percutaneous stabilization of unstable fractures of the humerus. J Bone Joint SUrg Am 1992;74:508-515.

[25] Kontakis G, Koutras C. Tosounidis T, Giannoudis P. Early management of proximal humeral fractures with hemiarthroplasty. J Bone Joint Surg (Br) 2008;90B(11):1407-1413.

[26] Lervick GN, Carroll RM, Levine WN. Complications after hemiarthroplasty for fractures of the proximal humerus. Instr Course Lect. 2003;52:3-12.

[27] Levine WN, Connor PM, Yamaguchi K, Self EB, et al. Humeral head replacement for proximal humeral fractures. Orthopedics 1998;21(1):68-73

[28] Martin TG, Iannotti JP. Reverse total shoulder arthroplasty for acute fractures and failed management after proximal humeral fractures. Orthop Clin North Am. 2008;39(4):451-7.

[29] Mighell MA, Kolm GP, Colinge CA, Frankle MA. Outcomes of hemiarthroplasty for fractures of the proximal humerus. J Shoulder Elbow Surg 2003;12:569-577.

[30] Moeckel BH, Dines DM, Warren RF, Altchek DW. Modular hemiarthroplasty for fractures of the proximal part of the humerus. J Bone Joint Surg Am 1992;74:884-889.
[31] Murachovsky J, Ikemoto RY, Nascimento LG, Milani C, Warner JJ. Pectoralis major tendon reference (PMT): A new method for accurate restoration of humeral length with hemiarthroplasty for fracture. J Shoulder Elbow Surg 2006;15(6):675-678.
[32] Neer CS. Fractures. In: Shoulder Reconstruction. Philadelphia, PA: WB Saunders Co. 1990:363-420.
[33] Neer CS. Displaced proximal humeral fractures, I: classification and evaluation. J Bone Joint Surg Am 1970;52:1077-1089.
[34] Neer CS. Displaced proximal humeral fractures, II: treatment of three-part and four-part displacement. J Bone Joint Surg Am 1970;52:1090-1103.
[35] Pijls BGCW, Werner PH, Eggen PJ. Alternative humeral tubercle fixation in shoulder hemiarthroplasty for fractures of the proximal humerus. J Shoulder Elbow Surg 2010;19:282-289.
[36] Plausins D, Kwon YW, Zuckerman JD. Complications of humeral head replacement for proximal humeral fractures. AAOS Instruc Course 2005;54:371-380.
[37] Reuther F, Mühlhäusler B, Wahl D, Nijs S. Functional outcome of shoulder hemiarthroplasty for fractures: A multicentre analysis. Injury. 2010;41(6):606-12.
[38] Robinson CM, Page RS, Hill RMF, Sanders DL, et al. Primary hemiarthroplasty for treatment of proximal humeral fractures. J Bone Joint Surg 2003;85A (7):1215-1223.
[39] Shrader MW, Sanchez-Sotelo J, Sperling JW, et al. Understanding proximal humerus fractures: image analysis, classification, and treatment. J Shoulder Elbow Surg 2005; 14(5): 497-505.
[40] Tanner MW, Cofield RH. Prosthetic arthroplasty for fractures and fracture-dislocations of the proximal humerus. Clin Orthop 1983;179:116-128.
[41] Voos JE, Dines JS, Dines DM. Arthroplasty for fractures of the proximal part of the humerus. J Bone Joint Surg Am. 2010 Jun;92(6):1560-7.
[42] Wall B, Walch G. Reverse Shoulder Arthroplasty for the Treatment of Proximal Humeral Fractures. Hand Clin 23,2007:425-430.
[43] Young TB, Wallace WA. Conservative treatment of fractures and fracture-dislocations of the upper end of the humerus. J Bone Joint Surg Br 1985;67:373-377.
[44] Zyto K. Non-operative treatment of comminuted fractures of the proximal humerus in elderly patients. Injury 1998;29(5):349-352.
[45] Young SW, Segal BS, Turner PC, Poon PC. Comparison of functional outcomes of reverse shoulder arthroplasty versus hemiarthroplasty in the primary treatment of acute proximal humerus fracture. ANZ J Surg. 2010;80(11):789-93.
[46] Zuckerman JD, Sajadi KR. Proximal Humerus Fractures: Hemiarthroplasty for Four-Part Fractures. Advanced Reconstruction Shoulder. AAOS 2007:30:283-98.

26

Postoperative Therapy for Metacarpophalangeal Arthroplasty

Nicola Massy-Westropp
School of Health Sciences, University of South Australia
Australia

1. Introduction

Since the earliest metacarpophalangeal (MCP) arthroplasties in the 1950s, numerous resurfacing and excisional arthroplasties, and a greater choice of surgical tools and techniques to implant the prostheses have become available. Of the excisional arthroplasties, one piece and two-piece hinge designs, constrained by screws or unconstrained, cemented and non-cemented, have been designed (1) Surgeons now perform these procedures as day surgery, and leave as much original bone as possible in the likelihood of replacing the prosthesis as the patient ages.

At the time of surgery, synovectomy and soft-tissue balancing procedures are often performed to increase lateral joint stability or enhance the biomechanical advantage of the tendons around the operated joint. These procedures may necessitate post-operative immobilisation, specific joint positioning and strict motion protocols to achieve the best soft tissue range of motion and stability around the prosthesis (2-6).

The efficacy of postoperative therapy regimens also requires research, as they affect patient outcome, and are time-consuming and expensive. The aim of this review is to determine which postoperative regimen are most effective in achieving freedom from pain and function, and if any particular regimen is best suited to a specific prosthesis or soft-tissue balancing procedure at the time of surgery.

2. Method

For inclusion in this review, studies had to evaluate the efficacy of a post-arthroplasty regimen for patients who had metacarpophalangeal or joint arthroplasty. Preferred study designs were metanalyses, systematic reviews, and randomised controlled trials, but all published literature except expert opinion was accepted. Patients may have received any type of implant and soft-tissue procedure, due to rheumatoid arthritis, osteoarthritis or trauma.

Electronic databases searched were the Cochrane Musculoskeletal Disease Group Register, The Cochrane Library of Systematic review, Google Scholar, and Scopus. Manual searches included of the Journal of Hand Therapy, Hand Therapy and the Journal of Arthroplasty. Search terms in all combinations included 'joint replacement, hand, wrist metacarpophalangeal, arthroplasty, rehabilitation, post-operative, occupational therapy, physical therapy'. The search included papers from 1990 onward, aiming to find research about currently used prostheses and not prostheses of older designs and materials.

Studies were appraised as described by the Cochrane Collaboration (7) for sources of methodological bias that could decrease the internal validity of a study. The types of methodological bias were in patient selection, equality of treatment, attrition of patients, and detection of all relevant outcomes. If the study could not be fully appraised from the publication, information was sought by writing to the authors.

3. Results

Sixteen studies described post-operative therapy for MCP joint replacement in enough detail to understand the treatment schedule. Four hundred and twenty-seven patients in these studies had rheumatoid arthritis, 19 had osteoarthritis and one had psoriatic arthritis. There were four randomised trials (one about post-operative therapy), three prospective cohort studies, three prospective case series (two about post-operative therapy), one case study about post-operative therapy, and the remaining were retrospective case series. Missing data was obtained from two authors, to assist in reviewing the rigour of the studies, but many authors could not be contacted.

The randomised controlled trial study found to specifically compare post-operative regimes for metacarpophalangeal arthroplasty (8) randomised patients into postoperative therapy groups that both included dynamic splinting, but the treatment group also included continuous passive motion. These researchers found no difference between treatment groups. Thomsen, Boeckstyns and Leth-Espensen(2003) (9) and retrospectively reviewed consectutive patients who had either dynamic MCP extension splinting, or had static splinting that was removed for exercises post-operatively. They found that residual extension lag was significantly less ($p = 0.002$) in the dynamically-splinted group, concluding that postoperative dynamic splinting was useful. Groth, Watkins and Paynter, (1996)(10) retrospectively compared patients who had dynamic flexion with those who had dynamic extension splinting, and found that those who had post-operative dynamic flexion splinting had greater post-operative MCP flexion. Burr, Pratt and Smith (2002)(11), Burr and Pratt (1999)(12) focussed their research on post-operative therapy, but neither study had a comparison treatment group. No further studies compared post-operative treatment regimes, therefore the results of the remaining studies can only be appreciated as a combination of surgery, implant and post-operative therapy.

One outcome common to nearly all postoperative patients in every study was the relief of pain once the diseased joint had been removed by surgery. Negative outcomes such as wound infection, implant loosening and migration were reported, in small proportions. Compliance with splinting and therapy was not discussed. Sixteen studies described the outcome of different implants and postoperative therapy regimes for MCP arthroplasty.

Features common to many regimens (Table 1) were postoperative avoidance of any hand activity for the first three to six weeks and long-term avoidance of ulnar forces on the fingers. Nearly all regimens began between the second and seventh postoperative day.

Regimens could be divided into two main categories with regard to splinting and exercise. Static splint regimens involved removal of the splint for active MCP range of motion exercises, and dynamic splint regimens involved active-assisted MCP extension and active MCP flexion exercises within the splint.

STUDY AND DESIGN	PARTICIPANTS	TREATMENT	OUTCOME	POTENTIAL FOR BIAS
Escott, Ronald, Judd and Bogoch 2010(13) Prospective cohort	N=33 with RA MCP flexion mean 89-91° extension lag mean 61-65°.	Treatment groups had Neuflex or Swanson joint prostheses. Day 4-6 Resting Splint, neutral wrist, 40° MCP flexion, 10-20° Week 1-3 MCP AROM flexion and extension and PROM for wrist and IP Patients were instructed to remove the splint only for ROM exercises during the next 3/52 3/52 PROM MCP flexion and extension of joints 4/52, splint removal for light ADL and ROM Splint wear at times of risk and at night. 6/52 splint at night only, and strengthening initiated Night splinting to minimum of 3/12 Patients educated to avoid positions of deformity.	One Year Outcomes: Both group showed significant improvement in mean Sollerman score and all 6 MHQ domains (p=.001), and MCP extension (mean ROM not provided) Both groups showed significant increases in grip strength improved significantly at the larger Jamar grip position 4 but not smaller positions 2&3 No significant differences between treatment groups, except those with Swanson implants demonstrated higher Michigan Hand Outcomes Questionnaire scores.	Patient selection included highly variable patients Detection of outcome may be inadequate at one year. Detection of outcome may not be powered Detection suffers from no comparison group
Harada, Okumura and Takahashi 2010(14) Retrospective case series	11 patients with RA mean AROM MP 52/95 Mean grip 5.1 kg	Patients had Swanson or Avanta silicone implants. Day 4–5: An outrigger splint was used for MPJ extension. Rubber band was pulled on an angle toward the radial-sided finger. Active flexion and passive extension of MPJ on the outrigger splint was started. 2/52 An outrigger splint was added for MP flexion. Outrigger splints for MP flexion and extension were used alternately every hour and alternately each night. 3–4 /52: Active and gentle passive motion of MPJ. 6 /52: Use of hand in light ADL.	mean follow-up 8.7/12 (4–14) mean AROM MP 5/65 Mean grip 4.9 kg	Patient selection included highly variable patients Detection of outcome may be inadequate at one year. Detection of outcome may not be powered Detection suffers from no comparison group Attrition of patients from series
Chung, Burns, Wilgis, Burke, Regan, Kim and Fox 2009.(15) Prospective cohort	N=70 with RA Michigan Hand Outcome Questionnaire mean score =37/100 (18) Grip=5.7(6) Key Pinch=3.5(2)	Patients had Swanson implants. Day 5-7 Dynamic MCP extension splint all times for 6/52 6/52 light ADL, splint worn in evening only 12/52 splint is discharged, normal ADL allowed.	One Year Outcomes: Michigan Hand Outcome Questionnaire mean score =59/100 (22) Grip=6.2(5) Key Pinch=3.1(2)	Patient selection included highly variable patients Detection of outcome may be inadequate at one year. Detection suffers from no comparison group

STUDY AND DESIGN	PARTICIPANTS	TREATMENT	OUTCOME	POTENTIAL FOR BIAS
Pettersson, Wagnsjo, Hulin 2006(16) Randomised trial	N=40 with RA Mean pain 3.5-4.5/10 Mean extension deficit 51-53° Mean MCP arc of motion = 33°	Patients randomly allocated to have NeuFlex or Sutter implants. Day 0-5 hand immobilised in plaster, only PIP joints free. Day 5 active mobilisation was started 3-5/24. Static splint allowed full PIP ROM, restricted MCP 0- 20°and stabilised the MCP in radial and ulnar deviation and gave volar support for t MCPs 6/52 splint replaced by night extension splint used for the first year to prevent ulnar deviation. Gradually increased motion initiated without radial and ulnar pressure 8/52, daily activities without weight bearing in ulnar direction were allowed. 3/12, no restriction except for ADL or work.	One Year Outcomes Mean pain 2.8-3.5/10 Mean extension deficit 20-21° Mean MCP arc of motion =49°	Patient selection included highly variable patients Detection of outcome may be inadequate at one year. Detection suffers from no comparison group
Nunez and Citron, 2005(17) Case series (uncertain if prospective)	N=seven patients, 10 implants with OA Mean pain = 68%, mean MCP arc of motion = 43°, patient-perceived strength 31%, patient-perceived satisfaction 44%	Patients had Ascension two piece unconstrained prosthesis. First 48 hours Patient asked to flex fingers in post-operative dressing After 48 hours, dressings are removed and patients may use passive assistance to achieve full ROM as soon as possible.	Follow-up one to four years one patient had a slight temporary wound inflammation Mean pain = 3%, mean MCP arc of motion = 52°, patient-perceived strength 86%, patient-perceived satisfaction 93%	Detection of outcome may be inadequate at one year. Detection of outcome may not be powered Detection suffers from no comparison group
Rettig, Luca and Murphy 2005(18) Retrospective case series	N=12 with OA Metacarpophalangeal joint flexion was 53° no excessive MCP ulnar deviation	Patients received Swanson implants, some had grommets over their implants. Day 0 to 3-7 Patients were placed in a bulky wrist, MCP PIP immobilization splint Day 3-7Gentle active extension and flexion commenced Until 6-8/52 night, static extension splint. 4/52 strengthening program.	6-8/52 MCP flexion 59° Nine patients noted excellent overall improvement, three said good overall improvement Nine patients stated excellent pain relief, one patient had good pain relief, and two had satisfactory pain relief. Nine patients 9 reported functional improvement > 75% Seven patients were able to perform the Jebsen-Taylor functional assessment within the normal time.	Detection of outcome may be inadequate at one year. Detection of outcome may not be powered

STUDY AND DESIGN	PARTICIPANTS	TREATMENT	OUTCOME	POTENTIAL FOR BIAS
Moller, Sollerman Geijer, Kopylov and Tagil 2005(19) Randomised trial	N=30 with RA, one psoriatic arthritis Active ROM =32° (range 8–58°) This was assumed to be MCP flexion. Mean MCP Extension deficit= 42-47 (2-85)	Patients randomised to Swanson or Avanta implants Day-7 hand mobilized in a dynamic extension splint, aiming to achieve 45° flexion. Night static palmar splint with MCP slightly flexed. PIP extension splint used if there was tendency to flex PIPs instead of MCPs. 4 /52goal was 70° flexion. If flexion was restricted, a dynamic flexion splint was used. 6/52 light loading permitted, dynamic extension splint weaned 12/52 Splints discharged and loading as permitted by pain.	Two year follow-up Active ROM improved to 42°(range 20–60°) after surgery (p= 0:04) in the Avanta group, whereas no significant improvement was seen in the Swanson group. Mean MCP Extension deficit= 16-19 (1-43)	Patient selection included highly variable patients Detection suffers from no therapy comparison group
Parkkila, Belt, Hakala, Kautiainen and Leppolahti 2005(20) Randomised trial	N=53 patients with RA, 58 hands operated.	Patients randomised to receive Sutter or Swanson prostheses. All received physiotherapy for 2/12, seven having continuous passive motion in and out of hospital. 2/12 five patients had finger manipulation if they were stiff	Four – Five year follow-up Five patients died, one was lost and two had strokes. Six patients (three from each group) had revision surgery. More patients showed osteolysis around the implant, if they had Sutter implants, over Swanson implants.	Patient selection included highly variable patients Attrition of patients Detection suffers from no therapy comparison group
Thomsen, Boeckstyns and Leth-Espensen 2003(21) Retrospective case series	N=22 Pre-operative measures not available	Patients received Swanson implants. **Group 1** Dynamic splint Day 6-4/52 dynamic extension and radial deviation splint used continuously active assisted flexion and passive extension exercises encouraged during the same period. Patients attended physiotherapy 3-5/7. Week 4-6/52 dynamic splint was night only **Group 2** No dynamic splint Day 0-5/7static splinting, exercises as described above were encouraged without the splint, static splint retained between exercises. 2/52 day time static splinting discontinued 2-4/52 night static splinting	**Group 1** Dynamic splint(n = 41) nearly 5 years follow up Extension lag 10 (0–50) Flexion 60 (5–90) Range of movement 45 (5–80) Ulnar deviation 10 (0–30) **Group 2** No dynamic splint (n = 29)) nearly 2 years follow up Extension lag 20 (0–45)* Flexion 60 (30–80) Ulnar deviation 10 (0–20) * p = 0.002	Patient selection may have included highly variable patients-no data Detection of difference in outcome may not be powered Attrition of patients high from both groups

STUDY AND DESIGN	PARTICIPANTS	TREATMENT	OUTCOME	POTENTIAL FOR BIAS
Radmer, Andresen and Sparman 2003 (22) Prospective Case series	N=eight women with RA marked ulnar deviation. mean active flexion = 30 (15–40°) mean extensor lag 55° (40–100)°.	Patients received WEKO hinged implants Day 0 – 2or 3 hand immobilized in palmar forearm plaster splint Day 2-3 – 6/52 dynamic splint. Position not described Exercises for the fingers were performed out of the splint, without restriction. Exercises not described.	One Year Outcomes: 20/28 prostheses had migrated mean active flexion = 30(22–35°) mean extensor lag 42° (40–48)°. average ulnar deviation 20° (0–50)°	Detection of outcome may be inadequate at one year. Detection of outcome may not be powered Detection suffers from no comparison group
Ishikawa, Murasawa and Hanyu 2002(23) Retrospective case series	N=64 with RA, 20 implants into the thumbs Mean MCP flexion= 72-73° Mean MCP extension lag=35-39° Pain=23-28/100	Patients received Swanson implants, some had grommets over their implants. Those with thumb implants received a 'flexible hinge toe implant'. Day0-5 a 'short arm splint' was worn Day 5 – 6/52 dynamic splint (assumed to be MCP extension) with AROM and PROM of MCP joints	Mean follow-up six years 12 revision surgeries Mean MCP flexion= 49-50° Mean MCP extension lag=15-28 Pain=0-6/100	Patient selection included highly variable patients Attrition of patients from series Detection suffers from no therapy comparison group
Burr, Pratt and Smith, 2002 (11) Prospective Case series	n = 15 with RA	Swanson prostheses Day 5-7 – 4/52:Two static splints, alternated 24 hourly, with MCP at 0° in one splint, and 60° flexion in the other. No ADL	Mean MCP flexion unchanged; improvements in pain, MCP extension, and power grip	Detection suffers from no therapy comparison group
Burr and Pratt, 1999 (12) Case study	n = One patient with RA	3/52 biofeedback to finger flexors and extensors no heavy lifting 4/52 IP ROM, MCP flexion , RD 3-10x hourly, 4/52 Light ADL 8/52 normal ADL 12/52 return to work, heavy lifting	At 8/52 0–15° MCP extension and 60–70° MCP flexion at 8/52.	ncies of studies reporting inadequate at 8/52
Ring, Simmons and Hayes, 1998 (8) RCT	n = 25 with RA	"Silicone arthroplasty" Day 2–7 Dynamic MCP extension splint with RD, until 6/52 Night MCP 0° for 12/52 MCP and IP ROM 3 10 every hour 2 hours in splint; RD at 4/52 Treatment group IP ROM, received MCP CPM No pinch for 12/52	at 5/12 CPM group did not achieve significant increases in ROM or strength	Detection of outcome may be inadequate at 5/12 Detection suffers from no therapy comparison group

STUDY AND DESIGN	PARTICIPANTS	TREATMENT	OUTCOME	POTENTIAL FOR BIAS
Groth, Watkins and Paynter, 1996 (10) Retrospective case series	n = 34 patients, 46 hands with RA	Timing not recorded **Treatment group** Dynamic MCP flexion splint Night static splint, MCP 20–30° flexion	Uncertain of follow-up duration Treatment group had significantly more MCP flexion than cohort, but similar MCP extension	Patient selection may have included highly variable patients Selection of patients not described. Attrition of patients from both treatment groups
Stothard, Thompson and Sherris 1991 (Prospective cohort	N=25 patients with RA Mean ulnar deviation preoperatively 34°	Thirteen patients had Swanson MCP implants and crossed intrinsic transfer, 12 patients had MCP implant only. Day 3 static resting hand splint with high ulnar borders for all patients, removed four times daily for active radial deviation, flexion and extension. Day 8-10 PROM ; no further details 3/52 splint worn at night only, light ADL 4/52 commenced occupational therapy, no further details	Follow-up 6-33/12 Five patients lost to follow-up Mean ulnar deviation 8° One infection occurred, one revision required Five patients in each treatment group had occasional pain or pain on use of their hand. Eighteen patients had improved or much improved function, three hand same function and three hand decreased function post-operatively. Crossed intrinsic transfer resulted in greater ROM	Patient selection included highly variable patients Detection of outcome may be inadequate at 6/12 Detection of outcome may not be powered Detection suffers from no therapy comparison group Attrition of patients from series

ADL=Activities of Daily Living, MCP= metacarpophalangeal, IP= interphalangeal joints; RD= radial deviation; RCT= randomized controlled trial; ROM= range of motion, RA=rheumatoid arthritis OA=osteoarthritis

Table 1. Studies reporting post-operative therapy for metacarpophalangeal arthroplasty, their design, treatment protocols, and outcomes.

4. Discussion

Sixteen studies described the outcome of different implants and postoperative therapy regimes for MCP arthroplasty. Two of these studies compared the efficacy of one regimen over another, one of these being prospective. Sambandam, Gul and Priyanka (2007)(25) state that 'most studies undermined the importance of this aspect (post-operative treatment) of the procedure' with regards to first carpometacarpal joint arthroplasty, but their claim could be expanded to arthroplasty of other joints of the hand. Post-operative protocols for splinting, activity and exercises are not always well-described, so although there were numerous studies about MCP arthroplasty, they are not included in this review.

Hand therapy for other conditions such as flexor tendon repair also offers multiple postoperative regimens. For example, healing tendons of the hand usually receive motion, but it may be passive, active, or a combination of all of these. The rationale for the various exercise regimens is based on biological healing of the tendon and the strength of the surgical repair, thus its ability to withstand stress without rupturing or gap formation (26,27). These patients usually have normal anatomy preoperatively, leaving few patient variables. Postoperative therapy regimens for MCP arthroplasty are also based on principles of healing and scar formation, but are not prescribed according to the patient's preoperative hand impairment, the type of implant used, or soft tissue balancing procedures performed. For example, patients having undergone extensor tendon rebalancing and recentralization may benefit from avoidance of passive flexion or avoidance of the extremes of flexion, much like a postoperative extensor tendon repair regime. The literature suggests that postoperative therapy for MCP arthroplasty has not been prescribed in this manner; rather, standard protocols have been designed and applied to consecutive patients.

To compare the efficacy of a new protocol, many patients would be required for allocation to various postoperative therapy groups. Their outcomes would have to be analyzed according to what protocol they received with the implant, surgery, and preoperative status as variables. The first difficulty in forming control or comparison groups lies in the infrequency of this procedure; for example Ring et al.(8) took three years to include 25 hands in their study.

The most common source of bias in the studies was selection bias, which occurs when patients are chosen for treatment or control groups as a result of characteristics that are expected to affect their outcome. Randomization is designed to control the confounding effects of differences between subjects at baseline, and the randomized trial is recommended as the best method of determining treatment efficacy. Here lies the second difficulty in forming control or comparison groups. Patients undergo MCP arthroplasty at all stages of their disease, evidenced by the wide range of motion deficits between the studies of Burr and Pratt, in which the case study patient had nearly normal preoperative MCP motion, and Burr et al., in which some patients had only 25° of MCP flexion, Measures of pain also varied widely in the latter study, ranging from "zero" to "eight out of ten." These baseline measurements demonstrate the difficulty in obtaining a homogeneous, comparable group of patients with rheumatoid arthritis.

The other three sources of bias described by the Cochrane Collaboration(7) were present in the reviewed studies. Performance bias occurs when patients receive a variation in duration, quality, or quantity of the treatment being studied, which was suspected in the continuous passive motion (CPM) study by Ring et al. Ring et al. describe the application of CPM in detail, except passive forces are described as "low" and treatment quantity is described as "as tolerated." As a result, the reader remains unsure of what amount of passive force is ineffective, as well as what quantity of treatment per day is ineffective.

Detection bias is determined if the timing of assessment, the outcome assessment used, or knowledge of the assessor of the patient's previous state could miss any relevant aspect of the outcome. This may have occurred in the study by Groth et al.,(10) in which some preoperative data were unavailable and patients were assessed at different postoperative time frames. Detection and comparison of outcomes between studies are only possible when the same outcome measures are used in a standardized manner. The researchers in this review all measured range of motion, but at different time frames (Table 1). Those who measured pain, cosmesis, and function applied different assessments at different time frames. The challenge of outcome measurement in rheumatology has led to the formation of focus groups such as OMERACT (Outcome Measures in Rheumatoid Arthritis Clinical Trials), who have made recommendations for outcome measures to be used in drug trials. OMERACT recommendations are not fully relevant to hand therapy research; however, the process of forming a focus group, and the development of assessment guidelines that allow comparison between homogeneous patients, is possible (28).

Attrition bias is determined if the loss of patients in the study is significant or varies between the treatment and control groups. This is common in long-term studies involving patients with rheumatoid arthritis, and was experienced by Groth et al.,(10) who were unable to obtain long-term follow-up of the patient group who received their extension protocol. Long-term follow-up is an issue with rheumatoid populations. These patients undergo numerous surgical and drug interventions, while their disease progresses and fluctuates, making the long-term effects of the MCP surgery and therapy difficult to define. Once more, large numbers of patients in each treatment group would be required to decrease the effects of attrition bias and to dilute the effects of subsequent interventions.

The difficulties of past studies guide the planning of future studies. Although the issues of low patient numbers, variable preoperative status, additional surgical and drug interventions, and chronic disease cannot be altered, study designs can. Large randomized trials may not be possible; however, samples of patients, paired according to preoperative status, may be allocated to different treatment protocols. Standardized measurement of pain, cosmesis, impairment, disability, and impact on the patient, made at similar postoperative time frames, would further assist in determining treatment efficacy.

5. Conclusion

This review suggests that *all* regimens contribute toward an increase in MCP motion and an increase in hand function, but despite the efforts of patients and clinicians, hand therapists remain unaware of the most effective postoperative protocol for MCP arthroplasty or the suitability of each regimen for specific implants and soft-tissue procedures. Difficulties in researching this topic include low patient numbers, highly variable preoperative status, lack of guidelines for outcome measures and time frames, and the effects of subsequent interventions received by the patient. The nature and size of the population with rheumatoid arthritis and MCP arthroplasty do not readily fit the randomized, controlled trial design. Paired sample designs are suggested, as well as the formation of standard outcome measures, for better comparison of results between patients.

6. References

[1] Krishnan J. The Biomechanical and Anatomical Basis for the Design of a New MCP Joint Prosthesis: [doctoral thesis], Australia: Flinders University School of Biomedical Engineering, 1998.

[2] Beevers DJ, Seedhom BB. Metacarpophalangeal joint prostheses. J Hand Surg. 1995;20B:125-36.

[3] Swanson AB. Silicone rubber implants for replacement of arthritic or destroyed joints in the hand. Surg Clin North Am. 1972;48:1113-27.

[4] Beiber EJ, Weiland AJ, Violenec-Dowling S. Silicone-rubber implant arthroplasty of the metacarpophalangeal joints for rheumatoid arthritis. J Bone Joint Surg [Am]. 1986;68:206-9.

[5] Pereira JA, Belcher HJCR. A comparison of metacarpophalangeal joint silastic arthroplasty with or without crossed intrinsic transfer. J Hand Surg. 2001;26B:229-34.

[6] Madden JW, De Vore G, Arem AJ. A rational post-operative program for metacarpophalangeal joint implant arthroplasty. J Hand Surg. 1977;2A:358-66.

[7] Clarke M, Oxman AD (eds). Cochrane Reviewers' Handbook 4.1.4. Oxford: The Cochrane Library, issue 4, update software, 2001.

[8] Ring D, Simmons BP, Hayes M. Continuous passive motion following metacarpophalangeal joint arthroplasty. J Hand Surg. 1998;23A:505–11.

[9] Thomsen NOB, Boeckstyns MEH and Leth-Espensen P. Value of dynamic splinting after replacement of the Metacarpophalangeal joint in patients with rheumatoid arthritis. Scand J Plast Reconstr Surg Hand Surg 2003; 37: 113–116.

[10] Groth G, Watkins M, Paynter P. Effect of an alternative flexion splinting protocol on mid-joint ROM [letter]. J Hand Ther. 1996;9:68-9.

[11] Burr N, Pratt AL, Smith PJ. An alternative splinting and rehabilitation protocol for metacarpophalangeal joint arthroplasty in patients with rheumatoid arthritis. J Hand Ther. 2002;15:41-7.

[12] Burr N, Pratt AL. MCP joint arthroplasty case study: the Mount Vernon static regime. Br J Hand Ther. 1999;4:137-40.

[13] Escott B, Ronald K and Judd M. NeuFlex and Swanson Metacarpophalangeal Implants for Rheumatoid Arthritis: Prospective Randomized, Controlled Clinical Trial Journal of Hand Surgery Volume 35, Issue 1, 2010, Pages 44-51.

[14] Harada Y, Okumura S and Takahashi Y. Hand Therapy After Metacarpophalangeal Joint Implant Arthroplasty in Rheumatoid Hand. Journal of Hand Therapy 2010Volume 23, Issue 4, Pages e2-e3.

[15] Chung KC, Kotsis SV, and Kim HM, A Prospective Outcomes Study of Swanson Metacarpophalangeal Joint Arthroplasty for the Rheumatoid Hand. J Hand Surg Am. 2004 July; 29(4): 646–653.

Pettersson K, Wagnsjo P, Hulin E. NeuFlex compared with Sutterprostheses: a blind, prospective, randomized comparison of Silastic metacarpophalangeal joint prostheses. Scand J Plastic Reconstr Surg 2006;40:284 –290.

[16] V.A. Nuñez and N.D. Citron. Short-term results of the Ascension™ pyrolytic carbon metacarpophalangeal Joint replacement arthroplasty for osteoarthritis. Chirurgie de la Main. Volume 24, Issues 3-4, June-August 2005, Pages 161-164.

[17] Rettig LA, Luca L and Murphy MS. Silicone Implant Arthroplasty in Patients With Idiopathic Osteoarthritis of the Metacarpophalangeal Joint J Hand Surg 2005;30A:667–672.

[18] Moller K, Sollerman C, Geijer M, Kopylov P, Ta¨gil M.Avanta versus Swanson silicone implants in the MCP joint -a prospective, randomized comparison of 30 patients followed for 2 years. J Hand Surg 2005;/30B:/8-13.

[19] Parkkila T , Belt EA, Markku Hakala M, Kautiainen H and Leppilahti J. Comparison of Swanson and Sutter Metacarpophalangeal Arthroplasties in Patients With Rheumatoid Arthritis: A Prospective and Randomized Trial Journal of Hand Surgery Volume 30, Issue 6, 2005, Pages 1276-1281

[20] Thomsen NOB, Michel E. H. Boeckstyns MEH and Leth-Espensen P. Value of dynamic splinting after replacement of the metacarpophalangeal joint in patients with rheumatoid arthritis. Scand J Plast Reconstr Surg Hand Surg 2003; 37: 113–116

[21] Radmer S, Andresen S and Sparmann M. Poor experience with a hinged endoprosthesis (WEKO) for the metacarpophalangeal joints. *Acta Orthop Scand* 2003; 74 (5): 586–590.

[22] Ishikawa H, Murasawa A, Hanyu T (2002). The effects of activity andtype of rheumatoid arthritis on the flexible implant arthroplasty ofthe metacarpophalangeal joint. Journal of Hand Surgery, 27B (2):180–183.

[23] Stothard J, Thompson AE and Sherris D. Correction of ulnar drift during silastic metacarpophalangeal joint arthroplasty. J Hand Surg (British Volume) 16B: 61-65.

[24] Sambandam SN Analysis of methodological deficiencies of studies reporting surgical outcome following cemented total-joint arthroplasty of trapezio-metacarpal joint of the thumb. Int Orthop 2007 31:639-45.

[25] Zhao C, Amadio PC, Zobitz ME, Momose T, Couvreur P, An K-N. Effect of synergistic motion on flexor digitorum profundus tendon excursion. Clin Orthop. 2002;396:223-30.

[26] Tang JB, Wang B, Chen F, Chen Zhong Pan, Xie RG. Biomechanical evaluation of flexor tendon repair techniques. Clin Orthop. 2001;386:252-9.

[27] Tugwell P, Boers M. OMERACT conference on outcome measures in rheumatoid arthritis clinical trials: conclusion. J Rheumatol. 1993;20:590-1.

Humeral Hemiarthroplasty with Spherical Glenoid Reaming: Theory and Technique of The Ream and Run Procedure

Moby Parsons
Seacoast Orthopedics and Sports Medicine
Somersworth, NH
USA

1. Introduction

Despite improvements in glenoid prosthesis design, materials and surgical techniques, complications related to the glenoid component continue to be a leading cause of failure after total shoulder arthroplasty. Although previously felt to be of little clinical significance, radiolucent lines around the glenoid prosthesis are now recognized as a sign of impending mid and long term fixation problems. While much attention in shoulder prosthesis design has focused on anatomical reconstruction of the humerus through increasing modularity, comparatively little progress has been made in solving the problems of glenoid wear and fixation failure. Resolving these issues on the socket side of the equation remains a challenge for the shoulder arthroplasty surgeon as the population ages, as young patients present with terminal shoulder arthritis and as patients demand higher performance from their implant.

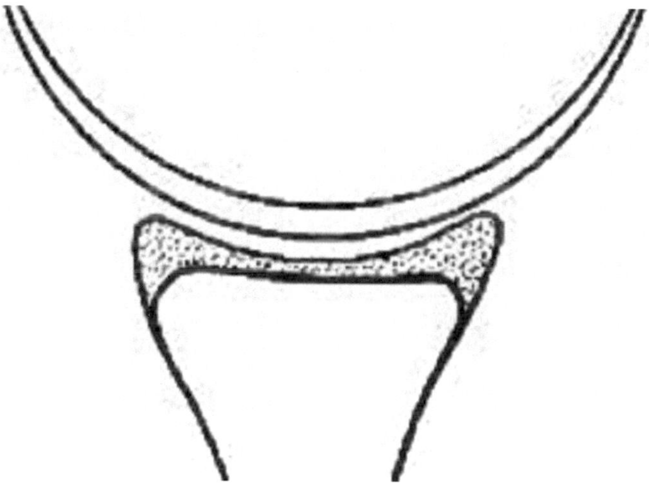

Fig. 1. In the normal glenohumeral joint, the compliance of the articular cartilage and the labrum provide for conforming surfaces which optimize stability and load distribution.

In the normal shoulder, the compliance of the articular cartilage and labrum allow the mating surfaces to conform under applied loads throughout a wide range of motion (Figure 1). Thus, normal, physiological glenohumeral translations can occur between congruent surfaces without introducing a kinematic conflict caused by excessive constraint. Because polyethylene glenoids are not compliant, they cannot instantly deform to remain congruent as normal translations occur. To resolve the potential conflict between conformity and constraint, total shoulder systems have introduced mismatch between the radii of curvature of the head and glenoid to permit small translations that increase range of motion and resolve some of the stresses transmitted to the fixation interface.

While mismatch has proven to reduce earlier fixation failure, it also facilitates eccentric loading by allowing the center of rotation of the humerus to translate away form the center of the glenoid concavity. As the contact point on the prosthetic glenoid surface changes, there are corresponding marked changes in the cement mantle stress than ultimately result in micromotion at the bone cement interface.[1] Oosterom and colleagues performed biomechanical studies looking at the effect of varying degrees of conformity on rim loading and found that mismatch increases rim displacement.[2] Furthermore, mismatch results in abrasive wear at the prosthetic surface and a higher likelihood of material failure under eccentric loading conditions.[3] Retrieval studies of failed glenoids that have radial mismatch, have repeatedly shown characteristic changes in the prosthetic surface including edge deformation, rim fracture, broad surface irregularity and wear to conformity (Figure 2).[4,5]

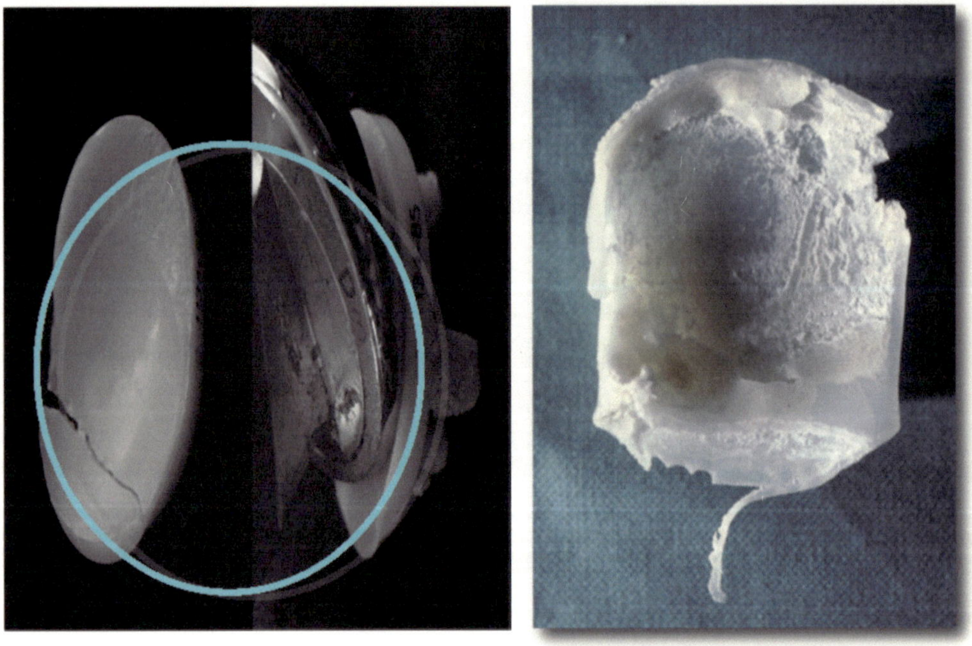

Fig. 2. Wear to conformity (left), broad surface abrasion and rim wear (right).

Modes of damage have been found most commonly in the inferior quadrant suggesting calcar impingement with the humerus.[6] Braman et al further showed that alterations in the surface geometry of the damaged prosthesis compromised its intrinsic stability, thus exacerbating the pathomechanics that result in surface damage to begin with.[4]

Several studies have looked at glenoid prosthesis design parameters and at cementation and bone preparation techniques seeking to optimize fixation to the host bone and resist tensile stresses imparted by eccentric loading conditions.[8-10] There is general consensus that pegged glenoid components tend to outperform keeled components and that third generation cementation techniques have reduced the incidence of early radiolucent lines. While most outcome studies show survivorship of the prosthesis at midterm, clinical outcome studies demonstrate deterioration in glenoid component longevity as the time interval from surgery increases. Walch and colleagues in a multicenter study of 333 shoulder arthroplasties performed with the same cemented convex-backed glenoid component showed that nearly 50% were radiographically loose at 10 years.[11] The need to eccentrically ream the glenoid to correct posterior erosion was associated with a higher rate of loosening. Young et al performed a similar multicenter study looking at long-term survivorship of a cemented flat-backed, keeled all-polyethylene glenoids and found radiographic loosening of 20% at 10 years and 67% at 15 years.[12] Kasten et al similarly noted at 9% rate of loosening at 5 years, which increased to 33% at 9 years. Radiolucent lines were noted to progress over time.[13] As with arthroplasty of other joints that rely on cement fixation, progressive radiolucency is an "at risk" sign for eventual loosening and though mid-term data show little correlation between lucency and revision, it is expected that longer follow-up will bear out eventual clinical failure. Bartelt et al followed a cohort of patients younger than age 55 years who underwent total shoulder arthroplasty and found a 30% rate of radiographic loosening at a mean of 6.6 years.[14] The implant survival rate in this group was only 92% at 10 years.

In light of these sobering data, there have been historical and resurging attempts to improve fixation durability by capitalizing on the proven success of bone ingrowth into porous metal surfaces. However, experience with early metal-backed designs demonstrated failure rates much higher than for cemented polyethylene components.[15] Taunton et al reported on revision or radiographic failure for a metal-backed, bone-growth glenoid of 20% at 5 years and 48% at 10 years.[16] Unacceptably high rates of radiographic failure have also been reported for cemented metal backed glenoid components.[17] Although some cases of fibrous ingrowth have been documented, many of these failures were not related to fixation problems between the metal and the bone, rather to excessive polyethylene wear, locking mechanism problems and severe osteolysis.[18] Tensile stress seems to be transferred to the fixation between the polyethylene and metal baseplates leading to the potential for excessive wear, fracture and dissociation of the components. While much of this experience is based on implants used in the 1980's to 1990's, there is renewed interest in metal-backed designs given the success of metal base plates in reverse shoulder arthroplasty and the desire to have modularity on the glenoid side facilitating conversion between primary and reverse shoulder replacement. Clinical outcome studies on newer designs have yet to prove their merit versus their historical counterparts and the current standard set by cemented all polyethylene designs, albeit a fair standard compared to survivorship data for hip and knee arthroplasty.

These data are alarming considering the growing epidemic of degenerative conditions in younger patients, the higher expectations of patients who wish to remain physically active into their older years and the general aging of the population. The conclusion one can draw from the current clinical and basic science literature is that modern prosthetic glenoid components are destined to fail by wear and loosening with repeated eccentric loading. Thus, for younger patients or those whose life-expectancy is greater than 15 years there is a high likelihood that revision surgery will be necessary to address glenoid component failure. In many of these cases, reimplantation of a glenoid component is not possible due to structural deficiency of the remaining glenoid vault, and functional outcomes are often uncertain.[19,20] Studies on structural grafting of bone deficits have shown a high rate of short-term reconstitution but long-term subsidence indicating that durable and reliable solutions for the failed glenoid are not yet available for this growing cohort of patients.[21,22]

To address the need for surgical options to treat shoulder arthritis in younger patients, biological resurfacing procedures using a number of different interposition materials have been evaluated with largely varying short and mid-term success. Autogenous fascia lata, Achilles tendon[23-24] and glenohumeral capsule,[25,26] allograft lateral meniscus[27,28] and dermal scaffolds,[29] and xenographic tissues patches[30] have all been used to resurface the worn glenoid. Both arthroscopic and open techniques have been reported and techniques have included humeral chondroplasty, humeral prosthetic surface replacement versus stemmed humeral hemiarthroplasty.[23] While some of these reports demonstrate initial improvement in pain and function, progressive joint space narrowing and glenoid erosion are common and consequent eventual revision to definitive arthroplasty. Gerber has nicely summarized the literature on this field, stating "Biologic resurfacing of the glenoid has hitherto failed to adequately restore the geometry and biology of the glenoid."[31] It is fair to say that lesser invasive approaches such as the arthroscopic techniques can be used as an interval step to delay arthroplasty but durable long-term results from these procedures seem to be the exception rather than the rule.

Hemiarthroplasty without glenoid resurfacing or reshaping is yet another alternative to total shoulder replacement which avoids the risk of glenoid failure. There has been extensive comparison between hemiarthroplasty and total shoulder arthroplasty in the literature looking at comparative outcomes. It is fairly well-established based on these studies including a meta-analysis of the existing literature, that total shoulder arthroplasty provides superior pain relief and range of motion over time.[32-34] Nevertheless, some series do show comparable outcomes recognizing that some patients with progressive glenoid erosion do require conversion to total shoulder arthroplasty.[35] Levine et al have shown that results of hemiarthroplasty are inferior if preoperative glenoid erosion or posterior wear exists.[36] This highlights the importance of recentering the humeral head and restoring proper load-bearing mechanics at the glenohumeral joint after prosthetic reconstruction. Sperling and colleagues studied long-term results of hemiarthroplasty versus total shoulder in patients 50 years or younger.[33] While glenoid wear after hemiarthroplasty was present in 72% of cases, radiolucencies around the glenoid prosthesis were present in 76% of patients. The risk of painful glenoid erosion necessitating revision glenoid replacement lead to the conclusion that patients with total shoulder replacement have superior clinical outcomes. The authors also concluded however based on survivorship of total shoulders in this cohort that "great care must be exercised, and alternative methods of treatment considered before either hemiarthroplasty or total shoulder arthroplasty is offered to patients aged 50 years or younger."

Based on this background, a definitive treatment option for young and physically demanding patients with end-stage shoulder arthritis remains both a need and a challenge. Experience with the failure modes of both hemiarthroplasty and total shoulder arthroplasty, along with a better understanding of glenohumeral biomechanics have laid a foundation on which such a treatment must be based to provided a lasting solution that withstands the rigors in which many of these patients wish to engage. In 1992, Frederick A. Matsen, III, MD began investigating the technique of humeral hemiarthroplasty with spherical glenoid reaming to restore a concavity to the glenoid and to reorient the worn glenoid perpendicular to the centerline of the scapular body. This technique has hence become known as the Ream and Run procedure. As follows is an in-depth description of basic science and clinical support for this technique, the principles of its application, patient selection, surgical technique, recovery and results.

2. Basic science and clinical support

According to Matsen, "glenoid components fail as a result of their inability to replicate essential properties of the normal glenoid articular surface to achieve durable fixation to the underlying bone, to withstand repeated eccentric loads and glenohumeral translation, and to resist wear and deformation."[37] The Ream and Run seeks to address these deficiencies by stimulating a biological response at the glenoid surface that can adapt to the applied stress through the process of healing and remodeling. Interest in this potential came from observations on retrieval studies of mold arthroplasty of the hip. Observations on this historical technique showed that the reamed acetabular bone was often covered with a smooth fibrous tissue layer that amounted to a biological resurfacing.[38] In addition, histologic studies demonstrated a relatively normal subchondral bony architecture that had remodeled according to the loads born on the surface.[39, 40] Failure of this technique was often due to loosening and bone resorption on the femoral side.[41] These results suggest that reamed bone has a regenerative potential to yield a durable joint surface when articulating with a convex metallic prosthesis.

Laboratory studies were then undertaken to determine if the reamed glenoid concavity was comparatively stable to either the native or a prosthetic glenoid. Weldon et al, using a cadaveric model, demonstrated that the intrinsic glenoid stability was compromised by loss of articular cartilage and that this stability could be restored to levels comparable to a prosthetic glenoid through spherical reaming.[42] In other words, the surface geometry of the bone predicts its influence on glenohumeral kinematics. To further characterize the healing process that occurs at the reamed glenoid surface, Matsen and colleagues performed histologic analysis of retrieved glenoids at serial follow-up intervals in a canine model of the Ream and Run.[43] At 24 weeks post-surgery specimens consistently showed growth of a thick fibrocartilaginous tissue covering and firmly attached to the glenoid surface.(Figure 3) This progressive maturation between 3 and 6 months and remained congruent with the articulating humeral hemiarthroplasty.

The implication of these findings are: 1) healing and remodeling of the reamed bone is a progressive process demonstrating continued biological activity in response to the mechanical environment; and 2) progressive maturation of the regenerative surface suggests its ability to withstand its mechanical environment.

Based on this background, the Ream and Run procedure been in clinical application now for well over a decade, and its indications and techniques have been refined with increasing experience. As the length of follow-up continues for these patients, the foundations for sustained positive outcomes and the modes of failure have become clearer. These foundations are anchored in the principles behind this technique all of which relate to replicating the anatomical relationships of the glenohumeral joint and the biomechanical properties these relationships engender.

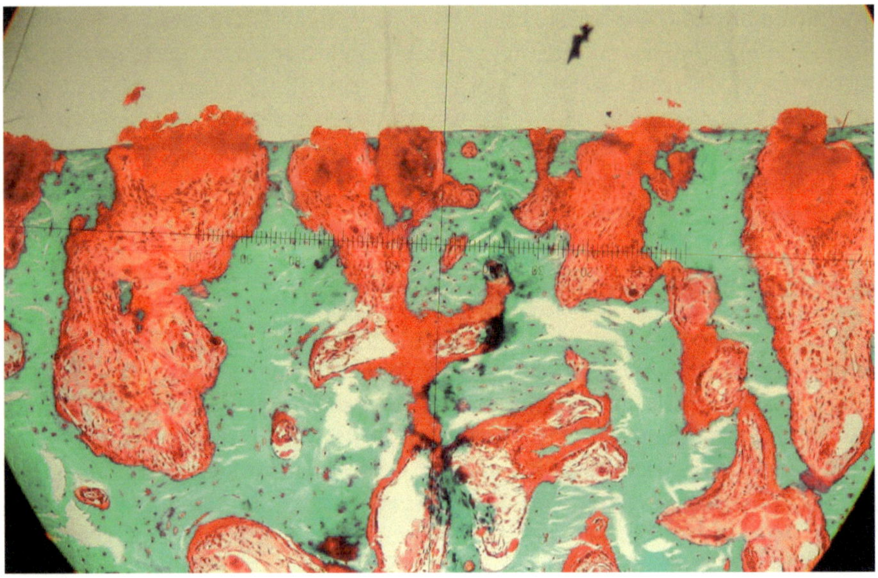

Fig. 3. Fibrocartilage growth between reamed boney trabeculae.

3. Principles

The key principles behind the Ream and Run which the surgeon must consider in reestablishing a lasting articulation that can withstand wear can be remembered as the 4 Cs: concavity, conformity, centerline and center of rotation. These are further discussed as follows.

3.1 Concavity

Stability of the glenohumeral joint in the midrange relies on dynamic centering of the humeral head into the glenoid concavity by the force couples generated by the rotator cuff. Coordination between the rotator cuff and periscapular stabilizing muscles ensures that the net reaction force at the glenohumeral joint is directed within the confines of the glenoid concavity. The depth and shape of this concavity can affect stability by altering the glenoids ability to contain the resultant force from shoulder motion. This can be measured as the balance stability angle (BSA) - the maximal angle the net humeral reaction force vector can make with the glenoid centerline before the head dislocates.[42] Both the width and the depth of the glenoid factor into the intrinsic stability and these, in turn, can be affected both by pathologic changes from arthritis as well as by corrective reaming.

Reestablishing a smooth concavity with sufficient depth and surface area is a central goal of the successful Ream and Run. Because reaming affects both depth and width, depending on the degree of necessary correction to recenter the humeral head, careful attention must be paid through preoperative planning and precise surgical technique to restore a sufficient concavity without compromising other principles as will be subsequently discussed. In cases where there is severe posterior glenoid wear, as can occur from capsulorraphy arthropathy, corrective reaming to restore glenoid version may sacrifice too much surface area in order to restore a sufficient concavity thus obviating the benefit of this procedure. Prosthetic glenoid resurfacing may be necessary in such cases despite the inherent risks of eventual failure.

3.2 Conformity

Although the boney anatomy is not conforming between the humeral head and glenoid concavity, the compliance afforded by the articular cartilage and glenoid labrum provide for conformity and congruency as the humeral head is centered and compressed. It is this conformity and compliance that permits load distribution over the glenoid face. Because bone and polyethylene are not as compliant as cartilage and labrum, some degree of mismatch between the diameter of curvature of the humeral head and glenoid has become a convention in total shoulder arthroplasty to avoid excessive constraint and allow physiologic translations. While historically mismatch seems to improve the longevity of prosthetic glenoid fixation, translations also allow eccentric glenoid loading, which contributes to eventual fixation failure. Mismatch also affects load distribution by concentrating loads over a smaller surface area on the glenoid surface.

In principle, the Ream and Run procedure must respect the biomechanical principles on which glenohumeral stability and load transfer are based while simultaneously reconciling the kinematic conflict that occurs between conformity and constraint as is seen with prosthetic glenoids. Stability is afforded by creation of a concavity into which the head can be centered after appropriate releases have been performed. Preservation of the labrum further deepens the socket and improves congruency between the ball and socket. Load distribution is optimized by choosing a mismatch of 2mm, which reduces point contact but allows some forgiveness in terms of constraint. It also provides some forgiveness in allowing the prosthetic humeral head to chose a centering point about which adaptive remodeling of the glenoid surface can define the final shape that optimizes joint kinematics and load transfer.

3.3 Centerline

In the normal shoulder, the glenoid is retroverted on average 10 degrees. The glenoid centerline (the line perpendicular to the glenoid face) thus normally points 10 degrees posterior to the axis of the scapular body. This line exits the scapula anteriorly at the base of the glenoid vault between the superior and inferior subscapularis crurae. Recentering the humeral head within the glenoid concavity is essential for shoulder mobility, stability and load transfer. The pathomechanics of primary and secondary arthritis often lead to posterior subluxation of the humerus and consequent posterior glenoid wear and erosion. These pathologic changes must be corrected to optimize load-bearing mechanics at the joint after prosthetic reconstruction. As will be discussed later, careful planning is necessary to determine the amount of correction that will restore the orientation of the glenoid.(Figure 4)

Reorientation of the glenoid concavity through corrective reaming can diminish the surface area of the articulation because the glenoid vault narrows as one moves medially. In addition, corrective reaming to "bring down the high side" may result in significant penetration of the subchondral bone, which is softer and less tolerant of bearing significant loads when articulating with a convex metal prosthesis. Medialization of the glenoid may also increase the reaction force at the glenohumeral joint by reducing the lever arm of the rotator cuff muscles and may result in secondary impingement by bringing the tuberosity underneath the lateral acromion. Thus, preoperative planning must assess the degree of necessary correction and whether this will exceed the anatomical parameters necessary to achieve the other principles and goals of the Ream and Run.

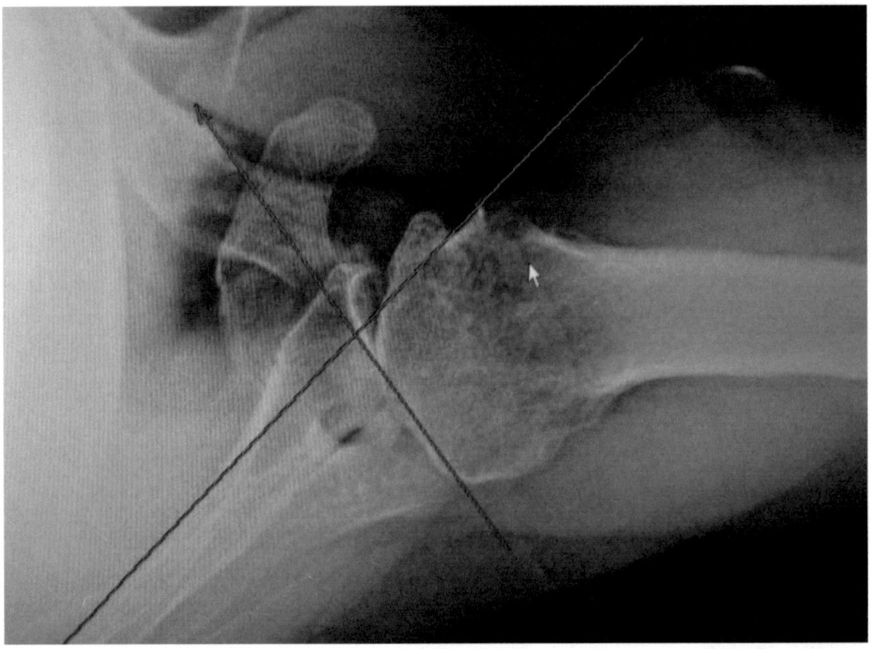

Fig. 4. Axillary lateral radiograph showing double concavity, posterior glenoid erosion and posterior humeral subluxation. Preoperative planning can determine the degree of corrective reaming needed to restore proper glenoid orientation relative to the axis of the scapula

In cases where significant correction is required, precontouring the glenoid with a burr and then using a relatively flatter conventional reamer to start may allow reorientation without as much medialization and subchondral penetration. Some surgeons have advocated under correction of the posterior erosion to maximize the articular surface area of the reamed glenoid.[44] While undercorrection risks recurrent posterior instability and consequent wear, excessive reaming risks reduced surface area for load distribution. Ultimately, the surgeon needs to make a judgment call intraoperatively after corrective reaming as to whether the concavity can sufficiently replicate the mechanical properties of a normal glenoid to provide lasting pain relief, stability and unrestricted function.

3.4 Center of rotation

Because the humeral head is nearly spherical, it has a center of rotation, which is slightly medially and posteriorly offset from the axis of the humeral shaft. In the normal shoulder this rotation center is aligned with center of the glenoid concavity. This phenomenon has been termed glenohumeral register.[44] This center of rotation actually exists within a larger arc of a sphere created by the coracoacromial arch and coracoid process - a boundary which partially constrains glenohumeral motion and helps define the path of rotation.(Figure 5) The motion of the humeral articular surface on the glenoid face can actually be described as slippage of the surfaces relative to one another. The centering point on the glenoid can thus be thought of as a slippage point. In the normal shoulder, this point is slightly inferior and anterior to the midpoint of Saller's line which bisects the glenoid along its superior to inferior axis.

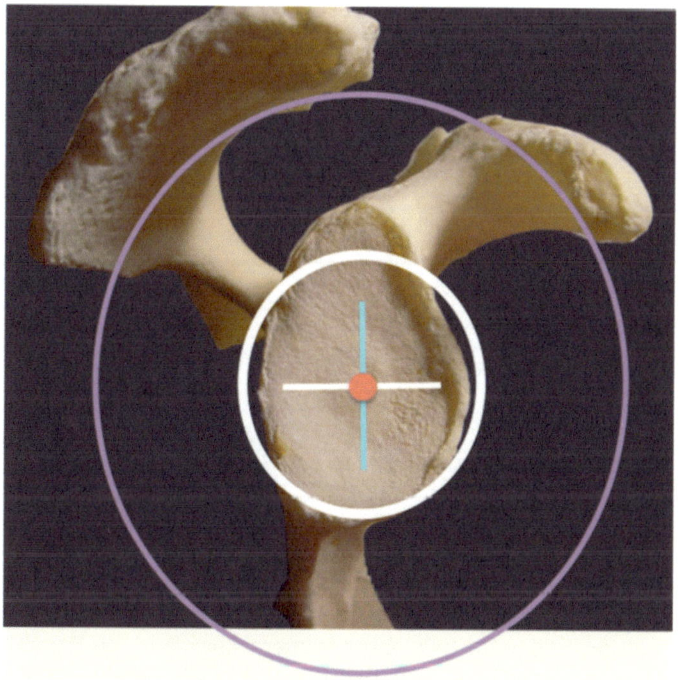

Fig. 5. The centering point on the glenoid is defined by the larger sphere created by the coracoacromial arch. The point is slightly inferior to the center of a line connecting the superior and inferior margins of the glenoid.

Anatomical reconstruction of the proximal humerus seeks to reestablish the head to tuberosity and head to shaft relationships and to replace a head of similar diameter and thickness. In a perfect world, this should restore the proper center of rotation though prior studies have shown that there can be significant displacement of the rotation center depending on how the chosen system fits relative to a given patient's anatomy. [45, 46] (Figure 6) This displacement has the potential to affect the location of the slippage point on the glenoid face and how the motion of the glenohumeral joint is defined by its location with fornix humeri.

When the glenoid is spherically reamed, the surgeon is effectively choosing a centering point for slippage of the humeral prosthesis. Much of the time in conventional shoulder arthroplasty, this point is chosen by looking at what appears to be the deepest point of the existing concavity. Current techniques and technology do not allow the reconstructed center of rotation of the humerus to chose it's proper slippage point that the surgeon can then use as the centering point for the reaming. The finding on failed glenoid retrievals that wear to conformity occurs at a point other than the geometric center of the prosthetic glenoid concavity, suggests that the humeral head is seeking ball and socket kinematics as defined by placement of the reconstructed humeral rotation center within the fornix humeri. Thus, one can presume that optimal registration between the rotation center of the humeral arthroplasty and the center of the reamed glenoid concavity would result in a blend of kinematics, stability and load distribution that would lend itself to long-term maintenance of pain relief and function.

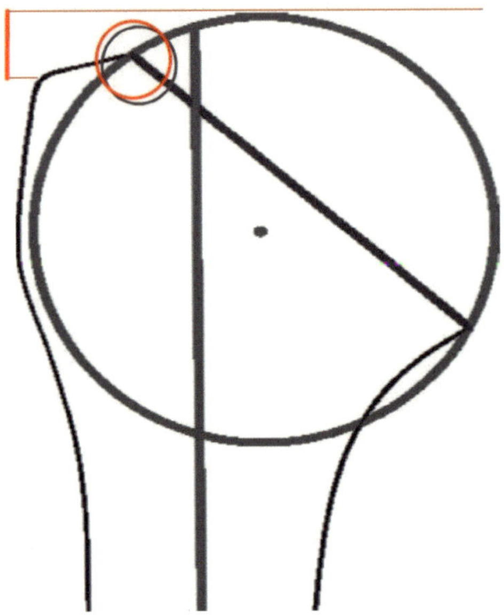

Fig. 6. Anatomical prosthetic reconstruction of the proximal humerus should seeks to restore the center of rotation relative to the axis of the humeral shaft and the transition between the superior articular surface of the head with the insertion of the articular side of the rotator cuff on the greater tuberosity

In the absence of a scientific method to register the humeral reconstruction with the slippage point on the reamed glenoid, the shoulder arthroplasty surgeon must resort to preoperative planning, intraoperative observation, precise surgical technique and perhaps a bit of good fortune. While the reamed glenoid bone is not as compliant as articular cartilage, it does have the capacity to adapt and remodel according to its mechanical environment and thus, over time there may be some forgiveness to a small margin of error through a process of bedding-in wear.

4. Indications

Proper patient selection is critical to achieving desired results after this procedure. Selection is based both on anatomical and physiological considerations as well emotional and social aspects of the patient. Foremost, patients with inflammatory arthritis are not candidates for this technique as the absence of a prosthetic glenoid will result in continued glenoid erosion following humeral hemiarthroplasty. Female patients also tend to have less predictable results. This likely relates to having lower bone density and its effect on the potential for continued glenoid pain after reaming and humeral resurfacing. For male patients with osteoarthritis, the following selection criteria must be carefully considered for optimal results:

4.1 Patient factors

1. *Age*: there are no strict age limitations. This technique is ideally suited for younger patients whose age and activity level predict glenoid failure relative to their average life expectancy. For patients older than 65 years, standard total shoulder arthroplasty is more likely to yield a predictable good to excellent result and is the preferred operation

unless patients specifically request to forgo glenoid resurfacing after discussion of the options. For the occasional older patient in this category who remains physically very active and engaged in "at risk" activities, non-prosthetic glenoid arthroplasty may be an option if other criteria are met.

2. *General Health Status*: optimal health is critical to good results after any procedure but particularly the Ream and Run. Patients with multiple comorbidities, especially those that may impair tissue healing are likely not suitable candidates for this procedure. Poorly controlled diabetes, poor nutritional status and medical problems that require the use of immunosuppressive drugs are contraindications. If there is concern about general health and nutritional status, blood work including absolute lymphocyte count (<1500 cells/mm3), serum transferrin level (<200 mg/dL) and albumin level (<3.5 g/dL) can be used to screen patients who may benefit from further optimization or consultation with a nutritionist prior to the procedure. For patients with diabetes the glycosylated hemoglobin (HgA1C) can be used to screen for glycemic control, which correlates with risk for infection and healing potential. Ideally this value should be below 7.0 for optimal healing potential. If patients are well above this mark, surgery should be delayed until their diabetes can be better controlled throughout the perioperative period
3. *Expectations*: experience has shown that recovery after this procedure generally takes longer than for a standard shoulder arthroplasty as healing of the reamed bone may progress and mature for 6 months or more and range of motion can improve for up to a year in motivated individuals. Achieving good range of motion is critical to outcomes for the Ream and Run as residual stiffness can lead to altered glenohumeral kinematics due to obligate capsular mediated translations - similar to the pathomechanics of primary shoulder osteoarthritis. Thus, patients who wish to pursue this alternative must be willing to accept a more prolonged recovery and must be sufficiently motivated to comply with the rehabilitation program including maintenance home exercises. Patients should also have exhausted all conservative measures and demonstrate sufficient pain, disability and joint degeneration to justify arthroplasty.
4. Social History:

a. *Smoking*: the dystrophic effect of smoking on tissue healing makes this a contraindication to the Ream and Run. Patients who wish to undergo this operation must be in optimal physical and nutritional health. Serum cotinine levels can be used as a method to ensure smoking cessation.

b. *History of narcotic habituation or chronic pain*: patients with a history of heavy regular use of narcotic medications are less likely to have a desirable outcome after the Ream and Run due to the potential for a more prolonged recovery process. These patients need to be appropriately counseled and advance and provisions should be made in advance of surgery to enlist a pain management specialist who can help steadily wean patients from narcotics as the healing progresses.

c. *Worker's Compensation claim or litigation*: as has been documented with many other conditions and surgeries, patients involved in a compensation claim or those litigating an injury invariably have worse outcomes after a surgical procedure. To the extent that the salvage of a failed Ream and Run requires prosthetic glenoid resurfacing, the results which are itself inferior in the revision setting, primary total shoulder arthroplasty or other surgical alternatives should be considered.

5. *Emotional History*: patients with ongoing poorly controlled mental health issues are not optimal candidates for this procedure. If patients have symptoms and disability out of proportion to the clinical scenario, have fibromyalgia or a significant poorly defined myofascial component to their pain or if patients have fallen victim to the disease construct of their condition, they are not likely to fair well with the Ream and Run procedure. The optimal patient has demonstrated a balanced self-management approach to their condition, has continued to remain active and engaged despite their physical limitation, and has demonstrated the emotional capacity to deal with the pain and life-altering nature of their diagnosis. Self-assessment scores can sometimes provide a useful window on a patient's emotional state. For instance, those patients who circle "No" on all 12 questions of the Simple Shoulder Score have a self-perceived disability that likely supersedes their actual physical limitation and their outcome after the Ream and Run will be uncertain. If a patient enters a "12" on a 0-10 Visual Analog Pain Scale, one should be concerned about the potential success of the Ream and Run.

4.2 Anatomy factors

1. *Glenoid Erosion and Morphology*: the success of Ream and Run hinges on the ability of the surgeon to achieve a smooth concavity that is oriented perpendicular to the native glenoid centerline. Preservation of subchondral bone leads to more predictable outcomes. In cases with preoperative posterior glenoid erosion, double concavity and/or posterior humeral subluxation, careful preoperative templating must be performed based on CT imaging to determine whether corrective reaming will compromise the aforementioned goals. Moderate correction often results in medialization of the glenoid, which not only reduces the surface area of the concavity but also may penetrate into the cancellous bone of the glenoid vault. In such cases, placement of a prosthetic glenoid component is recommended as hemiarthroplasty alone may result in postoperative erosion into the softer bone with consequent persistent glenoid pain. Patients noted to have decentering of the humeral head with glenoid erosion must be counseled preoperatively about the possible need for standard total shoulder arthroplasty pending the appearance of the glenoid after corrective reaming.
2. *Soft-tissue balance*: because younger patients with glenohumeral arthritis may have a variety of different arthritis types including post-traumatic and post-capsulorraphy arthropathy, there may be alteration of the soft-tissue anatomy from prior anatomy altering surgery. This is particularly the case for patients who may have undergone a prior Bristow or Latarjet type coracoid transfer in whom there can be significant scarring in the subscapularis and conjoint tendon region. If surgical releases are not able to result in a balanced soft tissue envelope that permits a wide range of motion, persistent postoperative stiffness may result in obligate translations that cause recurrent eccentric glenoid wear. Thus, a careful understanding the patients pre-operative anatomy and prior surgical history is critical to forecasting the success of the Ream and Run.
3. *Proximal humeral anatomy*: achieving an anatomical reconstruction of the proximal humerus is equally important to recentering the humeral head into a properly oriented and shaped concavity. A modern arthroplasty system that allows accurate and reliable reproduction of the native shoulder anatomy is essential and care must be taken to restore the proper relationships between the head, tuberosities and shaft in terms of the joint center of rotation and cuff insertion. A resurfacing cap may be used as an

alternative if surgeons are capable of achieving adequate glenoid exposure without humeral head osteotomy. If sequelae of prior trauma have resulted in alteration of the normal proximal humeral anatomy, specifically the head-tuberosity relationship, the surgeon must understand through appropriate imaging how this may affect the goal of achieving an anatomical reconstruction in terms of the position of the arc of the humeral convexity, center of rotation and soft-tissue balance.

5. Necessary equipment

In order to restore proper load bearing mechanics at the glenohumeral articulation, the reamed glenoid must be sufficiently concave to ensure stability, and sufficiently conforming to avoid load concentration over a small area. Thus, custom-made reamers are necessary so that there is a corresponding reamer for each humeral head diameter.(Figure 7) In order to avoid too much constraint and permit physiological glenohumeral translations, a 2mm mismatch between head diameter and reamer diameter has become the convention, as previously discussed. Thus, if the chosen head size is 52mm, a custom reamer with a diameter of curvature of 54mm is used for glenoid reaming. These reamers should enlarge in circumference as their diameter enlarges in order to contact the surface area of the native glenoid. Cannulated reamers are preferable in that they can follow a pre-drilled K-wire oriented along the glenoid centerline. This greatly improves the accuracy of the reaming process when correction is needed. An open blade reamer design is also beneficial since it allows the surgeon to see the area of bone that has been reamed during version correction.

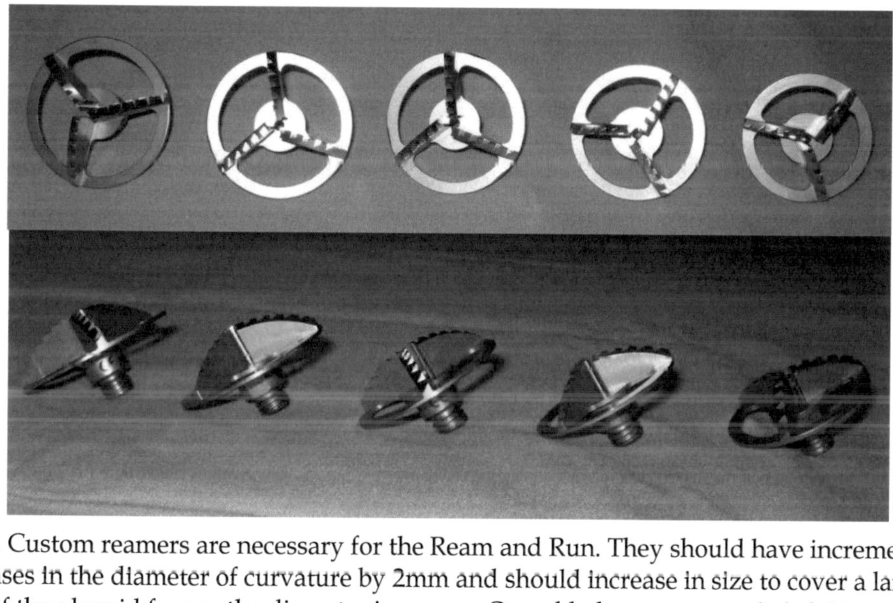

Fig. 7. Custom reamers are necessary for the Ream and Run. They should have incremental increases in the diameter of curvature by 2mm and should increase in size to cover a larger area of the glenoid face as the diameter increases. Open blade reamers are helpful in following the degree of correction during the reaming process.

An arthroplasty system of the surgeon's choice can be used with the stipulation that the chosen system allows reliable and reproducible anatomical reconstruction of proximal humeral anatomy. The author currently uses the Synthes EPOCA shoulder system (Synthes,

Westchester, PA), which includes press-fit and cemented stem options and a dual eccentricity design that allows precise placement of the humeral head on the humeral osteotomy surface. This precision improves the accuracy of restoring the humeral center of rotation and head-tuberosity relationship, which is critical in defining soft-tissue balance and proper rotator cuff function.

6. Surgical technique

The patient is positioned in a low beach chair position with the head supported in a cerebellar headrest. The body is shifted toward the operative side so the arm can be extended over the edge of the bed for humeral exposure. A rolled towel is placed beneath the medial scapular border to help orient the glenoid toward the operative field. Unless contraindicated, sterile preparation of the field should employ Choraprep solution, which has demonstrated superior bacteriocidal efficacy relative to other preparations. In addition, circumferential biodrape should be used to occlude the axillary region and cover all exposed skin. Receipt of prophylactic antibiotics must be ensured along with availability of necessary instruments and implants and confirmation of the correct patient, procedure and side.

A standard deltopectoral incision is used though some surgeons prefer a more vertical Bankart type incision in Langer's lines. The cephalic vein is taken laterally with the deltoid and the interval is developed from the clavicle to the pectoralis tendon. We do not routinely take down the pectoralis tendon unless necessary for exposure. The deltoid should be reflected off the coracoacromial ligament to facilitate exposure. The clavipectoral fascia should be excised en bloc from the inferior edge of the CA ligament superiorly to the superior edge of the pectoralis major tendon inferiorly and from the lateral border the conjoint tendon medially to the medial border of the anterior deltoid laterally. This opens the humeroscapular motion interface. A curved deltoid retractor such as a Browne's or delta Fukuda is placed behind the humeral head and a right-angle retractor such as Army Navy beneath the conjoint tendon.

The bicipital groove is opened and the biceps is sutured to the traversing pectoralis major tendon to maintain proper length and tension. It is then tenotomized in the rotator interval. The superior and inferior borders of the subscapularis are then dissected out, cauterizing or ligating the circumflex vessels. The author prefers a lesser tuberosity osteotomy for management of the subscapularis. This is done with a broad curved osteotome and started at the deepest portion of the bicipital groove. The tendon-bone fragment is tagged with suture. A curved blunt Hohman retractor is then placed along the anterior inferior humeral head and this is used to tension the humeral insertion of the inferior glenohumeral capsule-ligamentous complex. This is then released subperiosteally with progressive external rotation, and this release can be follow around to the humeral bare area posteriorly. This release greatly facilitates surgical dislocation of the humeral head.

Prior to dislocation of the humeral head, a lamina spreader type instrument can be used to distract the glenohumeral joint. This tensions the posterior capsule allowing superior visibility for thorough capsulotomy along the length of the posterior glenoid. A thorough release of the posterior capsule facilitates posterior humeral subluxation during glenoid exposure. Although some surgeons advocate selective capsular releases depending on the degree of preoperative humeral posterior subluxation, the author does not feel that capsular tissues play a role in glenohumeral stability except during the extremes of range of motion provided an adequate concavity is restored along the axis of the scapula and proper humeral retrotorsion is selected. In the author's personal series, circumferential capsular releases have never resulted in postoperative posterior instability but do improve range of motion during the early recovery. If there is a concern about posterior laxity, the rotator interval can be closed slightly more medially to provide a checkrein against posterior translation at the conclusion of the case.

The humeral osteotomy is then made along the anatomical neck generally in 25-30 degrees of retrotorsion. It is critical that this cut is flush with the articular-sided insertion of the supraspinatus tendon fibers so the anatomical reconstruction of the head-tuberosity relationship can be properly achieved.(Figure 8) Once the cut is made and refined, osteophytes around the margins of the anatomical neck can be removed, particularly those inferiorly which can cause calcar impingement with the inferior glenoid if not cleared out. A head diameter that best covers the osteotomy surface is then chosen. It is best to err toward the smaller size assuming there will be no uncovered bone that would impinge during glenohumeral rotation.

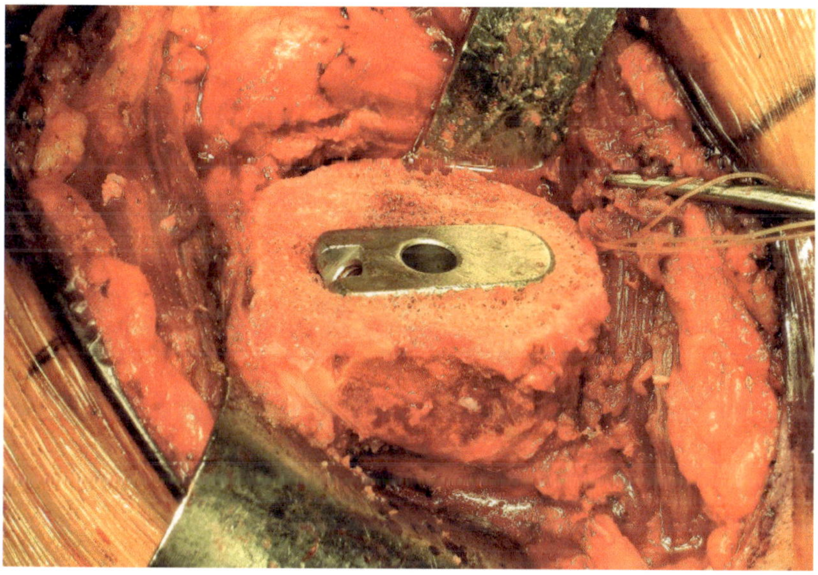

Fig. 8. The humeral osteotomy should be flush with the insertion of the supraspinatus tendon to restore the head-tuberosity relationship. The trial stem should be positioned to restore humeral retrotorsion of approximately 25-30 degrees.

If a stemmed arthroplasty is to be used, the humeral canal can then be prepped via the conventions of the given system and a trial stem placed. If a cap prosthesis is chosen, then the head can be reamed and the cap sized according to the system's technique.

The humerus is then subluxated posteriorly using a Fukuda or similar retractor. A complete circumferential release of the subscapularis can now safely be performed. The interval between the anterior capsule and inferior muscular fibers of the subscapularis is developed with Metzenbaum scissors allowing safe release of the anterior capsular from the glenoid rim and release of adhesions to the coracoid base. All adhesions should be released so that external rotation can be restored. The surgeon should feel a soft bounce when the subscapularis is pulled laterally. A blunt Hohman or spiked ribbon retractor can then be placed medially within the subscapularis fossa with the tendon and lesser tuberosity tucked medially behind it. This should allow full visualization down the anterior face of the scapular body, which is critical for restoring orientation of the glenoid concavity.

The inferior capsule is then release sharply in an extra labral fashion keeping the knife parallel to and against bone. Care should be taken to completely release the insertion of the anterior inferior and posterior inferior glenohumeral ligament from its glenoid-sided insertion. The author believes that selective capsular releases are never indicated assuming that the glenoid version is properly corrected and an adequate concavity is restored. The Fukuda retractor ring can be twisted off of the inferior glenoid rim to facilitate release of the posterior inferior capsule. Once a sufficient release has been performed, adequate glenoid exposure should permit insertion of the glenoid reamers. Internal rotation (rather than the conventional external rotation) can sometimes facilitate posterior humeral subluxation. Release of the coracohumeral ligament is sometimes necessary to improve glenoid exposure by further allowing the humerus to translate posteriorly.

The center of the existing glenoid concavity is then determined. The author uses a curved backed drill guide to help find the centering or slippage point. If there is a double concavity present, or if there is significant posterior glenoid erosion, the centering point often needs to be shifted somewhat anteriorly to properly restore glenoid version by reaming the high side. Any central ridges can be burred in advance to provisionally restore a concavity. In cases of significant posterior glenoid wear or double concavity, a flatter reamer can be used for provisional reshaping prior to definitive reestablishment of the concavity.

Once the centering point has been determined, a threaded-tipped Steinmann pin is drilled parallel to the glenoid centerline.(Figure 9) Because the scapular is a curved structure, this pin

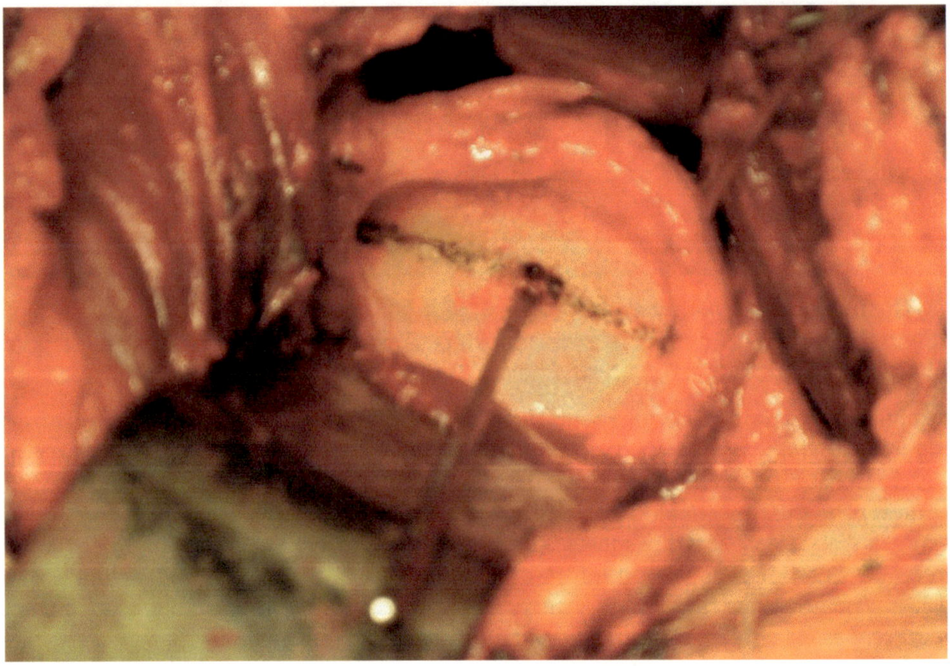

Fig. 9. The glenoid labrum is preserved during glenoid exposure and capsular releases. The centering point for the is determined and a threaded-tipped Steinmann pin is drilled to reorient the glenoid so that it is retroverted roughly 10 degrees relative to the axis of the scapular body.

should exit the anterior glenoid neck between the upper and lower crurae of the subscapularis fossa. The author uses the convention of being able to palpate the pin tip when the PIP joint of the index finger is placed against the anterior glenoid rim. If it exists too anteriorly then reaming will result in persistent retroversion that can lead to posterior instability.

Once the pin is properly positioned, the cannulated reamer can be introduced. The blades should be spinning prior to contact with the bone and the glenoid should be progressively reamed until circumferential contact occurs and a full concavity is achieved. (Figure 10) The goals of reaming are: 1) to restore glenoid version; and 2) to restore a smooth concavity. Once these goals are achieved, the surgeon must inspect the glenoid surface, the bone quality, the surface area and the degree of medialization that occurs from correction. If corrective reaming results in significant medialization, exposure of cancellous bone within the glenoid vault or loss of surface area as the glenoid narrows, placement of a glenoid prosthesis may be necessary. Ideally, there should be firm subchondral bone to support the humeral prosthesis.

Next a small drill is used to make multiple perforations in the reamed glenoid face. This serves two purposes.(Figure 11) Firstly, it decompresses the venous congestion than can occur in arthritic bone, which may improve pain relief. Secondly, it permits egress of bone marrow stem cells to help reform a fibro-cartilaginous coating on the reamed glenoid face.

The final humeral prosthesis is then inserted according to the specifications of the system. It is critical that the humeral head be optimally positioned to restore the center of rotation of the joint and to restore the proper head-tuberosity relationship.(Figure 12)

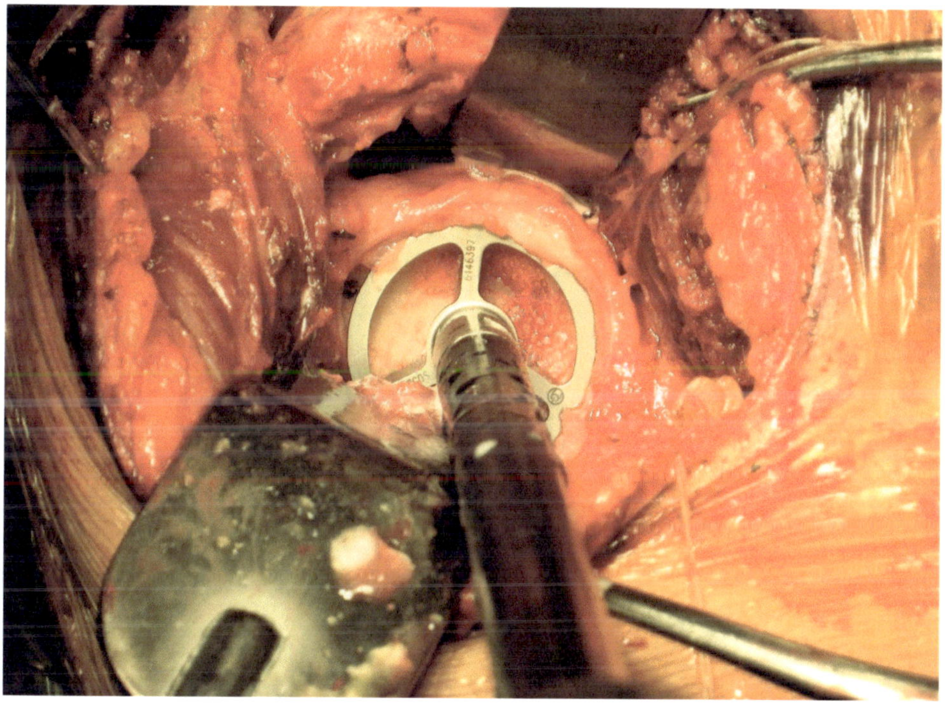

Fig. 10. The chosen reamer is introduced and the glenoid reamed until a smooth concavity is achieved.

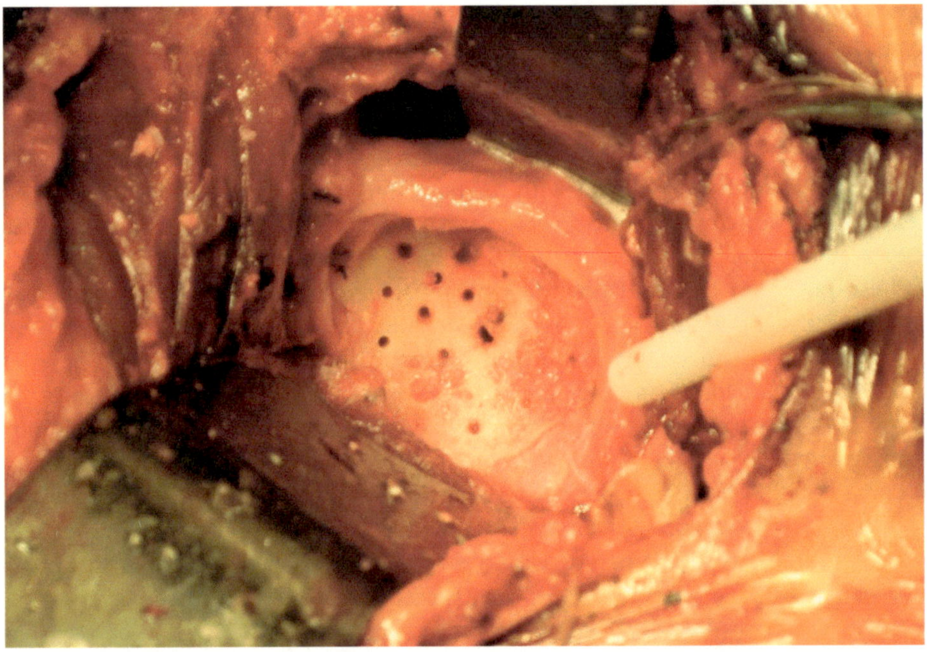

Fig. 11. Multiple holes are drilled into the reamed glenoid to decompress venous congestion and promote egress of stem cells to promote fibrocartilage formation.

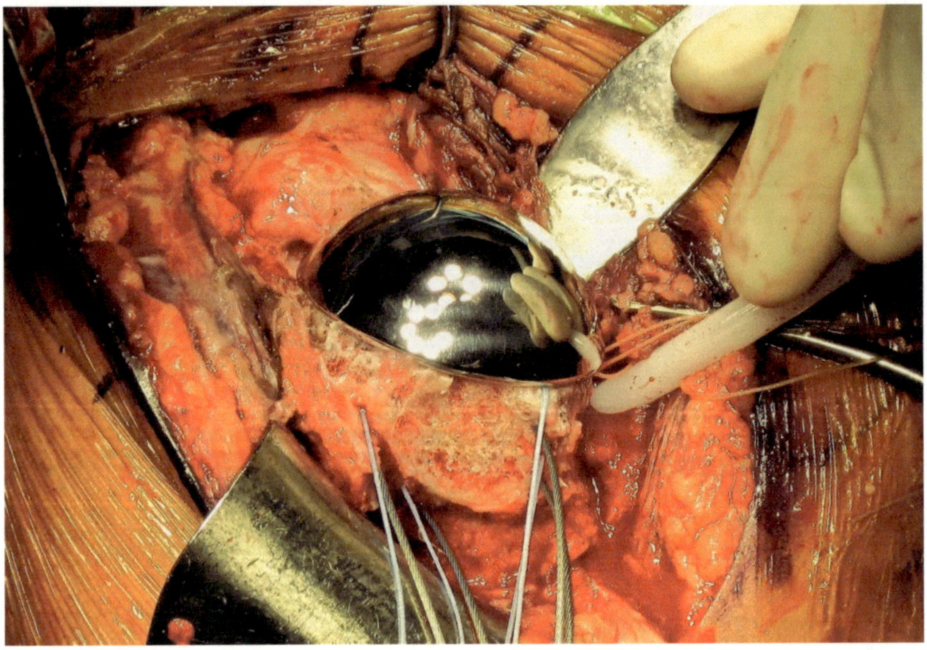

Fig. 12. The humeral head must achieve anatomical reconstruction with regard to coverage of the osteotomy and restoration of the head-shaft and head-tuberosity relationship. The head should have an anatomical height that does not overstuff the joint.

Excess anterior and posterior overhang must be avoided and there should be smooth transition at the calcar that prevents boney impingement in this region. A head thickness that corresponds to normal anatomy should be chosen. If the system used provides 3 offset options for each diameter, it is best to choose the middle size to prevent over or under stuffing of the joint. Conventional on-table measurements of passive translation are not helpful in determining proper soft tissue tension as they do no correlate with dynamic stability in the mid range of motion after surgery. It is best to err toward the looser side with the Ream and Run as it facilitates recovery of motion which is critical to outcomes and it does not correlate with postoperative instability assuming the glenoid has been properly corrected.

A secure subscapularis repair is essential to permit early range of motion. The author currently uses the technique described by Millett et al using cerclage sutures looped around the humeral stem.[47] If a porous ingrowth stem is used, the author uses two 1mm cables instead because micromotion of the sutures against the stem coating will result in suture rupture.(Figure 13) These cables are supplemented by a suture tension band construct tied over a cortical button lateral to the bicipital groove. If cables are used, the crimps are positioned in the bicipital groove and covered over by the biceps tendon to prevent soft-tissue irritation. The lateral part of the rotator interval is then closed. If there is concern about posterior instability, additional interval sutures can be placed more medially though this may compromise external rotation and potentially decentralize the humeral head.

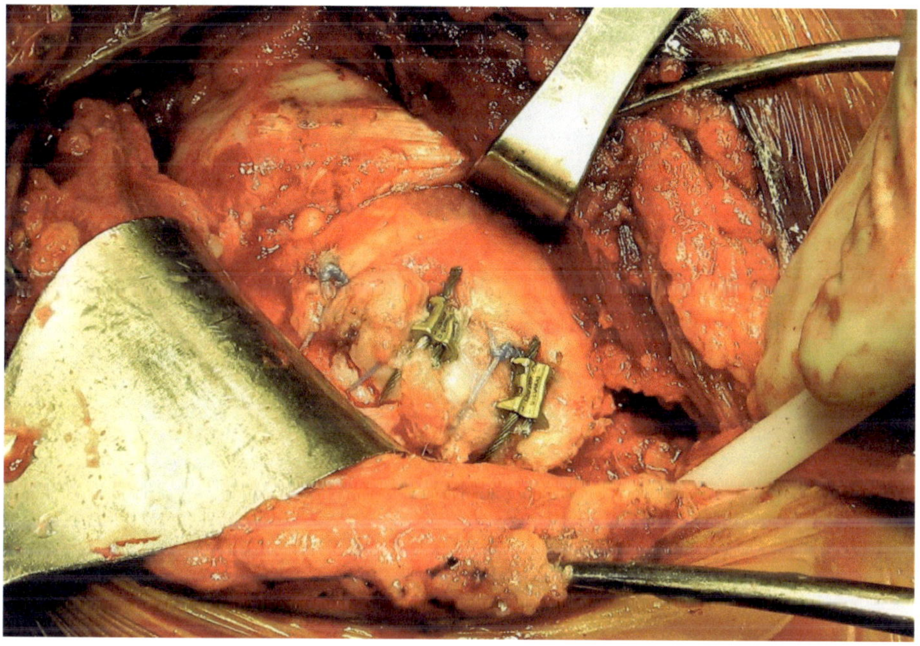

Fig. 13. A secure repair of the subscapularis is essential regardless of the technique. In this picture, horizontal cerclage cables have been used to compress the lesser tuberosity fragment to its osteotomy bed.

7. Post-operative protocol

Immediate range of motion exercises are begun under the supervision of the therapist. Forward elevation to 140 degree and external rotation to 40 degree is allowed along with external rotation isometrics, scapular pinches and cervical and elbow range of motion. Patients are instructed on how to perform active-assisted range of motion exercises and encouraged to do so several times daily. Positional exercises, such as placing the arm on the rest of a couch are also permitted. This holds a static position of stretch for a period of time that does not jeopardize the repair. Most patients are discharged from the hospital with home services and transition to outpatient therapy after their first postoperative visit around 10-14 days.

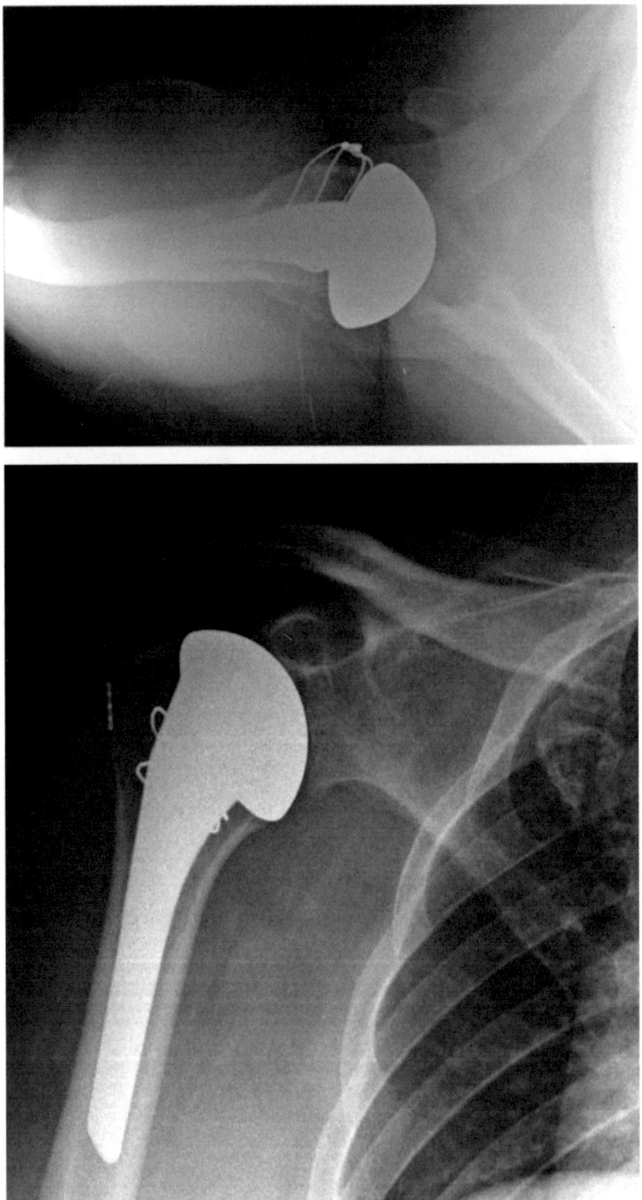

Fig. 14. A and B: Postoperative AP and axillary lateral radiographs demonstrating anatomical reconstruction of the humerus with creation of a smooth concavity.

Around 4 weeks, progressive return to maximal range of motion is permitted and exercises such as wall walks can be added. Active internal rotation is discouraged to protect the subscapularis. Patients are instructed to still limit use of the arm for physical activities and focus on flexibility.
At 8 weeks, the focus continues on maximizing range of motion. The subscapularis repair must still be protected from active internal rotation but patients can begin some posterior capsular stretching and light deltoid, trapezius and periscapular strengthening.
Assuming adequate progress and a negative belly-press test at 12 weeks, patients can start internal rotation strengthening and progressive use of the arm for normal daily activities. Return to physically demanding activities and sports requires at least 4 or more months to ensure and adequately healed subscapularis
In the author's experience in trying to accelerate the rehabilitation protocol, the subscapularis must be protected at all costs. Rupture can occur all the way out to three months despite what appears to be a very durable repair at the time of surgery. Rupture tends to occur from overzealous therapy or patient non-compliance and thus both parties must be educated about realistic goals and expectations during the early recovery.
By six months after surgery a full range of activities are permitted as tolerated by the patient's comfort and demands. Given the absence of concern about failure of a prosthetic glenoid, no specific restrictions are placed on patients activities. Maintenance stretching and strengthening exercises are strongly encouraged for up to 2 years as pain relief, motion and function see to go hand-in-hand in their potential to improve throughout this prolonged interval.

8. Complications

Complications of shoulder arthroplasty are well-documented and the Ream and Run is no exception to the conventional and well-accepted adversities that can occur from any open shoulder surgery such as infection and axillary nerve injury. The following discussion will focus on complications that are particularly pertinent though not exclusive to the Ream and Run procedure.

8.1 Glenoid wear and erosion

As has been previously discussed, overzealous reaming or the need for excessive glenoid version correction can result in penetration of the subchondral plate and exposure of cancellous bone in the glenoid vault. It can also result in narrowing of the anterior-posterior dimensions of the glenoid concavity, which reduces the overall surface area for contact stress distribution and predisposes to instability. In these situations, patients will continue to experience pain following humeral hemiarthroplasty and may demonstrate recurrent glenoid erosion both medially and posteriorly. Thus patient selection and work-up are critical to predicting who is the ideal candidate likely to have a good outcome and all patients must be counseled about the potential need for glenoid replacement if the principles and goals of non-prosthetic glenoid arthroplasty cannot be met intraoperatively. Rhee and colleagues have shown that the results of salvage glenoid replacement after failed hemiarthroplasty are inferior to primary total shoulder arthroplasty.[48] This highlights the importance of doing the right operation the first time around.

8.2 Subscapularis rupture

Despite the added security afforded by lesser tuberosity osteotomy, failure can still occur if undue stress is placed on the repair. While the contention maintains that lesser tuberosity osteotomy allows bone to bone healing, this is not guaranteed in all cases. Micromotion at the repair site may stimulate a fibrous union, and release of the subscapularis intraoperatively may disrupt the blood supply to this fragment resulting in avascular necrosis of the lesser tuberosity and inability to heal directly by bony union. While this has not been previously reported in the literature, the author has had occasion to explore 4 cases in which the lesser tuberosity repair ruptured after surgery as detected clinically and radiographically. In all cases, the bone was sclerotic and devoid of any bleeding when drilled at the time of re-repair. Future studies will need to better determine the biology of lesser tuberosity healing but until more is known about how to optimize this process, erring on the side of caution is the safest route to avoid the devastating complication of subscapularis failure. This fact is true regardless of the method of tendon repair used. Because these patients tend to be more active and aggressive in terms of lifestyle pursuits, they need to be educated in terms of recovery expectations so that their ambitions do not compromise their compliance with the recovery protocol.

8.3 Stiffness

Recovery of range of motion is critical to outcomes after the Ream and Run procedure. Residual stiffness will result in obligate, capsular-mediated translations that equate to the same pathomechanics resulting in posterior humeral subluxation and glenoid erosion. The author believes that in all cases, aggressive circumferential capsular releases are necessary to restore motion and selective releases for fear of instability are never indicated. Capsular-mediated stability only occurs at the terminal range of motion, which is never a concern in the first 3 months after surgery when the capsule is reforming around the prosthetic joint. Stability in the mid-range is a function of a properly oriented glenoid concavity of sufficient area and a functional rotator cuff. Surgeons should not rely on intraoperative tests of joint stability that measure capsular tension as they are largely irrelevant assuming a properly performed reconstruction.

Given the prior discussion about subscapularis failure, range of motion exercises must be a graduated process that focuses more on frequency than exertion for the first several weeks. Patients must take an active but responsible and educated role in their own recovery and they must understand the potential consequences of noncompliance. This is a delicate balance that requires pre and postoperative education from both the surgeon and therapist. The author has also found it invaluable to identify one or two therapists who take an interest in shoulder arthroplasty and have a better understanding of how to achieve desired results. As with any discipline, frequency, volume and practice beget experience and results in this regard.

9. Results

When patient selection is combined with surgical technique that achieves the principles of Ream and Run, outcomes can be comparable to total shoulder arthroplasty in terms of pain relief, range of motion and function. Given that no specific restrictions are placed on patients postoperatively, results in terms of return to physically demanding leisure time physical activities can be outstanding. Patients have returned to sports such as water skiing, weight lifting, competitive tennis, and other outdoor pursuits. As many of these patients previously engaged in activities that may have contributed to early glenohumeral degenerative disease, the ability to return to similar activities, albeit in a modified setting, is a significant improvement in their health-related quality of life.

The author currently performs the Ream and Run procedures in roughly 8% of all arthroplasty cases. Generally, it is reserved for male patients aged 65 or less who meet the criteria previously discussed and who understand and accept the longer recovery in favor of the absence of restrictions. Between 2004-2010, 55 Ream and Run cases have been performed in 52 patients ranging in age from 42-68 years (average 56 years). This series has included 50 males and 2 females. Although formal outcome measures have not been performed on this consecutive series, 5 patients have required additional surgery. Two patients underwent revision glenoid resurfacing for recalcitrant pain with recurrent posterior erosion at 16 and 26 months after the index procedure. One of these patients was female. The other was subsequently determined to have inflammatory osteoarthritis. Two patients underwent repair of a partial subscapularis rupture both of whom were noted to have a smooth, remodeled concavity with rests of fibrocartilage at the time of exploration 3 and 47 months postoperatively. One patient underwent explantation of the humeral prosthesis due to deep infection with Staph. Epidermidis. This patient was subsequently revised to a standard total shoulder arthroplasty after interval placement of an antibiotic cement spacer and parenteral antimicrobial treatment. Two additional patients have complained of persistent pain but have elected not to undergo further surgery. Neither of these patients has demonstrated significant glenoid erosion to suggest that the cause of pain is in fact due to wear at the articulation.

Lynch et al have reported on outcomes of the Ream and Run procedure at mid-term follow-up. In the initial report, 32 of 35 patients demonstrated improved function regaining an average of 4.5 functions on the Simple Shoulder Test (SST).[49] Overall average SST score improved from 4.7 to 9.4 at 2-4 years follow-up. Sequential improvement in function was noted all the way up to 36 months after surgery. Patients who had radiographic evidence of a joint space on postoperative x-rays had better outcomes indicating that presumed formation of a fibrocartilage interface correlates with better pain relief and improvement in function. Clinton et al in a similar series demonstrated outcomes comparable to a matched set of patients undergoing total shoulder arthroplasty.[50] Again, functional outcomes for those patients undergoing the Ream and Run were noted to improve sequentially out to 3 years postoperatively.

Recently, Saltzman et al reported on outcomes of the Ream and Run in patients aged 55 years or younger. In terms of pre versus postoperative comparative SST, 53 of 56 patients were improved to a degree comparable to patients who underwent a total shoulder arthroplasty by the same surgeon.[51] Patients with mild preoperative glenoid erosion did not demonstrate progression while one patient with moderate erosion progressed to severe erosion. Average medial glenoid erosion measured 1.1 mm at an average of 44 months with the worst case measuring 6.3mm. Nine of 65 shoulders required revision including 4 (6%) conversions to a total shoulder for painful glenoid wear. Patients who underwent revision surgery tended to have a more complicated preoperative course including more severe functional deficits to overcome and a higher incidence of multiple prior surgeries.

Collectively, these results are comparable or superior to previously discussed literature looking at hemiarthroplasty alone or biological resurfacing techniques in this age cohort.[23, 25, 29, 33, 52] As our experience with this technique grows, patient selection criteria, indications and techniques have been refined to reflect potential modes of failure and their risk factors. As with all of orthopedics, the right operation for the right problem in the right patient is the key to success. The shoulder arthroplasty surgeon must carefully evaluate each candidate clinically, radiographically and in terms of compliance and expectations. When proper surgical technique is applied to right clinical setting the results of the Ream and Run can be both impressive and lasting and should be a tool in the shoulder surgeons armamentarium for management of advanced arthritis in the young and active patient.

10. References

[1] Farron A, Terrier A, Buchler P. Risks of loosening of a prosthetic glenoid implanted in retroversion. *J Shoulder Elbow Surg*. 2006;15:521-526.

[2] Oosterom R, Rozing PM, Verdonschot N, Bersee HE. Effect of joint conformity on glenoid component fixation in total shoulder arthroplasty. *Proc Inst Mech Eng H*. 2004;218:339-347.

[3] Hopkins AR, Hansen UN, Amis AA et al. Wear in the prosthetic shoulder: association with design parameters. *J Biomech Eng*. 2007;129:223-230.

[4] Braman JP, Falicov A, Boorman R, Matsen FAr. Alterations in surface geometry in retrieved polyethylene glenoid component. *J Orthop Res*. 2006;24:1249-1260.

[5] Hertel R, Ballmer FT. Observations on retrieved glenoid components. *J Arthroplasty*. 2003;18:361-366.

[6] Nho SJ, Nam D, Ala OL, Craig EV, Warren RF, Wright TM. Observations on retrieved glenoid components from total shoulder arthroplasty. *J Shoulder Elbow Surg*. 2009;18:371-378.

[7] Arnold RM, High RR, Grosshans KT, Walker CW, Fehringer EV. Bone presence between the central peg's radial fins of a partially cemented pegged all poly glenoid component suggest few radiolucencies. *J Shoulder Elbow Surg*. 2011;20:315-321.

[8] Barwood S, Setter KJ, Blaine TA, Bigliani LU. The incidence of early radiolucencies about a pegged glenoid component using cement pressurization. *J Shoulder Elbow Surg*. 2008;17:703-708.

[9] Churchill RS, Zellmer C, Zimmers HJ, Ruggero R. Clinical and radiographic analysis of a partially cemented glenoid implant: five-year minimum follow-up. *J Shoulder Elbow Surg*. 2010;19:1091-1097.

[10] Groh GI. Survival and radiographic analysis of a glenoid component with a cementless fluted central peg. *J Shoulder Elbow Surg*. 2010;19:1265-1268.

[11] Walch G, Young AA, Melis B, Gazielly D, Loew M, Boileau P. Results of a convex-back cemented keeled glenoid component in primary osteoarthritis: multicenter study with a follow-up greater than 5 years. *J Shoulder Elbow Surg*. 2011;20:385-394.

[12] Young A, Walch G, Boileau P et al. A multicentre study of the long-term results of using a flat-back polyethylene glenoid component in shoulder replacement for primary osteoarthritis. *J Bone Joint Surg Br*. 2011;93:210-216.

[13] Kasten P, Pape G, Raiss P et al. Mid-term survivorship analysis of a shoulder replacement with a keeled glenoid and a modern cementing technique. *J Bone Joint Surg Br*. 2010;92:387-392.

[14] Bartelt R, Sperling JW, Schleck CD, Cofield RH. Shoulder arthroplasty in patients aged fifty-five years or younger with osteoarthritis. *J Shoulder Elbow Surg*. 2011;20:123-130.

[15] Fox TJ, Cil A, Sperling JW, Sanchez-Sotelo J, Schleck CD, Cofield RH. Survival of the glenoid component in shoulder arthroplasty. *J Shoulder Elbow Surg*. 2009;18:859-863.

[16] Taunton MJ, McIntosh AL, Sperling JW, Cofield RH. Total shoulder arthroplasty with a metal-backed, bone-ingrowth glenoid component. Medium to long-term results. *J Bone Joint Surg Am*. 2008;90:2180-2188.

[17] Tammachote N, Sperling JW, Vathana T, Cofield RH, Harmsen WS, Schleck CD. Long-term results of cemented metal-backed glenoid components for osteoarthritis of the shoulder. *J Bone Joint Surg Am*. 2009;91:160-166.

[18] Boileau P, Avidor C, Krishnan SG, Walch G, Kempf JF, Mole D. Cemented polyethylene versus uncemented metal-backed glenoid components in total shoulder arthroplasty: a prospective, double-blind, randomized study. *J Shoulder Elbow Surg*. 2002;11:351-359.

[19] Cheung EV, Sperling JW, Cofield RH. Reimplantation of a glenoid component following component removal and allogenic bone-grafting. *J Bone Joint Surg Am*. 2007;89:1777-1783.

[20] Cheung EV, Sperling JW, Cofield RH. Revision shoulder arthroplasty for glenoid component loosening. *J Shoulder Elbow Surg*. 2008;17:371-375.

[21] Neyton L, Walch G, Nove-Josserand L, Edwards TB. Glenoid corticocancellous bone grafting after glenoid component removal in the treatment of glenoid loosening. *J Shoulder Elbow Surg*. 2006;15:173-179.

[22] Phipatanakul WP, Norris TR. Treatment of glenoid loosening and bone loss due to osteolysis with glenoid bone grafting. *J Shoulder Elbow Surg*. 2006;15:84-87.

[23] Burkhead WZJ, Hutton KS. Biologic resurfacing of the glenoid with hemiarthroplasty of the shoulder. *J Shoulder Elbow Surg*. 1995;4:263-270.

[24] Burkhead WZJ, Krishnan SG, Lin KC. Biologic resurfacing of the arthritic glenohumeral joint: Historical review and current applications. *J Shoulder Elbow Surg*. 2007;16:S248-53.

[25] Elhassan B, Ozbaydar M, Diller D, Higgins LD, Warner JJ. Soft-tissue resurfacing of the glenoid in the treatment of glenohumeral arthritis in active patients less than fifty years old. *J Bone Joint Surg Am*. 2009;91:419-424.

[26] Lee KT, Bell S, Salmon J. Cementless surface replacement arthroplasty of the shoulder with biologic resurfacing of the glenoid. *J Shoulder Elbow Surg*. 2009;18:915-919.

[27] Wirth MA. Humeral head arthroplasty and meniscal allograft resurfacing of the glenoid. *J Bone Joint Surg Am*. 2009;91:1109-1119.

[28] Nicholson GP, Goldstein JL, Romeo AA et al. Lateral meniscus allograft biologic glenoid arthroplasty in total shoulder arthroplasty for young shoulders with degenerative joint disease. *J Shoulder Elbow Surg*. 2007;16:S261-6.

[29] de Beer JF, Bhatia DN, van Rooyen KS, Du Toit DF. Arthroscopic debridement and biological resurfacing of the glenoid in glenohumeral arthritis. *Knee Surg Sports Traumatol Arthrosc*. 2010;18:1767-1773.

[30] Savoie FHr, Brislin KJ, Argo D. Arthroscopic glenoid resurfacing as a surgical treatment for glenohumeral arthritis in the young patient: midterm results. *Arthroscopy*. 2009;25:864-871.

[31] Gerber C, Snedeker JG, Krause AS, Appenzeller A, Farshad M. Osteochondral glenoid allograft for biologic resurfacing of the glenoid: biomechanical comparison of novel design concepts. *J Shoulder Elbow Surg*. 2011

[32] Bryant D, Litchfield R, Sandow M, Gartsman GM, Guyatt G, Kirkley A. A comparison of pain, strength, range of motion, and functional outcomes after hemiarthroplasty and total shoulder arthroplasty in patients with osteoarthritis of the shoulder. A systematic review and meta-analysis. *J Bone Joint Surg Am*. 2005;87:1947-1956.

[33] Sperling JW, Cofield RH, Rowland CM. Minimum fifteen-year follow-up of Neer hemiarthroplasty and total shoulder arthroplasty in patients aged fifty years or younger. *J Shoulder Elbow Surg*. 2004;13:604-613.

[34] Edwards TB, Kadakia NR, Boulahia A et al. A comparison of hemiarthroplasty and total shoulder arthroplasty in the treatment of primary glenohumeral osteoarthritis: results of a multicenter study. *J Shoulder Elbow Surg*. 2003;12:207-213.

[35] Lo IK, Litchfield RB, Griffin S, Faber K, Patterson SD, Kirkley A. Quality-of-life outcome following hemiarthroplasty or total shoulder arthroplasty in patients with osteoarthritis. A prospective, randomized trial. *J Bone Joint Surg Am*. 2005;87:2178-2185.

[36] Levine WN, Djurasovic M, Glasson JM, Pollock RG, Flatow EL, Bigliani LU. Hemiarthroplasty for glenohumeral osteoarthritis: results correlated to degree of glenoid wear. *J Shoulder Elbow Surg*. 1997;6:449-454.

[37] Matsen FAr, Clinton J, Lynch J, Bertelsen A, Richardson ML. Glenoid component failure in total shoulder arthroplasty. *J Bone Joint Surg Am*. 2008;90:885-896.

[38] Milgram JW, Rana NA. Pathologic evaluation of the failed cup arthroplasty: a review of 32 cases. *Clin Orthop Relat Res*. 1981;158-179.

[39] Milgram JW, Rana NA. Roentgenologic and clinical evaluation of vitallium mold arthroplasty of the hip. *Surg Gynecol Obstet*. 1968;127:1042-1050.

[40] Enneking WF, Singsen ET. Pathologic changes in the idiopathic painful cup arthroplasty. *Clin Orthop Relat Res*. 1974;236-253.

[41] D'Ambrosia RD, McClain EJ, Wissinger HA, Riggins RS. Resorption of the femoral head beneath the vitallium mold. *Surg Forum*. 1972;23:465-467.

[42] Weldon EJr, Boorman RS, Smith KL, Matsen FAr. Optimizing the glenoid contribution to the stability of a humeral hemiarthroplasty without a prosthetic glenoid. *J Bone Joint Surg Am*. 2004;86-A:2022-2029.

[43] Matsen FAr, Clark JM, Titelman RM et al. Healing of reamed glenoid bone articulating with a metal humeral hemiarthroplasty: a canine model. *J Orthop Res*. 2005;23:18-26.

[44] Clinton J, Warme WJ, Lynch JR, Lippitt SB, Matsen FAr. Shoulder hemiarthroplasty with nonprosthetic glenoid arthroplasty: The Ream and Run. *Techniques in Shoulder and Elbow Surgery*. 2009;10:43-52.

[45] Pearl ML, Kurutz S. Geometric analysis of commonly used prosthetic systems for proximal humeral replacement. *J Bone Joint Surg Am*. 1999;81:660-671.

[46] Pearl ML, Kurutz S, Postachini R. Geometric variables in anatomic replacement of the proximal humerus: how much prosthetic geometry is necessary? *J Shoulder Elbow Surg*. 2009;18:366-370.

[47] Ponce BA, Ahluwalia RS, Mazzocca AD, Gobezie RG, Warner JJ, Millett PJ. Biomechanical and clinical evaluation of a novel lesser tuberosity repair technique in total shoulder arthroplasty. *J Bone Joint Surg Am*. 2005;87 Suppl 2:1-8.

[48] Rhee PC, Sassoon AA, Schleck CD, Harmsen WS, Sperling JW, Cofield RH. Revision total shoulder arthroplasty for painful glenoid arthrosis after humeral head replacement: the posttraumatic shoulder. *J Shoulder Elbow Surg*. 2011

[49] Lynch JR, Franta AK, Montgomery WHJ, Lenters TR, Mounce D, Matsen FAr. Self-assessed outcome at two to four years after shoulder hemiarthroplasty with concentric glenoid reaming. *J Bone Joint Surg Am*. 2007;89:1284-1292.

[50] Clinton J, Franta AK, Lenters TR, Mounce D, Matsen FAr. Nonprosthetic glenoid arthroplasty with humeral hemiarthroplasty and total shoulder arthroplasty yield similar self-assessed outcomes in the management of comparable patients with glenohumeral arthritis. *J Shoulder Elbow Surg*. 2007;16:534-538.

[51] Saltzman MD, Chamberlain AM, Mercer DM, Warme WJ, Bertelsen AL, Matsen FAr. Shoulder hemiarthroplasty with concentric glenoid reaming in patients 55 years old or less. *J Shoulder Elbow Surg*. 2011;20:609-615.

[52] Krishnan SG, Reineck JR, Nowinski RJ, Harrison D, Burkhead WZ. Humeral hemiarthroplasty with biologic resurfacing of the glenoid for glenohumeral arthritis. Surgical technique. *J Bone Joint Surg Am*. 2008;90 Suppl 2 Pt 1:9-19.

28

Development of Proprioception After Shoulder Arthroplasty

Michael W. Maier[1] and Philip Kasten[2]
[1]*Department of Orthopedics, Trauma Surgery and Paraplegiology, University of Heidelberg, Heidelberg*
[2]*Carl-Gustav Carus University of Dresden, Dresden*
Germany

1. Introduction

Since the introduction of shoulder arthroplasty in 1893 by the French surgeon Jule-Émile Péan [18], the indications for shoulder replacement have expanded. Today shoulder arthroplasty is a common treatment for glenohumeral osteoarthritis [2]. Shoulder arthroplasty can significantly improve the function of osteoarthritic shoulders [7, 13, 19, 27]. Comparing the results, TSR offers better short- and mid-term results, but has the risk of long-term problems as the glenoid loosening [2]. In our practice patients with glenohumeral osteoarthritis will receive a total shoulder arthroplasty. As an exception patients with osteoarthritis which is limited to the humeral head without eccentric erosion of a stable sclerotic glenoid (Typ A1 glenoid according to Walch [28]) can be treated with hemiarthroplasty (HA). If the glenoid shows eccentric posterior wear (> A1), a TSR is recommended.

The use of total shoulder replacement in the setting of rotator cuff-tear arthropathy (CTA) has led to poor outcomes because of early glenoid implant failure [17]. These failures were the result of early glenoid loosening caused by altered biomechanics in the cuff-deficient shoulder. The treatment of choice for most used to be hemiarthroplasty. Although good relief from pain has usually been obtained, most patients with CTA and subsequent hemiarthroplasty had a limited range of movement, leading to difficulties with the activities of daily living. These poor results let to the development of the reverse shoulder prosthesis, as a new method for treating CTA. Using the reverse prosthesis in CTA, favorable outcomes have been reported [15, 17].

In order to use the replaced shoulder for ADLs the concerted function of the active stabilizers and the passive restraints of the replaced shoulder joint is necessary.

2. Shoulder proprioception

In 1906, Charles Scott Sherrington published his work about proprioception [26]. He defined the term proprioception as the awareness of movement derived from muscular, tendon, and articular sources. Since then physiologists and anatomists are searching for specialized nerve endings that transmit data on joint capsule and muscle tension [11, 30]. It is known that joint proprioception plays a considerable role in stabilization of the normal healthy shoulder by helping to control muscular action [1]. However, there is little data available about proprioception of the replaced shoulder before and after surgery [6, 12, 16]. Parameters routinely examined in previous studies include pain, satisfaction, range of motion, and strength [5].

3. Proprioception after shoulder arthroplasty

By reason that the shoulder joint is balanced and centered by the rotator cuff and the glenohumeral ligaments, it can be postulated that proprioception plays an important role in the postoperative outcome and rehabilitation. However, to date there are only three studies analyzing proprioception after shoulder replacement [6, 12, 16]. Two of these studies [6, 12] have a short follow-up period, in both cases six months. Cuomo et al. [6] performed a passive and guided angle-reproduction test in 20 patients with shoulder osteoarthritis before and six months after total shoulder arthroplasty (TSA) with only one degree of freedom at a time and reported improvement of proprioception [6]. Kasten et al. [12] found out, six months after shoulder arthroplasty, proprioception remained unchanged or deteriorated, as assessed by an active and unlimited angle-reproduction test with 3D motion analysis [12]. It was assumed that this finding was most likely attributable to the relatively short rehabilitation period of six months. Therefore, the purpose of the third study by Maier et al. [16] was to examine the patients from the study described by Kasten et al. [12, 14] again three years postoperatively to find out whether proprioception changes after a longer rehabilitation period of three years. In the present study, the same active and unlimited angle-reproduction test with 3D motion analysis was used as described before [12]. The present study firstly describes the results of proprioception development in a cohort of different shoulder arthroplasties, including patients with reverse prosthesis.

4. Measurement of proprioception

Because proprioception is a complex system that relies on central integration of various afferent and efferent elements, it is difficult to measure proprioceptive performance. Up to now, there is no consensus on how proprioception should be measured because the different components of proprioception are difficult to examine at the same time. For clinical purposes, most authors differentiate between static proprioception and dynamic proprioception [21]. Static proprioception is usually defined as the position sense, what means conscious perception of the orientation of different parts of the body with respect to another. Dynamic proprioception is defined as kinesthesia and the sense of rates of movement [11].

4.1 Joint angle analysis with the Heidelberg Upper Extremity Model (HUX)

In our studies [12, 16], we used the Heidelberg Upper Extremity Model (HUX) to measure joint angles as described before [23]: Therefore a twelve-camera motion analysis system (Vicon 612; Vicon, Lake Forest, USA) working at 120 Hz was used to monitor the patients' movements. The spatial resolution of the system was approximately 1 mm. The underlying model consisted of seven segments: thorax, clavicles, upper arms, and forearms. The sternoclavicular joint and the glenohumeral joint were treated as a ball-and-socket joint, whereas the elbow was treated as a hinge joint. Translational degrees of freedom were not considered in any of these joints.

For the measurement, the patients were prepared with four markers placed on the trunk as recommended by the International Society of Biomechanics [31]. Four markers were placed on each forearm: one at the radial and one at the ulnar styloid process of the wrist and two, connected with a wand, on the ulna close to the elbow joint. One marker was placed laterally on the upper arm and one on the acromion. After a static trial, the patient was asked to perform isolated movements of elbow flexion/ extension, shoulder flexion/ extension and shoulder abduction/ adduction to determine the shoulder joint position and the location of the elbow joint axis. Specifically, in these shoulder calibration trials the sternoclavicular joint was treated as a cardan joint. Technical coordinate systems for the ulna/ forearm, humerus, clavicle, and thorax were not deduced by optimization methods as was done for marker clusters [3]. Instead, they were based directly on marker trajectories, i.e. the direction vectors between them, using cross-products as reviewed by Chiari et al. [4]. The technical coordinate system of the clavicle was based on the four thorax markers and the shoulder marker. This coordinate system was used only for dynamic calibration movements, which were limited to a range of shoulder motion of 0-40° flexion and abduction to assume constant glenohumeral movement and exclude skin motion artefacts. Constraint least squares optimization according to Gamage et al. was then used for joint centre determination [9].

The anatomical co-ordinate system for the ulna/ forearm, humerus, and thorax were based on the technical coordinate systems of these segments and on the joint axes and joint centers previously determined. A static trial was used to define the neutral position of the thorax. Angles of flexion and abduction were expressed as projection angles relative to the proximal anatomical coordinate system, while internal/ external rotation was defined according to the globe convention [8]. Elbow flexion was defined as the projected angle to the elbow axis. Custom software written in Java (Sun Mircosystems, USA) was used to calculate each joint angle in each trial of the angle-reproduction tasks.

The system and biomechanical model was validated with the manual goniometer and intraclass correlation coefficients of 0.989 for intrasubject variability, 0.996 for intersubject variability, and 0.998 for intertester variability were found [22]. Differences of more than 10° between the two methods were found for shoulder flexion of more than 160° [22, 23].

4.2 Active angle reproduction test

As described before [12, 16], our study group used an active angle reproduction test to measure proprioception: Test person sat on a chair with the arm hanging in 0° abduction and rotation. They were blindfolded to eliminate visual clues and wore sleeveless shirts. We ensured that the arm did not touch the trunk and, consequently, skin contact was minimized. The arm was moved to the desired position by the examiner with visual control of a manual handheld goniometer. In detail, the positions were 30° and 60° abduction, 30° and 60° flexion, and 30° external (and afterwards 30° internal rotation) in 30° abduction (total six joint positions). In the target position the subjects were told to maintain the position for ten seconds, and then the initial position with the arm hanging was resumed. Afterwards, the subject was asked to move the arm back into the target position and the mean value of the joint position was measured. Standardized instructions were given to all subjects, and a test trial was conducted to acquaint them with each test condition. All tests were randomized for side and movement. Two test trials were performed at each angle, and the mean value was used for further analysis. The total proprioception performance (total) was defined as the mean value of all single measurements (six joint positions) to have one quality to compare proprioceptive ability.

5. Patients and controls

Patients receiving three different types of shoulder arthroplasties in 2007 were examined from 2007 to 2010:

i. Ten consecutive patients underwent third-generation total shoulder arthroplasty (TSA) (Aequalis Shoulder; Tournier, Lyon, France) for degenerative osteoarthritis of the humeral head and glenoid with a mean age of 75 years (standard deviation [SD] 4.7 years). There were seven women and three men (mean height 167.0 cm [SD 11.0]; mean weight 81.0 kg [SD 15.9]), with four right shoulders and six left shoulders. In all cases the deltopectoral approach was used with detachment of the subscapularis tendon and release of all three glenohumeral ligaments. At the end of the surgery the subscapularis was reattached to the humeral bone. Primary osteoarthritis was found in eight cases and secondary posttraumatic osteoarthritis in two cases. The dominant side was involved in eight cases.

ii. Eleven consecutive patients underwent hemiarthroplasty (HEMI) for degenerative changes limited to the humeral head and a stable/ minimally deformed glenoid of type A1 or A2 according to Walch [29]. There were nine women and two men, with five right shoulders and six left shoulders, four on the dominant sides and seven non-dominant sides. In all cases the deltopectoral approach was used as described above. Osteoarthritis was primary in nine cases and post-traumatic in two cases. The mean age was 64 years (SD 13.8), mean height was 167.0 cm (SD 8.1), and the mean weight was 79.0 kg (SD 18.8).

iii. In five patients a reversed prosthesis was implanted for cuff tear arthropathy (REVERSE). All were women, their mean age was 73 years (SD 4.6), mean height was 160 cm (SD 7.3), and mean weight was 73.6 kg (SD 7.4). In all cases the dominant right shoulder was treated. For all patients the anterior lateral approach was used with partial detachment of the anteriorlateral deltoid muscle and refixation in the end of the surgery. The subscapularis tendon and the glenohumeral ligaments at the glenoid were released.Consecutive patients were enrolled in the study which resulted in uneven numbers in the different groups of arthroplasties implanted. The main focus and outcome measure were not on comparing the groups (especially no comparison with the REVERSE group), but to monitor proprioception over time within the groups.

iv. A matched control group consisted of five women and five men. Matched controls (n=10; NORM) had a mean age of 64.5 years (SD 7.3). The mean height was 170.3 cm (SD 9.3), and the mean weight was 78.2 kg (SD 11.6). All controls were right-hand dominant, healthy, and had normal shoulders according to medical history, physical examination and radiographs. In this group the test persons were also examined twice, over the period of three years.

6. Statistics

The statistical analysis was performed using SPSS Version 16.0 (SPSS Inc., Chicago, IL, USA). Group mean values (MV) and standard deviations (SD) were calculated. P values <0.05 were considered significant. The distribution of the data was checked with the

Shapiro-Wilk test, and the homogeneity of variance was assessed using the Levene test. The angle between the long axis of the humerus and the trunk position was determined. Differences in shoulder joint angles between target and reproducted position were compared between the pre- and postoperative examination with a Wilcoxon-test for the groups TSA, HEMI, and REVERSE. Afterwards as a second outcome measure differences among these groups and the controls were examined by a Mann-Whitney *U* test.

7. Results of proprioception measurement three years after shoulder arthroplasty

The hemioarthroplasty (HEMI) subgroup revealed significant lower AAR at 30° of external rotation before surgery with 3.1° [SD 3.5] as compared to three years after surgery 12.8° [SD 10.7]; (p=0.031) (fig. 1). By trend, in the TSA subgroup the AAR deteriorated from 7.1° [SD

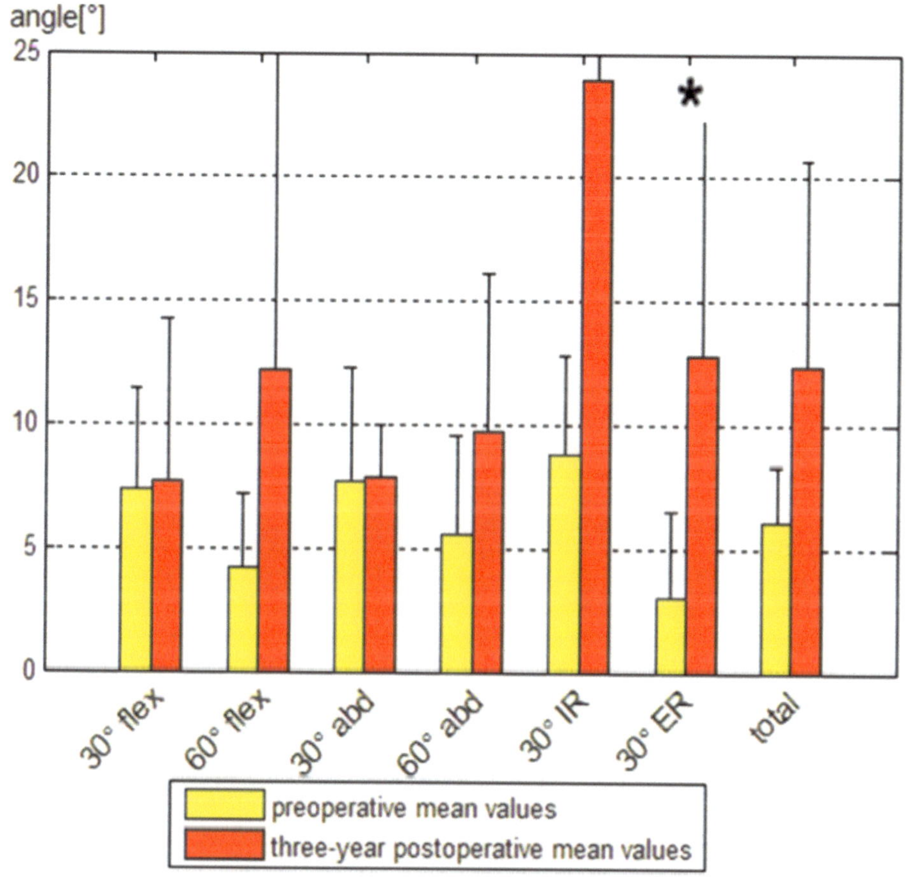

Fig. 1. The hemioarthroplasty (HEMI) group showed significant lower AAR at 30° of external rotation three years after surgery (3.1° [SD 3.5] vs. 12.8° [SD 10.7]; (p=0.031)). Otherwise there were no significances between pre- and postoperative AAR, although the total proprioception performance (total) almost reached significance (p=0.063). Graphically, there is a deterioration in all movements.

3.1] to 8.6° [SD 1.4] (fig. 2), in the HEMI subgroup from 6.1° [SD 2.1] to 12.4° [SD 8.3] (fig. 1) and in the reversed subgroup from 8.1° [SD 4.8] to 9.9° [SD 1.8] (fig. 3).
Although there are different underlying concepts and biomechanics between the TSA, HEMI and REVERSE group, the results were included in a combined analysis to get a general impression of the intervention of implantation of an arthroplasty: in all groups three years after shoulder arthroplasty the total proprioception performance (total) measured by the AAR deteriorated significantly (from 6.9° [SD 3.4] to 10.3° [SD 5.2]; p=0.018) (table 1). The internal rotation deteriorated significantly from 7.9° [SD 5.7] to 17.6° [SD 21.1] (p=0.039) (table 2). The comparison between the controls (NORM) and the three years postoperative values of all arthroplasty groups (TSA, HEMI and REVERSE) reveals a significant worse AAR in the arthroplasty group three years after shoulder arthroplasty (10.3° [SD 5.2] vs. 7.8° [SD 2.3]; p=0.030) (fig. 4).

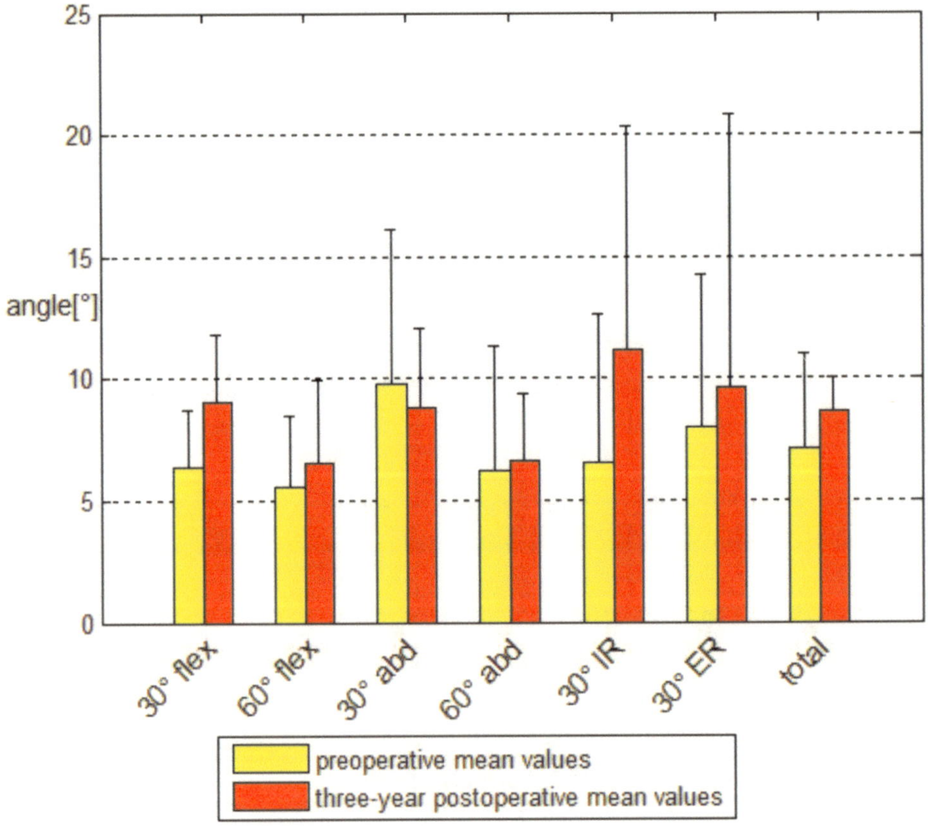

Fig. 2. The comparison pre- to postoperative values after implantation of a total shoulder arthroplasty (TSA) showed no significant differences between pre- and postoperative AAR. By trend, there is a deterioration of proprioception three years after surgery. The total proprioception performance (total) deteriorated by trend from 7.1° [SD 3.1] to 8.6° [SD 1.4].

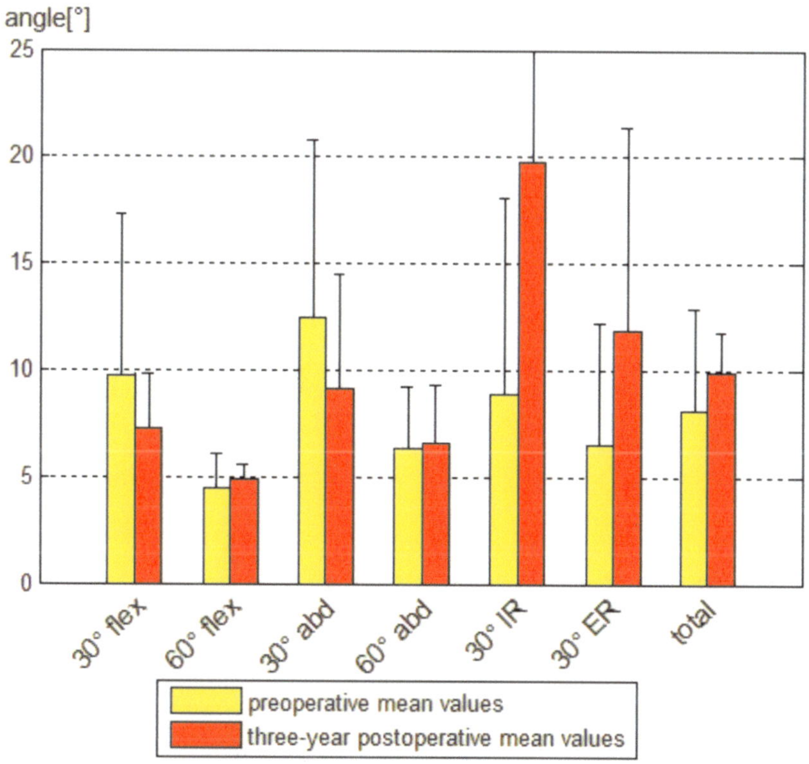

Fig. 3. The reversed shoulder arthroplasty (REVERSE) group graphically showed an improvement of the AAR at 30° of flexion and 30° of abduction. However, there is a deterioration for the other movements. The total proprioception performance (total) deteriorated by trend from 8.1° [SD 4.8] to 9.9° [SD 1.8].

	Preoperatively		**Three years postoperatively**		P value
Movement	Mean [°]	SD [°]	Mean [°]	SD [°]	
30° of flexion	7.4	± 4.1	8.2	± 4.3	0.669
60° of flexion	4.8	± 2.7	8.4	± 8.7	0.211
30° of abduction	9.5	± 5.7	8.5	± 3.1	0.562
60° of abduction	6.1	± 4.1	7.8	± 4.5	0.144
30° of external rotation	5.7	± 5.4	11.2	± 10.1	0.065
30° of internal rotation	7.9	± 5.7	17.6	± 21.1	**0.039**
Total	6.9	± 3.4	10.3	± 5.2	**0.018**

TSA total shoulder arthroplasty, *Hemi* hemiarthroplasty, *REVERSE* reversed arthroplasty, *SD* standard deviation;

Table 1. Active angle reproduction test (AAR) in all groups (TSA, HEMI and REVERSE) before operation and three years thereafter

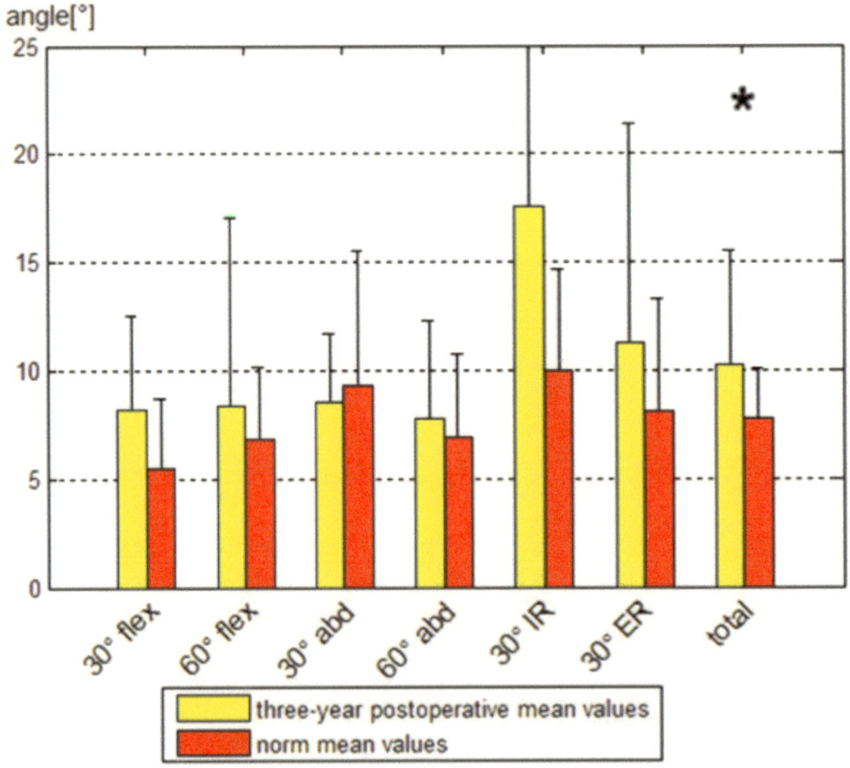

Fig. 4. The comparison between the controls and the three years postoperative values of all arthroplasty groups (TSA, HEMI and REVERSE) shows significantly better total proprioception performance (total) in the control (NORM) than in the arthroplasty group (10.3° [SD 5.2] vs. 7.8° [SD 2.3]; p=0.030).

8. Discussion of our findings with the literature

To our knowledge there are only three studies analyzing proprioception after shoulder arthroplasty [6, 12, 16]. Two are short-term studies with a six months follow-up [12, 16] and one is a middle-term follow up study [16]: Cuomo et al. [6] performed a prospective analysis of 20 consecutive patients with unilateral advanced glenohumeral arthritis who underwent total shoulder arthroplasty (TSA). Shoulder proprioception testing for passive position sense and detection of motion was performed one week before surgery and six months after TSA. Six months after TSA, position sense and the sensitivity of detection of motion were significantly improved ($p<0.05$) and did not differ significantly from the contralateral shoulder or the controls. Cuomo concluded that in patients with advanced glenohumeral arthritis after TSA there was a marked improvement in proprioception.

In our study group, Kasten et al. [12] assessed proprioception six months after shoulder arthroplasty by an *active* and unguided angle-reproduction test with 3D motion analysis. In contrast to Cuomo we found out that six months after surgery proprioception remained unchanged or deteriorated. Due to the fact that this is completely the different result as

Cuomo et. al., it was concluded, that this is either due to the different measurement methods (active versus passive) or the relatively short rehabilitation period of six months. Maybe an improvement would also be found in the mid-term follow-up. That's why we investigated the same patients three years after shoulder arthroplasty by the same active angle reproduction test to measure the development of proprioception [16]. The middl-term follow-up showed no improvement but rather a deterioration of proprioception over the course of three years after shoulder arthroplasty. How can we explain that?
Cuomo et al. used a hydraulic machine that passively moved the arm. The patient had to indicate when he or she noted movement ("detection of motion") and, in a separate approach, when he or she passively reassumed a joint position that was previously defined ("passive position sense"). Cuomo and colleagues thus measured two entities of proprioception separately. The outcome of the AAR test, used in our setting, can be influenced by some elements: The test person has to actively move the arm and is therefore not limited regarding the direction of movement. Consequently, a more comprehensive concept of proprioception is tested, comprising the elements of position sense, motion sense, and the muscle strength that is necessary to reassume the position.

9. Proprioception in shoulder instability

The AAR has been used to assess shoulder proprioception before, for example, in shoulder instability. Pötzl and colleagues examined the proprioceptive capabilities of 14 patients with recurrent anterior shoulder instability preoperatively and at least five years postoperatively using the AAR test [20]. In their series the joint position sense improved significantly in abduction, flexion, and rotation ($p<0.05$). They concluded that five years after surgical restoration of shoulder instability the joint position sense improved significantly to the same level as normal healthy shoulders. Having these results in mind we have to ask why proprioception measured with a comparable AAR deteriorates after shoulder arthroplasty, whereas it improves after surgery of shoulder instability?

10. Possible reasons why proprioception deteriorates after shoulder arthroplasty

In shoulder arthroplasty, the operative approach for implantation of a TSA and hemi-arthroplasty includes the cutting (and subsequent repair) of the subscapularis muscle and usually release of all glenohumeral ligaments. In cuff tear arthropathy the subscapularis is damaged from the beginning or released during surgery in our technique. However, these structures contain afferent and efferent structures important for proprioception. Therefore, concerning the influence on proprioceptive structures, the surgical procedures for shoulder instability and shoulder replacement are distinct. Since the approach in TSA and hemiarthroplasty is identical, a comparison seems to be valid. The different approach and the lack of the rotator cuff in cuff tear arthropathy limits a direct comparison with the other groups. However, the aim of this study was not the comparison of different types of implants that were implanted for different indications. The aim of this study was to assess proprioception changes three years after shoulder arthroplasty within the three groups. What we observed in our study is that nociceptors may also play an important role. During the repeat postoperative measurement, the patients mentioned that they were lacking the information input of pain sensation that they had usually during motion of the arm before surgery. The lacking of this afferent input might adversely influence the postoperative proprioception performance with the AAR.

11. What can we do to avoid postoperative deterioration of proprioception?

Another issue is how we could diminish the loss of proprioception after shoulder replacement. Certainly we have to take a look at the surgical procedure. In the cases of TSA and HEP the deltopectoral approach was used with detachment of the subscapularis tendon and release of all glenohumeral ligaments. In shoulder replacement different procedures exist for detachment of the subscapularis tendon. If the external rotation is > 20°, according to our concept the subscapularis tendon is divided 5-10 mm medial to its insertion at the lesser tuberosity. The lateral tendon stump will permit an end-to-end suture at the end of surgery. If the external rotation is <20°, the detachment of the subscapularis tendon from the lesser tuberosity is recommended, because this allows to gain length by medializing the tendon insertion after implantation of the prosthesis. At the end of the surgery, the subscapularis tendon is repaired in slight abduction and external rotation of the arm either with an end-to-end suture or, in the presence of joint contracture, reattached with the help of previously mounted transosseous sutures [10, 24]. This refixation is important, because otherwise it carries the risk of a later anterior instability of the prosthesis and loss of shoulder function.

This intraoperative soft tissue management could play an important role for the proprioceptive outcome according to a recently published study by Rokito et al. [25]. They investigated the degree to which surgical approach affects recovery of strength and proprioception. The recovery of strength and proprioception after open surgery for recurrent anterior glenohumeral instability was compared for two surgical procedures. Group 1 underwent an open inferior capsular shift with detachment of the subscapularis, and group 2 underwent an anterior capsulolabral reconstruction without detachment of the subscapularis. In group 1 the subscapularis was split horizontally at the junction of its upper two-third and lower one-third, and a glenoid-sided capsular shift was performed, followed by reapproximation of the split. At 6 months after surgery in group 1 patients there were still significant deficits in mean position sense and strength values. Rokito concluded that detachment of the subscapularis delays recovery of strength and proprioception. These findings can explain the deterioration of proprioceptive outcome in shoulder arthroplasty which usually implies the detachment of the subscapularis muscle. Another important issue is the release of the glenohumeral ligaments that play an important role in proprioception of the shoulder. Postoperative management with immobilizing in a Gilchrist sling or an abduction pillow, physiotherapy management including a temporary avoidance for rotational movements to allow for healing of the subscapularis muscle as well as proprioceptive neuromuscular facilitation exercises might play an important role for the individual proprioceptive outcome.

Performing shoulder arthroplasty did negatively affect one component of shoulder proprioception that was measured by the active angle-reproduction test. This might be related to the surgical approach that includes divison of the subscapularis muscle and the glenohumeral ligaments. In order to be able to diminish negative influences on postoperative proprioception further prospective studies will have to evaluate pre- and intraoperative variables to improve proprioception after shoulder replacement. Although proprioception does not improve three years after implantation of shoulder arthroplasty, a pain free increase of range of motion in activities of daily living, as we described in a previous study [13], is the main improvement for the patient after surgery.

Summary sentence
Shoulder proprioception deteriorates after shoulder arthroplasty.

Disclosures
All authors, their immediate family, and any research foundation with which they are affiliated did not receive any financial payments or other benefits from any commercial entity related to the subject of this article.

Source of funding
Research fund of the Department of Orthopaedic and Trauma Surgery of the Hospital of the University of Heidelberg.
The local ethics committee approved the study (S-305/2007) and all patients consented to the study.

12. Aknowledgements

We thank the research fund of the Department of Orthopaedic and Trauma Surgery of the Hospital of the University of Heidelberg for the financial support of the study. Furthermore, we would like to thank the motion analysis team of the University of Heidelberg, especially Petra Armbrust and Waltraud Schuster, for the practical support during the study.[Level of Evidence : Level III, Case-Control Study, Treatment Study.

13. References

[1] Blasier, R.B., J.E. Carpenter, and L.J. Huston, *Shoulder proprioception. Effect of joint laxity, joint position, and direction of motion*. Orthop.Rev., 1994. 23(1): p. 45-50.
[2] Boileau, P., et al., *Arthroplasty of the shoulder*. J.Bone Joint Surg.Br., 2006. 88(5): p. 562-575.
[3] Carman, A.B. and P.D. Milburn, *Determining rigid body transformation parameters from ill-conditioned spatial marker co-ordinates*. J Biomech, 2006. 39(10): p. 1778-86.
[4] Chiari, L., et al., *Human movement analysis using stereophotogrammetry. Part 2: instrumental errors*. Gait Posture, 2005. 21(2): p. 197-211.
[5] Constant, C.R. and A.H. Murley, *A clinical method of functional assessment of the shoulder*. Clin Orthop Relat Res., 1987(214). p. 160-164.
[6] Cuomo, F., M.G. Birdzell, and J.D. Zuckerman, *The effect of degenerative arthritis and prosthetic arthroplasty on shoulder proprioception*. J Shoulder Elbow Surg, 2005. 14(4): p. 345-348.
[7] Deshmukh, A.V., et al., *Total shoulder arthroplasty: long-term survivorship, functional outcome, and quality of life*. J Shoulder Elbow Surg, 2005. 14(5): p. 471-9.
[8] Doorenbosch, C.A., J. Harlaar, and D.H. Veeger, *The globe system: an unambiguous description of shoulder positions in daily life movements*. J Rehabil Res Dev, 2003. 40(2): p. 147-55.
[9] Gamage, S.S. and J. Lasenby, *New least squares solutions for estimating the average centre of rotation and the axis of rotation*. J Biomech, 2002. 35(1): p. 87-93.

[10] Habermeyer, P. and G. Engel, *Surgical technique for total shoulder arthroplasty.* Operat Orthop Traumatol, 2004. 16: p. 339-364.
[11] Jerosch, J. and M. Prymka, *Proprioception and joint stability.* Knee.Surg.Sports Traumatol.Arthrosc., 1996. 4(3): p. 171-179.
[12] Kasten, P., et al., *Proprioception in total, hemi- and reverse shoulder arthroplasty in 3D motion analyses: a prospective study.* Int Orthop, 2009. 33(6): p. 1641-7.
[13] Kasten, P., et al., *Can shoulder arthroplasty restore the range of motion in activities of daily living? A prospective 3D video motion analysis study.* J Shoulder Elbow Surg, 2010. 19(2 Suppl): p. 59-65.
[14] Kasten, P., et al., *Three-dimensional motion analysis of compensatory movements in patients with radioulnar synostosis performing activities of daily living.* J Orthop Sci, 2009. 14(3): p. 307-12.
[15] Loew, M., et al., *[Shoulder arthroplasty following rotator cuff tear: acquired arthropathy of the shoulder].* Orthopade, 2007. 36(11): p. 988-95.
[16] Maier, M.W., et al., *Proprioception three years after shoulder arthroplasty in 3D motion analysis: a prospective study.* submitted to Int Orthop, 2011.
[17] Matsen, F.A., 3rd, et al., *The reverse total shoulder arthroplasty.* J Bone Joint Surg Am, 2007. 89(3): p. 660-7.
[18] Nyffeler, R.W., et al., *Influence of humeral prosthesis height on biomechanics of glenohumeral abduction. An in vitro study.* J Bone Joint Surg Am, 2004. 86-A(3): p. 575-80.
[19] Orfaly, R.M., et al., *A prospective functional outcome study of shoulder arthroplasty for osteoarthritis with an intact rotator cuff.* J Shoulder Elbow Surg, 2003. 12(3): p. 214-21.
[20] Potzl, W., et al., *Proprioception of the shoulder joint after surgical repair for Instability: a long-term follow-up study.* Am.J.Sports Med., 2004. 32(2): p. 425-430.
[21] Proske, U. and S.C. Gandevia, *The kinaesthetic senses.* J Physiol, 2009. 587(Pt 17): p. 4139-46.
[22] Raiss, P., et al., *[Range of motion of shoulder and elbow in activities of daily life in 3D motion analysis].* Z.Orthop.Unfall., 2007. 145(4): p. 493-498.
[23] Rettig, O., et al., *A new kinematic model of the upper extremity based on functional joint parameter determination for shoulder and elbow.* Gait Posture, 2009. 30(4): p. 469-76.
[24] Rockwood, C.A., Jr., *The technique of total shoulder arthroplasty.* Instr Course Lect, 1990. 39: p. 437-47.
[25] Rokito, A.S., et al., *Recovery of shoulder strength and proprioception after open surgery for recurrent anterior instability: a comparison of two surgical techniques.* J Shoulder Elbow Surg, 2010. 19(4): p. 564-9.
[26] Sherrington, C.S., *On the proprioceptive system, especially in its reflex aspect.* Brain, 1906. 29: p. 1-28.
[27] van de Sande, M.A., R. Brand, and P.M. Rozing, *Indications, complications, and results of shoulder arthroplasty.* Scand J Rheumatol, 2006. 35(6): p. 426-34.
[28] Walch, G., P. Boileau, and P. Pozzi, *Glenoid resurfacing in shoulder arthroplasty.* In: Walch G, Boileau P, eds.: Shoulder arthroplasty.Berlin, Heidelberg, New York, Tokio: Springer, 1999: p. 177-181.
[29] Walch, G., et al., *Primary glenohumeral osteoarthritis: clinical and radiographic classification. The Aequalis Group.* Acta Orthop.Belg., 1998. 64 Suppl 2: p. 46-52.
[30] Warner, J.J., et al., *Static capsuloligamentous restraints to superior-inferior translation of the glenohumeral joint.* Am.J.Sports Med., 1992. 20(6): p. 675-685.
[31] Wu, G., et al., *ISB recommendation on definitions of joint coordinate systems of various joints for the reporting of human joint motion--Part II: shoulder, elbow, wrist and hand.* J Biomech, 2005. 38(5): p. 981-992.